Atlas of Three-Dimensional Echocardiography

Edited by

Navin C. Nanda, MD
Professor of Medicine and Director,
Heart Station/Echocardiography Laboratories
University of Alabama at Birmingham,
and
Director, Echocardiography Laboratory and The Kirklin Clinic
University of Alabama Health Services Foundation
Birmingham, Alabama

Vincent L. Sorrell, MD
Associate Professor of Medicine,
Sections of Cardiology and the Cardiovascular Center and
Medical Director of Graphics, and Exercise Physiology Labs,
East Carolina University Brody School of Medicine,
Greenville, North Carolina

FUTURA

Futura Publishing Company, Inc.
Armonk, NY

Library of Congress Cataloging-in-Publication Data

Atlas of three-dimensional echocardiography / edited by Navin C. Nanda, Vincent L. Sorrell.
p. ; cm.
Includes bibliographical references and index.
ISBN 0-87993-486-7 (hardcover : alk. paper)
1. Echocardiography—Atlases. 2. Three-dimensional imaging—Atlases. I. Nanda, Navin C. (Navin Chandar), 1937-II. Sorrell, Vincent L.
[DNLM: 1. Echocardiography, Three-Dimensional—Atlases. WG 17 A88455 2001]
RC683.5.U5 A87 2001
616.1′207543—dc21

2001051142

Futura Publishing Company, Inc.
135 Bedford Road
Armonk, New York 10504
www.futuraco.com

ISBN #:0-87993-486-7

Every effort has been made to ensure that the information in this book is as up to date and accurate as possible at the time of publication. However, due to the constant developments in medicine, neither the author, nor the editor, nor the publisher can accept any legal or other responsibility for any errors or omissions that may occur.

Printed in the United States of America on acid-free paper.

Preface

Echocardiography has become the most commonly used diagnostic tool in the evaluation of the patient with known or suspected cardiovascular disease. From its earliest inception using only M-mode techniques, clinically useful information has been obtained. After the development of two-dimensional (2D) echocardiography, even those who were initially skeptic of its incremental value became increasingly convinced of the advantage of imaging in multiple planes.

Three-dimensional (3D) echocardiography has been available for some time, and provides even greater anatomic knowledge over 2D echocardiography. The greatest disadvantage is related to reconstruction time, but this is constantly being shortened and is now only minutes. Progress is being made in refining and further developing the technique of real-time 3D echocardiography. The other commonly used noninvasive, diagnostic techniques—computed tomography and magnetic resonance imaging—have revealed the clinical impact of 3D anatomic data sets. These tools require much longer times for acquisition and reconstruction, and cannot image in real-time, providing a distinct advantage for 3D echocardiography. As these tools become more widely available, their impact in the diagnosis and management of cardiovascular disease will also increase. It is likely that 3D echocardiography using both reconstructed and real-time images will become an extremely useful noninvasive cardiac imaging technique in the near future.

Three-dimensional echocardiography utilizes the acquisition of digital images using standard ultrasound systems and usually a transesophageal echocardiographic transducer, although some newer transthoracic probes are in various stages of development. These digital images are gated to the electrocardiogram and through post-processing analysis, allow three spatial dimensions of anatomic, and more recently color flow, data to be stored. The addition of color Doppler flow 3D imaging has further enhanced its clinical impact.

Once the computer has a 3D data set, the cardiac anatomy may be viewed from any chosen position ("anyplane imaging"). This has been the greatest advantage of this technique. This has allowed, for example, the complex shape of the mitral valve to be characterized in greater detail. Ventricular and atrial septal defects can now be visualized from within the cardiac chambers giving *en face* views never before available. Coronary artery anatomy and complex aortic pathology may now be imaged in greater detail and abnormal left ventricular geometry does not prevent adequate assessment of left ventricular function.

The aim of this book is to provide a comprehensive, state-of-the-art review of this relatively new technique of 3D echocardiography in an atlas format, and to facilitate demonstration of numerous normal and pathologic cardiac findings. The Atlas contains nearly 700 illustrations.

The Atlas is organized into thirteen chapters. The first chapter provides an introduction to 3D echocardiography and reviews some historical aspects. The second chapter deals with normal anatomy, normal variants and artifacts, an extremely valuable background in beginning to understand images generated from reconstructed data sets. Valvular heart disease is extensively covered in the third chapter and is very clinically relevant. Chapter 4 deals with aortic pathology and reveals the marked difference in the appearance of dissection flaps on 3D echocardiography as compared to the 2D technique. Chapter 5 illustrates the usefulness of 3D echocardiography in the assessment of ischemic heart disease and its complications. Congenital heart disease is covered in a comprehensive manner in Chapters 6 and 7 and is valuable to both the adult and pediatric echocardiographer. Chapter 8 deals with cardiac masses and exemplifies the value of "anyplane imaging" in clarifying the exact anatomic relationships of these masses. Numerous miscellaneous lesions are covered in Chapter 9. Chapters 10 and 11 deal with the more recent innovations of 3D color Doppler flow imaging and it is easy to understand the clinical value of this development. The exciting new development of real-time 3D echocardiography is covered in Chapter 12. Finally, Chapter 13 deals with future directions in 3D echocardiography, leaving us with the probability that 3D imaging will likely evolve into a simple "touch pad" on all echo systems, similar to color flow Doppler and harmonic imaging adaptations.

The Suggested Readings Lists at the end of each chapter provide additional background reading material for the reader of the Atlas, and acknowledge the work of many echocardiographers and scientists who have contributed to the development of three-dimensional echocardiography. The Suggested Readings Lists were compiled by Rajasekhar Nekkanti, MD and Michelle White, from The University of Alabama at Birmingham's Echocardiography Laboratories, and we are grateful for their help.

Besides illustrations from our own Echocardiography Laboratories, numerous other well-known echocardiographers and scientists have contributed extensively to the Atlas. Their contributions are individually acknowledged in the Atlas and we are most grateful to them for all their help. They are: Drs. Rachele Adoriso, Masood Ahmad, Fause Attie, Raffaele De Simone, Stefano De Castro, Jaroslaw Drozdz, Nilda Espinola-Zavaleta, Andreas Franke, Annette Geibel, Gerald Glombitza, Ivan Godoy, Albert A. Hagege, Siegried Hagl, Michael Handke, Peter Hanrath, Jaroslaw D. Kasprzak, Harald P. Kühl, Jan Kulhanek, Roberto Lang, Alexsandra Lange, Rene Lerch, Hans Peter Meinzer, Francisco Javier Roldan, Angel Romero-Cardenas, Dietrich Markus Schäfer, Kirk T. Spencer, Lissa Sugeng, Christian Friedrich Vahl, Jesus Vargas-Barron, Clara Vazquez-Antona, Cedric Vuille, Xin-Fang Wang, Helmut Wollschläger, and Jim Bednarz, Bernhard Mumm, John Oxaal, Anja Schöchlin, and Lynn Weinert.

We must also thank several individuals in our Universities who have contributed directly or indirectly to the growth and development of 3D echocardiography in our Echocardiography Laboratories. First and foremost, we are grateful to all the present and past members of the Divisions of Cardiovascular Disease from both Universities for providing us full clinical support. Most of all, we are grateful to the Divisions of Cardiovascular Surgery, especially Dr. John W. Kirklin, Dr. Albert D. Pacifico, Dr. James K. Kirklin, Dr. George L. Zorn, Jr, Dr. William Holman, and Dr. David McGiffin, from the University of Alabama at Birmingham and Dr. W. Randolph Chitwood, JR, Dr. J. Mark Williams, Dr. Theodore C. Koutlas, Dr. Jon F. Moran, and Dr. Nicola A. Francalancia, MD, from the East Carolina University not only for facilitating the performance of intraoperative transesophageal echocardiography but also for providing us surgical correlation in the patients operated upon by them. We also thank Dr. PoHoey Fan, Assistant Professor of Medicine in the Division of Cardiovascular Disease at the University of Alabama at Birmingham for his help and support in performing 3D echocardiography. We are thankful to Photography and Instructional Graphics of the University of Alabama at Birmingham, especially J. Michael Strawn and Steven W. Wood for their support.

We are most grateful to the Clinical and Research Fellows, Medical Residents, and Observers, both past and present, from the Heart Station/Echocardiography Laboratories at the University of Alabama at Birmingham and East Carolina University who directly or indirectly helped in the performance of 3D echocardiography. From the University of Alabama at Birmingham they are: Dr. Srinivasa R. Aaluri, Dr. Dipak Agrawal, Dr. Gopal Agrawal, Dr. Ramesh Aggarwal, Dr. Kamlesh G. Ansingkar, Dr. Steve Bakir, Dr. Mahesh M. Bhambore, Dr. Robert W. Biederman, Dr. Sang-Man Chung, Dr. Francisco Costa, Dr. Sayed Mohammed Abd El-Rahman, Dr. Miguel Espinal Santos, Dr. Wen Ying Huang, Dr. Ming Hsiung, Dr. Farrukh Jamil, Dr. Ajay Jindal, Dr. Abraham S. John, Dr. Mohammad Kamran, Dr. Gaurav Kapur, Dr. Gajendra Khatri, Dr. Kee-Sik Kim, Dr. Zhi-An Li, Dr. Andrew Miller, Dr. Mohamed Moursi, Dr. Osman M.E. Mukhtar, Dr. Virenjan Kumar Narayan, Dr. Rajasekhar Nekkanti, Dr. Ozelem Ocak, Dr. Arnold Pasia, Dr. Luis Pinheiro, Dr. Virender Puri, Dr. Steven Rosenthal, Dr. Debasish Roychoudhury, Dr. Aditya Kumar Samal, Dr. Rajat Sanyal, Dr. Gamal M. Shoeb, Dr. Joao Baptista de Sousa, Jr, Dr. Abhash C. Thakur, (all Clinical or Research Fellows), Dr. Szilard Voros (Medical Resident), Dr. Sanjay Malhotra, Dr. R.J. Kottakoka, and Dr. Dilek Yesilbursa (all Observers). From the East Carolina University they are: Drs. John Viola, Ghassan Alkoutami, Steve Hunley, Nadim Geloo, Jerry Simpson, Sagir Ahmed, Sanjay Patel, Jan Kulhanek, Mahmoud Atieh, Shekar Kumar, Stacey Brewington, Nazim Khan, Srivani Ambati, and Angan-pally Rajeev.

We were also saddened by the passing of our very dear friend and colleague, Dr. William C. Reeves, who died prior to the completion of this project. He was an excellent cardiologist and superb echocardiographer and without his support, this book could not have been completed.

We deeply appreciate the help of Lindy Chapman, Administrative Associate at the University of Alabama at Birmingham, who provided excellent editorial and secretarial assistance. We would also like to thank our clinical sonographers who were responsible for data acquisition and storage of 3D images at ECU. They include Deena Carraway, Christopher Mann, Mary Erdmann, and Julia Campbell.

Finally, we are grateful to our families for their support during the innumerable hours we spent on this project: Dr. Nanda's family wife Kanta K. Nanda, MD, sons, Nitin Nanda, Anil Nanda, M.D. and daughter, Anita Nanda, M.D.; Dr. Sorrells' parents Dr. Meredith E. and Bonnie M. Sorrell, brother Duane E. Sorrell, and wife and family Amanda J., Zoe L. and Jack A. Sorrell.

Navin C. Nanda, MD
Vincent L. Sorrell, MD

Contributors

Rachele Adoriso, MD Research Fellow, Department of Clinical Medicine, "La Sapienza" University of Rome, Rome, Italy

Masood Ahmad, MD Professor of Medicine and Director, Echocardiography Laboratory, The University of Texas Medical Branch at Galveston, Galveston, Texas

Fause Attie, MD Instituto Nacional de Cardiologia, Ignacio Chavez, Juan Badiano Tlalpan, Mexico

Jim Bednarz, BS The University of Chicago, Department of Medicine, Section of Cardiology, Chicago, Illinois

Stefano De Castro, MD Assistant Professor of Cardiology, Department of Clinical Medicine and Associate Chief of the Echocardiography Laboratories, "La Sapienza" University of Rome, Rome, Italy

Raffaele De Simone, MD University of Heidelberg, Department of Cardiac Surgery, Heidelberg, Germany

Jaroslaw Drozdz, MD Department of Cardiology, Medical University of Lodz, Lodz, Poland

Nilda Espinola-Zavaleta, MD Instituto Nacional de Cardiologia, Ignacio Chavez, Juan Badiano Tlalpan, Mexico

Andreas Franke, MD Medicine Clinic I, University Hospital Aachen, Aachen, Germany

Annette Geibel, MD Assistant Professor of Medicine, Universitatsklinik Freiburg, Innere Medizin III—Kardiologie, Freiburg, Germany

Gerald Glombitza, PhD German Cancer Research Center, Heidelberg, Germany

Ivan Godoy, MD The University of Chicago, Department of Medicine, Section of Cardiology, Chicago, Illinois

Albert A. Hagège, MD Director, Echocardiographic Laboratory, Hôpital European Georges Pompidou, Paris, France

Siegried Hagl, MD University of Heidelberg, Department of Cardiac Surgery, Heidelberg, Germany

Michael Handke, MD Universitatsklinik Freiburg, Innere Medizin III—Kardiologie, Freiburg, Germany

Peter Hanrath, MD Professor of Medicine, Head of the Department, Medicine Clinic I, University Hospital Aachen, Aachen, Germany

Jaroslaw D. Kasprzak, MD Department of Cardiology, Medical University of Lodz, Lodz, Poland

Harald P. Kühl, MD Medicine Clinic I, University Hospital Aachen, Aachen, Germany

Jan Kulhanek, MD Adult Cardiovascular Fellow, East Carolina University Brody School of Medicine, Greenville, North Carolina

Roberto Lang, MD The University of Chicago, Department of Medicine, Section of Cardiology, Chicago, Illinois

Alexsandra Lange, MD Royal Hospital for Sick Children, Edinburgh, United Kingdom

Rene Lerch, MD Professor of Cardiology, Cardiology Center, University Hospital Geneva, Switzerland

Hans Peter Meinzer, PhD German Cancer Research Center, Heidelberg, Germany

Bernhard Mumm TomTec Imaging Systems, Gmbh, Munich, Germany

John Oxaal Volumetrics Medical Imaging, Inc. Durham, North Carolina

Francisco Javier Roldan, MD Instituto Nacional de Cardiologia, Ignacio Chavez, Juan Badiano Tlalpan, Mexico

Angel Romero-Cardenas, MD Instituto Nacional de Cardiologia, Ignacio Chavez, Juan Badiano Tlalpan, Mexico

Dietrich Markus Schäfer, MD Universitatsklinik Freiburg, Innere Medizin III—Kardiologie, Freiburg, Germany

Anja Schöchlin, MA Universitatsklinik Freiburg, Innere Medizin III—Kardiologie, Freiburg, Germany

Kirk T. Spencer, MD The University of Chicago, Department of Medicine, Section of Cardiology, Chicago, Illinois

Lissa Sugeng, MD The University of Chicago, Department of Medicine, Section of Cardiology, Chicago, Illinois

Christian Friedrich Vahl, MD University of Heidelberg, Department of Cardiac Surgery, Heidelberg, Germany

Jesus Vargas-Barron, MD Instituto Nacional de Cardiologia, Ignacio Chavez, Juan Badiano Tlalpan, Mexico

Clara Vazquez-Antona, MD Instituto Nacional de Cardiologia, Ignacio Chavez, Juan Badiano Tlalpan, Mexico

Cedric Vuille, MD Senior Cardiologist, Cardiology Center, University Hospital Geneva, Geneva, Switzerland

Xin-Fang Wang, MD Union Hospital, Wuhan, People's Republic of China

Lynn Weinert, BS The University of Chicago, Department of Medicine, Section of Cardiology, Chicago, Illinois

Ivo Wolf, PhD German Cancer Research Center, Heidelberg, Germany

Helmut Wollschläger, MD Professor of Medicine, Klinikum St. Marien Amberg, Amberg, Germany

Contents

Chapter 1

Technical Background and Current & Future Aspects of Three-Dimensional Echocardiography

Bernhard Mumm, Navin C. Nanda, MD, and Vincent L. Sorrell, MD

Introduction

Today's conventional transthoracic (TTE) and transesophageal (TEE) echocardiography provides only one-dimensional (M-Mode) information or two-dimensional tomographic slices (B-Mode) of a three-dimensional structure, the heart.

The cardiologist must perform a mental three-dimensional (3D) reconstruction based on his or her experience to understand the complex cardiac pathology from multiple two-dimensional (2D) slices displayed sequentially during the 2D echo examination. The ultrasound transducer has to be moved manually in order to get the tomographic slices necessary for the diagnosis. For example, if a study has been acquired by a sonographer, and has to be reviewed from a videotape, there is no chance to get additional diagnostic image information other than the 2D echo images on the tape. To get missing information, the patient has to be called in again.

Three-dimensional echocardiography can overcome such limitations. Here, the heart or any region of interest within it is recorded as a so-called digital 3D data set, containing all anatomic information in space and motion (often called dynamic 3D echo, or 4D echo).[1] Such a 3D data set can be acquired digitally in different ways utilizing 3D ultrasound systems as described later in this chapter.

The "digital data set" can contain the entire spatial or morphological information of the heart in one or multiple heartbeats. Thus, the dynamics of the heartbeat or valve motion, and optionally together with the color flow information, can be assessed in a three-dimensional way. Multiple dynamic 3D views of the heart or a structure of interest can be digitally produced in the 3D computer based on such a data set.

To answer a given clinical question, the relevant diagnostic information can be retrieved from this data set retrospectively. A cardiac surgeon for example could "open" the heart in the digital data set as if opening the heart in the operating room. He could digitally "vivisect" the heart in the computer to generate 3D views comparable to what he would see during the surgery. But in most surgeries, the patient's heart is not beating. All the dynamic information is missing. The heart is collapsed. In a computed 3D display, the entire heart motion or, for example, the dynamics of the valve leaflets, can be seen in a "virtual" surgical view (Figure 1). Providing these kinds of images helps to improve the communication between the echocardiographer and the cardiac surgeon.

History of Three-Dimensional Echocardiography

Medical 3D imaging has been mainly developed in the field of magnetic resonance imaging (MRI) and computed tomography (CT) since 1970. In this field, 3D is already a well established diagnostic tool. Magnetic resonance and CT are both—like ultrasound—tomographic imaging modalities. The imaging planes are acquired parallel to each other. For example, by moving the patient table orthogonal to the imaging plane in equidistant steps, an organ or even the entire body can be scanned in many parallel slices. These slices can then be stacked together to generate a volumetric data set for further 3D reconstructions.

But both modalities are not well suited for the as-

From Nanda NC and Sorrell VL: *Atlas of Three-Dimensional Echocardiography.* ©Futura Publishing Co., Inc, Armonk, NY, 2002.

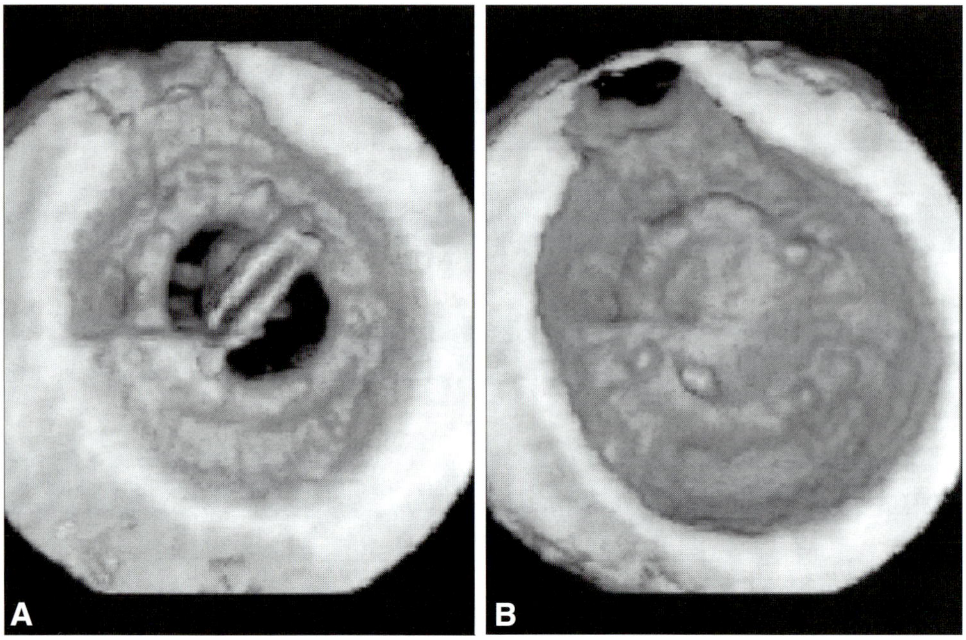

Figure 1. Prosthetic mitral valve (MV) seen from the left atrium in an open (**A**) and closed (**B**) position.

sessment of fast moving cardiac structures. Newly developed systems are now very much improved in temporal resolution, but are still not comparable to ultrasound, with its high frame rates and good spatial resolution, as a cost efficient, mobile, and well suited technology for cardiology.

The use of ultrasound to study the heart was first reported in 1953. In the beginning, only a one-dimensional beam could be used. Later, in the 1960s, multiple beams could be combined to form a 2D image. With the development of real-time 2D ultrasound systems and electronic phased array transducers, 2D echocardiography became the most widely used diagnostic imaging method in clinical cardiology.

The idea of combining the 3D concepts of MRI and CT with the benefits of ultrasound led to the development of 3D echocardiography.

Early research work in the field of 3D echocardiography was done by several investigators, including Dekker et al. in 1974,[2] Ghosh, Nanda, Maurer et al. in 1982,[3] Collins et al. in 1988,[4] Pini in 1989, Levine et al. in 1989[5] and others (Figures 2–8).[6–9]

One of the commercial approaches was to somehow "miniaturize" the parallel scanning of a CT into an esophagoscope.[10] Based on this concept, a special 3D TEE probe and commercial 3D ultrasound system was developed in 1990 (Echo-CT, TomTec Imaging Systems GmbH, Munich, Germany) to perform a parallel 3D scan of the beating heart. After the insertion of this TEE probe, the distal part of the probe could be

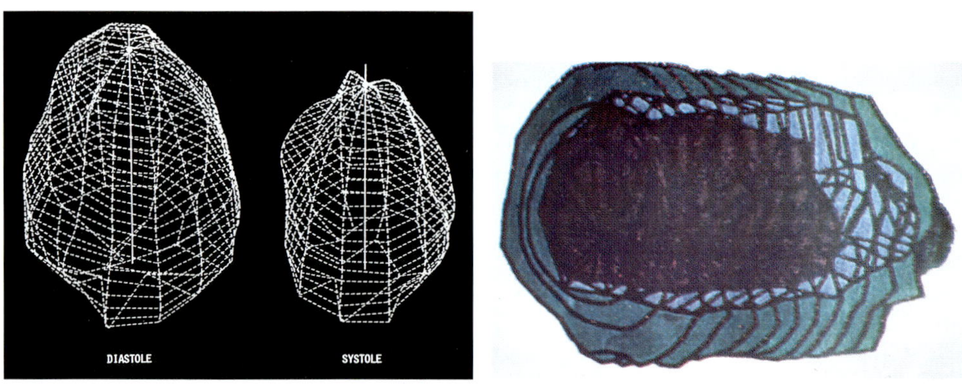

Figure 2. (**A**) Three-dimensional (3D) reconstruction of echocardiographic images using apical rotation method: 3D end-diastolic (left) and end-systolic (right) views of the left ventricle. These 3D views were obtained at a viewing angle of 45° from the apical axis. (**B**) Four-dimensional reconstruction of two-dimensional echocardiographic images: overlay of high-flow velocity isopleths and left ventricular (LV) endocardium. Green = LV endocardium; blue = low-velocity isopleth; red = high-velocity isopleth. Figure A is reprinted with permission from reference 3. Figure B is reprinted with permission from Raqueno et al. Four-dimensional reconstruction two-dimensional echocardiographic images. *Echocardiography* 1989;6:323–337.

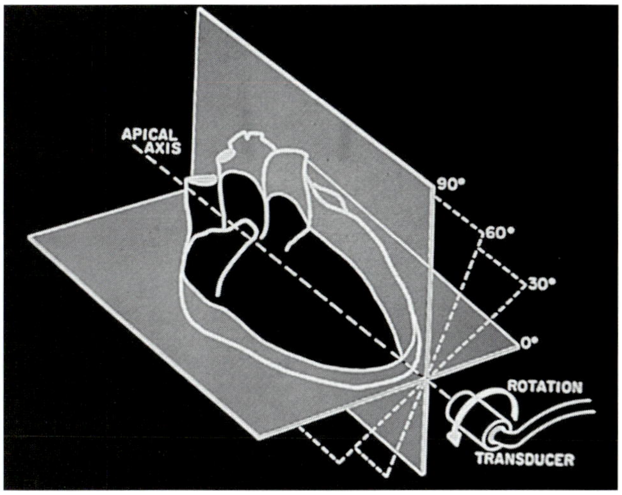

Figure 3. Three-dimensional reconstruction of echocardiographic images by apical axis rotation method. The transducer rotation and different planes intersecting the heart are shown here. Reprinted with permission from reference 7.

mechanically straightened to form a rigid tube. In this tube, the ultrasound crystal could be moved up and down on a sliding carriage. A stepper motor moved the crystal up in parallel equidistant steps controlled by an ECG- and respiration gating logic.[11] While such a system was installed in about 50 research institutes around the world and many papers were published, the special parallel scan 3D TEE probe was of limited value for routine application of this technology.

The use of standard transthoracic transducers and

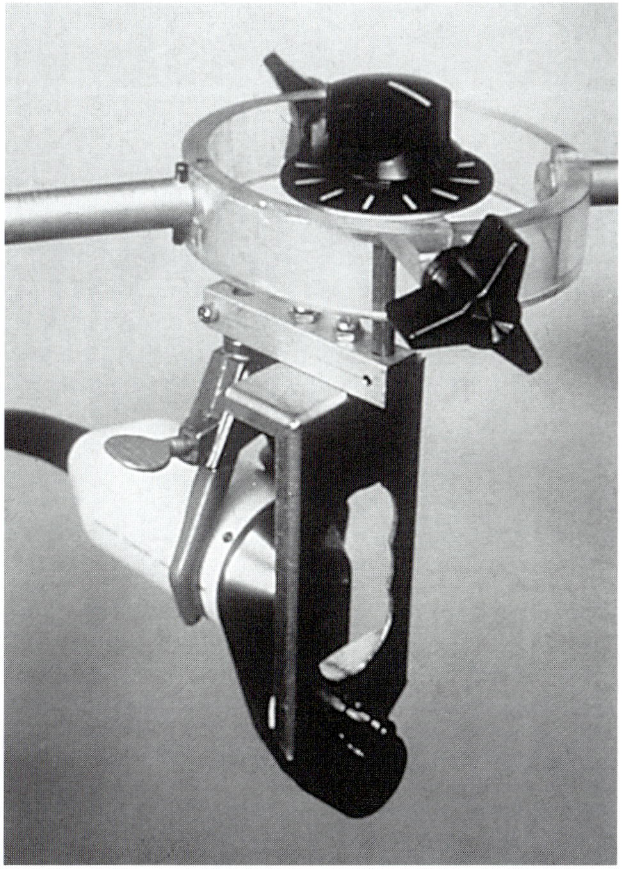

Figure 4. Three-dimensional reconstruction of transthoracic echocardiographic images. Transducer and the mechanical arm. The transducer is mounted on a mechanical arm which permits only 1° of freedom- rotation about its axis. Reprinted with permission from reference 7.

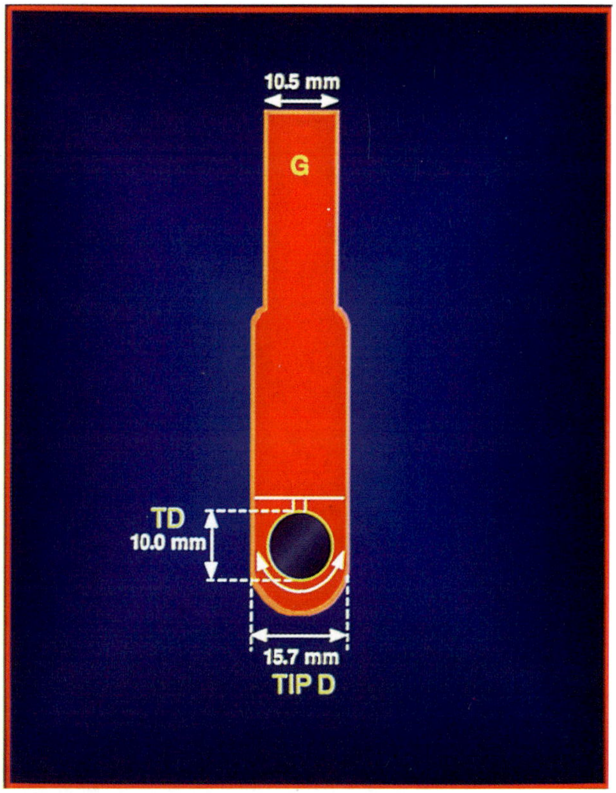

Figure 5. Schematic of the distal end of the currently utilized TEE probe. This is a standard TEE probe without any additional modification in size or appearance. G = gastroscope; TD = diameter of the transducer; TIP D = diameter of the tip of the probe. Reproduced with permission from Nanda et al. Multiplane transesophageal echocardiographic imaging and three-dimensional reconstruction. *Echocardiography* 1992;9:667–676.

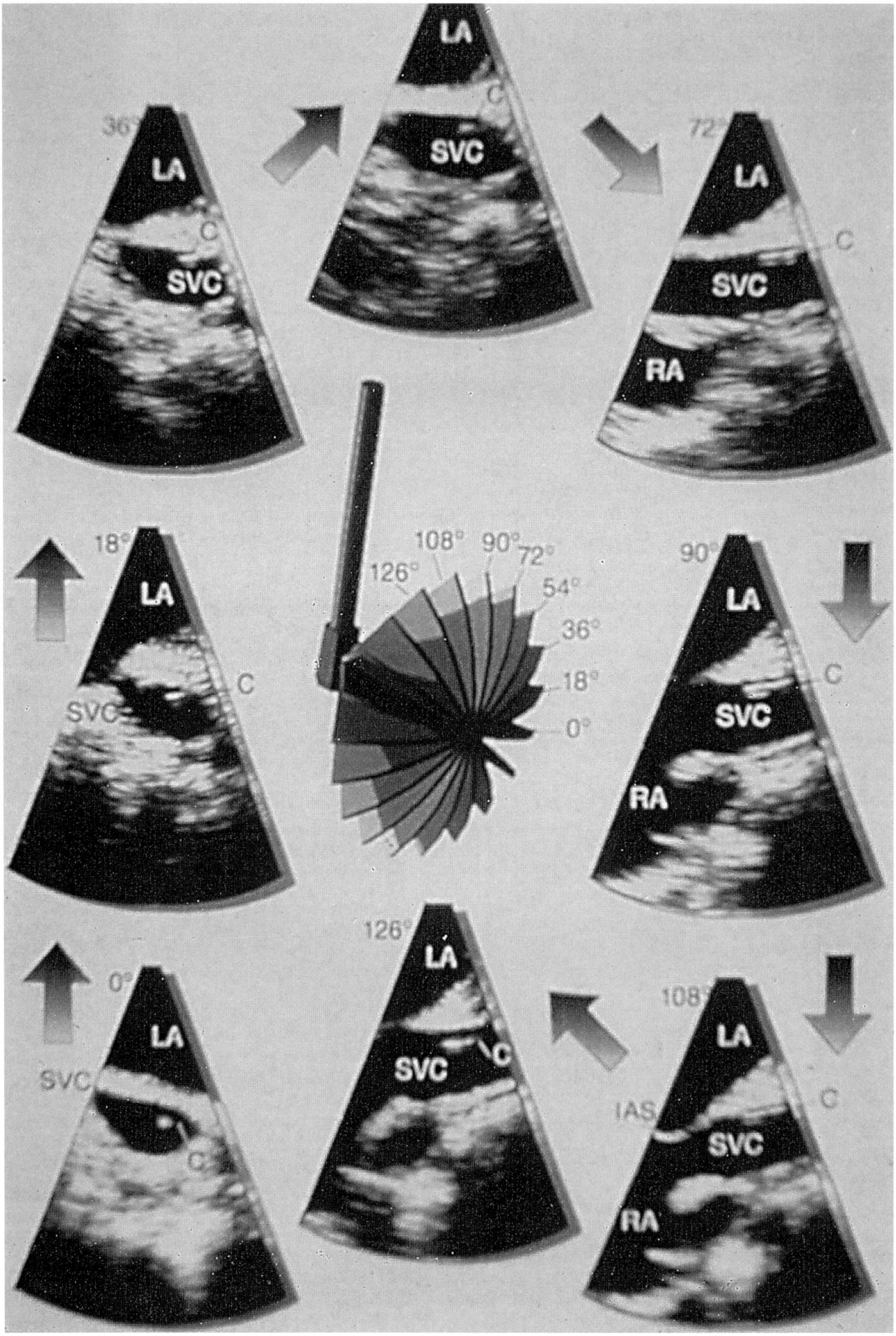

Figure 6. Multiplanar transesophageal two-dimensional images at the level of the superior vena cava (SVC). C = catheter; IAS = intra-atrial septum; LA = left atrium; RA = right atrium. Reproduced with permission from Nanda et al. Multiplane transesophageal echocardiographic imaging and three-dimensional reconstruction. *Echocardiography* 1992;9:667–676.

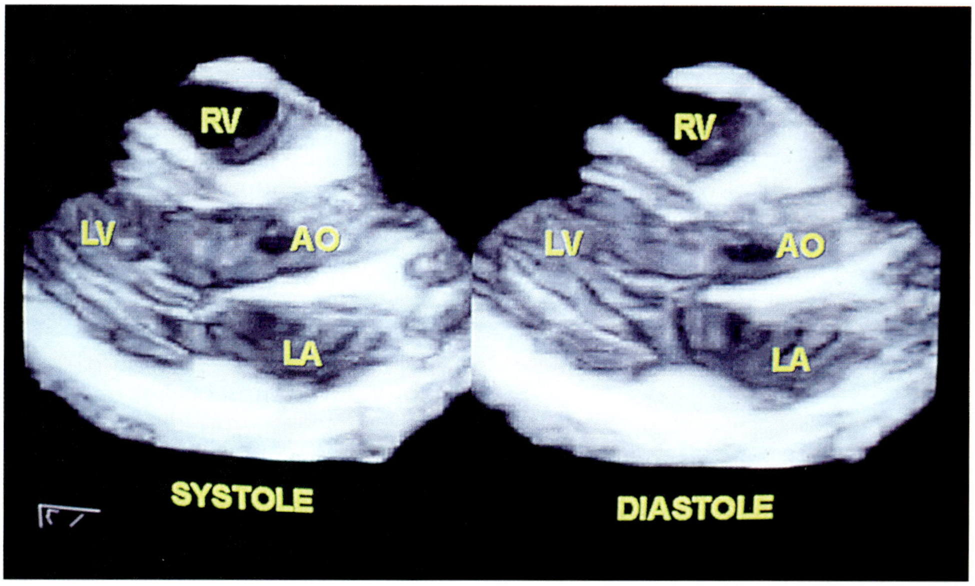

Figure 7. This three-dimensional (3D) echocardiogram was reconstructed from a transthoracic acquired data set and shows a conventional cut-plane image of a parasternal long axis in systole (**left**) and diastole (**right**). Dynamic 3D image of normal long-axis view obtained by TTE. Tomographic section and depths of left ventricular wall, and mitral and aortic valves can be visualized clearly. Left figure was taken in systole; mitral valve was closed and aortic valve was open. Right figure was taken in diastole; mitral valve was open and aortic valve was closed. Reproduced with permission from Wang XF et al. Four-dimensional echocardiography: Methods and clinical application. *Am Heart J* 1996;132:674.

transesophageal multiplane probes for the 3D acquisition was the major step forward for this motor-based methodical acquisition technique. As in a multiplane probe, the imaging plane is rotated around its middle axis in (for example) 2-degree steps, from 0° to 180°, done for the first time by Pini in 1989 and Roelandt.[12] This rotated 3D acquisition technique was first commercially implemented by TomTec Imaging Systems in 1994 as an add-on system to any standard 2D ultrasound unit, and by Hewlett-Packard (Andover MA) as an integrated 3D acquisition option. Up to now, this rotated TTE and TEE multiplane type 3D acquisition has been the most commonly used technique to acquire a cardiac 3D data set.

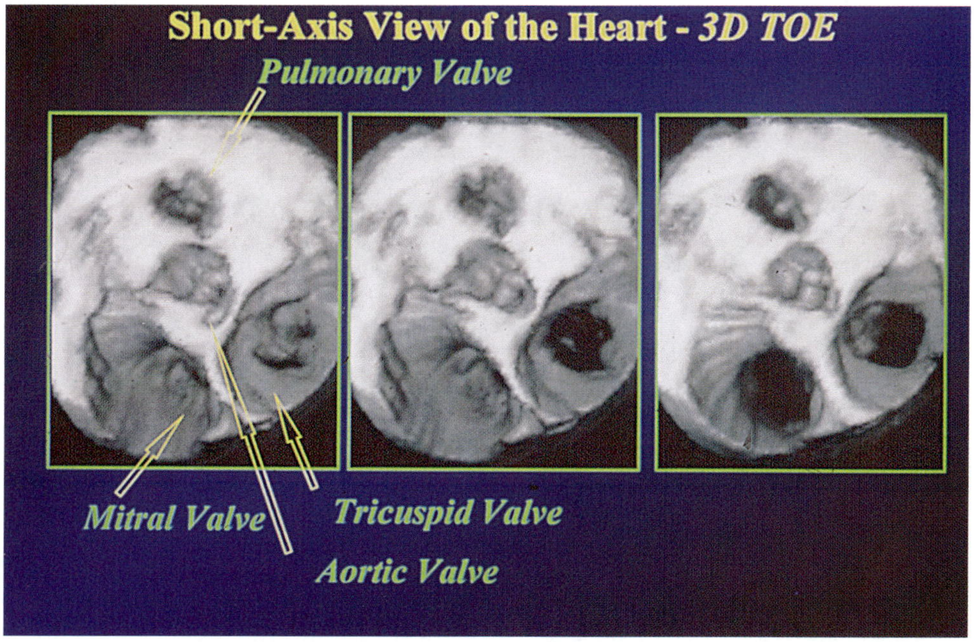

Figure 8. With three-dimensional echocardiography, additional information is routinely acquired as in this basal, short-axis cut-plane image showing all four cardiac valves. This image cannot be obtained with 2D-echo since the valve planes are in various locations. From Aleksandra Lange, MD.

In parallel, other methods have been developed. A real-time 3D echo system has been introduced by von Ramm et al.[13–14] This system is based on a Matrix (Volumetrics Medical Imaging, Inc., Durham, NC) array transducer and a complex highly parallel architecture for the signal processing. It can acquire a dynamic volumetric data set of the heart within one heartbeat in real-time. This system was commercially available from 1997–1999.

Another commercial approach was to use an acoustic spatial coordinate sensor (spark gap) to register the spatial position and movement of the 2D ultrasound probe for the acquisition of a three-dimensional data set.[15]

Most recently, the spatial coordinate sensor technique has been improved by use of small miniaturized electromagnetic position sensors in combination with the ECG- and respiration gating technique. With this method, transthoracic 3D data sets can be acquired in a user friendly and fast manner. More clinical studies have to be performed to prove the robustness of this method.

Theoretical Background of Three-Dimensional Echocardiography

In comparison to a 2D tomographic slice or B-mode image which is based on a matrix of its smallest image elements (the pixels), a 3D data set consists of spatial pixels—the so called voxels (Figure 9). If a complete heartbeat is stored within such a dynamic 3D image (dynamic volume – or "tolume"), we are talking about four-dimensional voxels – or "toxels."

These volume elements within a 3D-echo data set and their visual representation as a 3D reconstruction are generated by the following algorithm:

- Data acquisition
- Geometric resampling
- Image conditioning
- 3D visualization
- 3D quantification

Step 1: Three-Dimensional Acquisition

To utilize 3D display techniques for cardiac structures, it is necessary to acquire a cubic data set of the beating heart. This can be achieved by scanning the volume of interest methodically in equidistant steps, nonsystematically (e.g., by using position sensor systems), or in real-time utilizing a matrix array probe.

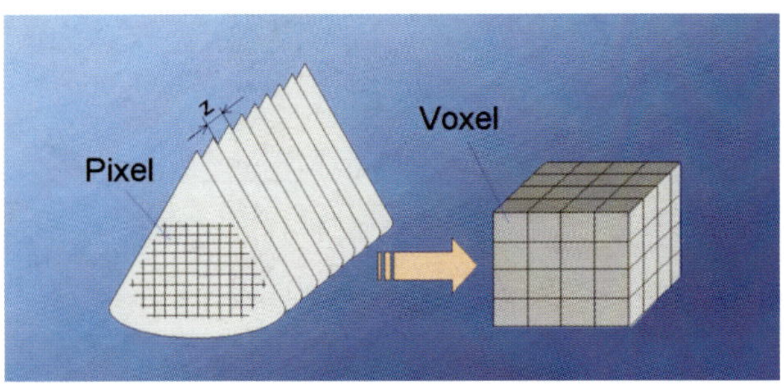

Figure 9. Pixel and voxel.

Most of the methodical 3D acquisition techniques used today are based on a motor to precisely move either the ultrasound crystal within a 3D probe in predefined steps, or to move the entire transducer with so called "probe carriage devices." Such a device holds the entire conventional 2D transducer and performs the predefined movement (in most cases a rotation) of the probe.

Three different methodical acquisition methods are possible: parallel scanning, fan like scanning, and rotational scanning (Figure 10).

Parallel scanning is similar to the scanning technique used for MRI or CT. The image plane is moved, for example, in multiple 1-mm steps perpendicular to itself to acquire the volume of interest. From a theoretical aspect, parallel scanning has the most benefits. It creates equidistant planes in which the voxels close to the transducer have the same distance from each other, like those in in the farfield. This is not the case for fan like or rotational scanning. In addition, it is the less sensitive method for motion artifacts. A later geometric reformation of the parallel scanned 3D data set is not necessary. One disadvantage is the need for a large acoustic window; therefore it is not best suited for scanning of the heart, but peripheral vessels, the carotid, or abdominal structures.

Fan Like Scanning

In fan like scanning, the image plane is swept in a fan to acquire a sector shaped data set. This method combines the benefits of parallel scanning and rotational scanning without the disadvantages of both. Theoretically, a small echo window is sufficient, as for rotational scanning. But a small intracostal space could become a problem if the tilt angle is too big. Another disadvantage is that the color Doppler angle is dependent on the sweep angle, and therefore not constant as with parallel or rotational scanning. An advantage is that the 3D scanning process can be stopped if the target area is acquired. This is not the case with rotational scanning.

Rotational Scanning

Rotational scanning is the most used method of acquiring a 3D study. A multiplane or TTE probe is used to acquire image planes from 0° to 180°, typically in 2° or 3° step angles, which leads to a cone-shaped data set. A motor rotates nearby the attached probe around the middle axis of the ultrasound plane. Thus, the necessary acoustic window is only as big as the diameter of the transducer footprint. A disadvantage is the nonisotropic resolution of the data set, with an over-sampling near the rotation axis and an under-sampling in the areas with a bigger radius from the

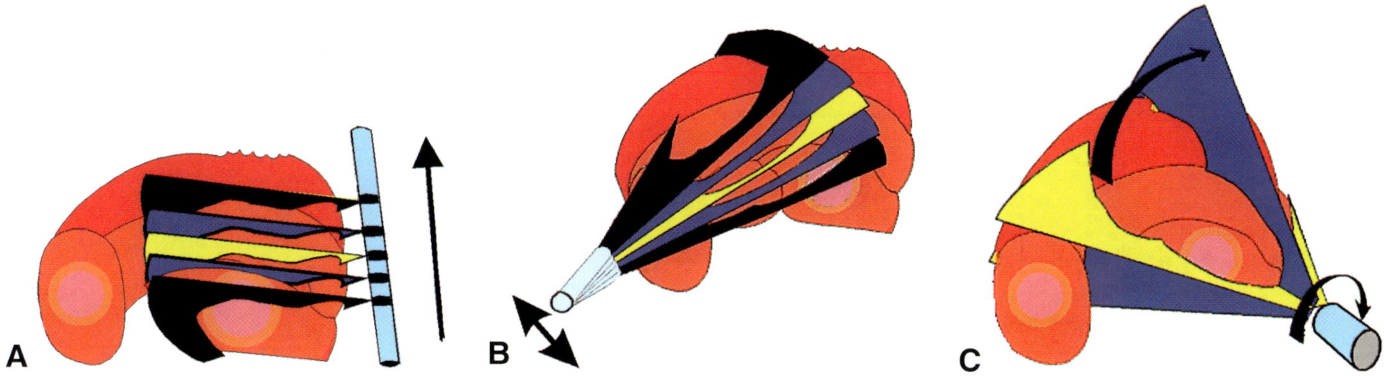

Figure 10. **(A-C)** Parallel scanning, fan like scanning, rotational scanning.

middle axis. This needs to be compensated with interpolation techniques. Another disadvantage is that each movement of the rotation axis during the scan generates a so-called middle artifact. Ideally, all image data along the rotation axis should be identical through all rotated planes. If the middle axis was moved during the scan, this is then no longer the case. Compared to parallel or fan like scanning, the rotational scan must always be completed (from 0° to 180°), otherwise the data set cannot be used, because of missing structures through the entire object.

Nonsystematical Scanning with Position Sensors

Beside these methodical scans, a 3D position sensor, such as an acoustic spark gap device[15] or electromagnetic sensors, can be used for a random or freehand acquisition. The user can freely move the echo transducer by hand, e.g., in a fan like way by slowly sweeping it or in a combination of sweep, shift, and rotation. With each acquired 2D-image, the spatial (x,y,z) coordinates as well as the tilt angle of the probe are recorded and later used to generate a Cartesian data set by storing the images into a 3D cube according to their position. This approach is limited to transthoracic acquisitions today. Typically, about 90 image planes are recorded in about 2 minutes acquisition time. The acquisition can always be stopped by the user if the interesting region has already been acquired. Due to the user-dependent acquisition, the data set can contain gaps or missing information and does not create an isotropic volume. This has to be created by the postprocessing step. Gaps have to be filled with interpolated data.

The limitations of the freehand technique are the position sensor systems themselves. The electromagnetic sensor, for example, is sensitive to electromagnetic disturbances like those generated from strong power supply cables or ferromagnetic material between the sensor and the transmitter. Therefore, the clinical experience is rather small today compared to the other methods mentioned, but this technique will get its application area.

The "Gating technique" for a Dynamic Three-Dimensional Acquisition

For all the above listed dynamic 3D acquisition methods, the heart must be somehow frozen in time to eliminate motion artifacts by using an ECG- and respiration trigger and gating logic (Figure 11). After placing the ECG electrodes and the respiration sensor onto the patient, the 3D acquisition system analyzes the ECG R-wave to R-wave interval time and respiration signals for a learning period (e.g., 30 seconds) to calculate a representative heart cycle. Based on that, the system defines the limits for acceptable heart cycles automatically. However, the user can interactively change or adapt these presettings.

After the 3D acquisition has started, the system 'digitally' records images of a complete heart cycle at each scanning plane. The currently used 3D add-on systems are connected to the video output of a standard 2D echocardiography system. This video signal is then digitized by a frame grabber with a maximum frame rate of 60 frames/second (in NTSC), typically into 8-bit voxel information.

If the first heart cycle is accepted by the gating logic based on the R-R interval length and the respiration phase, the motor moves the probe to the next plane position, e.g, by rotating the transducer 2°. If the heart cycle is not accepted, then the system is rejecting this cycle and is waiting for the next acceptable heartbeat. This automatically continues until the entire volume of interest is scanned. This typically takes 2 to 4 minutes.

Different sensor systems are currently used to register the patients respiration signal:

Chest Impedance.

Here, the impedance is measured between two electrodes, mounted on the right and left side of the

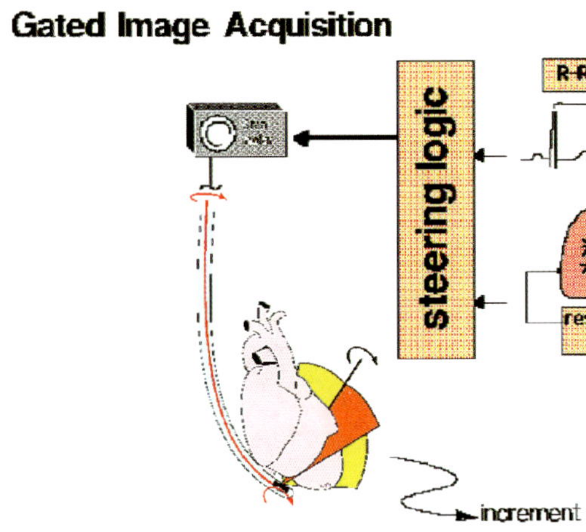

Figure 11. ECG and respiration gating.

chest. Between the inspiratory and expiratory phase, the impedance changes. An electronic circuit then converts this signal into a computer readable form.

Nasal Thermistor.

The nasal thermistor sensor measures the temperature change during inspiration (decreasing temperature) and expiration (increasing temperature) directly in or on the nose.

Acquisition with a Matrix Array Probe

Compared to these "gated 3D acquisition techniques," a new technique is now coming up to acquire one or more heartbeats as a 3D data set in real-time utilizing a 3D matrix array probe. Such a transthoracic matrix array transducer and a special ultrasound system has been initially developed by von Ramm[13] and previously commercialized by Volumetrics Inc. Two-dimensional and 3D color flow as well as a matrix array multiplane probe will follow in the future. This technique cannot be used with a conventional ultrasound system.

Step 2: Digital Reformatting

After image acquisition, a Cartesian data volume must be generated. Depending on the acquisition method, different functions have to be used. In example, a dataset acquired with rotational scan must be converted from a cylindrical into a Cartesian coordinate system. Gaps in the acquired volume must be filled using 3D interpolation algorithms comparable to the 2D scan conversion in a conventional 2D ultrasound scanner. Here the gaps between the sector-shaped "beams" have to be filled with interpolated image data. In 3D space, the gaps are not between the one-dimensional beams but between the 2D planes.

Step 3: Image Processing

In an image conditioning step, image noise and motion artifacts will be reduced or eliminated. Special image processing filters have been developed for this purpose. The artifacts can be created by patient or probe movement during the scan or insufficient ECG/respiratory gating on, for example, patients with irregular heart beat. Other artifacts are based on a changing echo contact during the scan and inhomogenous grey value distribution within the 3D data set.

Step 4: Three-Dimensional Image Display

Cardiac 3D-images can be displayed in different ways, including reconstructed 2D cutplanes similar to MRI or CT (called "Ultrasound CT"), as dynamic 3D surface reconstructed images, or as wireframe-based 3D model of the heart.

Clinically Useful Two-Dimensional Cutplanes

Different standardizations (anyplane, paraplane, rotoplane, mainplane) of such computer generated 2D-images have been published.[12] Such artificial 2D images can show unique views of the heart retrospectively. It is possible to examine the patient's heart digitally in the computer.

In the anyplane mode, any desired cross-section of the heart which might be difficult or physically impossible to obtain from standard precordial or transesophageal acoustic windows can be computed from the data set and displayed in a cine loop of an entire heartbeat.

The paraplane mode provides a sequence of equidistant parallel cut planes through a structure, which are then displayed all together. This is comparable to a sequence of parallel CT images.

The rotoplane mode can provide images that are rotated around one middle axis, like images seen during a rotation of the transducer within a multiplane TEE probe. Therefore, most inexperienced 3D users are easily familiar with this kind of cut plane through a heart within the 3D data set.

In the mainplane mode, three cutplanes are orthogonal to each other, as in a technical drawing. This provides the best overview of a 3D structure, like a simultaneous display of a two-chamber, four-chamber, and short axis view of a left ventricle (LV).

Figure 12 shows an example of such reconstructed 2D planes. In this example, anyplane mode, six different views can be displayed side by side.

3D Surface Reconstructions

Before a 3D surface reconstruction can be generated, the structure of interest must be segmented. This means the user has to define the "surface" of the object. This can be done with different algorithms and methods, for example like a grey value thresholding. All image elements below a certain grey value intensity (threshold), like the blood pool within the heart chambers, are supposed to be fully transparent. The endocardiac wall and/or valve structures should then be adjusted to be the surface by having higher grey value intensities than the blood pool. After this, the user has to define his viewpoint within 3D space, e.g., whether he wishes to look from the left atrium (LA) onto the mitral valve or from the LV side. In order to look "inside" the heart, he has to somehow "open" the heart from one side. This is achieved by a cutplane through the 3D data set. To look down on the mitral valve from the LA side, the cut plane is a kind of "unroofing"of the LA. If the heart is now opened and the surface structure is determined, the surface itself can be visualized in different ways, giving it a different appearance. This process is called "shading technique." The surface appearance could be, for example, very similar to the 2D echo perception ("texture shading"), or more like an anatomic specimen with "distance-" or "gradient-shading."[16–17]

An optimal 3D image can be the mixture of such different shading methods.

Texture Shading.

With this approach, the surface point is displayed with the intensity of the grey value at this particular point in space. This gives the characteristic appearance of the 2D echo image on the surface, but a rather poor 3D impression.

Distance Shading.

This is the simplest shading technique with the least "3D impression." A surface point is displayed very bright if it is close to the virtual light source (or viewer) and very dark if it is far away.

Gradient Shading.

Gradient shading gives the most realistic impression. Here the normal surface vector (or grey value gradient within, for example, a $3 \times 3 \times 3$ cube) is detected and then used for the illuminating model (Phong shading). The light reflection from the surface is calculated according to the normal surface as a direct reflection and a diffuse portion.

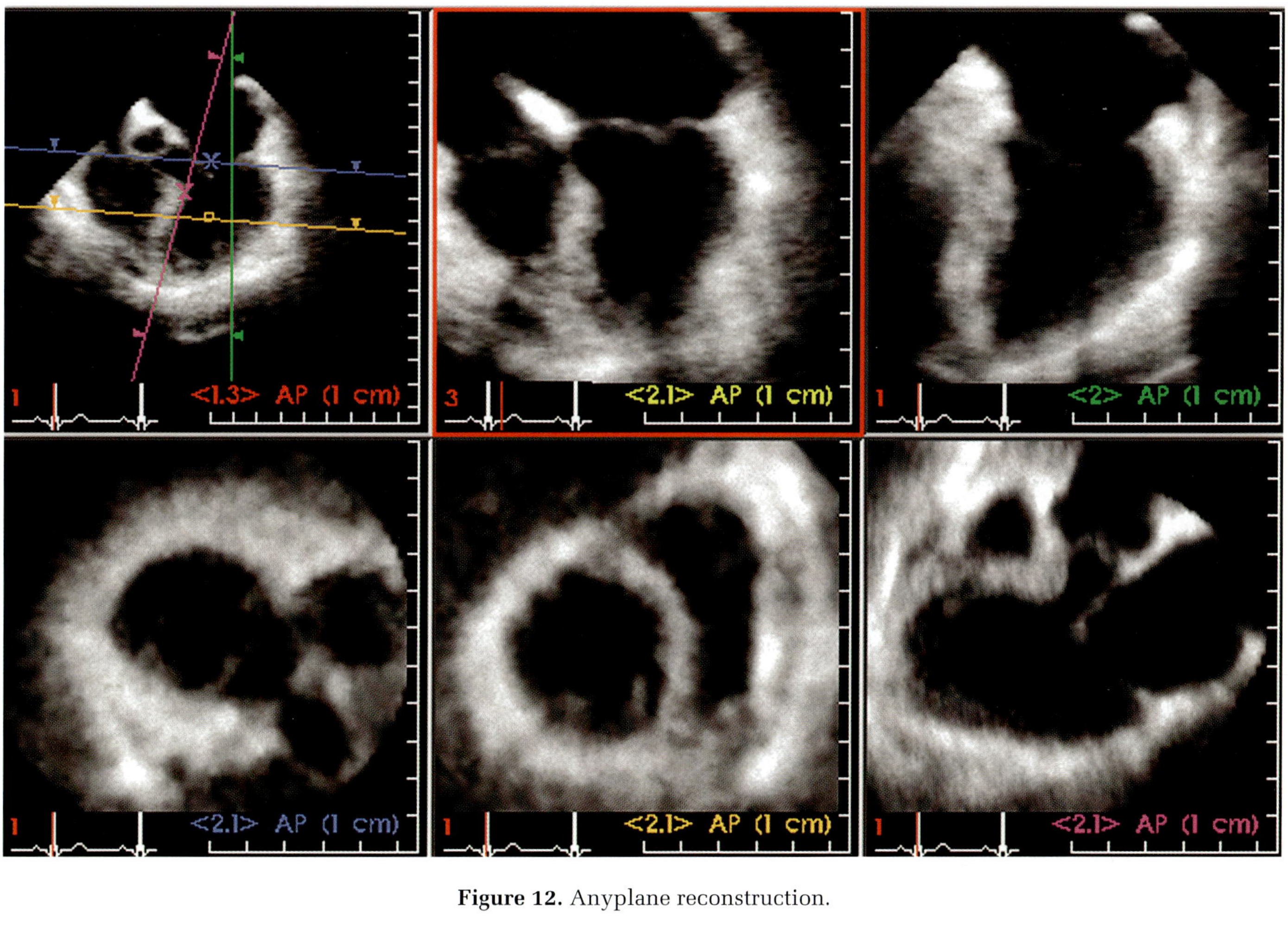

Figure 12. Anyplane reconstruction.

The 3D reconstruction itself is done with the so-called ray casting (or sometimes called ray tracing) algorithm, where rays are sent out from the viewer's perspective through the digital 3D data set to determine the surface along each of the rays based, for example, on the grey value threshold. If the surface is detected, this surface is then displayed, applying one of the above described shading techniques. An even more photorealistic appearance can be achieved by applying additional shadowing or different light sources and positions, virtually illuminating the scene.

Wireframe-Based Three-Dimensional Surface Reconstructions

A so-called surface-based 3D display is generated by manual tracing of, for example, the endocardial border of the LV. This method was originally designed for computer-assisted design and manufacturing (CAD/CAM). No internal structures can be seen, except for the ventricle, which appears like an "empty bag" (Figure 13). This visualization is well suited for LV wall motion display, but not for valvular structures.

Cardiac 3D echo images can be displayed in different ways:

- As 3D surface reconstructions (voxel based) as in the accompanying example of a Mitral Valve (Figure 14).
- As perspective 3D views (endoscopic views) like "sitting" in the heart or "flying" through the heart or coronary vessels (Figure 15).
- As B-mode like computer generated "artificial 2D cut planes" (Figure 16) similar to multiplanar reconstructions (MPR) in MRI or CT.[18]
- As a wireframe based 3D model of the heart (Figure 17). A sequence of 2D contours is extracted from 2D echo planes within a 3D data set. These contours can be combined together to form a 3D shape, visualizing for example the shape of a LV as a wireframe or solid object.

These 3D visualization tools allow "computation" of unlimited new views of the heart out of one 3D data set. Conventional TTE or TEE approaches could never achieve the same views because of the echo window limitations.

Three-dimensional echo is not only a very helpful tool to visualize anatomy or improve the diagnosis of pathology, but it also enables more precise quantification of spatial structures or hemodynamic parameters without using geometric assumptions. Examples are the measurement of right or left ventricular volumes, ejection fraction (EF),[19] quantification of cardiac masses,[20,21] atrial septal defect size and shape, 3D distances and angles, valve opening areas, or (for example) the size of a prolapsing portion of a valve leaflet. Thus, 3D echo helps to get a better understanding of complex cardiac anatomy. This is especially important for the assessment of adult and pediatric congenital heart disease.[22]

But 3D echo should not only be seen as a tool to get improved answers to the same clinical questions which can already be answered with 2D echo today. Three-dimensional echo is a very powerful tool to ask *new* clinical questions which cannot be addressed

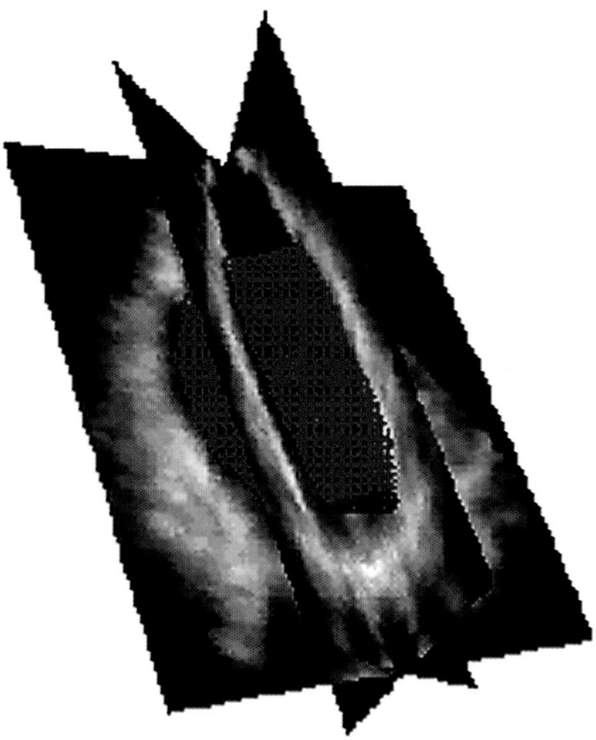

Figure 13. CAD/CAM like contour based three-dimensional display of a left ventricle.

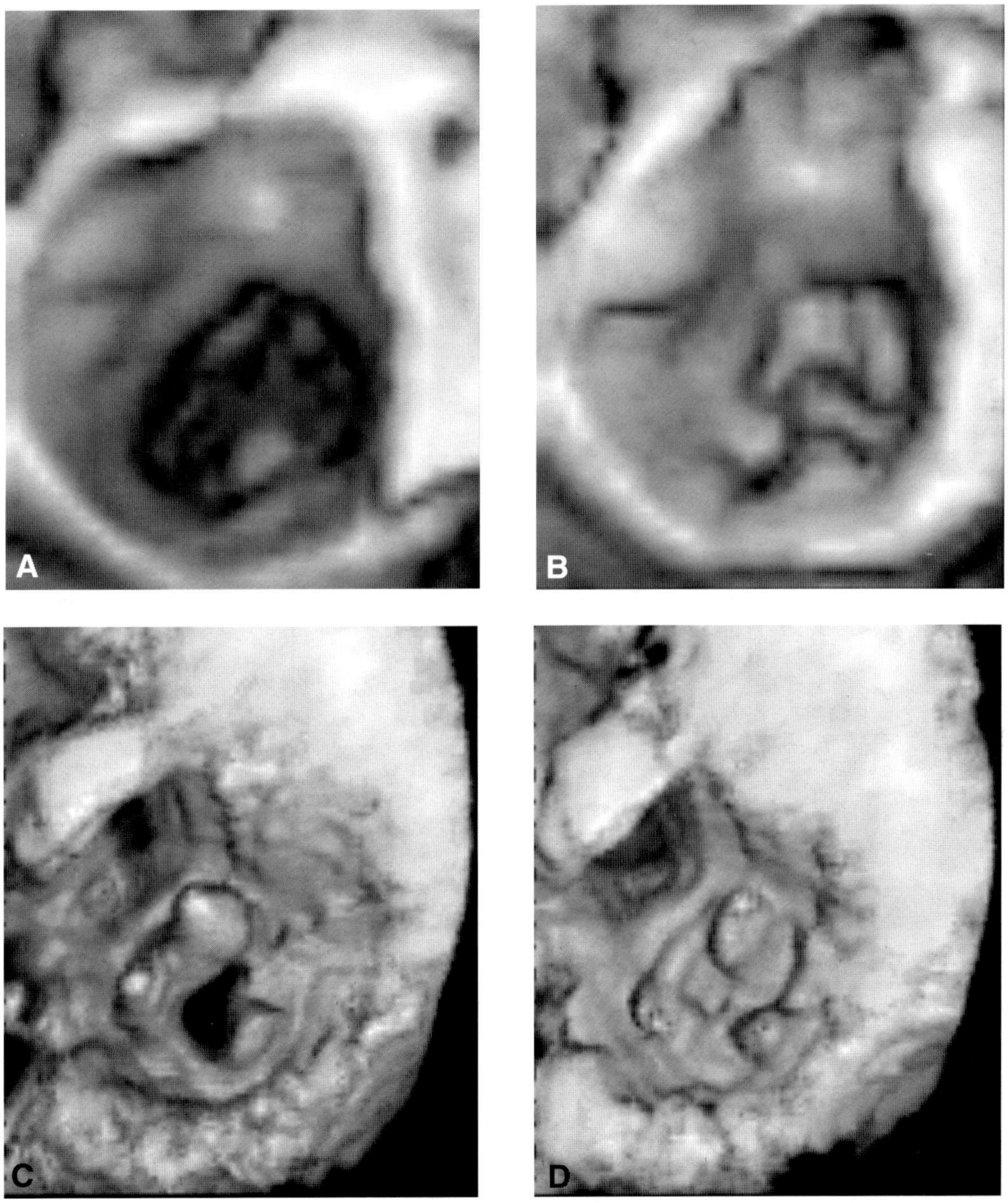

Figure 14. Three-dimensional reconstruction of a bioprosthetic mitral valve viewed from the left atrium in diastole (**A**) and systole (**B**) and from the left ventricle in diastole (**C**) and systole (**D**).

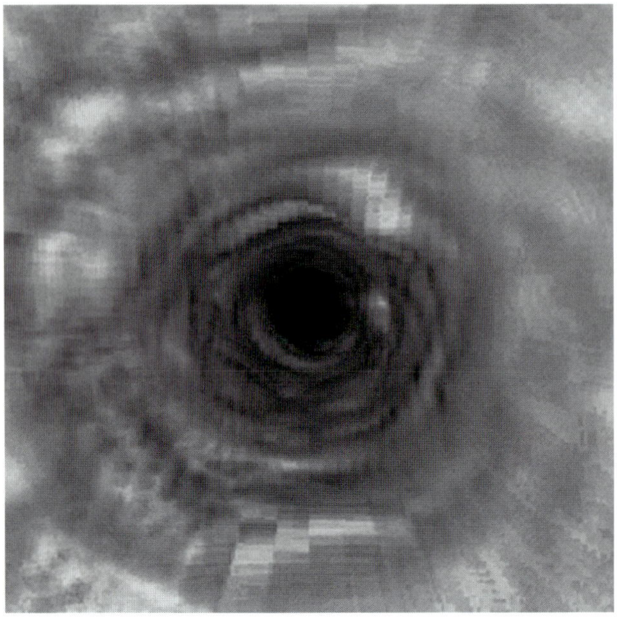

Figure 15. "Endoscopic view" into a coronary vessel based on three-dimensional intravascular ultrasound (courtesy of Professor Roelandt, Thorax Center Rotterdam, The Netherlands).

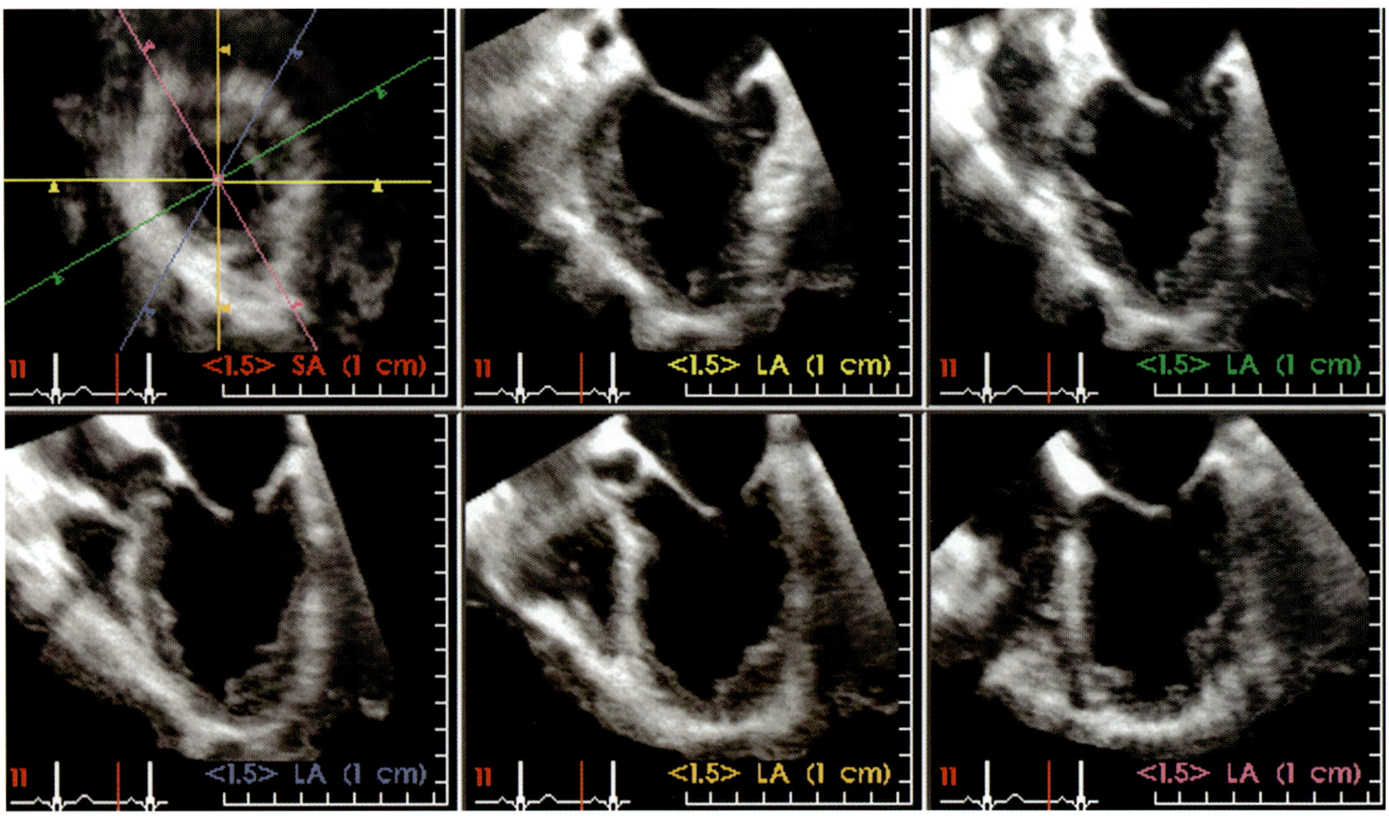

A

Figure 16. (A-D) Computer generated two-dimensional images or cutplanes through the heart.

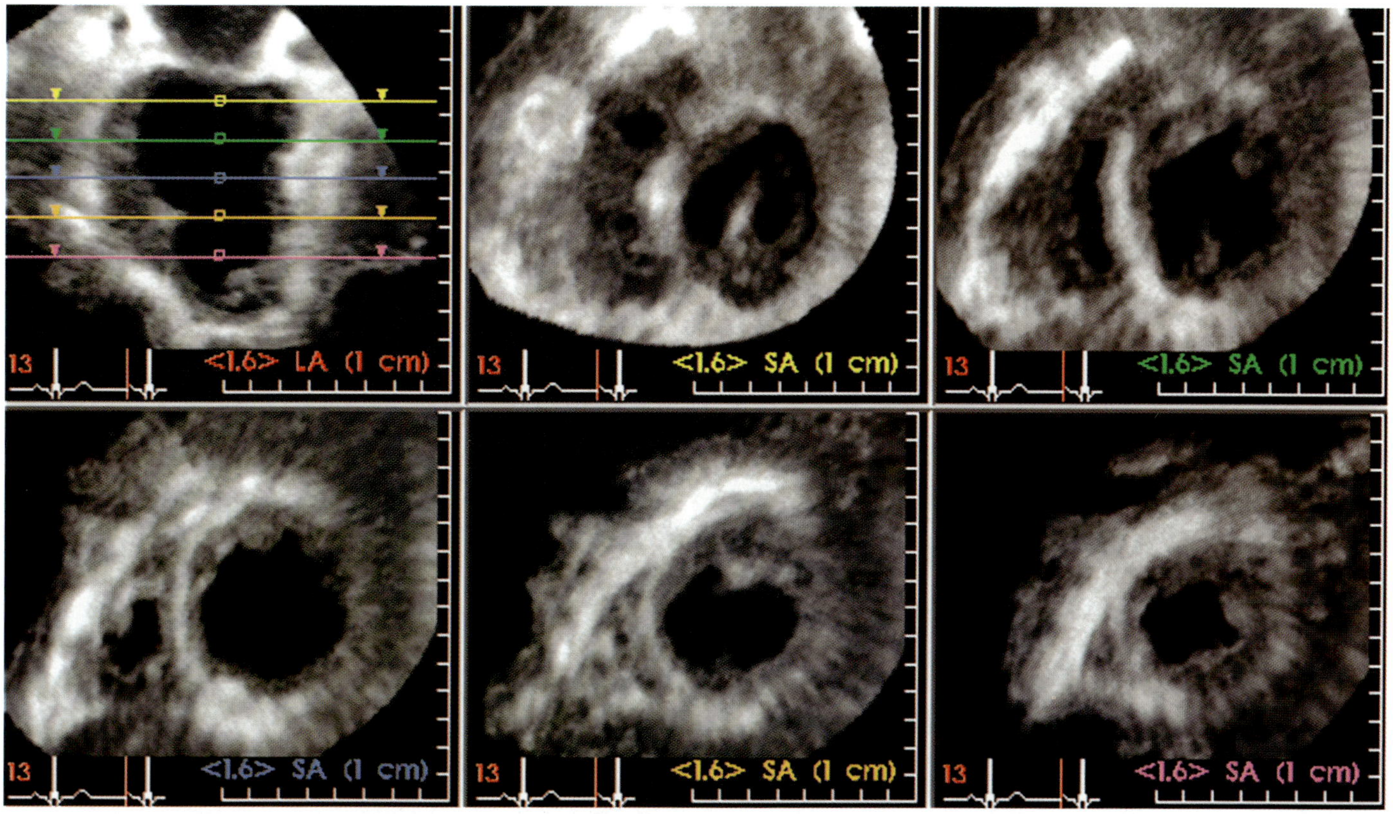

B

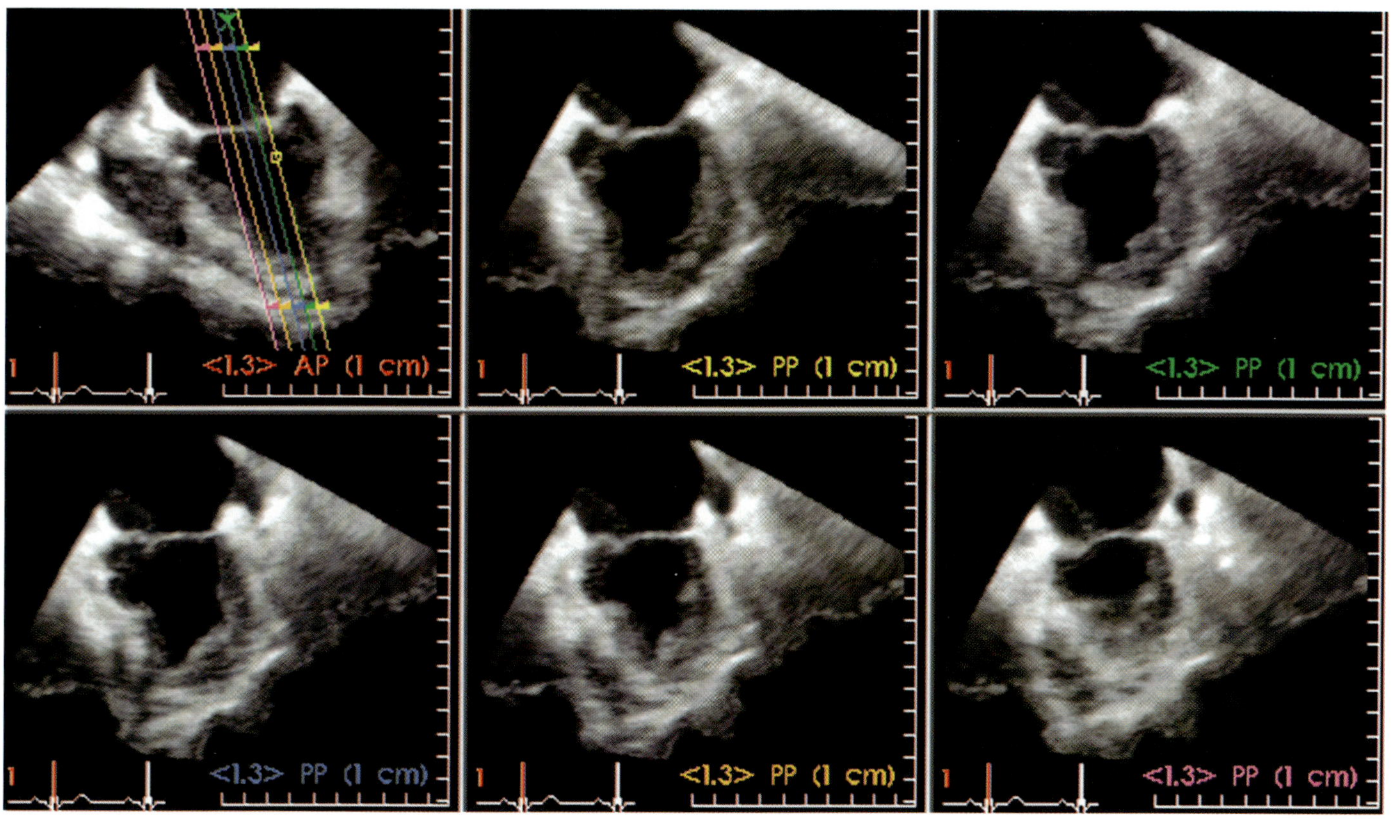

C

Figure 16. **(B-C)** Continued.

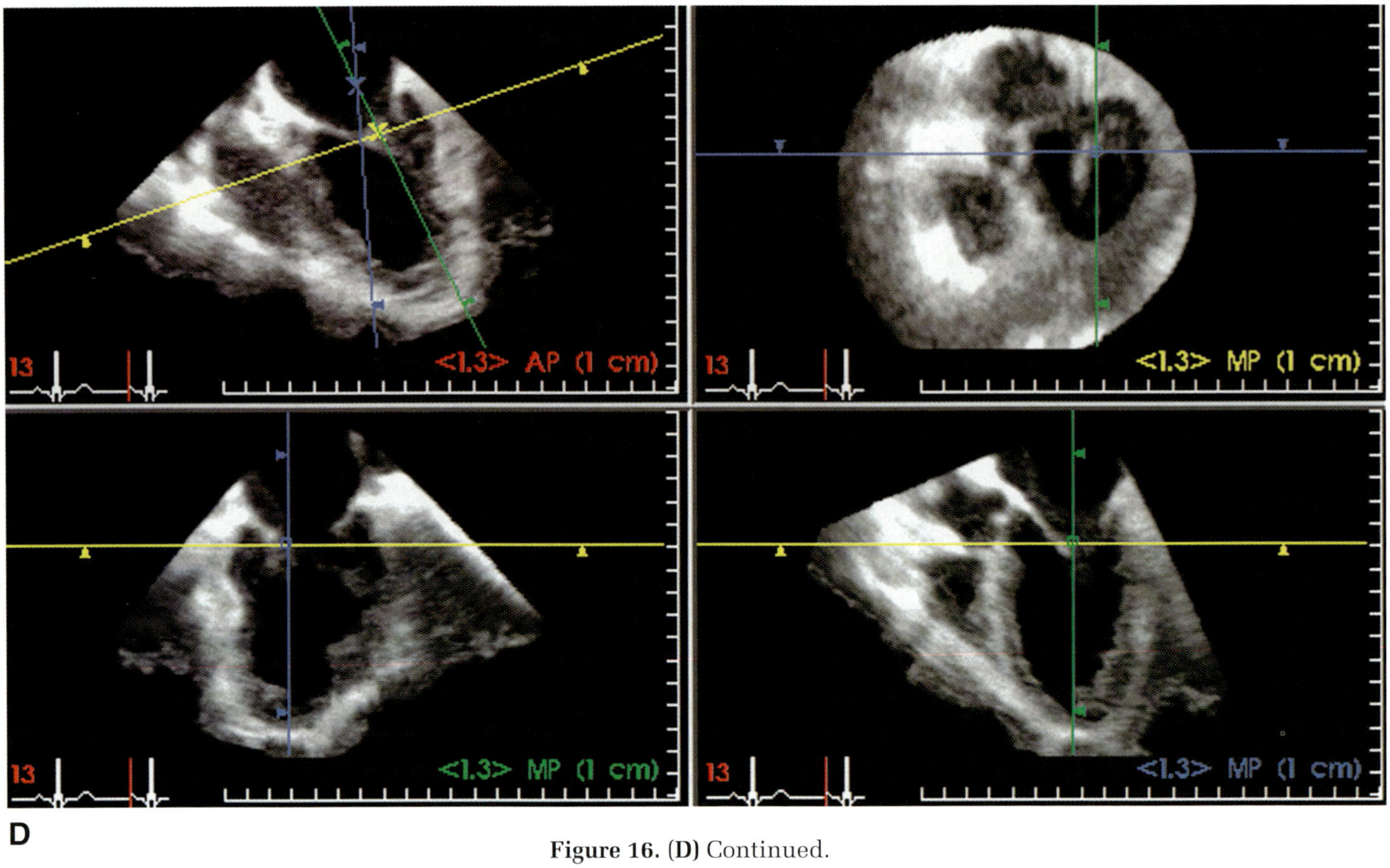

Figure 16. **(D)** Continued.

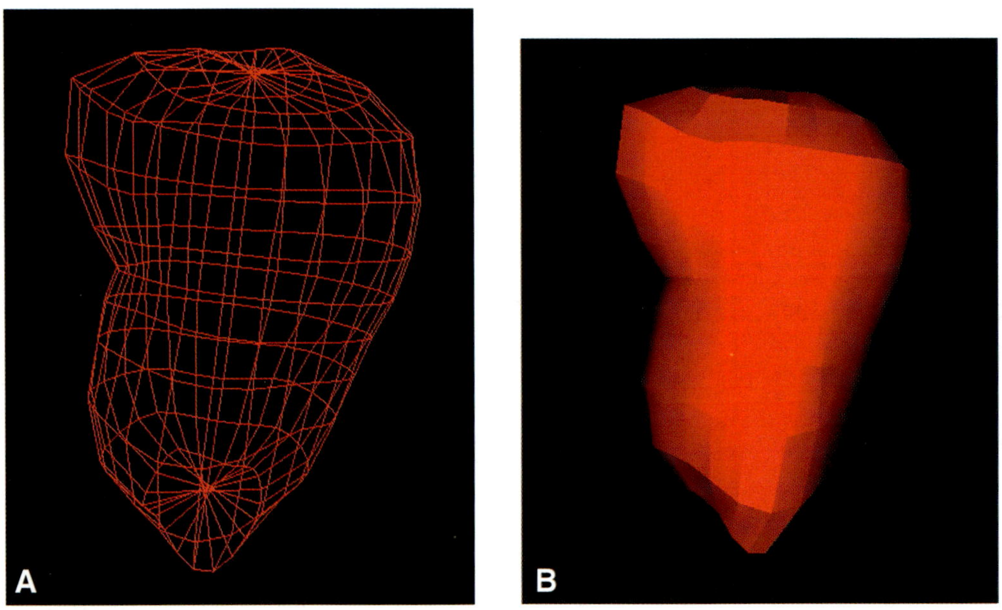

Figure 17. Contour based three-dimensional reconstruction of the left ventricle as a wireframe (**A**) and wireframe based surface visualization (**B**).

with 2D echo. Rapid technological developments over the past few years have helped 3D echo evolve from a research oriented procedure to a clinically applicable diagnostic tool.

Step 5: Three-Dimensional Quantification

Three-dimensional echo is very helpful to visualize pathology. This will enable precise quantification of 3D distances, angles, areas like atrial or ventricular septal defects, the valve opening area, or the precise volume of the atria or ventricles, etc., without making any geometric assumptions. For a 3D-based volume quantification, different methods have been developed. The most commonly used one is the segmentation in a "slice by slice" way. Here, an object is traced slice by slice in space by manual contour tracing or automatic/semiautomatic border detection algorithms. These contours can be traced on a stack of parallel cut planes (disk summation method), rotated cut planes (rotoplane method), or even freely double oblique oriented cut planes. Out of these contours, a wireframe can be generated to precisely define the surrounding volume.

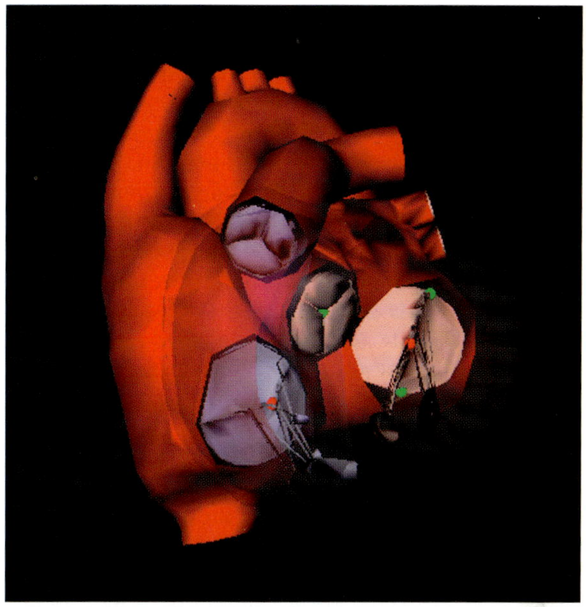

Figure 18. Virtual reality heart model.

Future Outlook

Today, 3D echo is mainly clinically applied with add-on systems. In the future it will be seamlessly integrated into the ultrasound platform itself. Three-dimensional echo will be a mode, like M-Mode, B-Mode or color flow. This will lead to a 100% digital signal processing and will improve the overall image quality. Special 3D-transducers, like the real-time 3D acquisition matrix array probe or the recently developed concept of a fast rotating 2D-transducer,[12] will ease and speed up the acquisition to just seconds, and will be initiated by a simple push-button tool. Not only will this change the practice of echocardiography in the future by making it less operator dependent,[12] but such rapid 3D scanning techniques will facilitate the acquisition of 3D contrast echo studies (e.g., for the quantification of three-dimensional myocardial perfusion[23,24] or for 3D stress echo and 3D wall motion analysis studies).

A real-time 3D reconstruction as well as "online" interaction and navigation within the 3D data is already possible with high performance computer systems. The rapid developments and improvements in standard computer technology, mainly driven by the gaming industry, will dramatically speed up the reconstruction time to be completely "online."

The digital data exchange standard DICOM 3 will get a 3D extension to support digital 3D echo data sets. Thus, such a data set can be transferred digitally via local or remote area network to offline review workstations, for example to facilitate a 3D telemedicine diagnosis. A remote echocardiography specialist could interactively review the study on a 3D computer in his office for a teleconsultation. These concepts are starting to be developed for use in battlefield situations. Here, a 3D data set will be acquired with a portable 3D ultrasound system, then transferred via satellite to a remote diagnostics center.

Another concept is to use a 3D data set for reproducing a solid model of the heart (e.g., with Stereolithography). Such a model could then be used by the cardiac surgeon for surgical planning, e.g., to prepare the right type and size of a prosthetic valve.

The use of DICOM standards for 3D data from different modalities like MRI, CT, nuclear, or ultrasound will lead to the creation of "multimodality" or "multidimensional" data sets. The physician could then decide using a "multidimensional workstation" which information he needed for the diagnosis.

Virtual reality tools will help to improve the navigation within 3D data sets.[25] Here the real 3D data set of the patient's heart is "linked" in space and time with a computer graphics-based virtual model of the heart. Virtual reality technology can then be used to "walk" or "fly" through the heart as a teaching or training tool as well as a diagnostic tool (Figure 18). Most monitors or displays today only provide a 2D, flat representation of a 3D structure. This can be changed with stereographic glasses or stereo display monitors.

Even the education, training and examination of students and sonographers can be done on a kind of "virtual patient" by the use of recently developed ultrasound simulator systems (UltraSim system, MedSim Ltd., Ft. Lauderdale, FL). The concept is to train for invasive procedures (like TEE) or difficult pathology on a simulator, like training airline pilots in an airplane simulator for approaching difficult airports or for flying in severe weather conditions.

With all the above listed potential for improvements and future developments of 3D echo, this exciting new technology will become a standard diagnostic tool of each high-end ultrasound system. There will no longer be the question of whether a diagnosis should be done by 2D *or* 3D echo. Three-dimensional echo will not replace 2D echo. It will be used in addition to it, as color flow is used today. Therefore, the future will be 2D *and* 3D echo. In some aspects of echocardiography, 3D echo can provide new clinical parameters. One important example—the global and regional assessment of ventricular function—should be added here.

The measurement of LV function based on 2DE can only provide results based on geometric assumptions. Here, 3D echo has big advantages. The LV cavity can be detected in all three dimensions (Figure 19) based on a sequence of 2D slices out of a 3D data set. An automatic border detection algorithm can be applied to detect the endocardial border more reliably and reproducibly than by a hand tracing approach (Figures 20 and 21). Such a dynamic LV model of one cardiac cycle (Figure 22) contains all information required for a global and regional assessment of LV function. Several new functional parameters can be retrieved out of this information. For example, regional volumes or regional EF can be measured or displayed as color coded on the LV model (Figures 23 and 24).

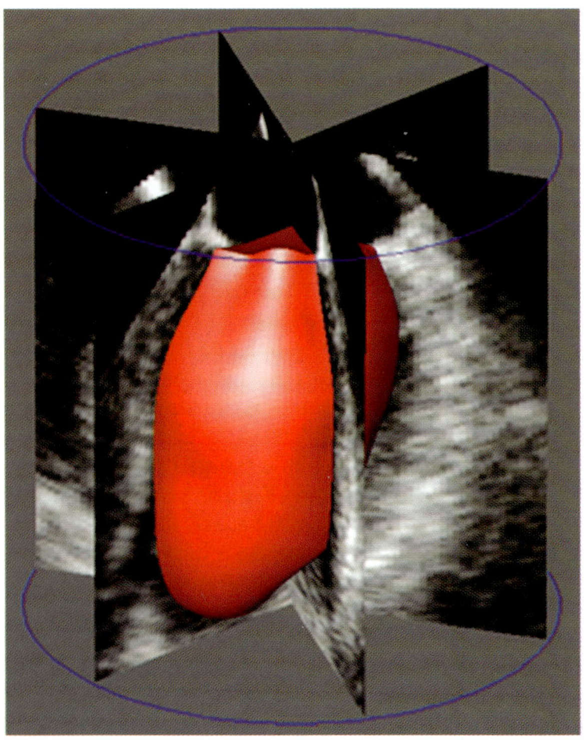

Figure 19. A sequence of equidistant rotated multiplane TEE images is used to generate a three-dimensional model of the left ventricular cavity.

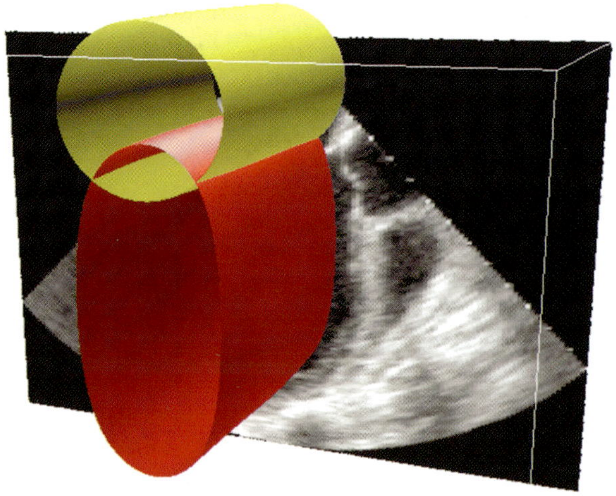

Figure 20. The endocardial left ventricular border can be found automatically based on a special "time tube" approach.

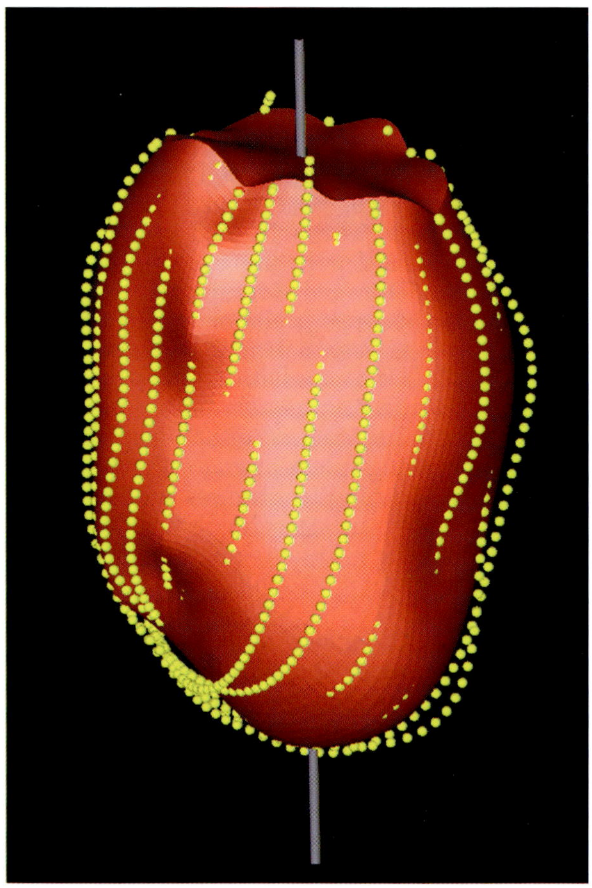

Figure 21. Automatic border detection based on three-dimensional echocardiography provides a more robust method to delineate the endocardial border by interpolating the contours in a spatial and temporal neighborhood (four dimensions).

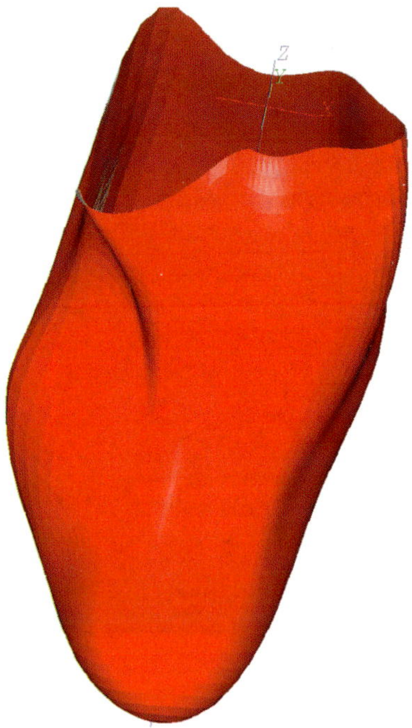

Figure 22. One phase of a dynamic left ventricular model.

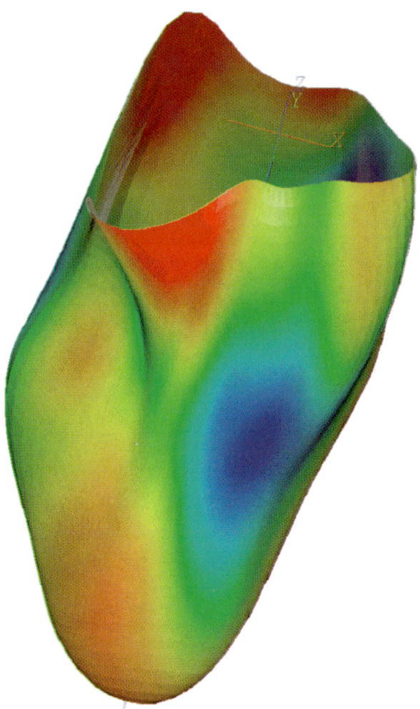

Figure 23. Regional parameter of the left ventricular (LV) function like regional ejection fraction can be displayed as color-coded information on the LV model.

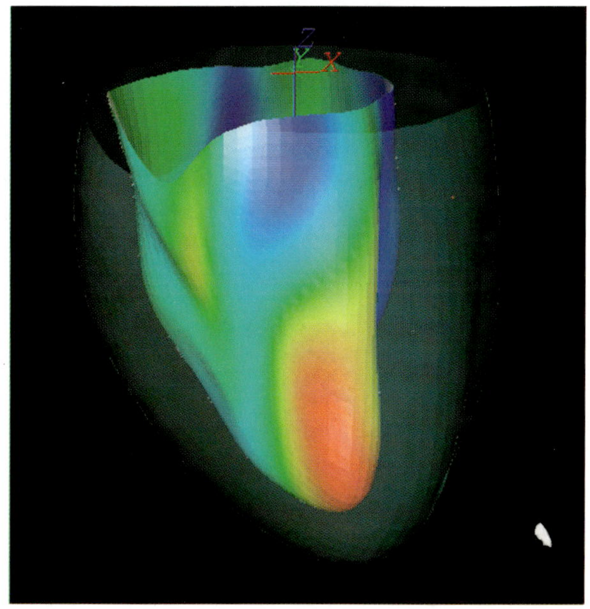

Figure 24. Regional parameter of the left ventricular (LV) function like regional ejection fraction can be displayed as color-coded information on the LV model.

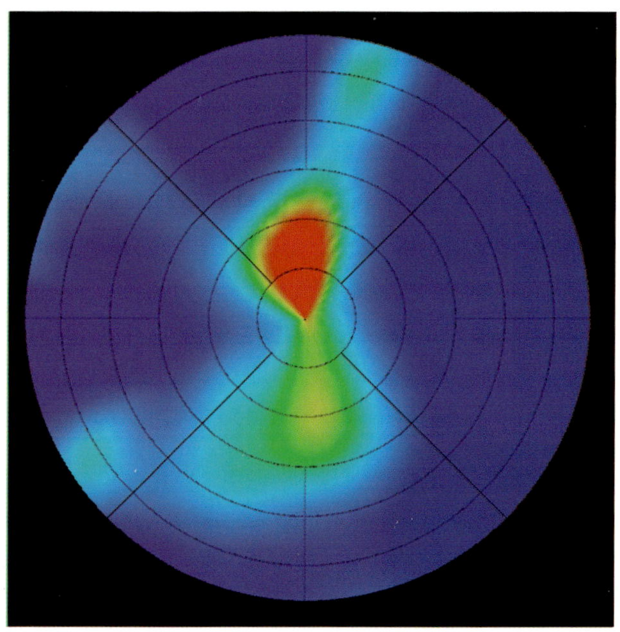

Figure 25. Bulls-eye display of regional left ventricular function.

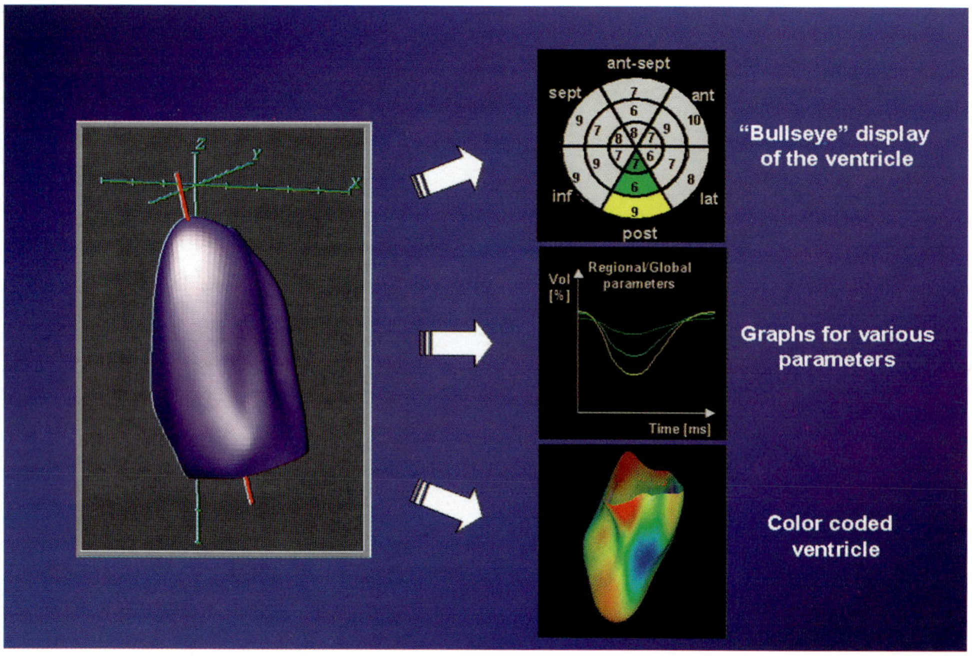

Figure 26. Left ventricular quantitation software features.

The same regional information can be plotted in a "bulls eye" view commonly used in nuclear medicine (Figure 25). New quantitative software packages are under development[26] to automatically generate new information like regional volumes, regional EF or stroke volume, regional wall thickening, regional ejection and filling function, or regional endocardiac wall motion (Figure 26).

References

1. Pandian NG, Nanda NC, Schwartz SL, et al. Three-dimensional and four-dimensional transesophageal echocardiographic imaging of the heart and aorta in humans using a computer tomographic imaging probe. *Echocardiography* 1992;9:677–687.
2. Dekker DL, Piziali RL, Dong E Jr. A system for ultrasonically imaging the human heart in three dimensions. *Computer Biomed Research* 1974;7:544–553.
3. Ghosh A, Nanda N, Maurer G. Three-dimensional reconstruction of echocardiographic images using the rotation method. *Ultrasound Med Biol* 1982;6:655.
4. Collins S, Chandran KB, Skorton DJ. Three-dimensional cardiac imaging. *Echocardiography* 1988;5:311.
5. Levine RA, Handschumacher MD, Sanfilippo AJ, et al. Three-dimensional echocardiographic reconstruction of the mitral valve with implications of the diagnosis of the mitral valve prolapse. *Circulation* 1989;80:589–598.
6. Geiser EA, Ariet M, Conetta DA, et al. Dynamic three-dimensional echocardiographic reconstruction of the intact human left ventricle. Techniques and observation in patients. *Am Heart J* 1982;103:1056–1065.
7. Moritz WE, Pearlman AS, Mccabe DH, et al. An ultrasonic technique for imaging the ventricle in three dimensions and calculating its volume. *IEEE Trans Biomed Eng* 1983;30:482–492.
8. Nixon JV, Saffer SI, Lipscomb K, et al. Three-dimensional echoventriculography. *Am Heart J* 1983;106:435–442.
9. Raichlen JS, Trivedi SS, Herman GT, et al. Dynamic three-dimensional reconstruction of the left ventricle from two-dimensional echocardiograms. *J Am Coll Cardiol* 1986 8(2):364–370.
10. Wollschläger H, Zeiher AM, Klein HP, et al. Transesophageal echocomputer tomography: A new method for dynamic 3-D imaging of the heart. *Circulation* 1989; 80:II-569.
11. Pandian NG, Roelandt JRTC, Nanda NC, et al. Dynamic three-dimensional echocardiography: Methods and clinical potential. *Echocardiography* 1994;11:237–259.
12. Roelandt JRTC, Salustri A, Vletter W, et al. Precordial multiplane echocardiography for dynamic anyplane, paraplane and three-dimensional imaging of the heart. *The Thoraxcentre Journal* 1994;6:4–13.
13. Von Ramm OT, Smith SW, Pavy HG Jr. High speed ultrasound volumetric imaging system. Part II. Parallel processing and image display. *IEEE Trans Ultrason Ferroelec Freq Contr* 1991;38:109–115.
14. Sheikh KH, Smith SW, Von Ramm O, et al. Realtime three-dimensional echocardiography: Feasibility and initial use. *Echocardiography* 1991;8:119–125.
15. King DL, King Dl Jr, Shaeo MY. Three-dimensional spatial registration and interactive display of position and orientation of realtime ultrasound images. *UI Ultrasound Med* 1990;9:525.
16. Höhne HH, Bernstein R. Shading 3D images from CT using gray level gradients. *IEEE Trans Med Imaging MI-5* 1986;1:45–47.
17. Coatrieux JL, Barillot C. A survey of 3D display techniques to render medical data. In NATO ASI Series, Vol. F 60: *3D Imaging in Medicine*. Heidelberg, Springer Verlag, 1990:175–195.
18. Barillot C, Gilbaud B, Luo LM, et al. 3-D Representation of anatomic structures from CT examinations. *Biostereometrics 85, Proc. SPIE* 1985;602:307–314.

19. Nosir Y, Salustri, Kasprzak JD, et al. Left ventricular ejection fraction in patients with normal and distorted left ventricular shape by two three-dimensional echocardiographic methods. A comparison with radionuclide angiography. *J Am Soc Echocardiography* 1998;11(6):620–630.
20. Nanda NC, Abd-el Rahman SM, Khatri G, et al. Incremental value of three-dimensional echocardiography over transesophageal multiplane two-dimensional echocardiography in qualitative and quantitative assessment of cardiac masses and defects. *Echocardiography* 1995; 12:619–628.
21. Kühl HP, Franke A, Frielingsdorf J, et al. Determination of left ventricular mass and circumferential wall thickness by three-dimensional reconstruction: In vitro validation of a new method that uses a multiplane transesophageal transducer. *J Am Soc Echocardiogr* 1997; 10:107–119.
22. Vogel M, Pandian N, Marx G, et al. Thransthoracic realtime three-dimensional echocardiography in 100 pediatric and adult patients with heart disease: Clinical utility of unique new views unavailable in two-dimensional echocardiography. *Circulation* 1993;88:1868.
23. Delabays A, Sugeng L, Cao QL, et al. Three-dimensional echocardiographic delineation of myocardial perfusion teritories: Description of a new 3D-image processing approach with a new ultrasound contrast agent. (Abstract) *J Am Coll Cardiol* 1995;25:39A.
24. Kasprzak JD, Aiazian A, Vletter WB, et al. Three-dimensional myocardial perfusion using contrast echo. (Abstract) *Eur Heart J* 1995;16(Suppl):205.
25. Bruining N, Roelandt JRTC, Janssen M, et al. Virtual reality: A teaching and training tool or just a computer game? *The Thoraxccentre Journal* 1998;10:17–20.
26. Kuehl H, Schreckenberg M, Franke A, et al. Automatic quantification of volumes and function using 3-D echocardiography: In vitro validation in a pulsatile flow model. *Eur J Echocardiography* Euroecho 4 Abstracts, Dec. 2000.

Suggested Reading List

1. Maurer G, Ghosh A, Nanda NC. Volume determination and three-dimensional reconstruction of echocardiographic images using rotation method. (Abstract) *Circulation* 1981;64:IV–206.
2. Ghosh A, Nanda NC, Maurer G. Three-dimensional reconstruction of echocardiographic images using rotation method. *Ultrasound Med Biol* 8:1982;655–661.
3. Schott JR, Moos S, Raqueno R, et al. 4-dimensional reconstruction from 2-dimensional echocardiograms. (Abstract) *Circulation* 1986;74:11–144.
4. Wixson SE, Nanda NC. Display of 4-dimensional ultrasound data. (Abstract) *J Ultras in Med* 1986;5:(9) 136
5. Wixson SE, Nanda NC, Iliceto S, et al. Evaluation of aortic dissection by color Doppler echocardiography. (Abstract) Annual Scientific Assembly of Southern Medical Association, Nov. 1986, Atlanta, GA.
6. Ghosh A, Schott JR, Moos S, et al. Merging color Doppler imaging with 4-dimensional echocardiogram reconstruction. (Abstract) *J Am Coll Cardiol* III-A, 1987.
7. Ghosh A, Schott JR, Moos S, et al. New methods for displaying 3-dimensional echo images. (Abstract) *Clin Res* 1987;35:280A.
8. Schott JR, Moos S, Raqueno R, et al. Feasibility analysis of 3-dimensional reconstruction of color Doppler flow velocities. (Abstract) *J Am Coll Cardiol* 1987;III–214A.
9. Schott JR, Raqueno R, Moos S, et al. Successful merging of 3-dimensional color flow velocities and 3-dimensional reconstruction of the left ventricle. (Abstract) *Circulation* 1987;76:IV–527.
10. Schott JR, Raqueno R, Ghosh A, et al. Four-dimensional cardiac blood flow analysis using color Doppler echocardiography. In: Nanda NC (Ed), Textbook of Color Doppler Echocardiography. Philadelphia: Lea and Febiger 1989, pp. 332–341.
11. Nanda NC, Pandian N. Three and four dimensional transesophageal echocardiography. *Administrative Radiology* 1992;XI:56–59.
12. Nanda NC, Pinheiro L, Sanyal R, et al. Multiplane transesophageal echocardiographic imaging and three-dimensional reconstruction: A preliminary study. *Echocardiography* 1992;9:667–676.
13. Pandian NG, Nanda NC, Schwartz ST, et al. Three-dimensional and four-dimensional transesophageal echocardiographic imaging of the heart and aorta in humans using a computed tomographic imaging probe. *Echocardiography* 1992;9:677–687.
14. Azvedo J, Cao QL, Pandian N, et al. Simulation of intraoperative 3-dimensional visualization of cardiac structures in pre-operative 3-dimensional and 4-dimensional transesophageal echocardiograms acquired using a computerized tomographic imaging probe. (Abstract) *J Am Coll Cardiol* 1993;21:180A.
15. Azevedo J, Cao OL, Pandian N, et al. Simulation of intraoperative three dimensional visualization of cardiac structures in pre-operative three dimensional and four dimensional transesophageal echocardiograms acquired using a computerized tomographic imaging probe. (Abstract) *European Heart J* 1994;August:441.
16. Ofili EO, Nanda NC. Three dimensional and four dimensional echocardiography. *Ultrasound in Med & Biol* 1994;20:669–675.
17. Pandian N, Cao QL, Erbel R, et al. A comprehensive approach for image segmentation, cutting planes and display projections in three dimensional echocardiography: Suggested guidelines for clinically useful projections based on multicenter experience in 300 adult and pediatric patients. *J Am Coll Cardiol* 1994;23:9A.
18. Pandian NG, Roelandt J, Nanda NC, et al. Dynamic three dimensional echocardiography: methods and clinical potential. *Echocardiography* 1994;11:237–259.
19. Li Z, Wang X, Nanda NC, et al.Three-dimensional reconstruction of transesophageal echocardiographic longitudinal images. *Echocardiography* 1995;12:367–375.
20. Nanda NC, Abd-El Rahman SM, Khatri G, et al. Incremental value of three-dimensional echocardiography over transesophageal multiplane two-dimensional echocardiography in qualitative and quantitative assessment of cardiac masses and defects. *Echocardiography* 1995; 12:619–628.
21. Kanojia A, Kasliwal RR. Three dimensional echocardiography: From the realm of research to clinical reality. [Review] [38 refs]. *J Assoc Physicians India* 1996;44:649–652.
22. Binder T, Globits S, Zangeneh M, et al. Value of three-dimensional echocardiography as an adjunct to conventional transesophageal echocardiography. *Cardiology* 1996;87:335–342
23. Capineri L, Masotti L, Rocchi S, et al. Nearly real-time visualization of arbitrary two-dimensional sections from three-dimensional acquisition. [Review] [8 refs]. *Ultrasound Med Biol.* 1996;22:319–328.
24. Hagege A, Desnos M, Mirochnik N, et al. [Three-dimensional echocardiography. Principles and applica-

tions]. [Review] [27 refs] [French]. *Arch Mal Coeur Vaisseaux* 1996;89:1405–1411.
25. Kucera D, Martin RW. Segmentation of sequences of echocardiographic images using a simplified 3D active contour model with region-based external forces. *Comp Med Imaging Graphics* 1997;21:1–21.
26. Flachskampf FA, Franke A, Kuhl HP, et al. [3-D echocardiography: technical toy in search of a clinical application or logical evolution of diagnostic equipment?]. [Review] [53 refs] [German]. *Zeitschrift Kardiologie* 1997;86: 336–345.
27. Greco C, Salustri A, Romano P, et al. [Three-dimensional transesophageal echocardiography: a new cardiologic diagnostic tool. Initial experience with 150 patients]. [Italian]. *Giornale Italiano Cardiologia* 1997;27:55–63.
28. Vuille C, Sztajzel J, Hoffmann JL, et al. [Dynamic three-dimensional cardiac reconstruction by transesophageal echocardiography. A clinical experience apropos of 100 cases]. [French]. *Arch Mal Coeur Vaisseaux* 1997;90: 217–224.
29. Salgo IS. Three-dimensional echocardiography. [Review] [78 refs]. *J Cardiothoracic Vasc Anesthes.* 1997;11:506–516.
30. Pinto FJ, Veiga F, Lopes MG, et al. Dynamic three-dimensional echocardiography: A new era in ultrasound technology. [Review] [74 refs]. *Revista Portuguesa Cardiologia* 1997;16:786–787.
31. Meunier J. Tissue motion assessment from 3D echographic speckle tracking. *Phys Med Biol* 1998;43:1241–1254.
32. De Castro S, Yao J, Pandian NG. Three-dimensional echocardiography: clinical relevance and application. [Review] [29 refs]. *Am J Cardiol* 1998;81:96G–102G.
33. Yoshikawa J. [Forefront of cardiac ultrasonography]. [Review] [5 refs] [Japanese]. *J Japan Soc Int Med* 1998;87: 1910–1915.
34. Vrints CJ, Bosmans J, Claeys MJ, et al. User-friendly and low-cost computer system for immediate review, analysis, and reconstruction of intracoronary ultrasound images. *Cath Cardiovasc Diagn* 1998;43:357–362.
35. Roelandt JR, Yao J, Kasprzak JD. Three-dimensional echocardiography. [Review] [100 refs]. *Curr Opin Cardiol* 1998;13:386–396.
36. Roelandt JR. Three-dimensional echocardiography: The future today!. [Review] [100 refs]. *Acta Cardiologica* 1998; 53:323–336.
37. Pinto FJ, Veiga F, Lopes MG, et al. Three dimensional echocardiography. [Review] [12 refs]. *Revista Portuguesa Cardiologia.* 1998;17 Suppl 3:III59–63.
38. Matsumura M. [Current status and future of three-dimensional echocardiography]. [Review] [24 refs] [Japanese]. *Japan J Anesthesiol* 1998;47 Suppl:S118–125.
39. Berg S, Torp H, Martens D, et al. Dynamic three-dimensional freehand echocardiography using raw digital ultrasound data. *Ultrasound Med Biol* 1999;25:745–753.
40. Duann JR, Lin SB, Hu WC, et al. Computer system for four-dimensional transesophageal echocardiographic image reconstruction. *Comp Medical Imaging Graphics* 1999;23:173–179.
41. Godoy IE, Bednarz J, Sugeng L, et al. Three-dimensional echocardiography in adult patients: Comparison between transthoracic and transesophageal reconstructions. *J Am Soc Echocardiograph* 1999;12:1045–1052.
42. Veiga M, Lopes MG, Pinto FJ. Dynamic three-dimensional reconstruction of the heart by transesophageal echocardiography. *Arquivos Brasileiros Cardiologia* 1999;72: 559–568.
43. Sarti A, Mikula K, Sgallari F. Nonlinear multiscale analysis of three-dimensional echocardiographic sequences. *IEEE Transact Med Imaging* 1999;18:453–466.
44. Abdullah M, Maeno Y, Bigras JL, et al. Superiority of 3-dimensional versus 2-dimensional echocardiography for left ventricular volume assessment in small piglet hearts. *J Am Soc Echocardiograph* 2000;13(10.):918–923.
45. Fedele F, De Castro S, Volponi MC, et al. The echocardiography laboratory in the informatic era. [Review] [11 refs]. *Am J Cardiol* 2000;86(4A):33G–35G.
46. Franke A, Kuhl HP, Hanrath P. [Imaging techniques in cardiology: Three-dimensional echocardiography]. [Review] [30 refs] [German]. *Zeitschrift Kardiologie* 2000;89(3): 150–159.
47. Hozumi T, Yoshikawa J. Three-dimensional echocardiography using a muliplane transesophageal probe: The clinical applications. [Review] [18 refs]. *Echocardiograph* 2000;17(8):757–764.
48. Plein S, Williams GJ. Developments in cardiac ultrasound. [Review] [21 refs]. *Hosp Medicine (London)* 2000; 61(4):240–245.
49. Premawardhana U, Celermajer DS. Advances in echocardiography. [Review] [28 refs]. *Australian New Zealand J Med* 2000;30(3):360–366.
50. Sakas G, Walter S, Grimm M, et al. [Free hand acquisition, reconstruction and visualization of 3D and 4D ultrasound]. [German]. *Radiologe* 2000;40(3):295–303.
51. Weidenbach M, Wick C, Pieper S, et al. [Augmented reality in echocardiography. A new method of computer-assisted training and image processing using virtual and real three-dimensional data sets]. [German]. *Zeitschrift Kardiologie* 2000;89(3):168–175.
52. Boukerroui D, Basset O, Baskurt A, et al. A multiparametric and multiresolution segmentation algorithm of 3-D ultrasonic data. *IEEE Trans Ultrason Ferroelectr Freq Control* 2001;48(1):64–77.
53. De Castro S, Adorisio R, Azevedo J, et al. Current status of three-dimensional echocardiography. [Review] [30 refs]. *Revista Portuguesa Cardiologia* 2001;20(Suppl.1):9–16.
54. Zotz RJ, Trabold T, Bock A, et al. In vitro measurement accuracy of three-dimensional ultrasound. *Echocardiography* 2001;18(2):149–156.
55. Lees W. Ultrasound imaging in three and four dimensions. [Review] [74 refs]. *Seminars in Ultrasound CT & MR* 2001;22(1):85–105.

Chapter 2

Normal Anatomy, Normal Variants and Artifacts

Navin C. Nanda, MD and Vincent L. Sorrell, MD

Three-dimensional (3D) echocardiography will become the imaging modality of choice to obtain the most comprehensive anatomic and physiologic data regarding cardiac function, valve pathology and physiology, and myocardial, pericardial and vessel disease. A complete understanding of 2-dimensional (2D) echocardiographic anatomy is necessary to fully benefit from 3D data set acquisition. Therefore, the specific descriptions of normal anatomy are not reiterated in this atlas, but the reader is encouraged to utilize conventional echocardiographic textbooks for assistance when needed. Furthermore, since the 3D data set is vastly greater than routine 2D echo, we routinely utilize cardiac models, as well as surgical and anatomy textbooks, and encourage the beginning 3D echocardiographer to do so as well.

Any new diagnostic technique requires an extensive understanding of the appearance of the various normal anatomic structures before one can embark on diagnosing pathology. The development of transesophageal echocardiography (TEE) improved the visualization of structures seen with transthoracic echo (TTE), but also resulted in the imaging of structures not previously well understood, and increased the potential for misinterpretation. Combining 3D imaging with TEE further increases the potential for structural misinterpretation and requires frequent comparisons with the 2D cutplanes (obtained from the 3D data set). This chapter demonstrates the varied normal appearances of many of the common structures likely to be interrogated with 3D imaging. Whenever possible, 2D images are also displayed for optimal comparisons. The images highlighting the manifestation of Lambl's excrescences are a good example of a commonly misunderstood finding that is benign, but may result in further and unnecessary additional investigations.

Another potential for misinterpretation results from the numerous artifacts that are common with ultrasound techniques. Just as the evolution from M-mode to 2D echo initially reported artifacts directly resulting from the enhanced imaging capabilities, 3D artifacts are common and potentially misleading. With the requirement for computer-generated reconstruction of the 3D data set, additional processing artifacts are new to echocardiography. Many of these technical artifacts are included in this chapter to help demonstrate the appearance of the more common errors.

Lastly, the first few figures provide a framework for additional capabilities provided with 3D data sets. Two of the most important variables predicting mortality are the left ventricular (LV) function and the existence of LV hypertrophy (LVH). Despite the overwhelming prognostic value of these parameters, they are most commonly estimated by visual assessment. The visually estimated LV ejection fraction (LVEF) has been shown to be more accurate when a high volume, experienced interpreter is directly compared to a lower volume or less well-trained individual. Additionally, even the most experienced echocardiographers have a poor intra- and interobserver variability when the LVEF is not either normal or severely depressed. The same finding exists for documenting LVH. Numerous quantitative methods exist for deriving the LVEF or LV mass, but are frequently not utilized since these require geometric assumptions that are often not valid in patients with cardiac disease. Furthermore, these calculations are frequently time-consuming.

Three-dimensional echocardiography will provide an avenue to increase the accuracy of LVEF and LV mass calculations by providing an actual volume data set and thereby eliminating the need for geometric assumptions. The future of routine, clinical echocardiography will certainly be three-dimensional, and extensive progress has already been made towards a real-time, on-line 3D transducer and ultrasound system.

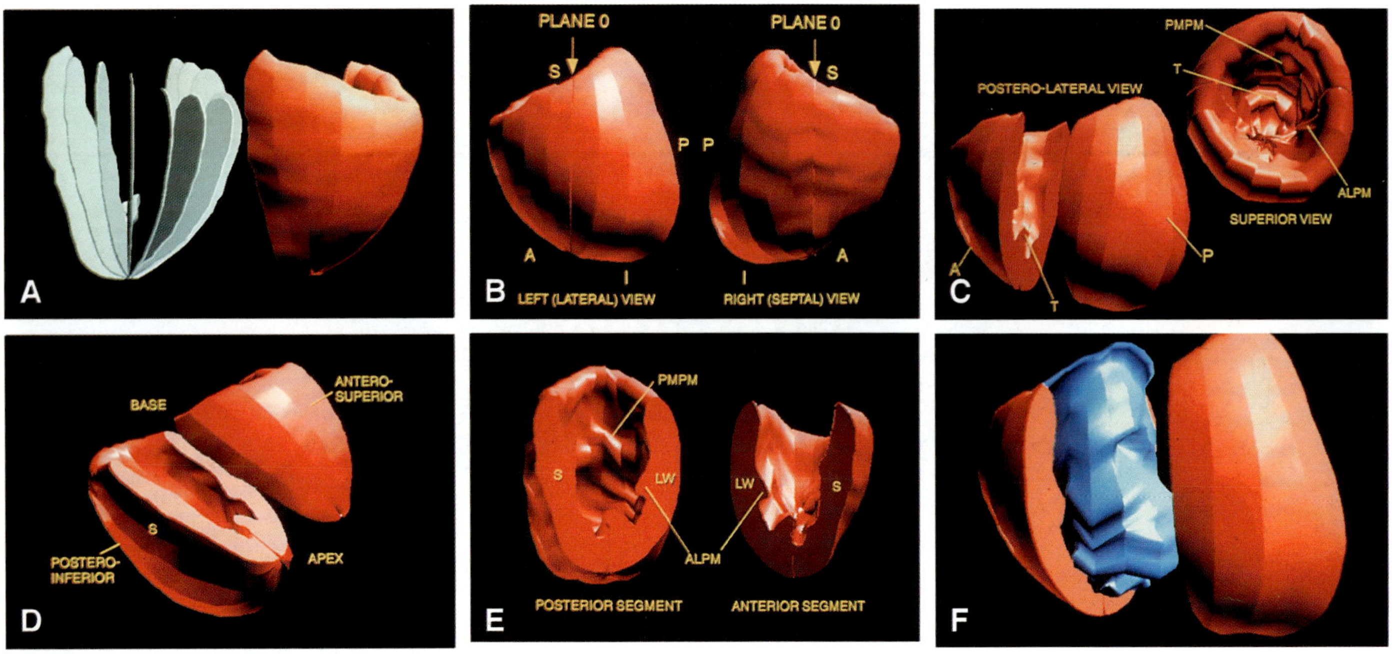

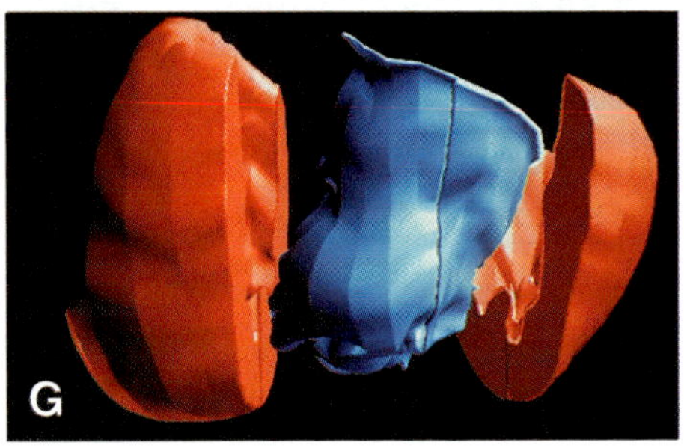

Figure 1. Three-dimensional (3D) reconstruction of the left ventricle (LV) using sequential planes obtained from multiplane transesophageal examination in a patient. For 3D reconstruction, all frames were obtained in mid-diastole using the mitral valve motion as the reference. **(A)** shows the "rib cage" on the left. **(F)** and **(G)** show the "volume cast" of the left ventricular cavity. A = anterolateral wall; ALPM = anteriolateral papillary muscle; I = inferior wall; LW = lateral wall; P = posterior wall; PMDM = posteromedial papillary muscle; S = ventrciular septum; T = trabeculation. (Reproduced with permission from Nanda et al. Multiplane transesophageal echocardiographic imaging and three-dimensional reconstruction. Echocardiography 1992;9:667–676.)

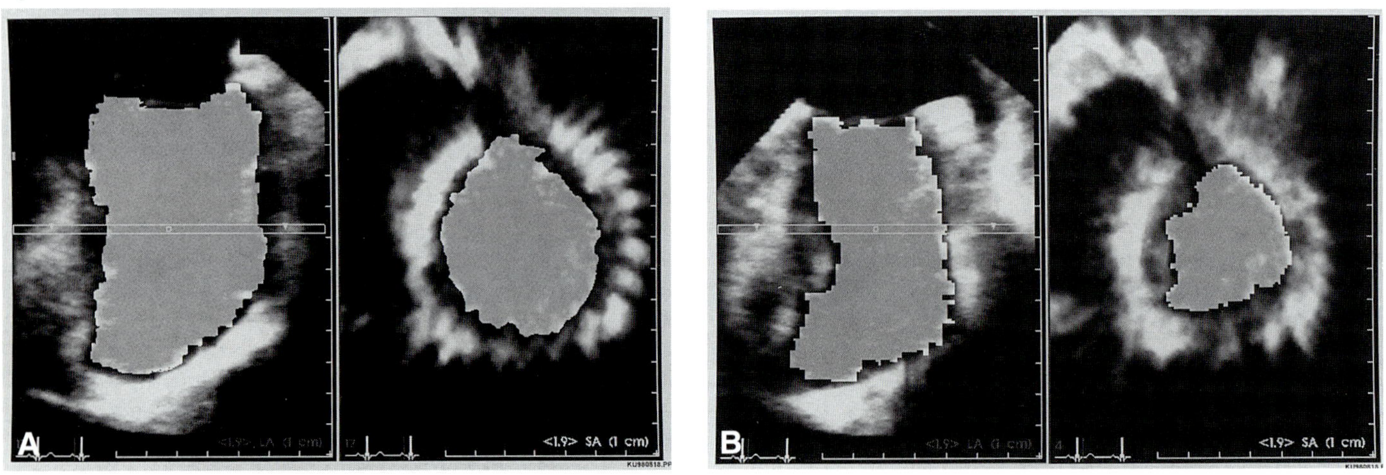

Figure 2. Assessment of left ventricular (LV) end-diastolic and end-systolic volumes, stroke volume and ejection fraction (EF) with transesophageal three-dimensional (3D) echocardiography. Diastolic (**A**) and systolic (**B**) stop-frame images showing a long-axis view and a short-axis view reconstructed from the 3D data set in a patient with an apical LV aneurysm. Manual contour tracing of endocardial borders is performed in reconstructed short-axis views, which are perpendicular to the long-axis images. These short-axis views represent slices of freely selectable thickness marked by the rectangle in the long-axis reference image. Total LV volume is calculated by the summation of the volumes of each slice covering the whole ventricle from base to apex. Stroke volume and EF are calculated from measured end-diastolic and end-systolic LV volumes. This method has been validated in-vitro and in-vivo in patients with normal and severely distorted hearts in comparison to biplane angiography and thermodilution methods. From Andreas Franke, MD, Harald P. Kühl, MD, and Peter Hanrath, MD, Aachen, Germany. (Reproduced with permission from Kühl et al. Three-dimensional echocardiographic determination of left ventricular volumes and function by multiplane transesophageal transducer: Dynamic In vitro validation and in vivo comparison with angiography and thermodilution. *J Am Soc Echocardiography* 1998;11:1113–1124).

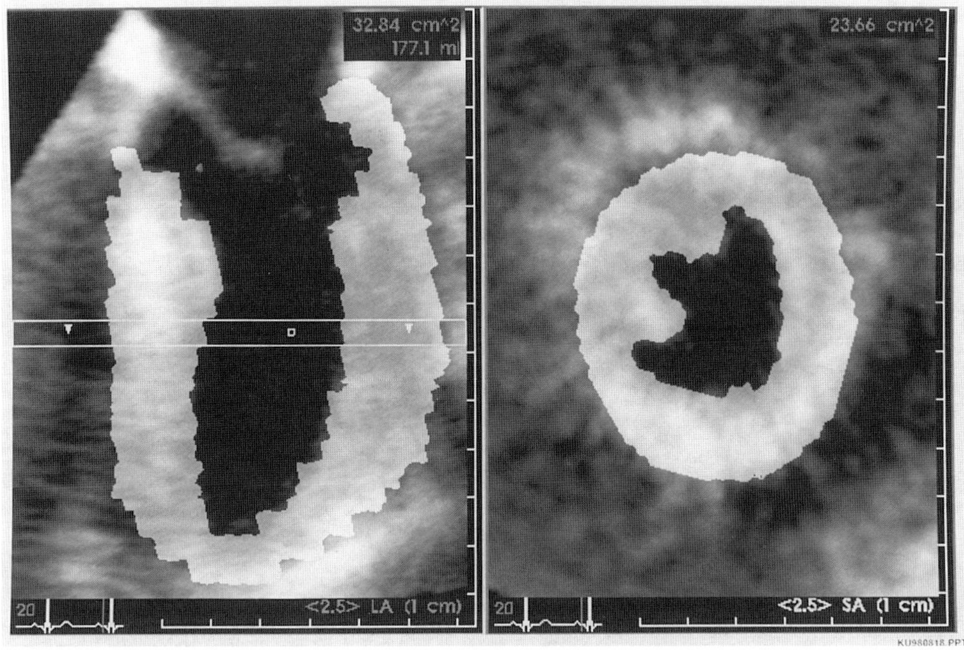

Figure 3. Assessment of left ventricular (LV) mass with transesophageal three-dimensional (3D) echocardiography. Diastolic stop frame image showing a long-axis view (left) and a short-axis view (right) reconstructed from the 3D data set. Manual contour tracing of endocardial and epicardial borders is performed in reconstructed short-axis views, which are perpendicular to the long-axis images. These short-axis views represent slices of freely selectable thickness marked by the rectangle in the long-axis reference image. Total LV mass is calculated by the summation of the myocardial volume of each slice covering the whole ventricle from base to apex and by multiplication of the resultant total myocardial volume with the density (1.05 g/cm^2). This method has been validated in-vitro with necropsy left ventricles and in-vivo in patients with normal and severely hypertrophied left ventricles. From Andreas Franke, MD, Harald P. Kühl, MD, and Peter Hanrath, MD, Aachen, Germany. (Reproduced with permission from Kühl et al, Determination of left ventricular mass and circumferential wall thickness by three-dimensional reconstruction; In vitro validation of a new method that uses a multiplane transesophageal transducer. *J Am Soc Echocardiography* 1997;10:107–119).

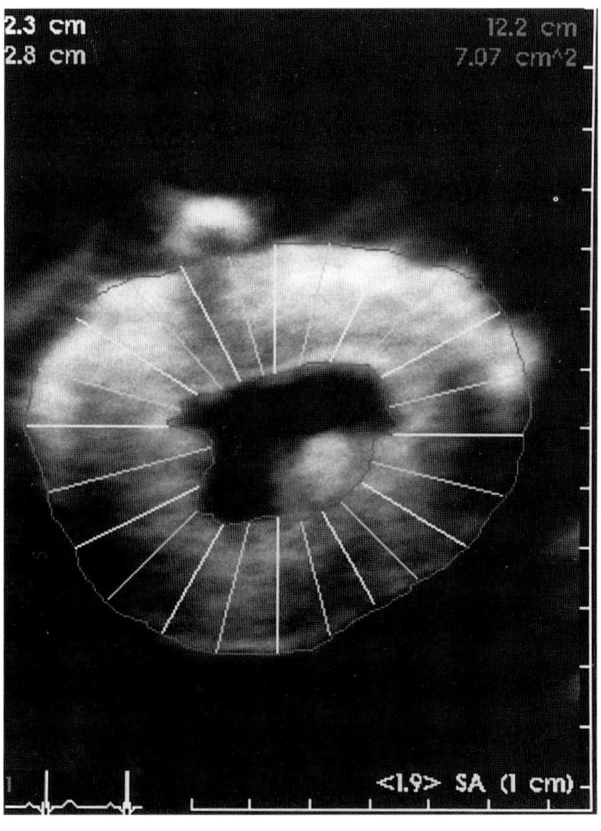

Figure 4. Assessment of wall thickness in-vitro: three-dimensionally reconstructed short axis view of a human necropsy left ventricle scanned in a water bath using a multiplane transesophageal transducer. Endocardial and epicardial boundaries were outlined manually excluding papillary muscles. Radial wall thickness measurements were validated using a transparent overlay comparing measurements to true wall thickness measurements in the necropsy specimens. Although the technique does not yield true three-dimensional wall thickness it can be used to assess relative wall thickening from base to apex in the three-dimensionally reconstructed left ventricles. From Andreas Franke, MD, Harald P. Kühl, MD, and Peter Hanrath, MD, Aachen, Germany. (Reproduced with permission from Kühl et al, Determination of left ventricular mass and circumferential wall thickness by three-dimensional reconstruction; In vitro validation of a new method that uses a multiplane transesophageal transducer. *J Am Soc Echocardiography* 1997; 10:107–119).

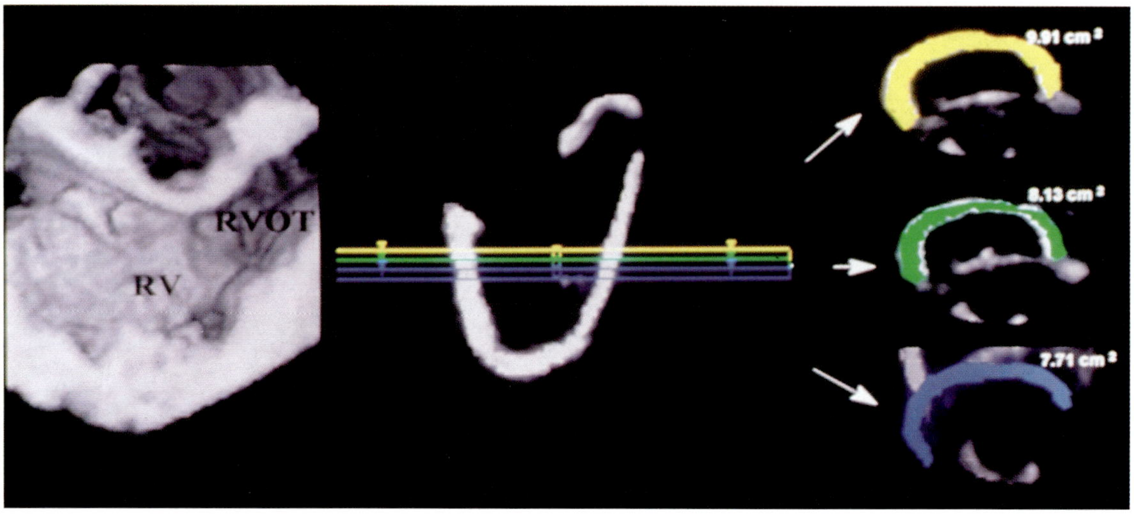

Figure 5. Three-dimensional echocardiographic images (**left**) of right ventricular (RV) cavity and outflow tract (RVOT). In the middle, a long-axis view and corresponding (**right**) multiple short-axis views of the right ventricle have shown. The right ventricle has been manually traced, labeled and automatically measured by the integrated software. From Stefano DeCastro, MD and Rachele Adoriso, MD.

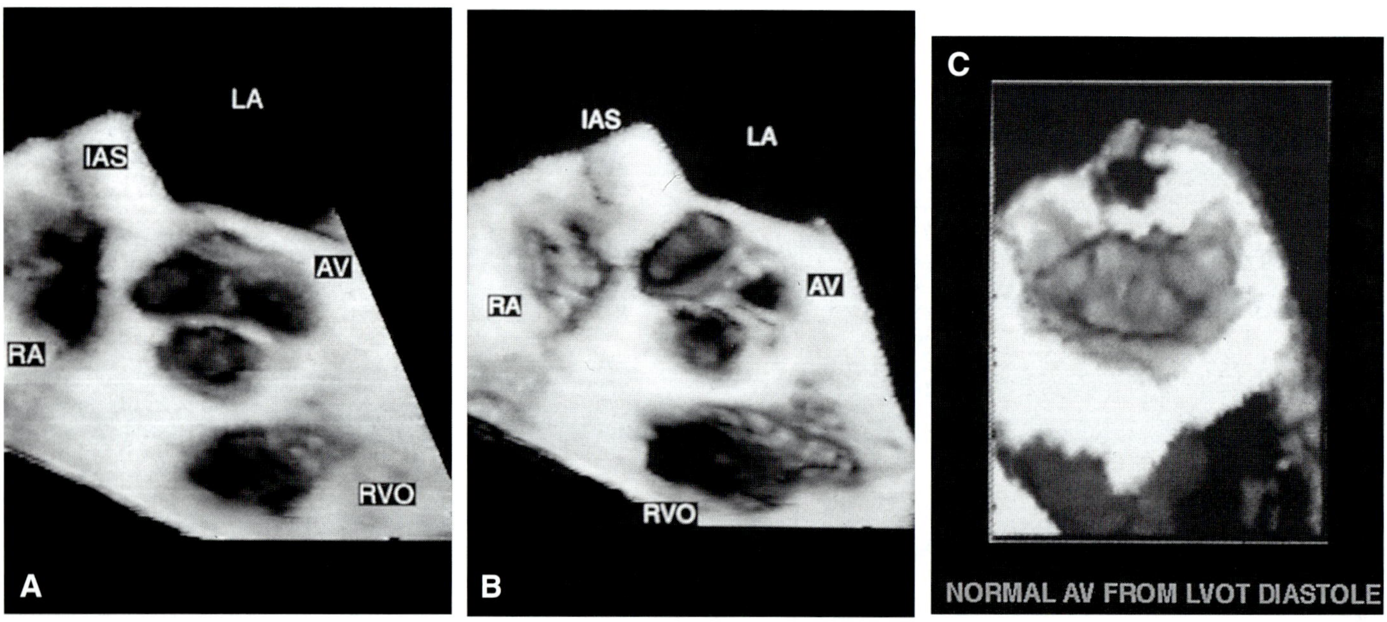

Figure 6. (**A**) Three-dimensional (3D) echo of the aortic valve in diastole. The image is viewed from the aorta. (**B**) 3D echo of the aortic valve in a slightly different plane. Note the larger right ventricular outflow tract (RVOT) and smaller right atrium. (**C, D**) The aortic valve can be viewed from any chosen reference point. In these images, the aortic valve is viewed from the left ventricular outflow tract (LVOT) in diastole and systole.

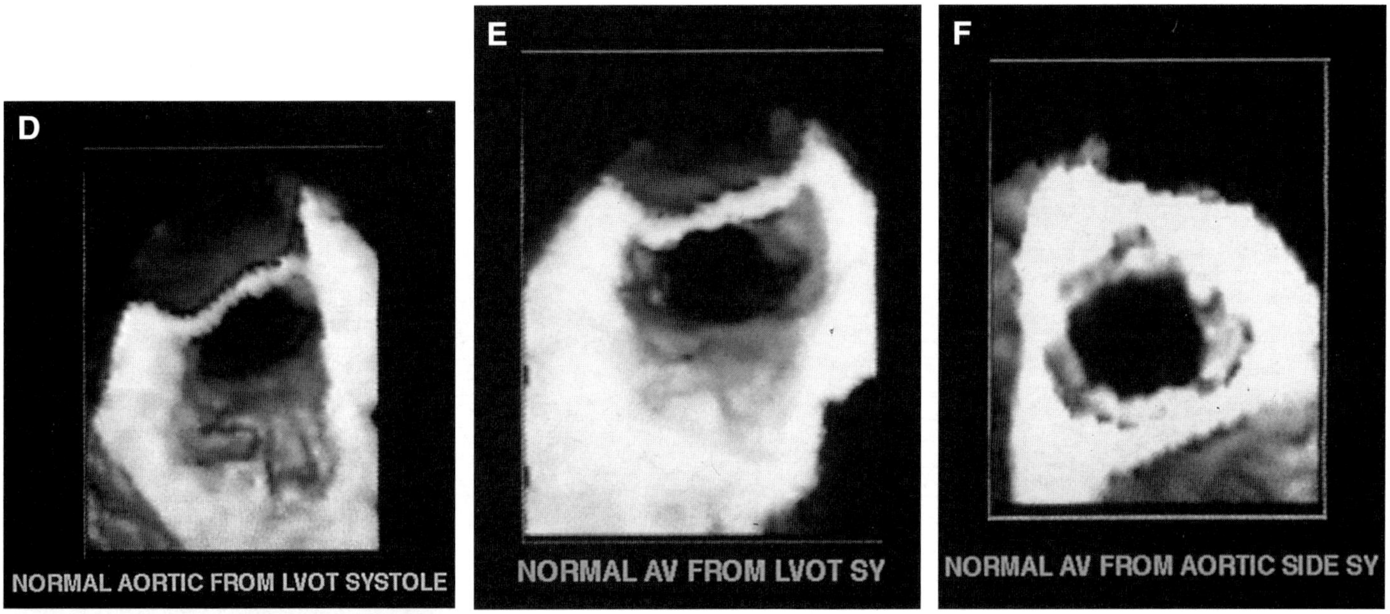

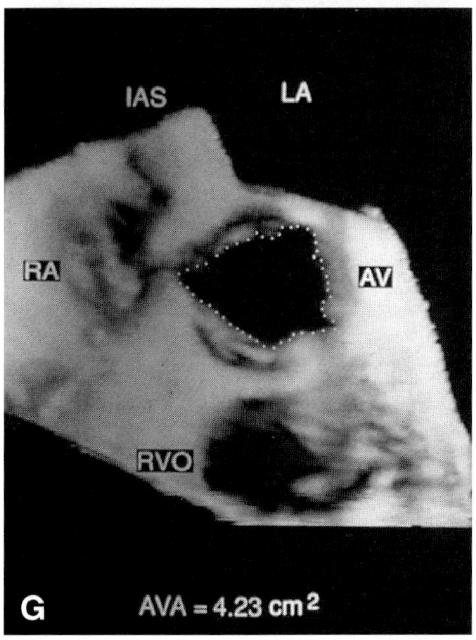

Figure 6. Continued. **(D)** The aortic valve can be viewed from any chosen reference point. In these images, the aortic valve is viewed from the left ventricular outflow tract (LVOT) in diastole and systole. **(E)** The aortic valve is now viewed in a slightly different plane. Note the smaller LVOT. **(F)** The aortic valve is now fully opened (systole) and is viewed from the aorta. **(G)** The aortic valve is viewed from the aorta in systole and allows optimal planimetry of the aortic valve area (AVA).

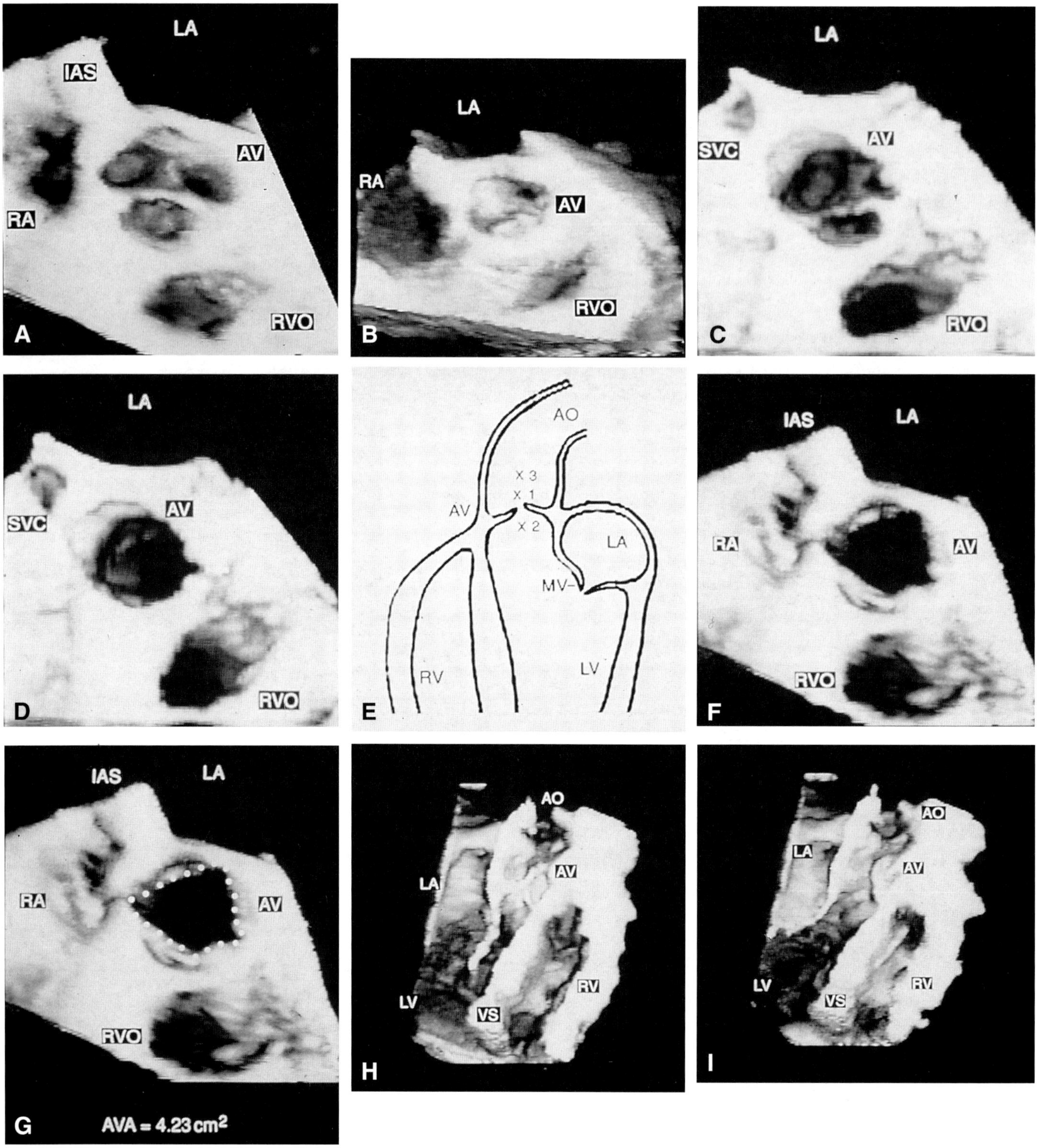

Figure 7. Transesophageal three-dimensional reconstruction of normal aortic valve. (**A**) When the aortic valve is viewed from the aortic side in short axis, the aortic sinuses appear as saucer-shaped depressions in the closed position in diastole. (**B**) When viewed from the left ventricle the bulge produced by the aortic sinuses in diastole is evident. (**C, D**) When the aortic valve is viewed from a position higher in the supravalvar aorta, the aortic valve is viewed together with a segment of the proximal ascending aorta in both diastole (**C**) and systole (**D**). The arrow points to the orifice of the left main coronary artery. (**E**) Schematic showing the three positions used by us to view the aortic valve. 1 = aortic root close to the aortic valve. 2 = left ventricle close to the aortic valve. 3 = supravalvar aorta. (**F, G**) Show the aortic valve in the open position in systole. The aortic orifice area obtained by planimetry (**G**) measured 4.23 cm^2, which is in the normal range. (**H, I**) The aortic valve and both left and right ventricles (RV) are viewed in long axis in diastole (**H**) and systole (**I**). IAS = interatrial septum; LA = left atrium; MV = mitral valve; RA = right atrium; RVO = right ventricular outflow tract; SVC = superior vena cava; VS = ventricular septum. Reproduced with permission from Nanda et al. Quantitative assessment of normal and stenotic aortic valve using transesophageal three-dimensional echocardiography. *Echocardiography* 1994;11:617–625.

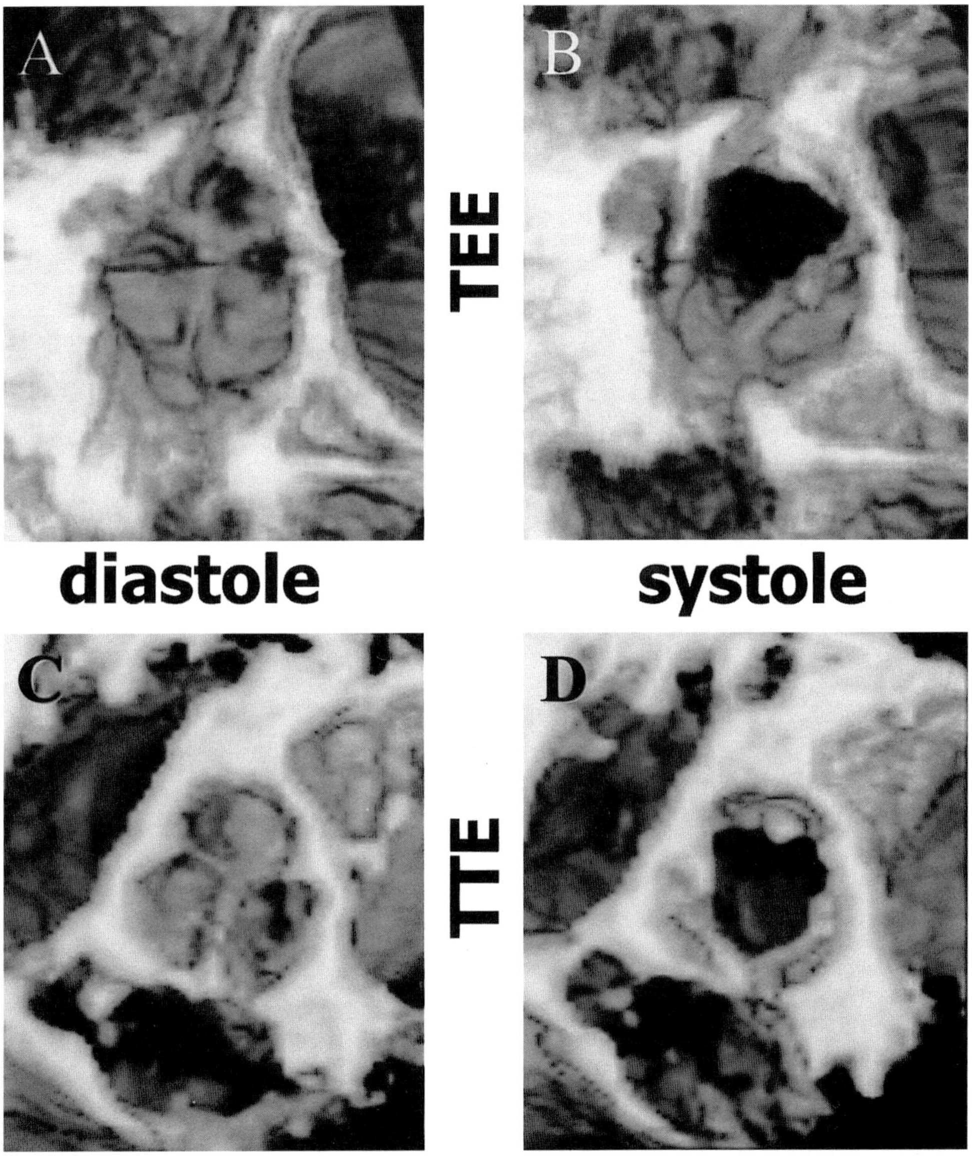

Figure 8. Diastolic (**A**) and systolic (**B**) frames of an aortic valve. This three-dimensional reconstruction was obtained from transesophageal images using a multiplane transducer. In the same patient the reconstruction was repeated from the transthoracic approach (**C, D**). Please note the similarity between both reconstructions. The ability to obtain accurate reconstructions from the transthoracic approach is important because it allows serial acquisitions in a noninvasive manner. From Lissa Sugeng, MD, Ivan Godoy, MD, Kirk T. Spencer, MD, Jim Bednarz, BS, Lynn Weinert, BS, and Roberto M. Lang, MD.

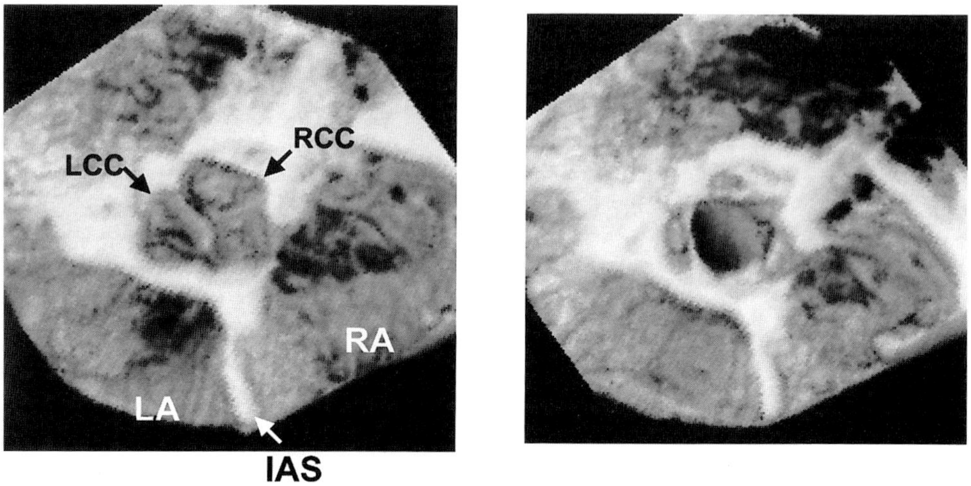

Figure 9. This is a transesophageal acquisition of a normal aortic valve. A cranial view of the aortic valve is seen in diastole (**left**) and systole (**right**). The right coronary cusp (RCC), left coronary cusp (LCC) and noncoronary cusp are well defined in diastole. The aortic valve opening during systole allows visualization of the left ventricular outflow tract. The left atrium (LA) and right atrium (RA) are separated by the intra-atrial septum (IAS). From Lissa Sugeng, MD, Ivan Godoy, MD, Kirk T. Spencer, MD, Jim Bednarz, BS, Lynn Weinert, BS, and Roberto M. Lang, MD.

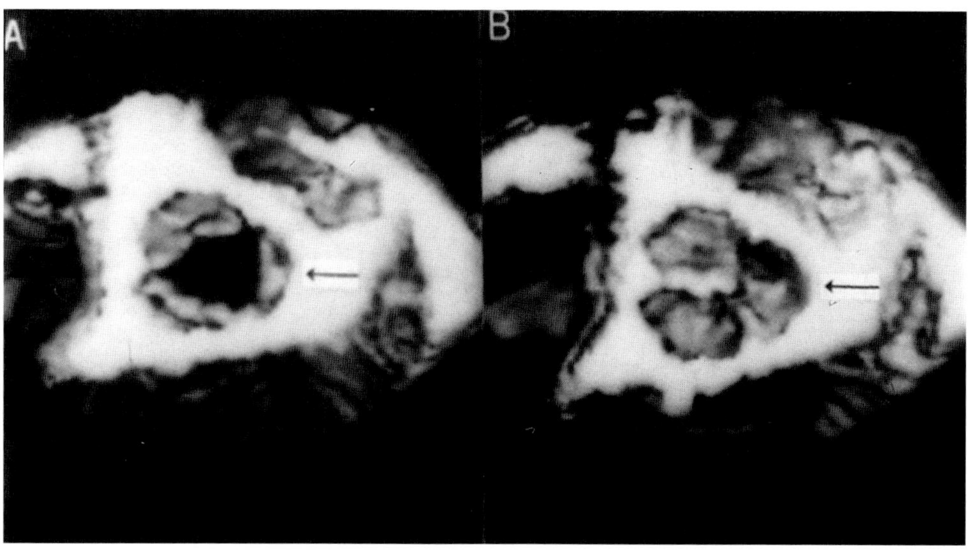

Figure 10. Birds' eye view of normal aortic valve. (**A**) Figure was taken in systole, aortic valve orifice was open. (**B**) Figure was taken in diastole, aortic valve was closed. The leaflets were thinner with good coaptation. From Xin-Fang Wang, MD.

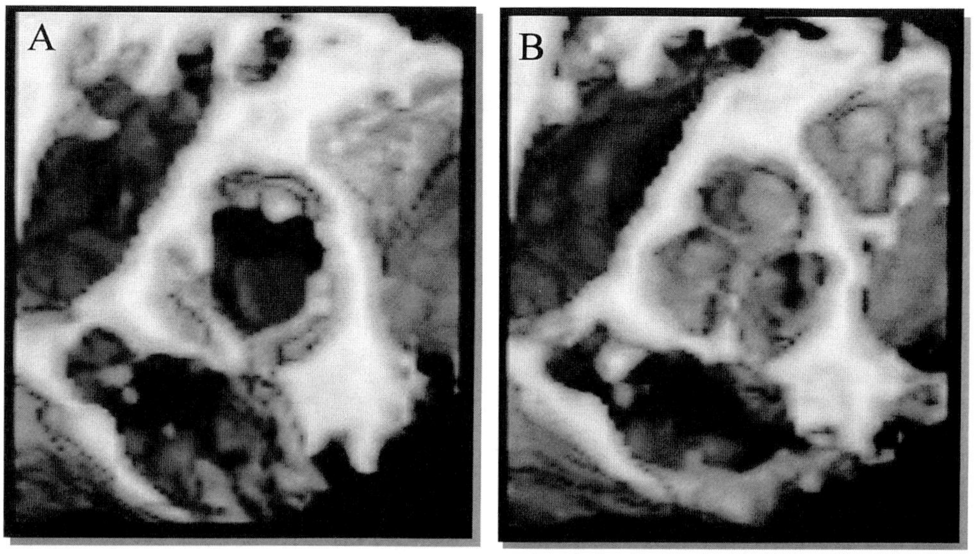

Figure 11. Systolic (**A**) and diastolic (**B**) frames of an aortic valve. This three-dimensional reconstruction was obtained from transthoracic images using a rotational transducer. The valve is viewed from the aorta. Note a small, calcified nodule on the right coronary cusp. From Lissa Sugeng, MD, Ivan Godoy, MD, Kirk T. Spencer, MD, Jim Bednarz, BS, Lynn Weinert, BS, and Roberto M. Lang, MD.

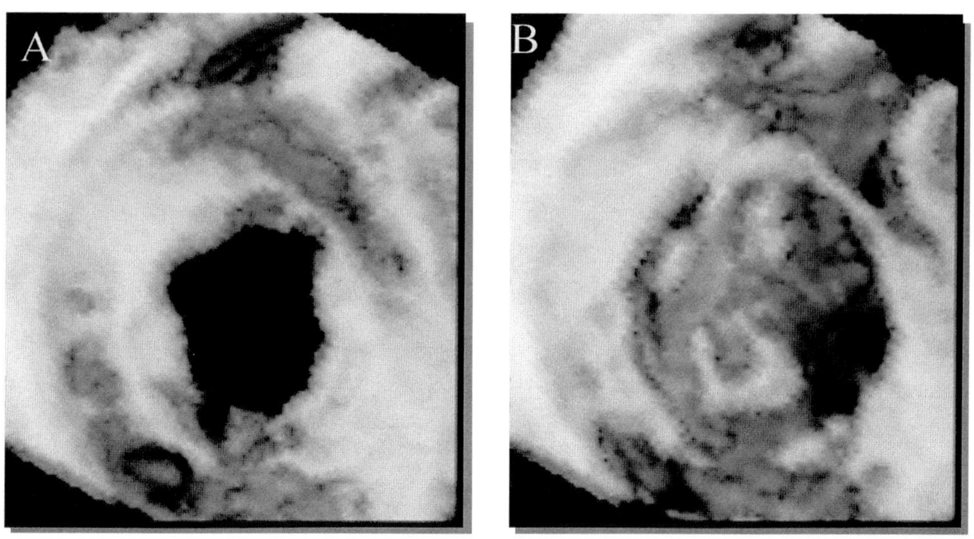

Figure 12. Diastolic (**A**) and systolic (**B**) frames of the mitral valve. This reconstruction was obtained from transthoracic images using a rotational transducer. The valve is viewed from the left ventricular apex. From Lissa Sugeng, MD, Ivan Godoy, MD, Kirk T. Spencer, MD, Jim Bednarz, BS, Lynn Weinert, BS, and Roberto M. Lang, MD.

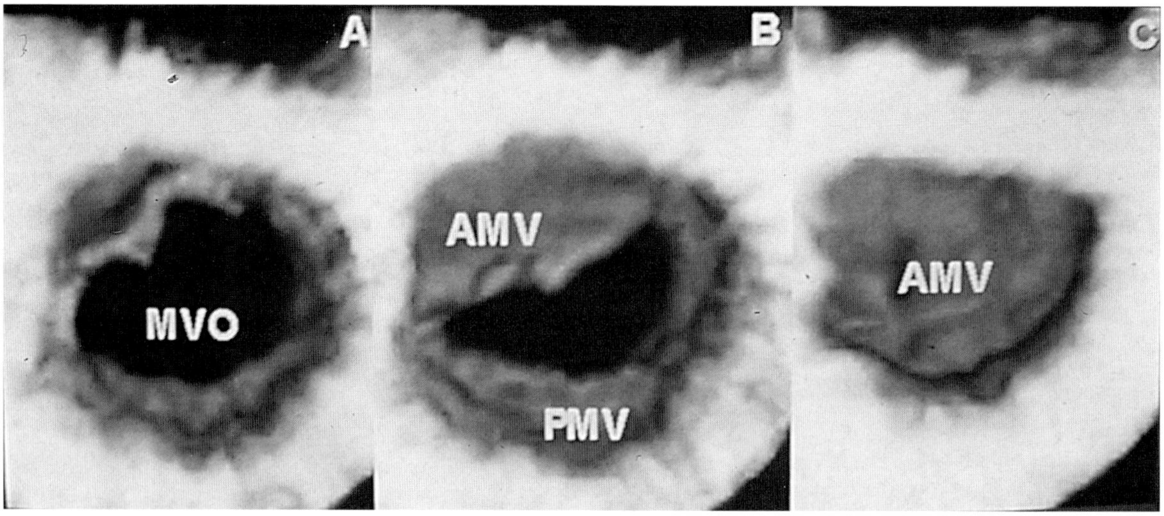

Figure 13. Dynamic three-dimensional bird's eye view of a normal mitral valve. (**Left**) In early diastole, mitral valve fully open. (**Center**) In middle diastole, area of mitral valve orifice reduced. (**Right**) In systole, mitral valve tightly closed. From Xin-Fang Wang, MD.

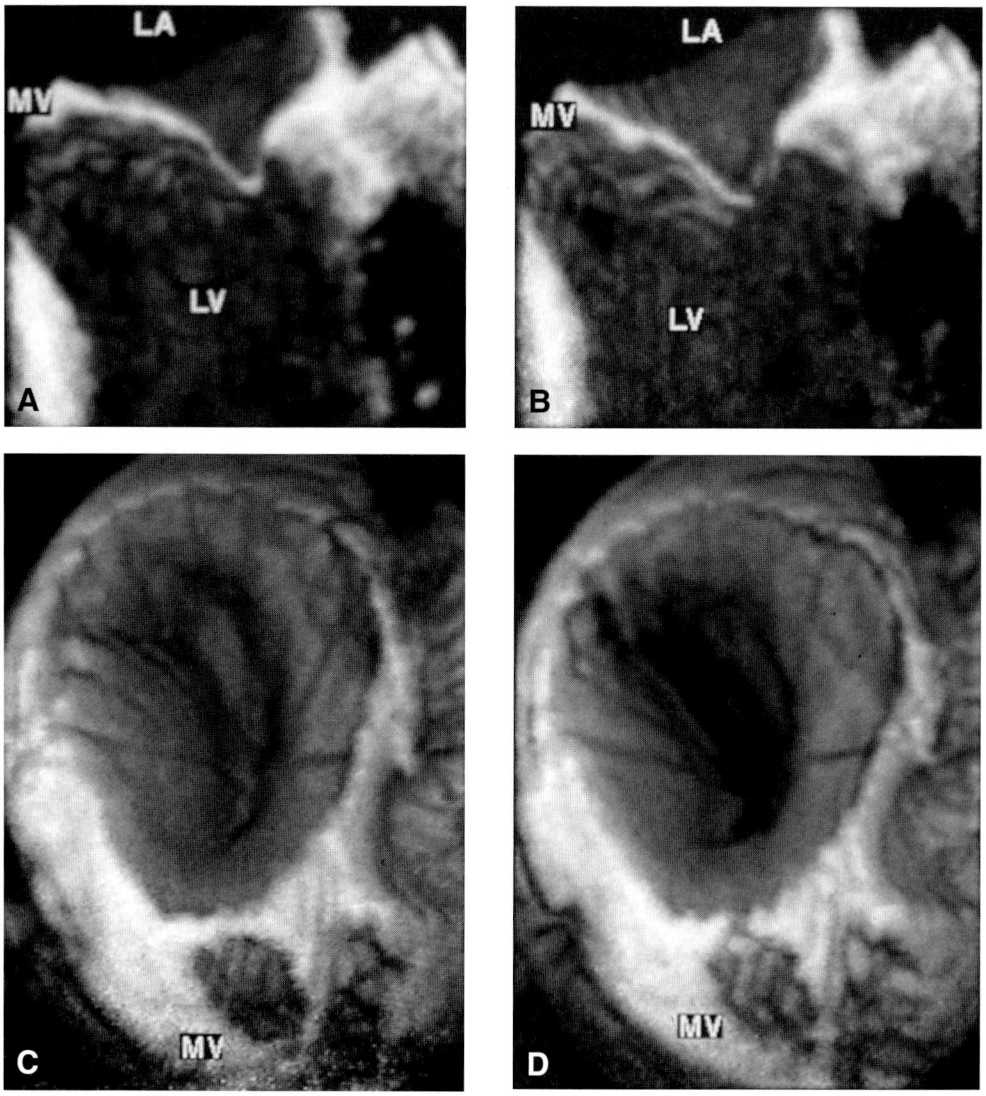

Figure 14. (**A**) This three-dimensional (3D) echocardiogram was reconstructed in the LAX plane, concentrating on the mitral valve (MV). There is normal coaptation and positioning in systole. (**B**) This 3D echo is from a slightly different cardiac cycle than the previous figure. Note the MV position is starting to open. (**C, D**) The MV may be reconstructed and imaged from any chosen point of reference. Here, the MV is viewed from the left atrial side in systole and diastole.

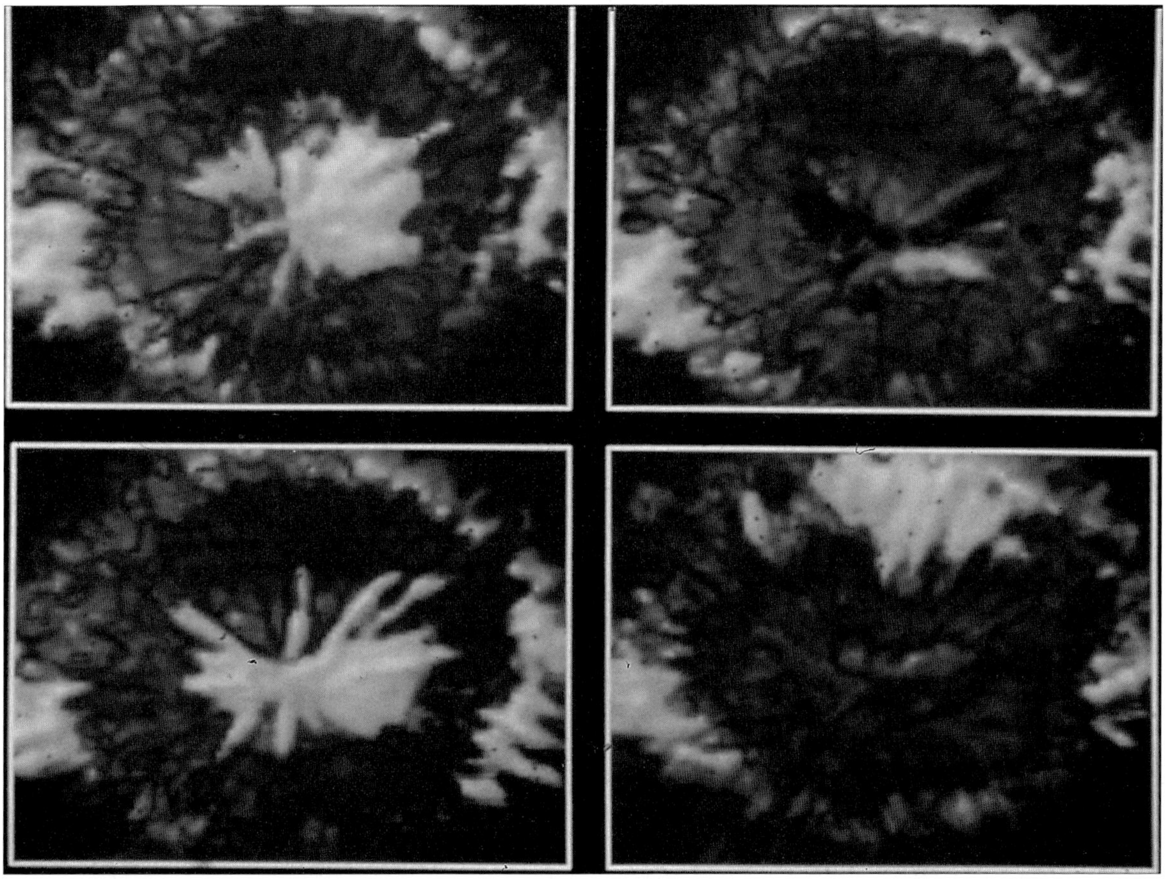

Figure 15. Flow through the mitral valve during the cardiac cycle. Black and white reconstruction from color-Doppler maps. Short-axis view of the left ventricle with anterior wall at top. **Top left:** Early filling flow (bright white) fills the open valve. **Top right:** In diastole almost no flow is seen between the leaflets. **Bottom left:** During atrial systole, flow is seen again. Acquisition and reconstruction artifacts create some oblique lines extending from the central flow. **Bottom right:** During ventricular systole, a small flow signal is detected along the closing line, corresponding to the converging mitral regurgitant flow. From Cedric Vuille, MD and Rene Lerch, MD.

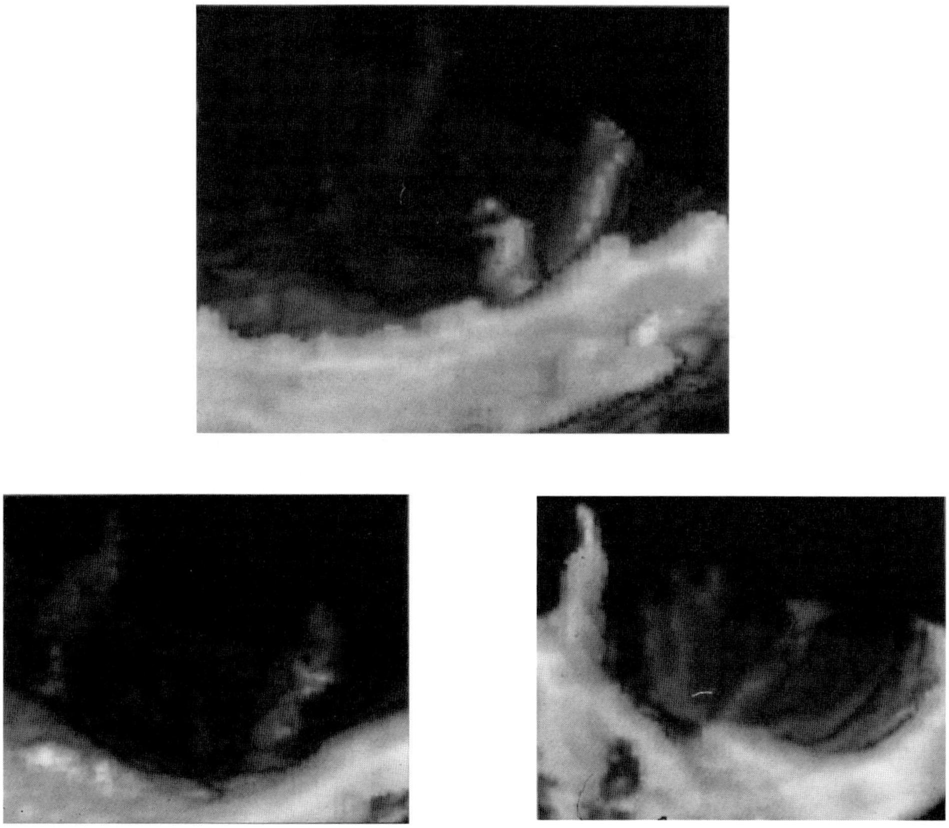

Figure 16. Normal regurgitant jets of a bileaflet mitral prosthesis. Black and white reconstruction from color-Doppler maps. Seen from the roof of the left atrium, four small jets are seen in systole, close to the hinge points. From Cedric Vuille, MD and Rene Lerch, MD.

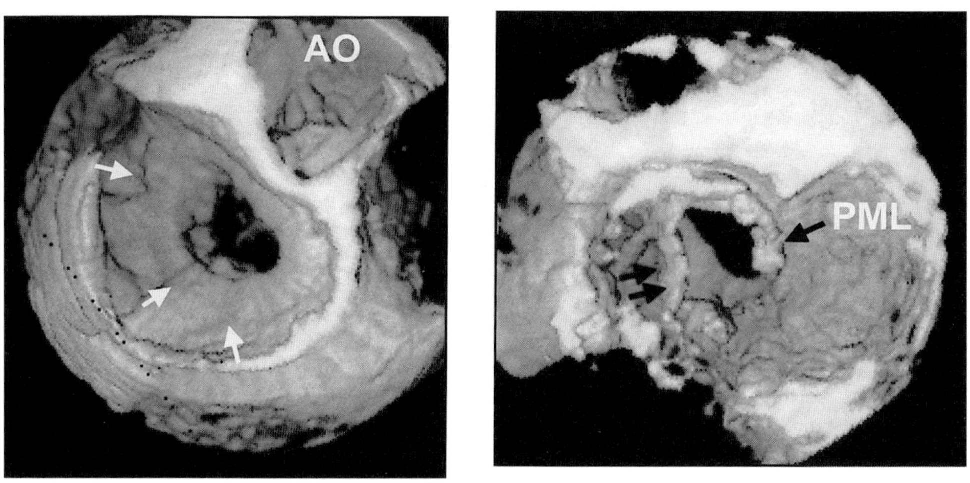

Figure 17. This patient with the posterior flail scallop received a mitral ring. A postoperative study was performed. **Left:** The ring (white arrows) is noted from a left atrial view. The size of the left atrium is notably smaller. **Right:** From a left ventricular view, the anterior mitral leaflet (double black arrows) and corrected posterior leaflet can be observed during diastole. From Lissa Sugeng, MD, Ivan Godoy, MD, Kirk T. Spencer, MD, Jim Bednarz, BS, Lynn Weinert, BS, and Roberto M. Lang, MD

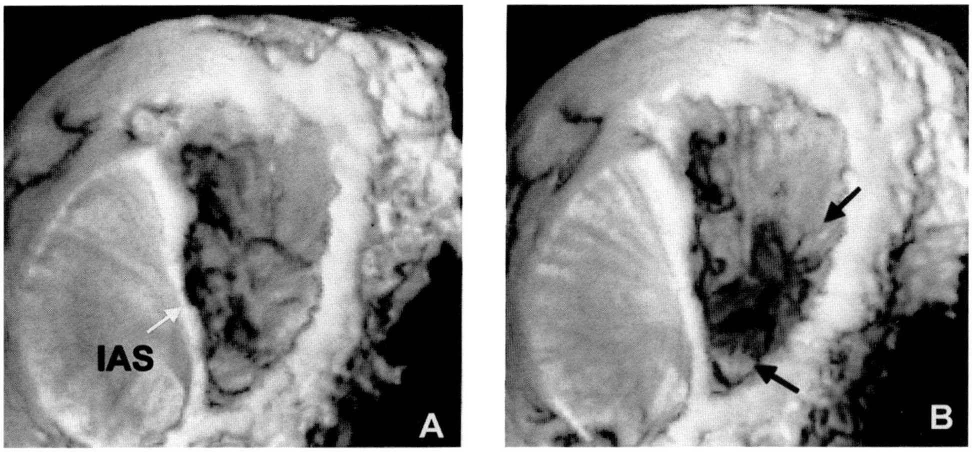

Figure 18. (**A**) In systole, a normal tricuspid valve is observed from an atrial view. (**B**) Separation of the three tricuspid valve leaflets in diastole can be appreciated. From Lissa Sugeng, MD, Ivan Godoy, MD, Kirk T. Spencer, MD, Jim Bednarz, BS, Lynn Weinert, BS, and Roberto M. Lang, MD.

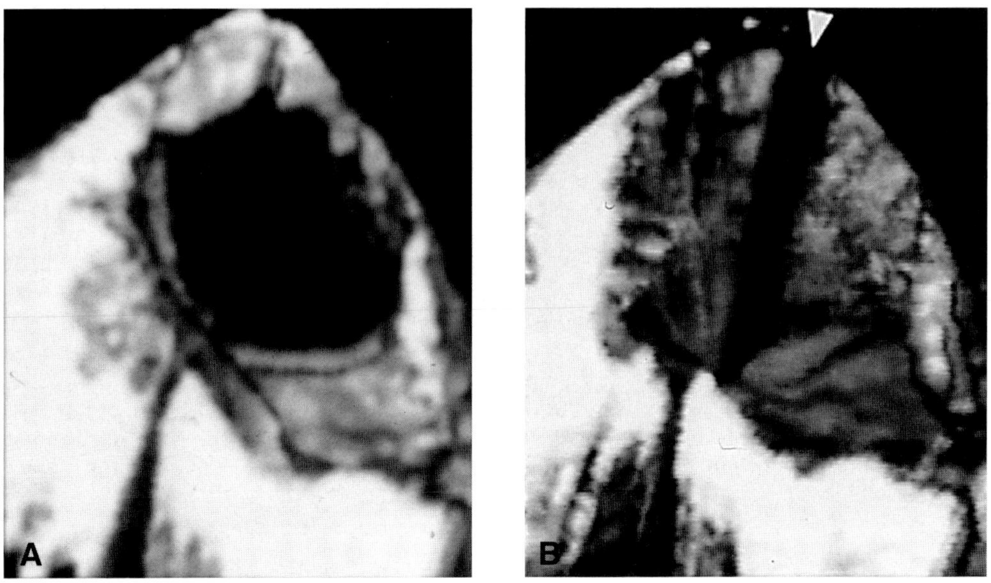

Figure 19. This three-dimensional echo reconstruction is of a normal triscupid valve in diastole as viewed from the right atrium. It was limited by prominent artifact related to tissue "drop-out" (**A**). In systole, the drop-out is even more severe, and should not be confused with pathology (**B**).

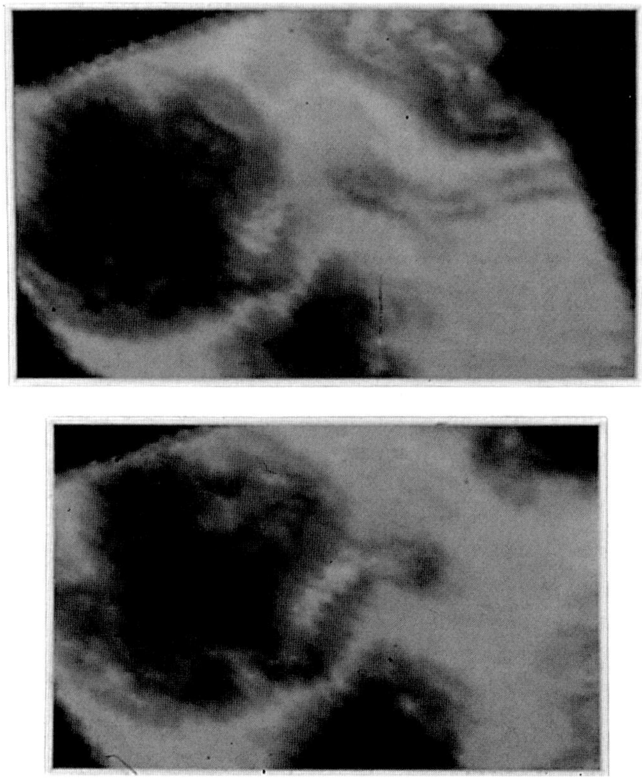

Figure 20. Two views (2 mm apart) of the left main (LM) coronary artery displayed in a conventional way (short-axis view of the aortic valve in two-dimensional echocardiography, with left atrium at the bottom and part of left atrial appendage seen just below the LM). **Top:** LM dividing into left anterior descending artery (running to the right of the image) and circumflex artery (running toward the bottom). **Bottom:** LM arising from the aorta. From Cedric Vuille, MD and Rene Lerch, MD.

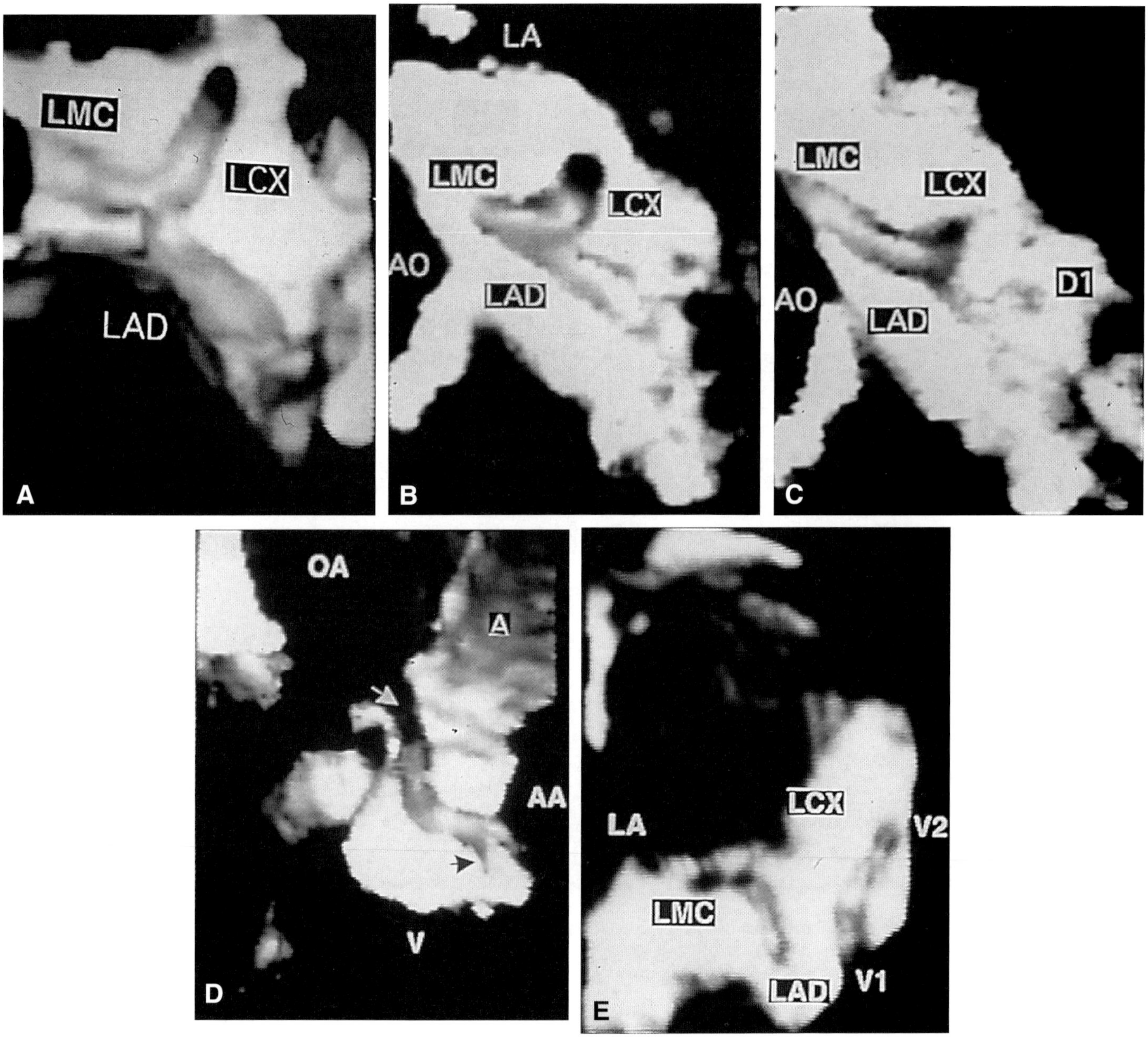

Figure 21. Transesophageal three-dimensional (3D) echocardiographic examination of coronary arteries. (**A**) The left main coronary artery (LMC) originating from the aortic root as well as the proximal left anterior descending (LAD) and circumflex (LCX) arteries are viewed in long axis in 3D. Note short-axis imaging of the more distal portion of the circumflex vessel. There is no evidence of stenosis (**B, C**). Both **A** and **B** represent two different 3D reconstructions of left-sided coronary arteries from the same dataset stored in the computer. **B** shows delineation of the first diagonal branch (D1), which is not visualized in **A.** (**D**) The right coronary artery (oblique arrow) is seen arising from the aortic root and coursing along the right atrioventricular groove adjacent to the right atrial appendage. The horizontal arrow points to a right ventricular branch. (**E**) Both interventricular (V1) and great cardiac (V2) veins are delineated accompanying the LAD and LCX coronary arteries. A = right atrium; AO = aortic root; LA = left atrium V = right ventricle. From Abd El-Rahman SM, et al. Transesophageal three-dimensional echocardiographic assessment of normal and stenosed coronary arteries. *Echocardiography* 1996;13:503–510.

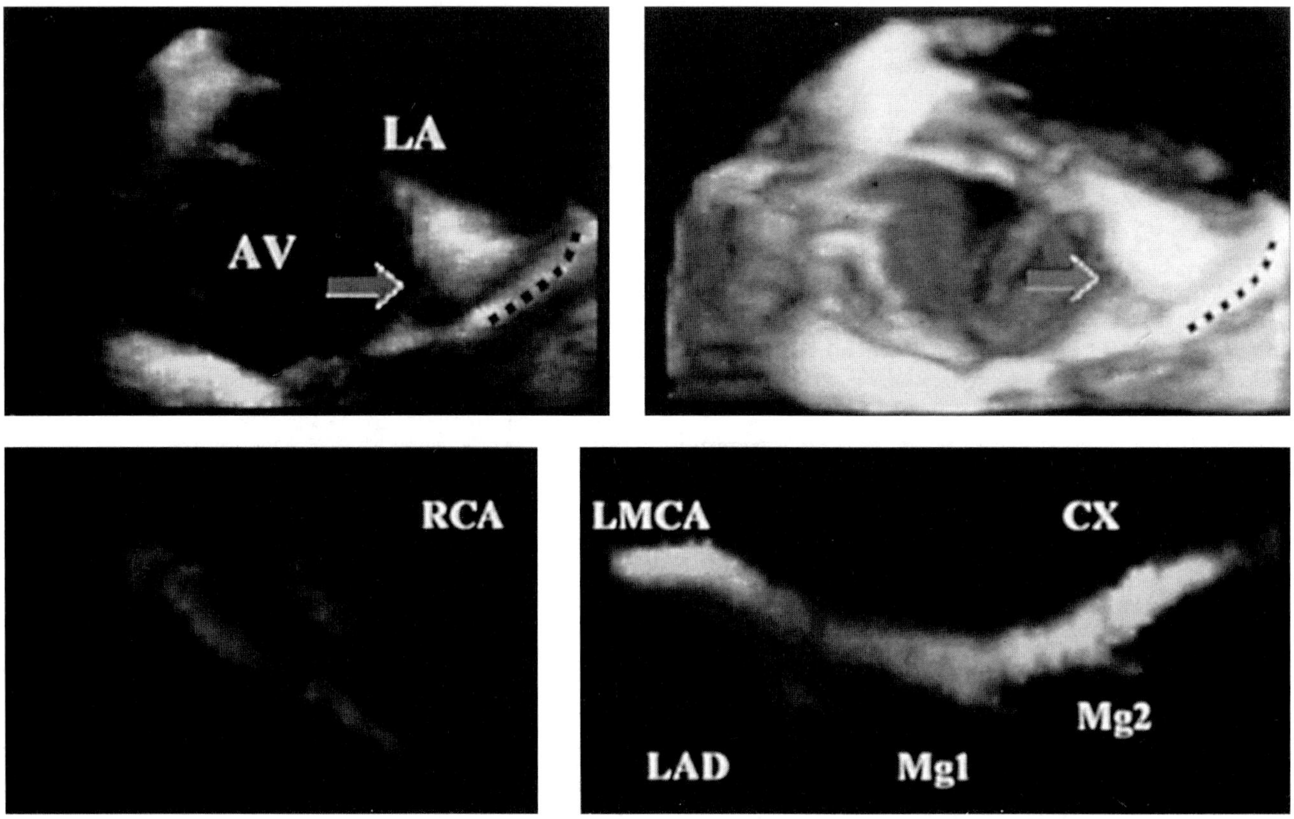

Figure 22. Three-dimensional echocardiographic imaging of proximal coronary arteries. Left upper panel is a reconstructed anyplane view across the aortic root and the right upper panel is a corresponding volume-rendered image. The origin of left main coronary artery from the left sinus of Valsalva is indicated with an arrow, and a dotted line marks the course of the proximal circumflex artery. The lower panels show extracted proximal segments of the right and left coronary artery. AV = aortic valve; CX = left circumflex artery; LA = left atrium; LAD = left anterior descending; LMCA = left main coronary artery; Mg = marginal branch; RCA = right coronary artery. From Jaroslaw D. Kasprazak, MD.

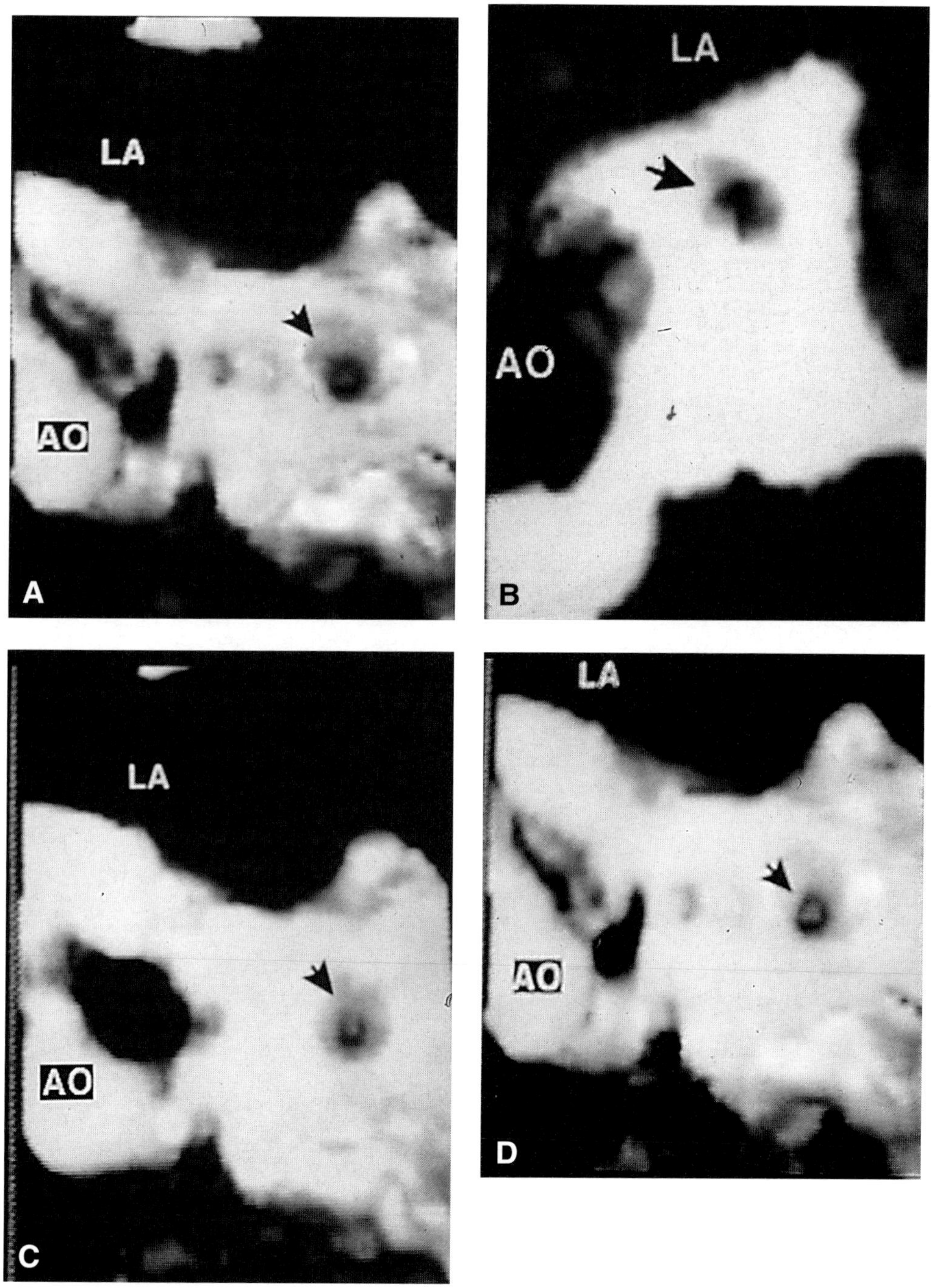

Figure 23 (A–D). The left circumflex coronary artery may be imaged in cross-sectional, short-axis views to obtain circumferential images at various locations. These four images were obtained at slightly different positions. Note the improved extent of visualization over conventional two-dimensional imaging and the ability to image in short-axis (**D**). This is thought to be one of the most significant advantages of three-dimensional echo.

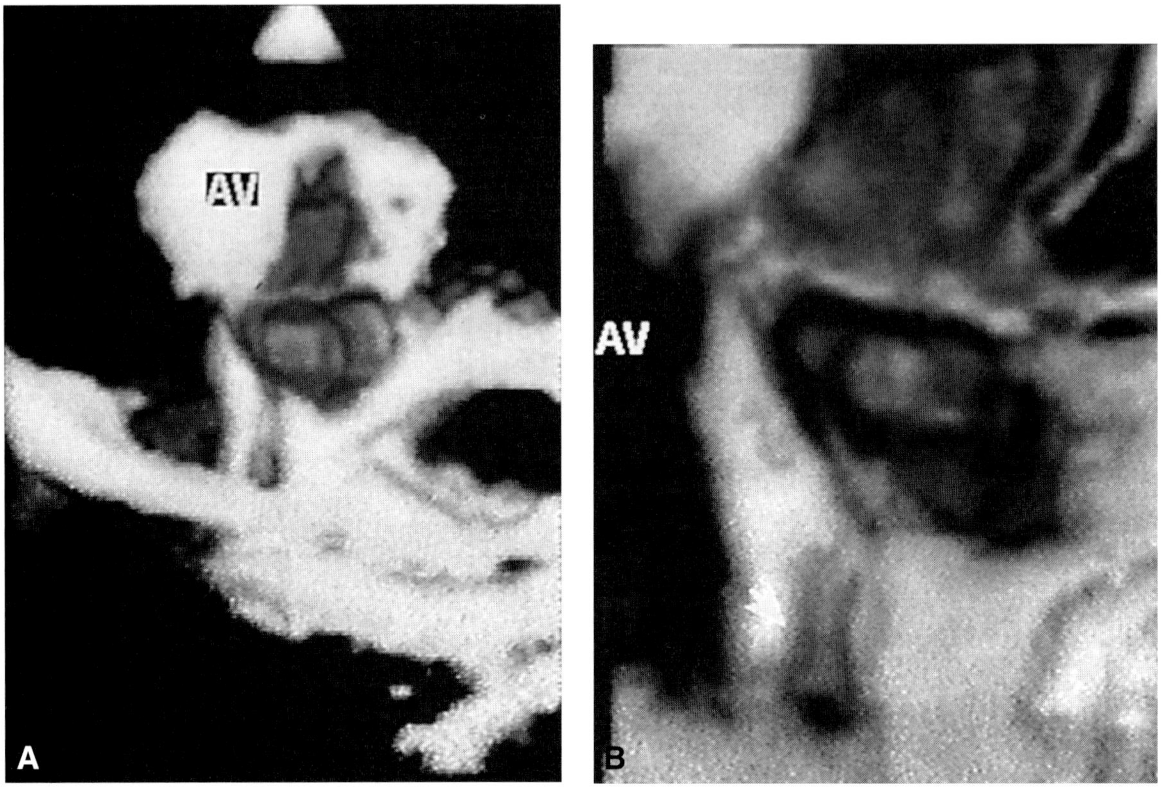

Figure 24. (**A**) A long portion of the proximal right coronary artery (RCA) is readily visualized in this reconstructed three-dimensional echo image during transesophageal echocardiography. (**B**) A zoom image of the same RCA at a slightly different cardiac cycle.

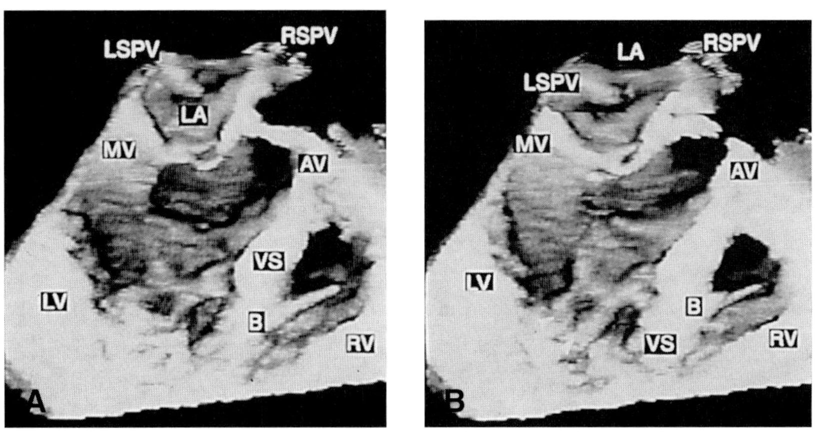

Figure 25. (**A, B**) Three-dimensional reconstruction of the left and right ventricles. The arrows denote papillary muscles in the left ventricle. AV = aortic valve; B = moderator band in the right ventricle; LA = left atrium; LSPV = left superior pulmonary vein; LV = left ventricle; MV = mitral valve; RSPV = right superior pulmonary vein; RV = right ventricle; VS = ventricular septum. Reproduced with permission from Nanda et al. Quantitative assessment of normal and stenotic aortic valve using transesophageal three-dimensional echocardiography. *Echocardiography* 1994;11:617–625.

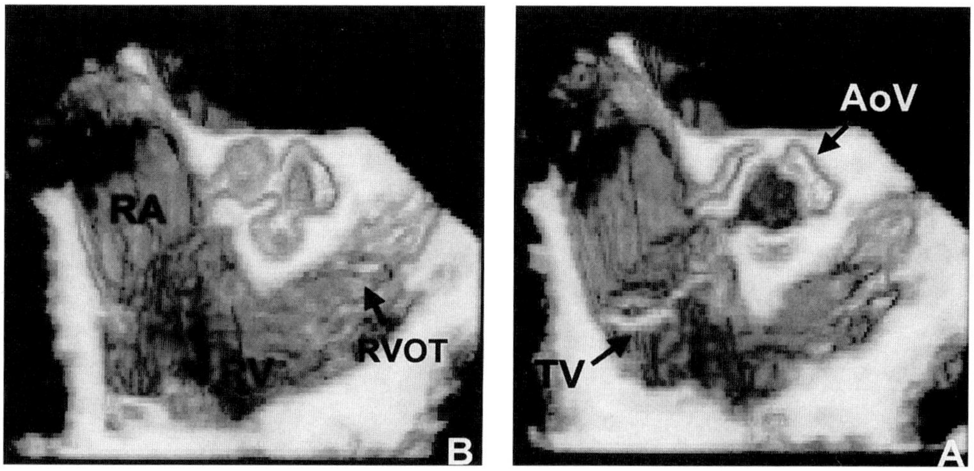

Figure 26. A long axis view of the right heart demonstrating the right atrium (RA), right ventricle (RV) and right ventricular outflow tract (RVOT). The tricuspid valve is seen in systole (**B**) however, not as well in diastole (**A**). The aortic valve can be observed in a short axis plane. From Lissa Sugeng, MD, Ivan Godoy, MD, Kirk T. Spencer, MD. Jim Bednarz, BS, Lynn Weinert, BS, and Roberto M. Lang, MD.

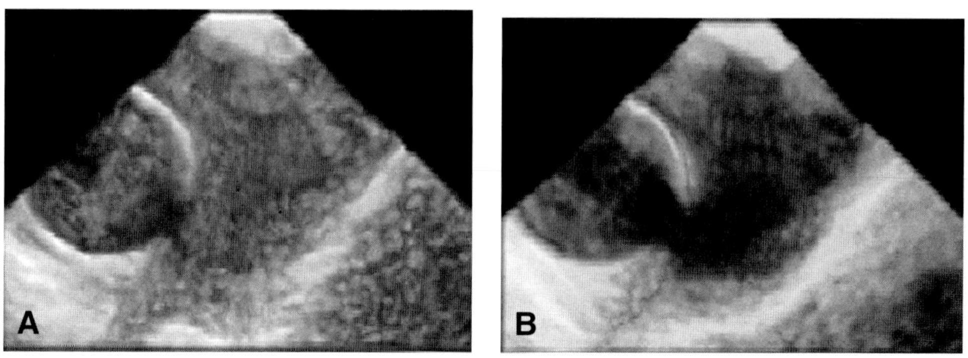

Figure 27. Normal pulmonary artery. Traditional imaging orientation processed in a three-dimensional (3D) display of the main pulmonary artery at its bifurcation into the proximal right and left branches. Note the variable detail and exchange of artifact location with more prominent shading (**A**) and less shading (**B**). These variables provide the 3D echocardiographer with additional image controls that at times improve and at others times degrade the chosen image. From Vincent L. Sorrell, MD.

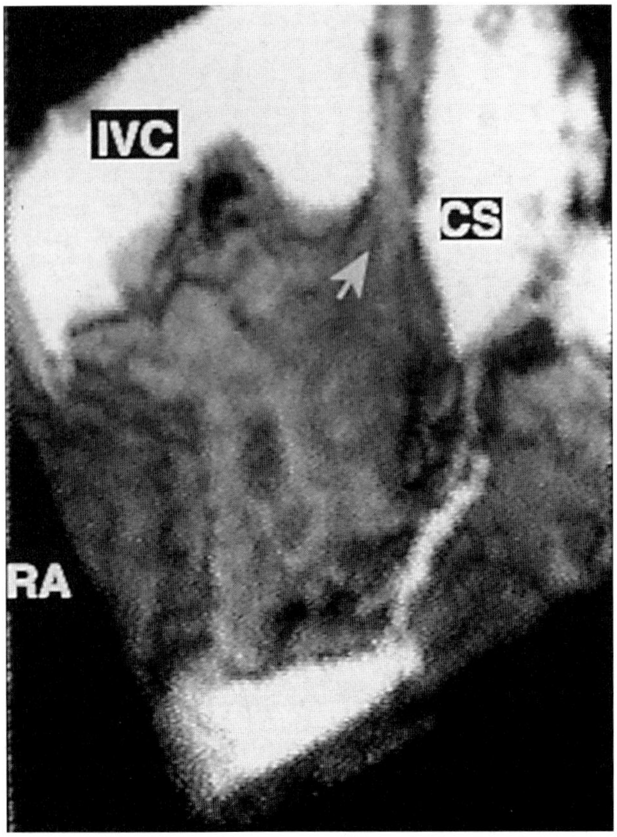

Figure 28. A transesophageal echocardiography-acquired, three-dimensional reconstruction of a normal coronary sinus entering into the right atrial cavity.

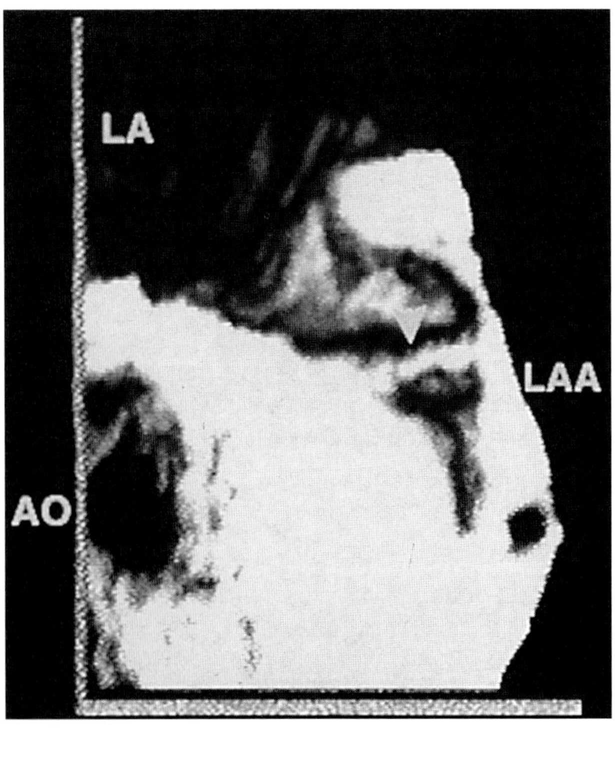

Figure 29. This reconstruction allows the details of the left atrium and its appendage to be visualized. Note the prominent pectinate muscle located in the body of the appendage (arrow).

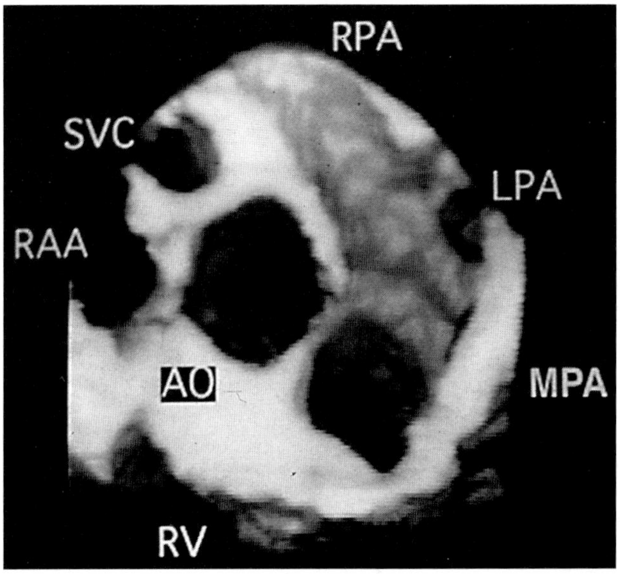

Figure 30. Transesophageal echocardiography acquired, three-dimensional data set allowing the reconstruction of the main pulmonary artery as it bifurcates into the proximal left and right pulmonary arteries.

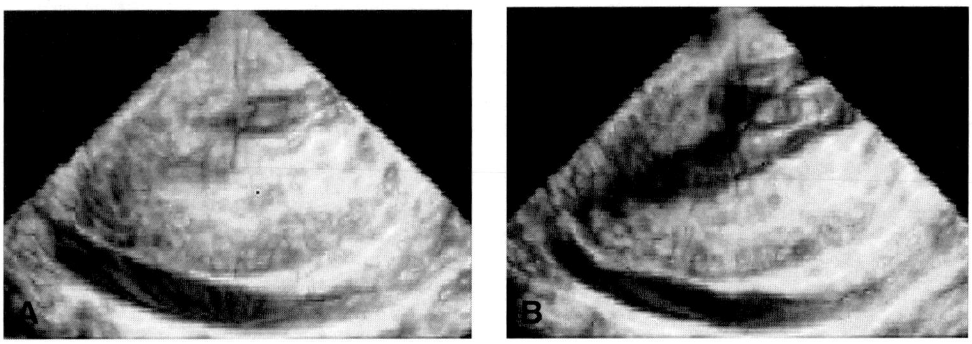

Figure 31. Left ventricular hypertrophy. (**A, B**) Transgastric transesophageal echocardiography, three-dimensional long-axis view of an elderly patient with long-standing hypertension and severe left ventricular hypertrophy (**A** = systole; **B** = diastole). A moderate sized pericardial effusion was also noted. From Vincent L. Sorrell, MD.

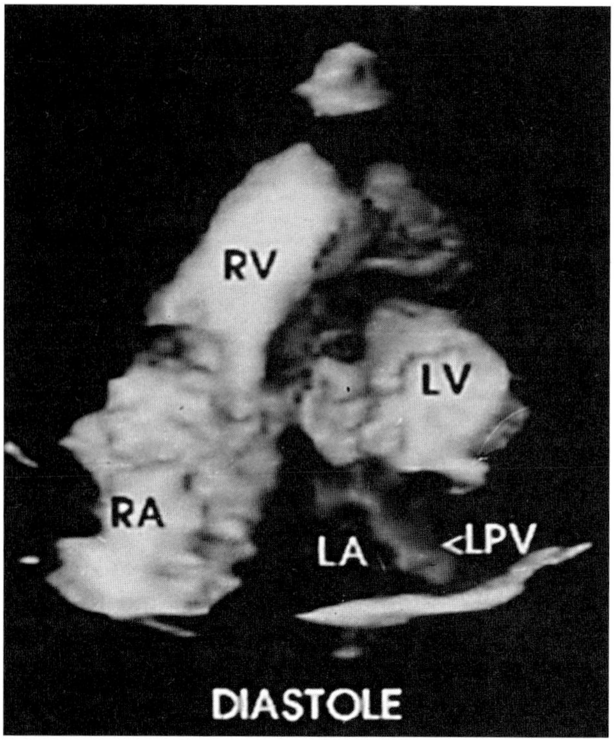

Figure 32. Dynamic three-dimensional Doppler flow imaging. Obtained in a normal subject by transesophageal echocardiography in diastole, showing blood flow passed through the tricuspid valve from the right atrium into the right ventricle; in the left heart, there was a stream of blood flow (arrowhead) from the left pulmonary vein (LPV) into the left atrium. Reproduced with permission from Wang XF. Four-dimensional echocardiography: Methods and clinical application. *Am Heart J* 1996;132:672–84.

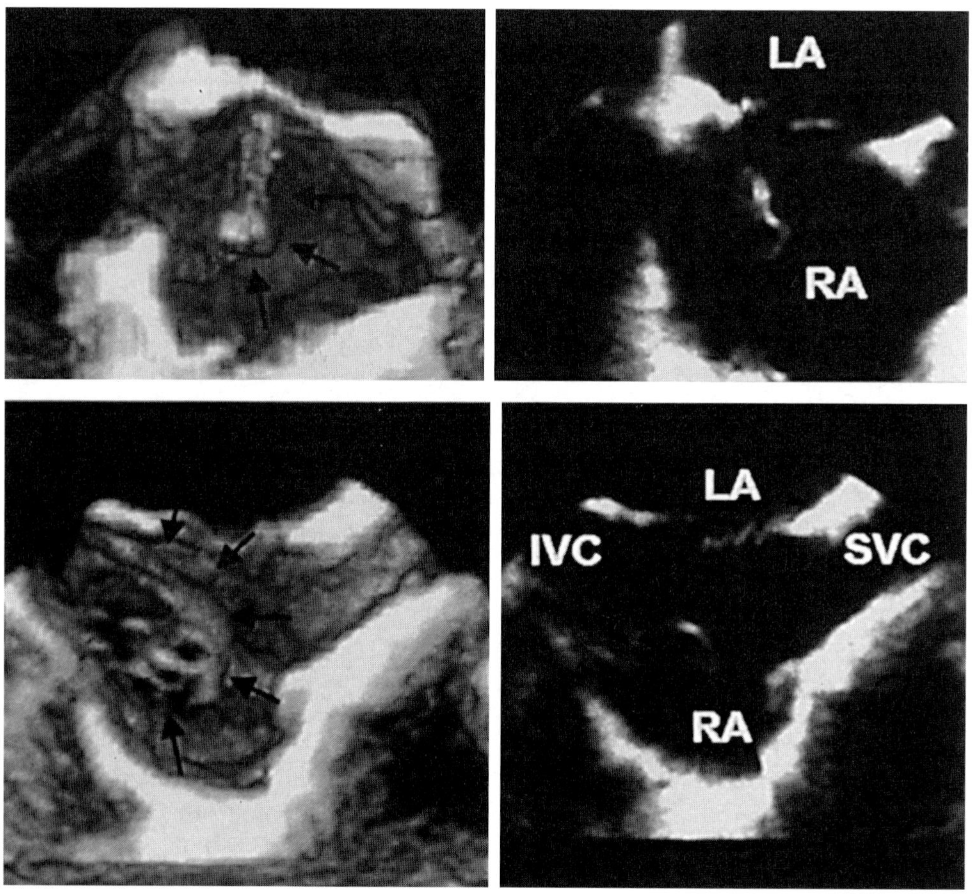

Figure 33. Chiari network (arrows) in a 24-year-old pregnant female with suspected right atrial mass. Reconstructed anyplane views (right) allow the display of attachment of the network to the orifice of the inferior caval vein and interatrial septum. Volume-rendering clearly demonstrates the fenestrated appearance of the network, which caused no inflow obstruction. IVC = inferior caval vein; LA = left atrium; RA = right atrium; SVC = superior vena cava. From Jaroslaw D. Kasprzak, MD and Jaroslaw Drozdz, MD.

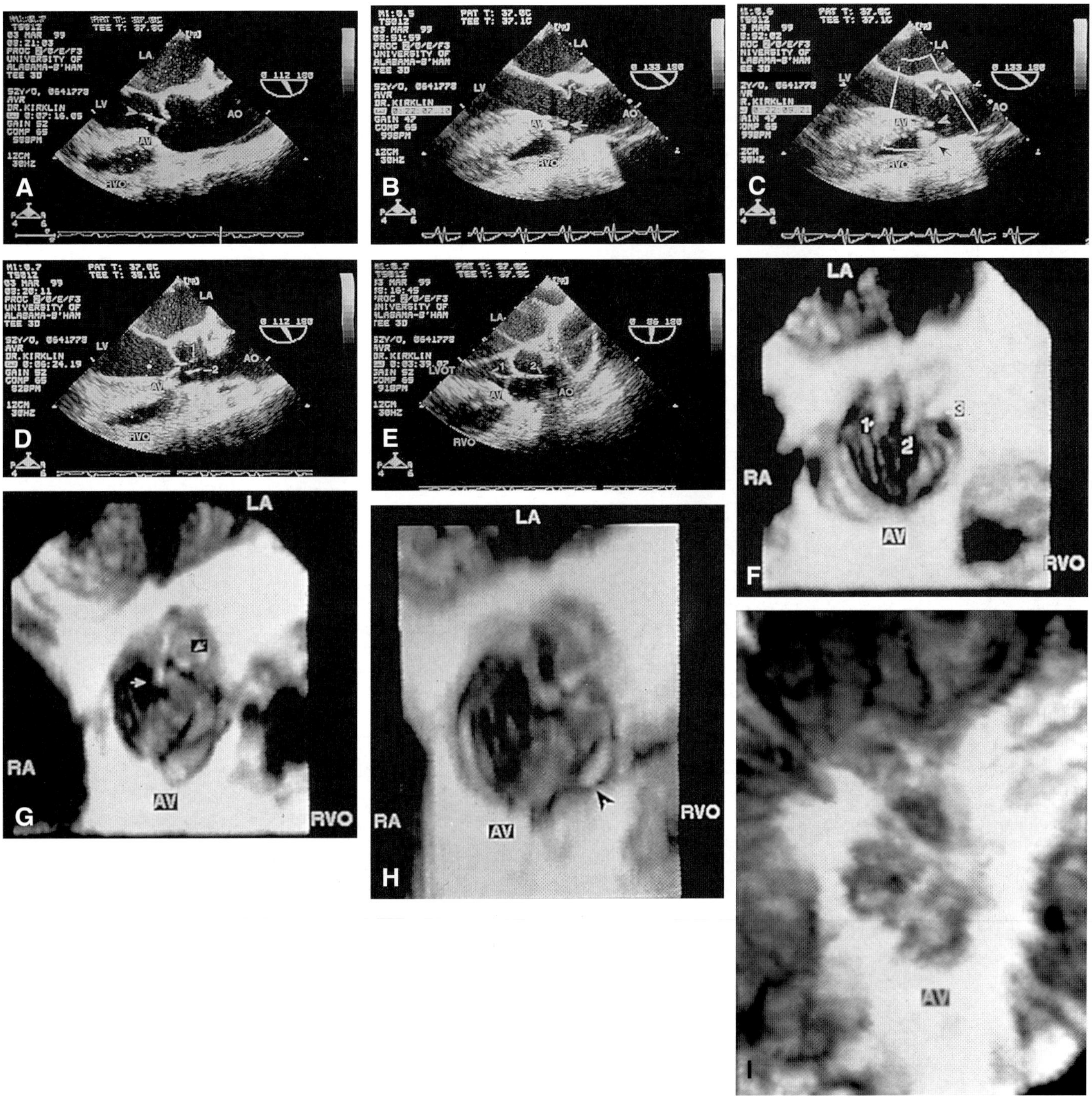

Figure 34. Lambl's excrescences on the aortic valve. Multiplane transesophageal two-dimensional (2-D) echocardiography. (**A**) The arrowhead points to a right coronary cusp excrescence protruding into the left ventricular outflow tract. (**B, C**) The top arrow points to an excrescence on the left coronary cusp, and the bottom arrow shows an excrescence on the right cusp of the aortic valve. Both excrescences show localized terminal thickening. The filled arrow in **C** points to the proximal right coronary artery. (**D**) Both excrescences (1 and 2) in the aorta (AO). (**E**) One excrescence (1) in the left ventricular outflow tract (LVOT) and the other one (2) in the aorta (AO). Transesophageal three-dimensional (3D) echocardiographic reconstruction. (**F–H**) Aortic valve viewed in short axis from the aortic side. (**F**) Three excrescences are noted: one on the noncoronary cusp (1) and two on the left cusp (2 and 3). (**G**) Two excrescences (arrows) on the left cusp. Clublike thickening of the terminal portions of the excrescences is clearly demonstrated. (**H**) Single excrescence (arrowhead) is visualized on the right cusp. Thus, a total of four excrescences were visualized by 3D echocardiography; 2D imaging showed only two. (**I**) Aortic valve viewed in short axis from the left ventricular side. No excrescences are attached on this surface. LA = left atrium; LV = left ventricle; MV = mitral valve; RA = right atrium; RV = right ventricle; RVOT = right ventricular outflow tract; VS = ventricular septum. Reproduced with permission from Samal AK et al. Three-dimensional echocardiographic assessment of Lambl's excrescences on the aortic valve. *Echocardiography* 1999;16:437–441.

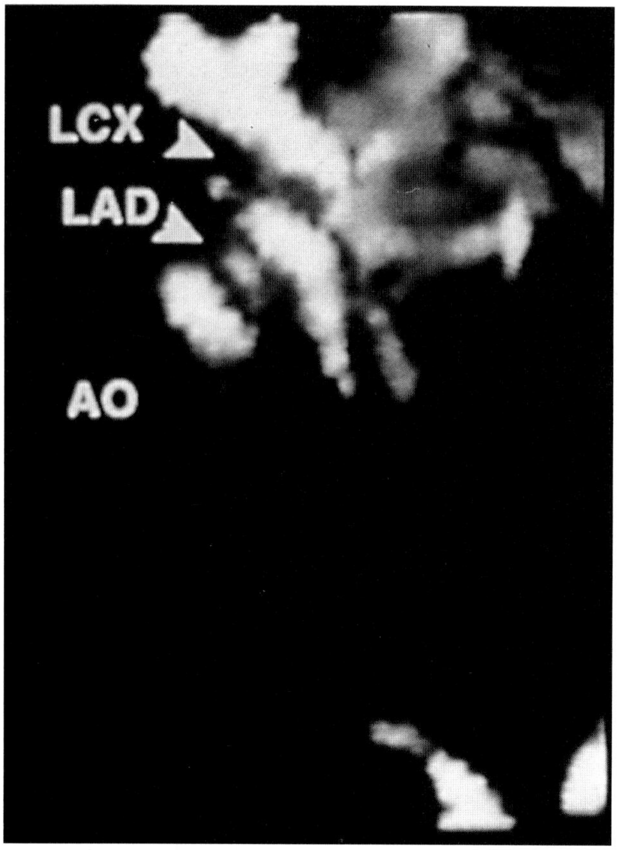

Figure 35. Transesophageal three-dimensional echocardiographic examination of coronary arteries. In this adult patient, the left main coronary artery is absent and both the left anterior descending (LAD) and circumflex (LCX) arteries originate separately from the aortic root (AO). Reproduced with permission from Abd El-Rahman SM et al. Transesophageal three-dimensional echocardiographic assessment of normal and stenosed coronary arteries. *Echocardiography* 1996;13:503–510.

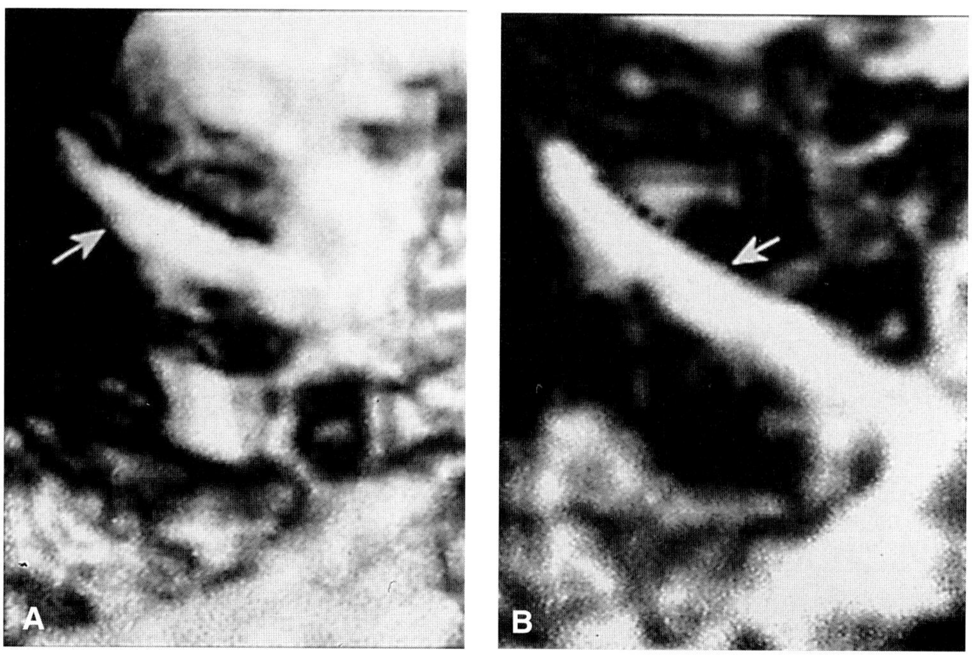

Figure 36. (**A**) Transesophageal three-dimensional echocardiographic image focusing on the right ventricle (RV), which has a catheter (arrow) within the cavity. (**B**) With a slightly different orientation and adjustment in the contrast, the catheter (arrow) can be further illustrated within the RV cavity.

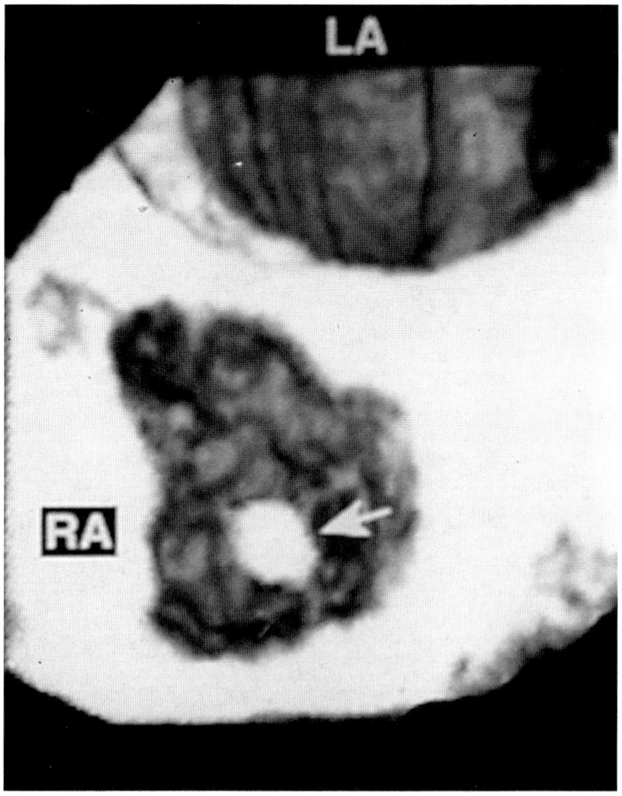

Figure 37. Short-axis, transesophageal three-dimensional echocardiographic image of the atrial septum in another patient with a highly visible catheter (arrow) noted within the right atrium.

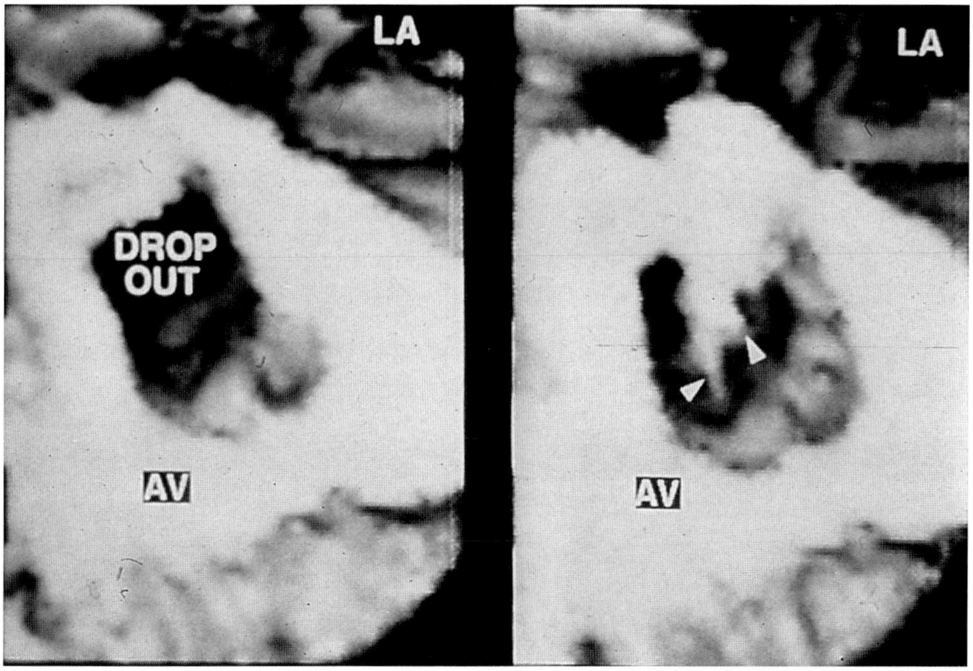

Figure 38. (**Left**) Large dropout because of a tangential cut through the aortic valve region in this patient with vegetations (arrows) involving the aortic valve (**right**). AV = aortic valve; LA = left atrium. Reproduced with permission from Nanda NC et al. Incremental value of three-dimensional echocardiography over transesophageal multiplane two-dimensional echocardiography in qualitative and quantitative assessment of cardiac masses and defects. *Echocardiography* 1995;12:619–628.

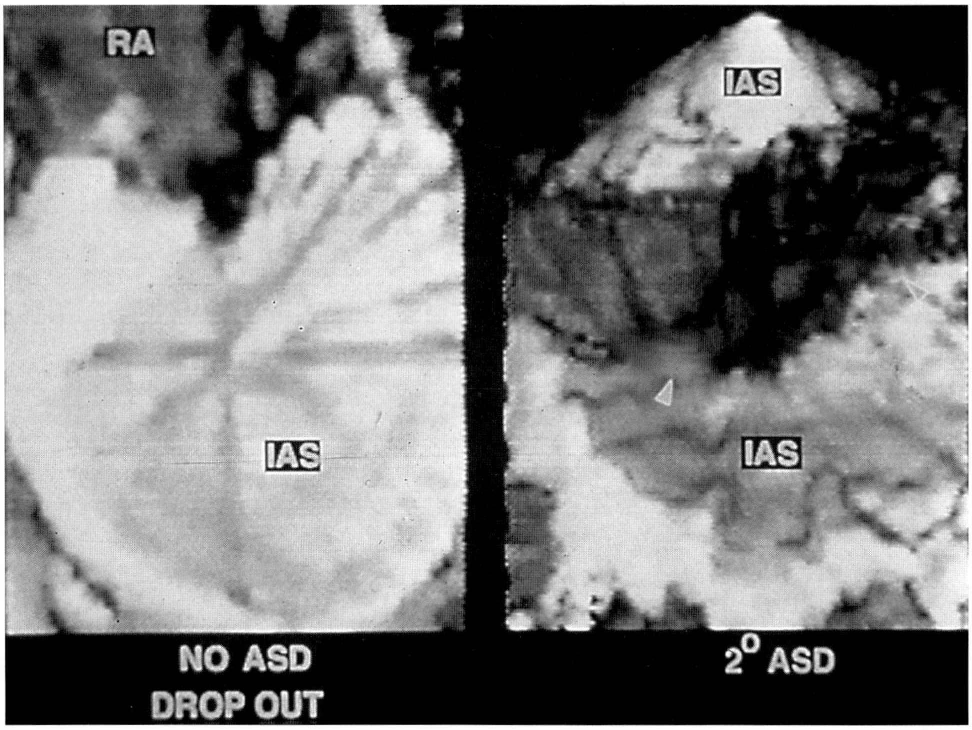

Figure 39. Left: Three-dimensional (3D) image of normal intact interatrial septum (IAS) with a dropout noted at the top of the image (viewed from the left atrial side). **Right:** Three-dimensional image of a huge secundum atrial septal defect (arrows) also viewed from the left atrial side. RA = right atrium. Reproduced with permission from Nanda NC et al. Incremental value of three-dimensional echocardiography over transesophageal multiplane two-dimensional echocardiography in qualitative and quantitative assessment of cardiac masses and defects. *Echocardiography* 1995;12:619–628.

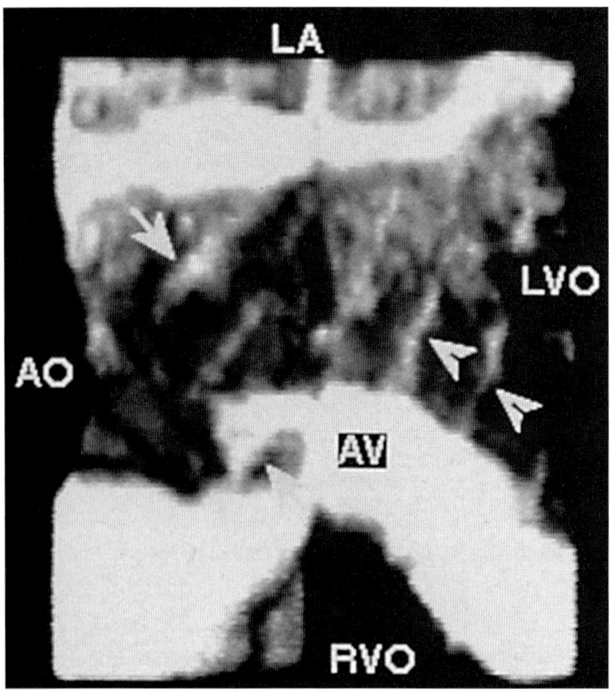

Figure 40. Intraoperative transesophageal echocardiographic evaluation performed during cautery to illustrate the linear artifacts (multiple arrows) generated when the surgeon attempts to use this device.

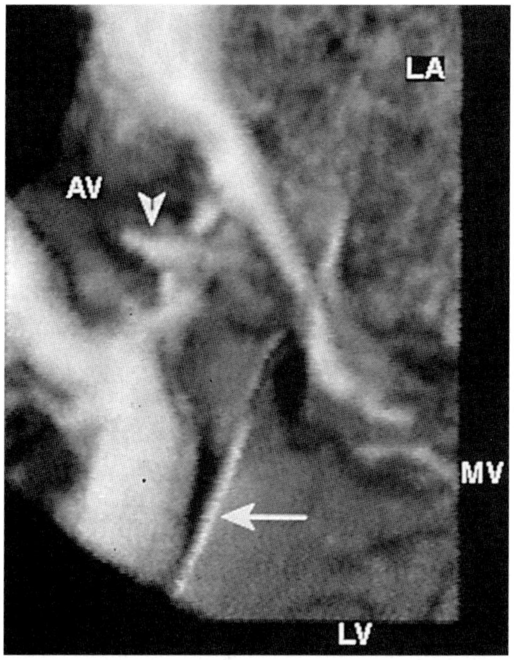

Figure 41. Transesophageal echocardiographic apical image in a patient with an aortic valve vegetation (arrowhead). Note the lengthy artifact (thin arrow) within the left ventricle. Linear or radial artifacts such as this are frequently related to motion during acquisition and are commonly multiple.

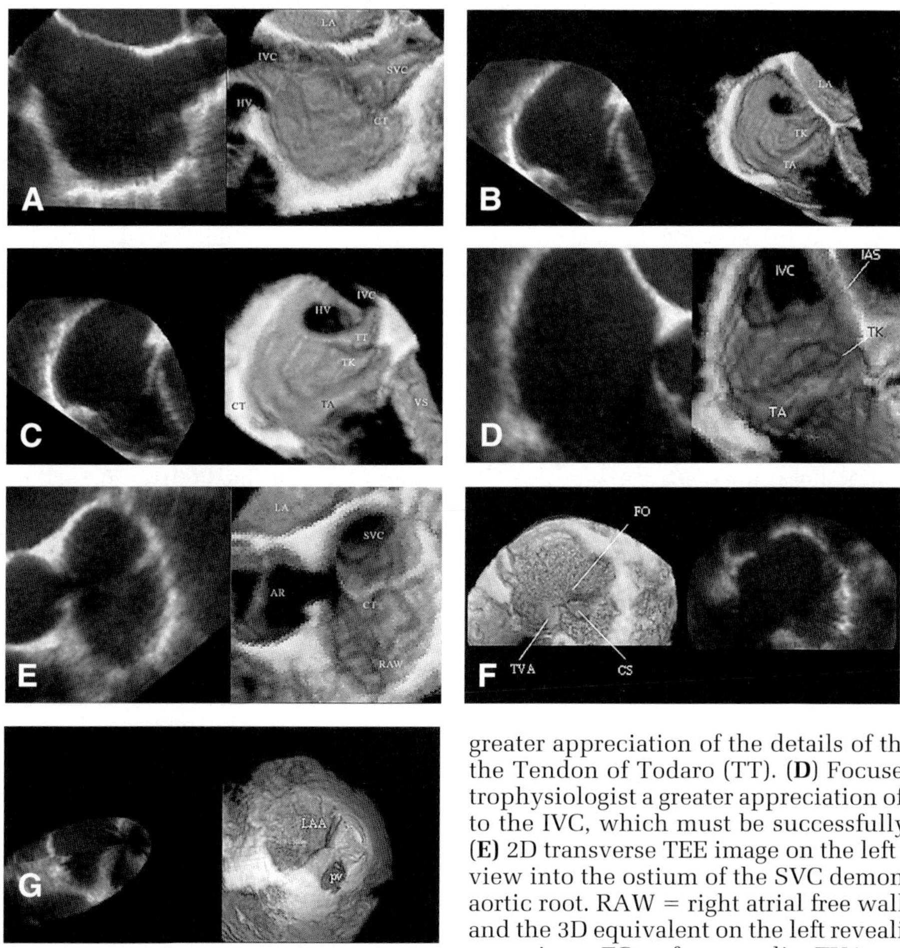

Figure 42. Detailed right atrial anatomy. With the additional shading capabilities available with three-dimensional (3D) imaging techniques, the contour of the right atrial (RA) free wall is seen to a much greater detail than conventional two-dimensional (2D) imaging. Numerous key intracardiac structures can be seen and appear to be vital to the electrophysiologist performing radiofrequency ablation of supraventricular arrythmias. (**A**) On the left, a conventional 2D transesophageal echocardiographic (TEE) longitudinal bicaval view. On the right, the corresponding 3D reconstruction. Note the enhanced visualization of the inferior (IVC) and superior vena cava (SVC), hepatic vein ostium (HV), and crista terminalis (CT). (**B**) On the left, conventional 2D tranverse image of the tricuspid valve annulus (TA) and atrial septum. On the right, the corresponding 3D-equivalent image. Note the improved visualization of the right atrial floor including the triangle of Koch (TK). (**C**) Same orientation as in **B.** With slight angulation, there is a greater appreciation of the details of the right atrial anatomy including the TK and the Tendon of Todaro (TT). (**D**) Focused orientation of this region allows the electrophysiologist a greater appreciation of the relationship of the anatomy from the TA to the IVC, which must be successfully "burned" for optimal arrhythmia ablation. (**E**) 2D transverse TEE image on the left and the 3D equivalent on the right. Superior view into the ostium of the SVC demonstrating the superior aspect of the CT. AR = aortic root. RAW = right atrial free wall. (**F**) 2D longitudinal TEE image on the right and the 3D equivalent on the left revealing the interatrial septum en face. CS = coronary sinus. FO = fossa ovalis. TVA = tricuspid valve annulus. (**G**) Very high cutplane 2D transverse TEE image on the left (not available with conventional 2D imaging) and the 3D equivalent on the right. This important image allows a comprehensive view of the left superior pulmonary vein (PV) ostium from the perspective of the lateral left atrial wall. This is the common location of radiofrequency ablation for atrial fibrillation. LAA = cross sectional view of the left atrial appendage. From Vincent L. Sorrell, MD and Jan Kulhanek, MD.

Suggested Reading List

1. Maurer G, Ghosh A, Nanda NC. Volume determination and three-dimensional reconstruction of echocardiographic images using rotation method. (Abstract) *Circulation* 1981;64:IV-206.
2. Schott JR, Moos S, Raqueno R, et al. 4-dimensional reconstruction from 2-dimensional echocardiograms. (Abstract) *Circulation* 1986;74:11–144.
3. Wixson SE, Nanda NC. Display of 4-dimensional ultrasound data. (Abstract) *J Ultras in Med* 1986;5:(9)136.
4. Wixson SE, Nanda NC, Iliceto S, et al. Evaluation of aortic dissection by color Doppler echocardiography. (Abstract) Annual Scientific Assembly of Southern Medical Association, Nov. 1986, Atlanta.
5. Ghosh A, Schott JR, Moos S, et al. Merging color Doppler imaging with 4-dimensional echocardiogram reconstruction. (Abstract) *J Am Coll Cardiol* III-A, 1987.
6. Ghosh A, Schott JR, Moos S, et al. New methods for displaying 3-dimensional echo images. (Abstract) *Clin Res* 1987;35:280A.
7. Schott JR, Moos S, Raqueno R, et al. Feasibility analysis of 3-dimensional reconstruction of color Doppler flow velocities. (Abstract) *J Am Coll Cardiol* 1987;III-214A.
8. Schott JR, Raqueno R, Moos S, et al. Successful merging of 3-dimensional color flow velocities and 3-dimensional reconstruction of the left ventricle. (Abstract) *Circulation* 1987;76:IV-527.
9. Raqueno R, Ghosh A, Nanda NC, et al. Four-dimensional reconstruction of two-dimensional echocardiographic images. *Echocardiography* 1989;6:323–337.
10. Nanda NC, Pandian N. Three and four dimensional transesophageal echocardiography. *Administrative Radiology* 1992;11:56–59.
11. Nanda NC, Pinheiro L, Sanyal R, et al. Multiplane transesophageal echocardiographic imaging and three-dimensional reconstruction: A preliminary study. *Echocardiography* 1992;9:667–676.
12. Pandian NG, Nanda NC, Schwartz ST, et al. Three-dimensional and four-dimensional transesophageal echocardiographic imaging of the heart and aorta in humans using a computed tomographic imaging probe. *Echocardiography* 1992;9:677–687.
13. Azvedo J, Cao QL, Pandian N, et al. Simulation of intraoperative 3-dimensional visualization of cardiac structures in pre-operative 3-dimensional and 4-dimensional transesophageal echocardiograms acquired using a computerized tomographic imaging probe. (Abstract) *J Am Coll Cardiol* 1993;21:180A.
14. Azevedo J, Cao OL, Pandian N, et al. Simulation of intraoperative three dimensional visualization of cardiac structures in pre-operative three dimensional and four dimensional transesophageal echocardiograms acquired using a computerized tomographic imaging probe. (Abstract) *European Heart J* August 1994, p. 441
15. Ofili EO, Nanda NC. Three dimensional and four dimensional echocardiography. *Ultrasound Med Biol* 1994;20:669–675.
16. Pandian N, Cao QL, Erbel R, et al. A comprehensive approach for image segmentation, cutting planes and display projections in three dimensional echocardiography: Suggested guidelines for clinically useful projections based on multicenter experience in 300 adult and pediatric patients. *J Am Coll Cardiol* 1994;23:9A.
17. Pandian NG, Roelandt J, Nanda NC, et al. Dynamic three dimensional echocardiography: Methods and clinical potential. *Echocardiography* 1994;11:237–259.
18. Li Z, Wang X, Nanda NC, et al. Three-dimensional reconstruction of transesophageal echocardiographic longitudinal images. *Echocardiography* 1995;12:367–375.
19. Nanda NC, Abd-El Rahman SM, Khatri G, et al. Incremental value of three-dimensional echocardiography over transesophageal multiplane two-dimensional echocardiography in qualitative and quantitative assessment of cardiac masses and defects. *Echocardiography* 1995;12:619–628.
20. Bates JR, Tantengco MV, Ryan T, et al. A systematic approach to echocardiographic image acquisition and three-dimensional reconstruction with a subxiphoid rotational scan. *J Am Soc Echocardiography* 1996;9:257–265.
21. Legget ME, Martin RW, Sheehan FH, et al. How positionally stable is a transesophageal echocardiographic probe? Implications for three-dimensional reconstruction. *J Am Soc Echocardiography* 1996;9:266–273.
22. Sadaniantz A, Burtt D, Nanda NC, et al. Three dimensional echocardiography of right heart pathology. *Echocardiography* 1998;15:795–806.
23. Samal AK, Nanda NC, Thakur AC, et al. Three-dimensional echocardiographic assessment of Lambl's excrescences on the aortic valve. *Echocardiography* 1999;16:437–441.
24. Nosir YF, Vletter WB, Kasprzak JD, et al. Optimal rotational interval for 3-dimensional echocardiography data acquisition for rapid and accurate measurement of left ventricular function. *J Am Soc Echocardiography* 2000;13(8):715–722.
25. Chuang ML, Hibberd MG, Beaudin RA, et al. Patient motion compensation during transthoracic 3-D echocardiography. *Ultrasound in Med & Biol* 2001;27:203–209.
26. Miller A, Mukhtar O, Aaluri Sret al. 2-D and 3-D TEE differentiation of lymphoma involving the atrial septum from lipomatous hypertrophy. *Echocardiography* 2001;18:205–209.
27. Nadkarni SK, Boughner DR, Drangova M, et al. In vitro simulation and quantification of temporal jitter artifacts in ECG-gated dynamic three-dimensional echocardiography. *Ultrasound in Med & Biol* 2001;27(2):211–222.

Chapter 3

Valvular Heart Disease

Navin C. Nanda, MD and Vincent L. Sorrell, MD

Using a transesophageal echocardiographic (TEE) approach provides the most consistent visualization of the mitral valve, since the image is displayed unimpeded through the adjacent left atrium. However, even with the increased detail available with TEE, the contour of the saddle-shaped mitral annulus limits the complete interrogation without significant manipulation of the probe. With images being obtained at variable times, the interpreter must mentally reconstruct these for optimal understanding of the anatomy and any pathology. Although the mitral valve has been the most studied to date, and provides the greatest number of images in this atlas as well as in the published literature, each valve has similar three-dimensional (3D) contours that are just beginning to be characterized. Through the continued advancements in 3D imaging, it is hoped that all valves and nearby structures will become as well understood as the mitral valve has become.

Three-dimensional data sets improve upon this greatly by providing the interpreter with the ability to directly image the 3D-contoured anatomy. This fact will likely enable the surgeon to better prepare for needed surgery. It allows a better appreciation of the spatial anatomy, which is often abnormal in patients with valvular heart disease and those who have undergone surgical procedures.

One of the major advantages of 3D echo is the ability to obtain two dimensional (2D) cutplanes using the 3D data set. This provides the interpreter the unique option of imaging at any chosen plane through any desired pathology ("anyplane" imaging). This chapter includes many of the common abnormalities one is likely to encounter in an active echocardiography lab and takes advantage of anyplane imaging by revealing many never-before-seen displays of such common diseases as mitral valve prolapse, mitral stenosis, and valvular endocarditis. Furthermore, some less common diseases are also displayed, such as paravalvular extension of infection as well as dehiscence of a mitral valvular ring.

Images previously not available with conventional 2D imaging are now readily obtained with 3D, and include detailed leaflet definition of mechanical prosthesis, optimal *en-face* delineation of valve stenosis for direct planimetry using anyplane methodology, and the ability to graphically display the image in any chosen orientation. This latter ability is enthusiastically supported by our surgical colleagues, who prefer to have the disease displayed from the "surgeon's perspective" for the most comprehensive preoperative assessment.

For the most accurate surgical comparisons, it is also important to be able to describe the location of any identified specific pathology in descriptive terminology understood by the surgeon. Describing the valves from the visualized anatomic perspective of the surgeon, using a standard clockface orientation, is a very helpful comparison; the following are provided for this purpose. When viewing the mitral valve, the left atrial appendage is at nine or ten o'clock in a surgeon's perspective. Therefore, describing important findings in relation to this will allow the surgeon to focus their attention directly in the same area. Other surgical landmarks include the left main coronary artery at eleven o'clock, and the interatrial septum at seven o'clock, when viewing the aortic valve.

Readers are encouraged to also view additional valve lesions within other sections of the atlas including: Normal Anatomy, Normal Variants and Artifacts (normal native and prosthetic valves; Lambls excrescences); Congenital Heart Disease (bicuspid aortic valve; subaortic membrane; Ebstein's anomaly); Masses (mitral valve myxoma); and the sections on 3D Color Flow Doppler.

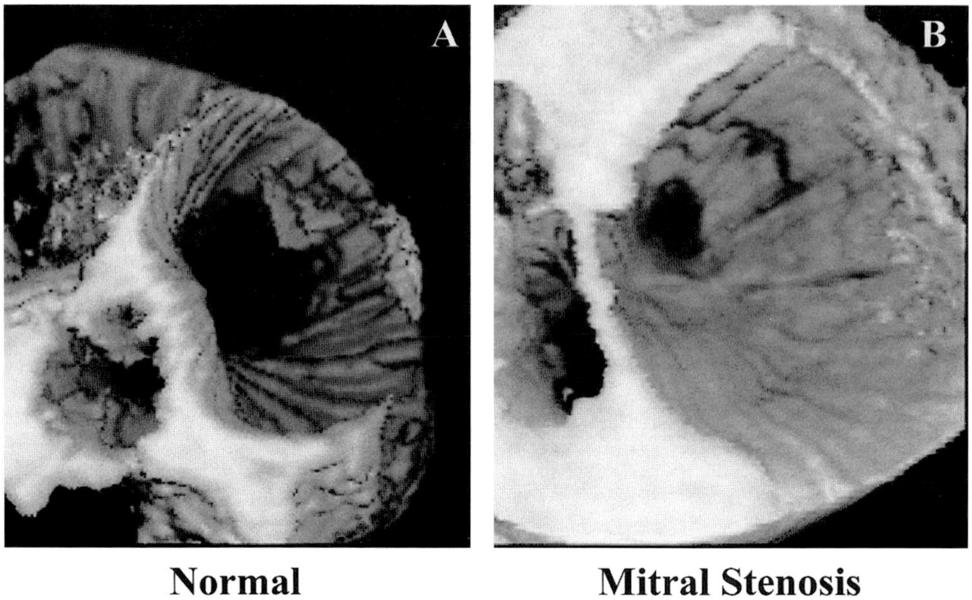

Figure 1. (**A**) Diastolic frame depicting a normal mitral valve as viewed from the left atrium. This reconstruction was performed from transesophageal images acquired with a multiplane transducer. (**B**) Diastolic frame depicting a rheumatically deformed mitral valve with severe mitral stenosis. This reconstruction was performed from transesophageal images acquired with a multiplane transducer. Note the reduced mitral area estimated at cardiac catheterization to be 0.8 cm^2. From Lissa Sugeng, MD, Ivan Godoy, MD, Kirk T. Spencer, MD, Jim Bednarz, BS, Lynn Weinert, BS, and Roberto M. Lang, MD.

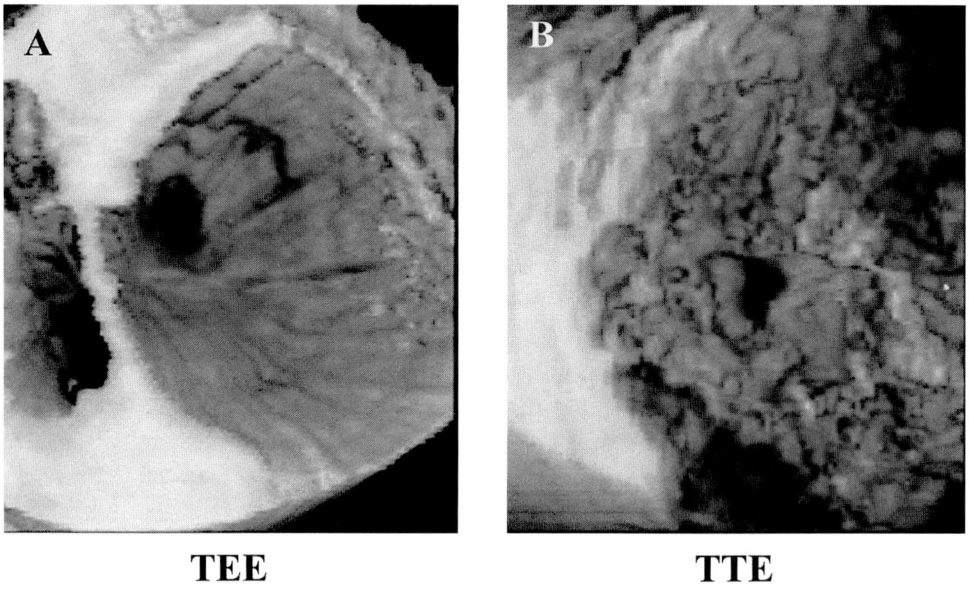

Figure 2. (**A**) Diastolic frame depicting a rheumatically deformed mitral valve with severe mitral stenosis. This reconstruction was performed from transesophageal images acquired with a multiplane transducer. Note the reduced mitral valve area estimated at cardiac catherization to be 0.8 cm^2. From Lissa Sugeng, MD, Ivan Godoy, MD, Kirk T. Spencer, MD, Jim Bednarz, BS, Lynn Weinert, BS, and Roberto M. Lang, MD

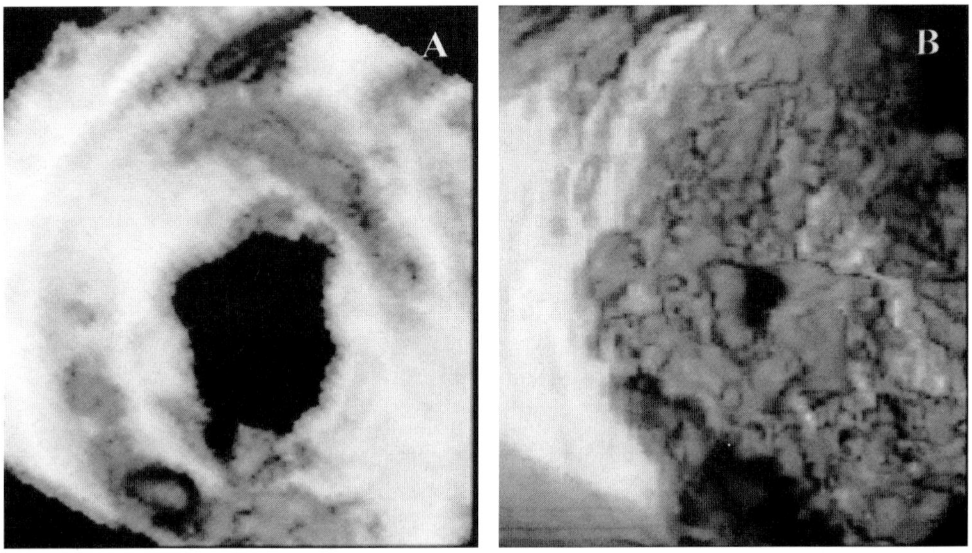

Figure 3. (**A**) Diastolic frames of a normal mitral valve. This reconstruction was obtained from transthoracic images using a rotational transducer. The valve is viewed from the left ventricular apex. (**B**) Diastolic frames of a rheumatically deformed mitral valve with severe mitral stenosis. This reconstruction was obtained from transthoracic images using a rotation transducer. The valve is viewed from the left ventricular apex. From Lissa Sugeng, MD, Ivan Godoy, MD, Kirk T. Spencer, MD, Jim Bednarz, BS, Lynn Weinert, BS, and Roberto M. Lang, MD

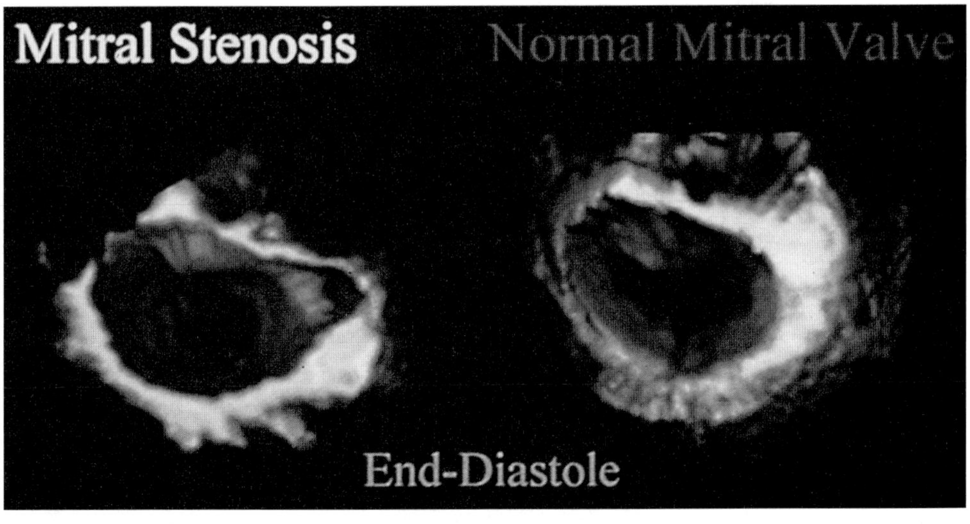

Figure 4. Left: A stenotic mitral valve is reconstructed from the point of reference of the left atrium. Note the extensively thickened and irregular surface with the small, eccentric opening. Three-dimensional echo allows optimal orientation for planimetry, which is most often from the left atrial perspective. **Right:** A normal mitral valve is reconstructed for comparison. From Aleksandra Lange, MD.

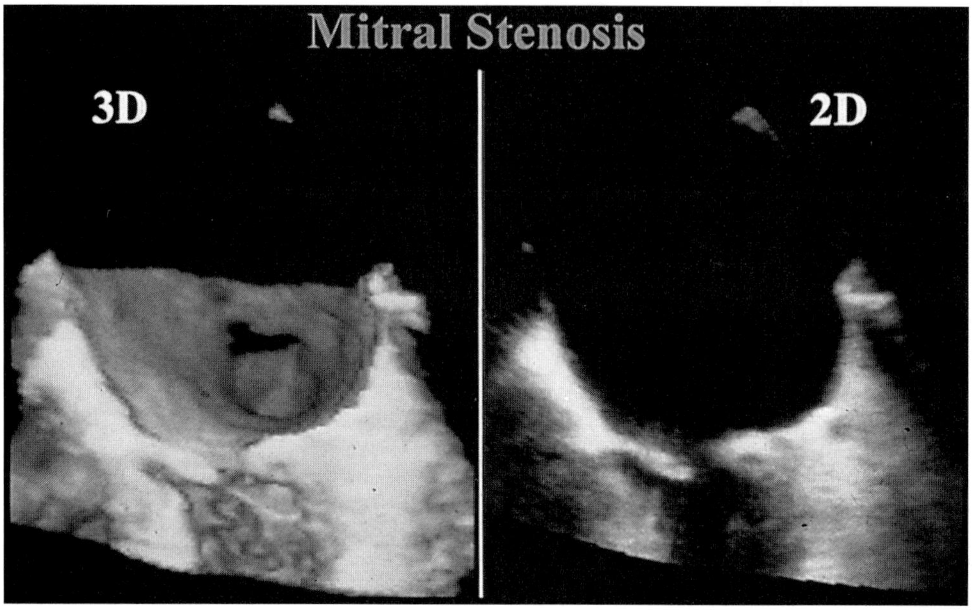

Figure 5. Left: A three-dimensional reconstruction of a very small orifice of a rheumatic mitral valve stenosis visualized from the left atrium. On the right, a two-dimensional apical 4-chamber view of the same patient for comparison. From Aleksandra Lange, MD.

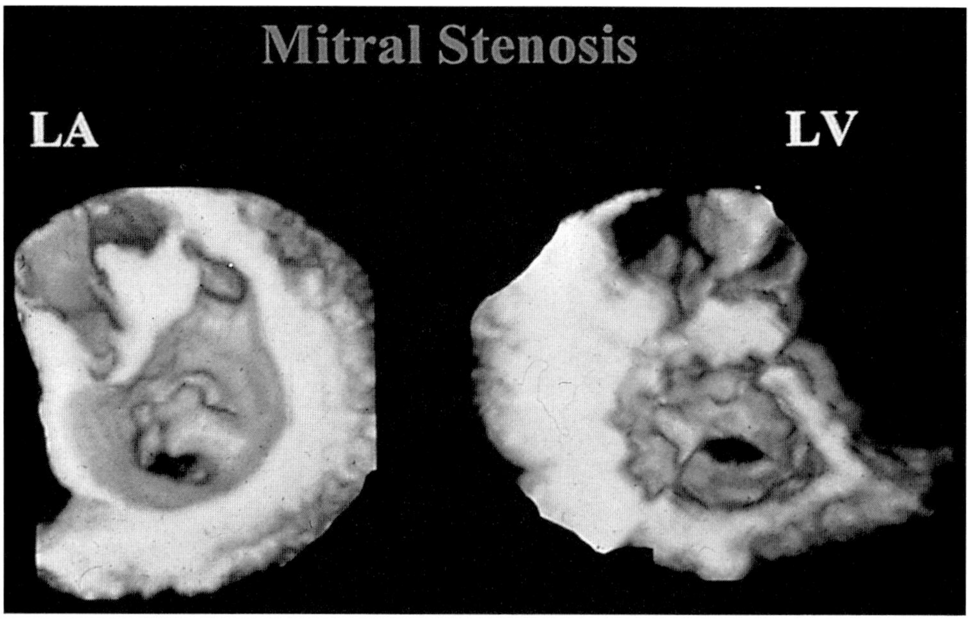

Figure 6. These images show a three-dimensional reconstruction of a critically narrowed mitral valve orifice from the perspective of the left atrium (**left**) and the left ventricle (**right**). From Aleksandra Lange, MD.

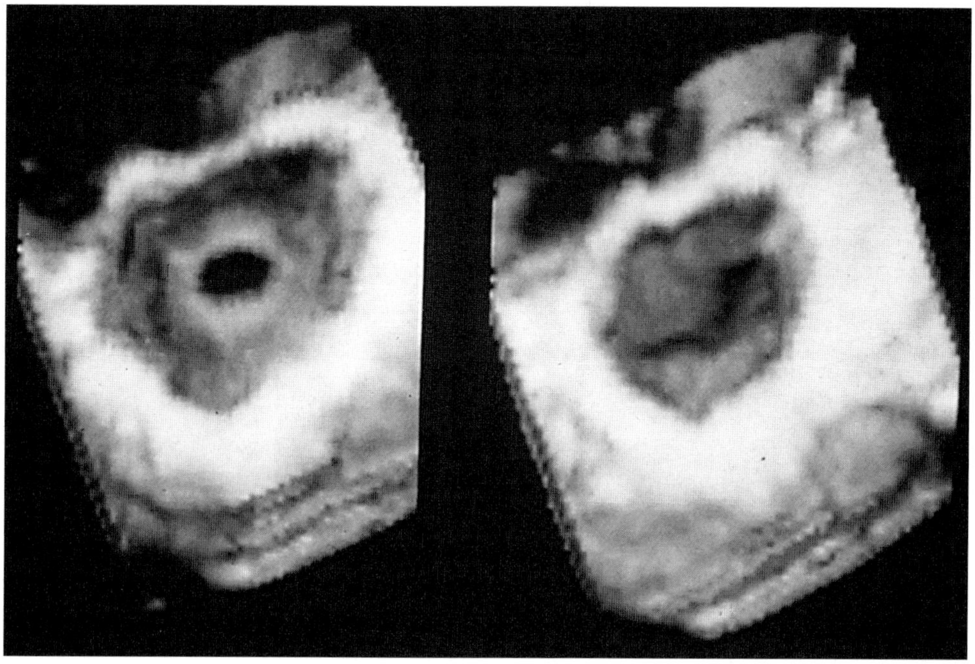

Figure 7. Transesophageal echo *en-face* image of the mitral valve from the perspective of the left ventricle (**left**) and the left atrium (**right**) in another patient with critical mitral stenosis. From Xin-Fang Wang, MD.

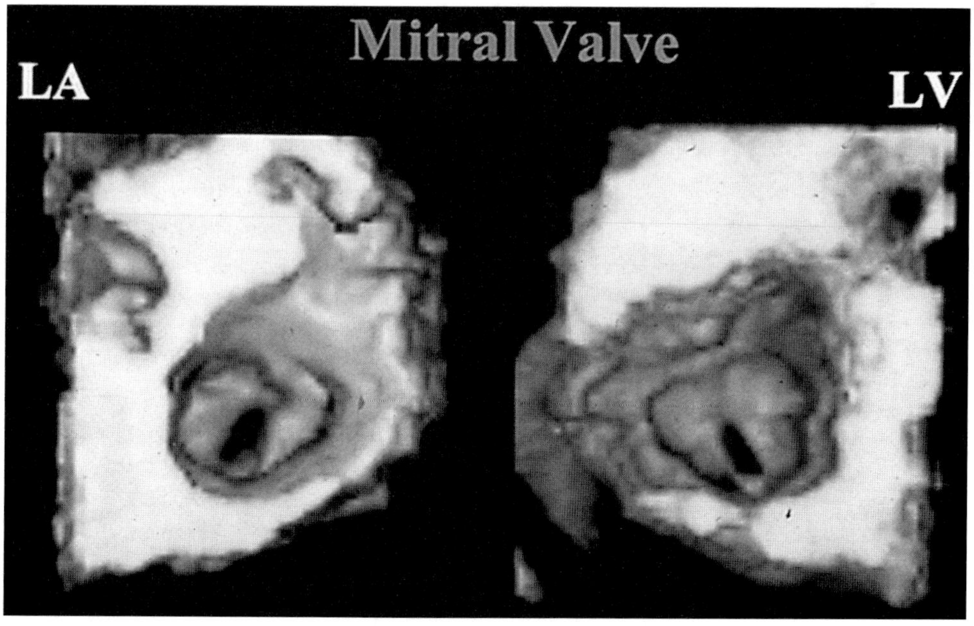

Figure 8. Stenotic mitral valve reconstructed *en face.* Also, corresponding left atrial (LA) and left ventricular perspective (LV). In this case, the orifice is also small but central (as opposed to Figure 7, where the orifice was eccentric) and with well-visualized outline of the extent of commissural fusion from both perspectives. From Aleksandra Lange, MD.

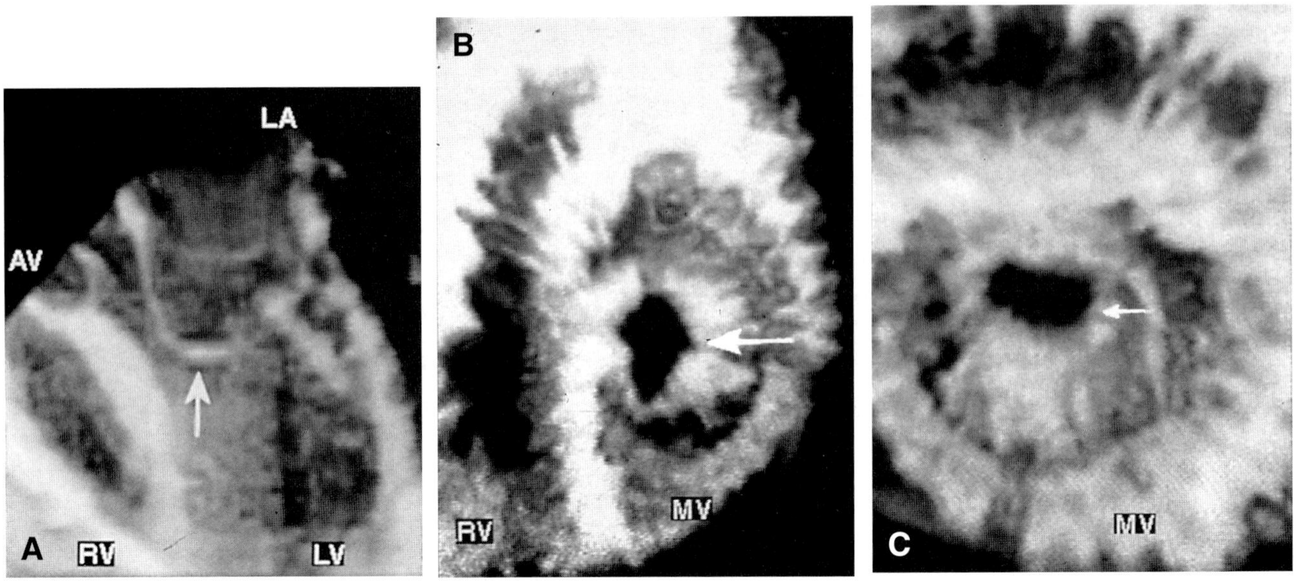

Figure 9. (**A**) Transesophageal echo (TEE) long-axis, apical 4-chamber image of a patient with mitral stenosis. Note the diastolic "bowing" of the anterior mitral valve leaflet (arrow) and thickened chordae tendinea. (**B, C**) TEE short axis image through the mitral annulus of the same patient as in **A**, oriented in the vertical (**B**) and horizontal (**C**) plane. (arrow = rheumatic mitral stenosis).

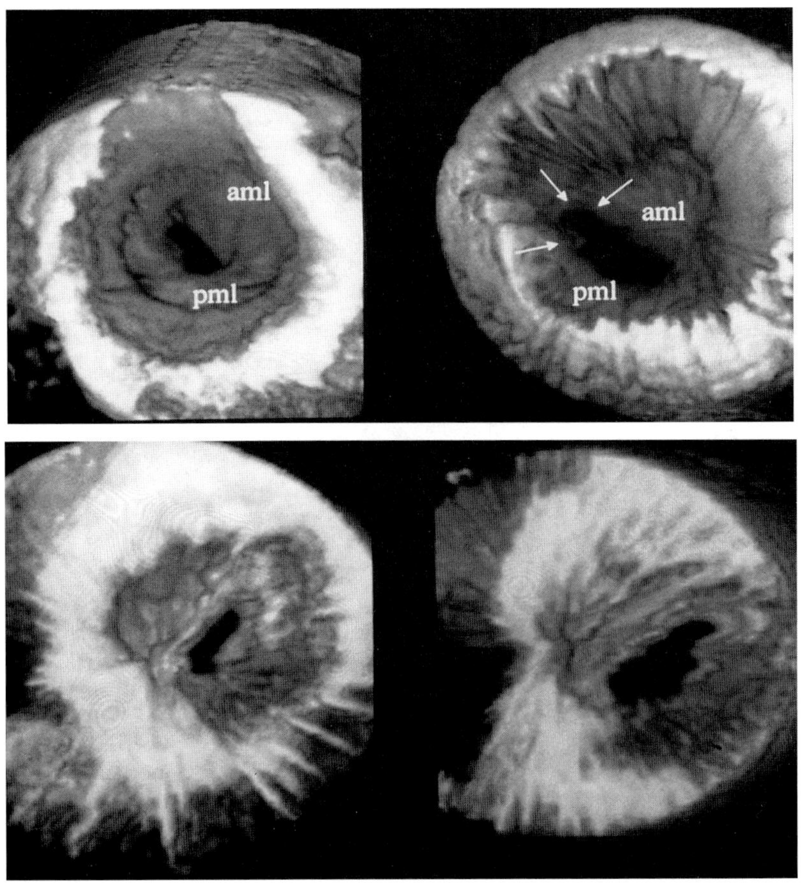

Figure 10. Transesophageal echo (TEE) image of the mitral valve before (left) and after (right) balloon valvuloplasty. Note the fractured commissure (arrows) that documents success of the procedure. This can be observed from the left atrium (**upper frames**) or the left ventricular perspective (**lower frames**). From Stefano De Castro, MD and Rachele Adorisio, MD.

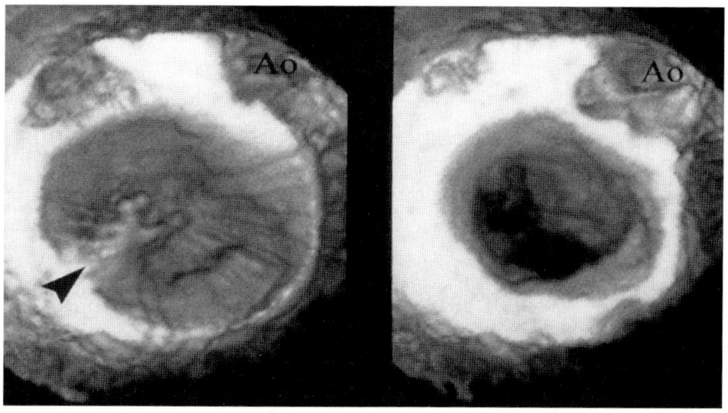

Figure 11. This image was obtained from a three-dimensional data set acquired during transesophageal echo and shows a prolapsing posterior mitral valve leaflet (PMVL—middle scallop) and attached chordae tendinea (arrow) in systole (**left**) and diastole (**right**) from the left atrial point of view. From Stefano De Castro, MD and Rachele Adorisio, MD.

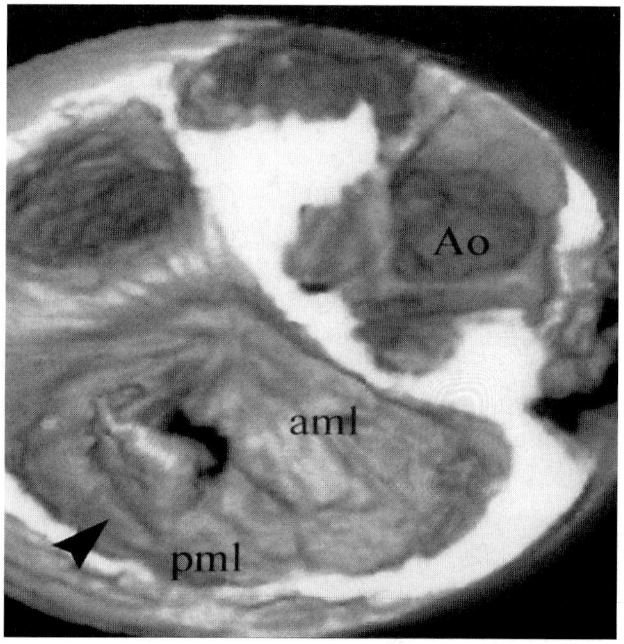

Figure 12. Basal, short axis transesophageal image of another patient with mitral valve prolapse of the middle scallop posterior mitral valve leaflet (arrow). From Stefano De Castro, MD and Rachele Adorisio, MD.

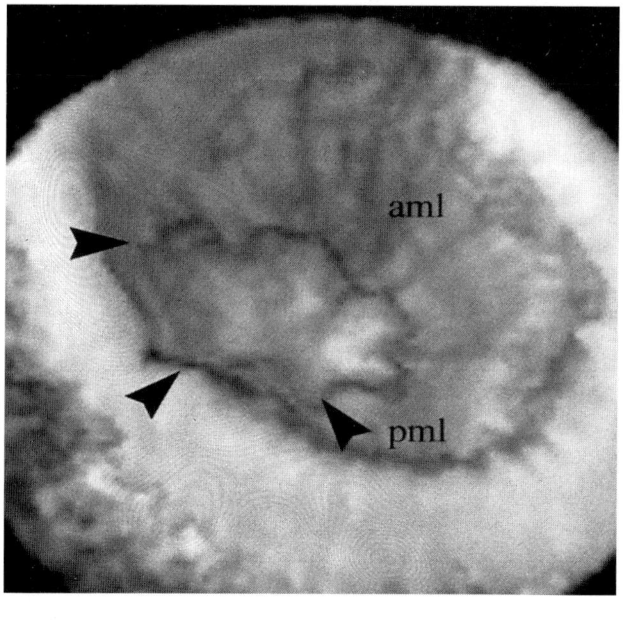

Figure 13. The exact size and morphologic shape of the abnormal myxomatous tissue (arrows) is easily determined with *en-face* views and may allow better surgical preparation, as seen in this three-dimensional reconstruction. From Stefano De Castro, MD and Rachele Adorisio, MD.

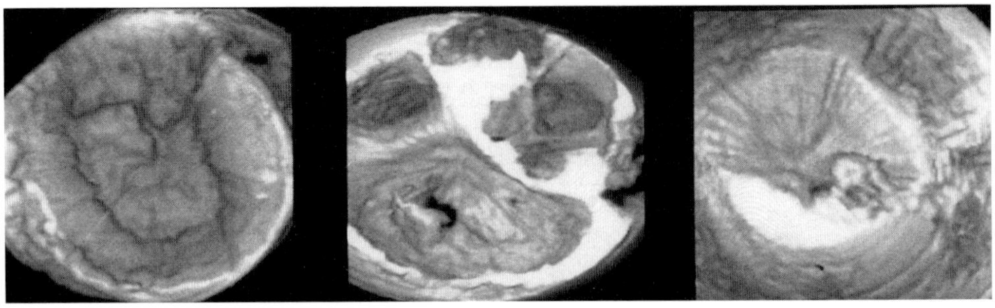

Figure 14. This series of images compares the various abnormalities that commonly involve the posterior mitral valve leaflet from the left atrial perspective. **Left:** P3 or Medial scallop prolapse; **Middle:** P2 or Middle scallop prolapse; **Right:** P1 or Lateral scallop prolapse. From Stefano De Castro, MD and Rachele Adorisio, MD.

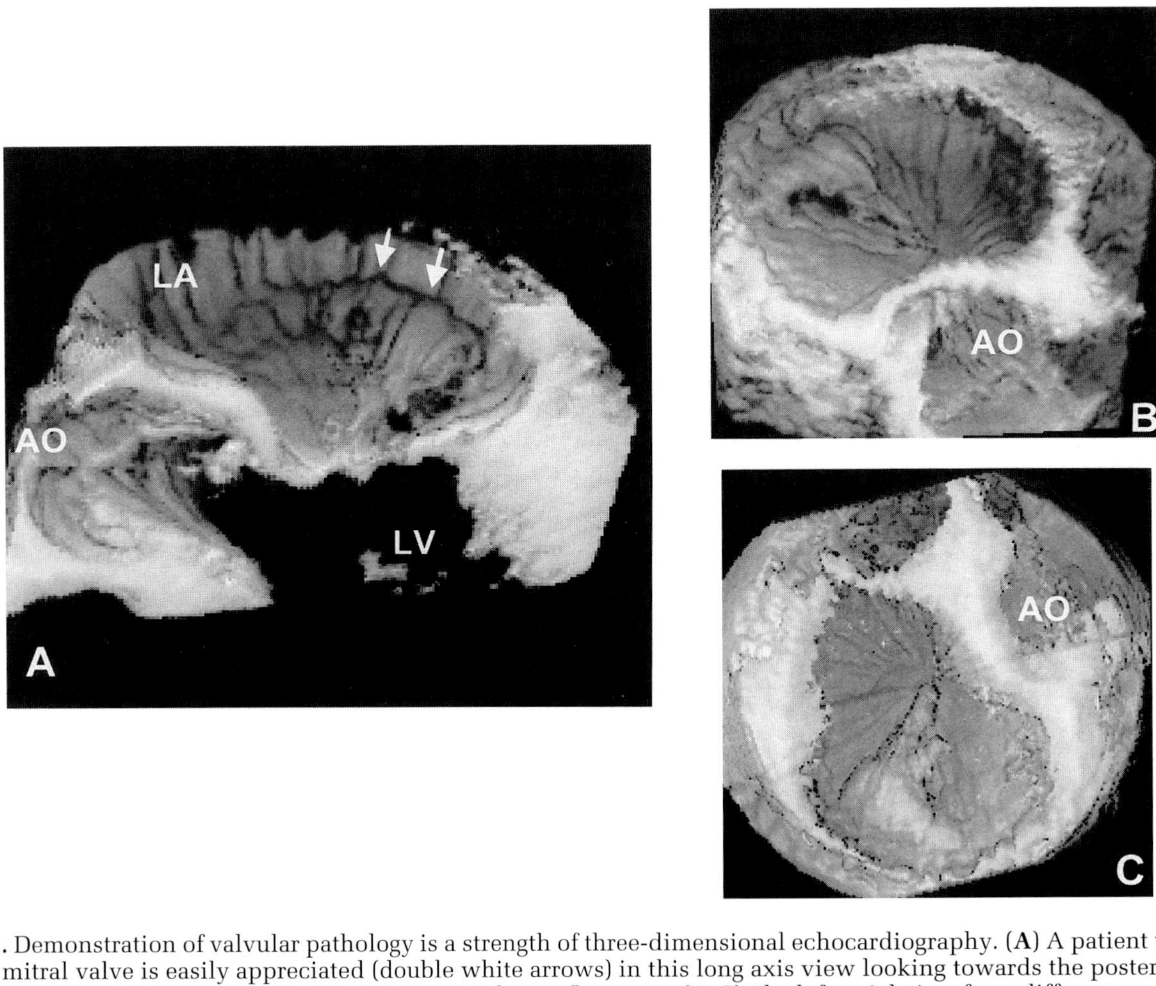

Figure 15. Demonstration of valvular pathology is a strength of three-dimensional echocardiography. (**A**) A patient with a flail posterior mitral valve is easily appreciated (double white arrows) in this long axis view looking towards the posterior wall of the left atrium (LA), left ventricle (LV) and left ventricular outflow tract. (**B, C**) The left atrial view from different angles clearly distinguishes the flail portion as well as the chordae attached to the tips of the leaflet. From Lissa Sugeng, MD, Ivan Godoy, MD, Kirk T. Spencer, MD, Jim Bednarz, BS, Lynn Weinert, BS, and Roberto M. Lang, MD.

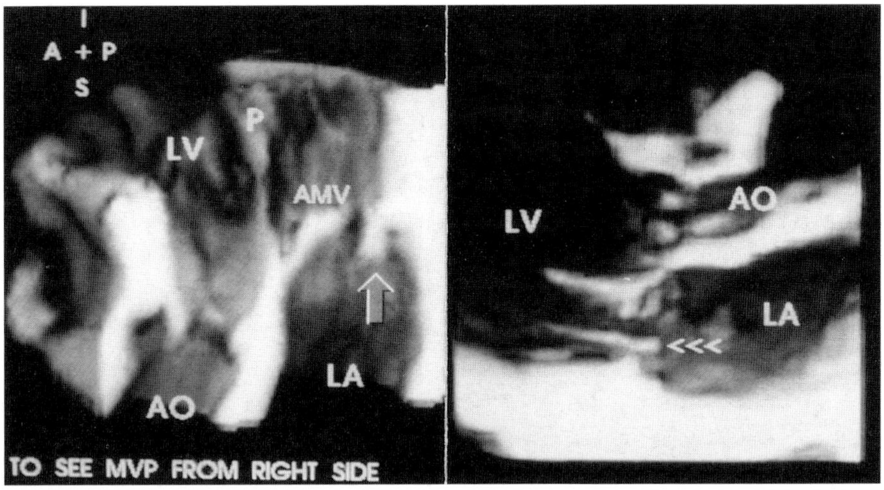

Figure 16. Dynamic three-dimensional images of ruptured chordae tendinae. **Left:** Long-axis view of mitral valve in systole, viewed from right side, showing flail posterior leaflet (arrow) inside left atrium. **Right:** Long-axis view of same patient as seen from left side, again showing flail posterior leaflet (arrow) lying partially in left atrium. Reproduced with permission from Cheng TO et al. Evaluation of mitral valve prolapse by four-dimensional echocardiography. *Am Heart J* 1997;133:120–125. From Xin-Fang Wang, MD

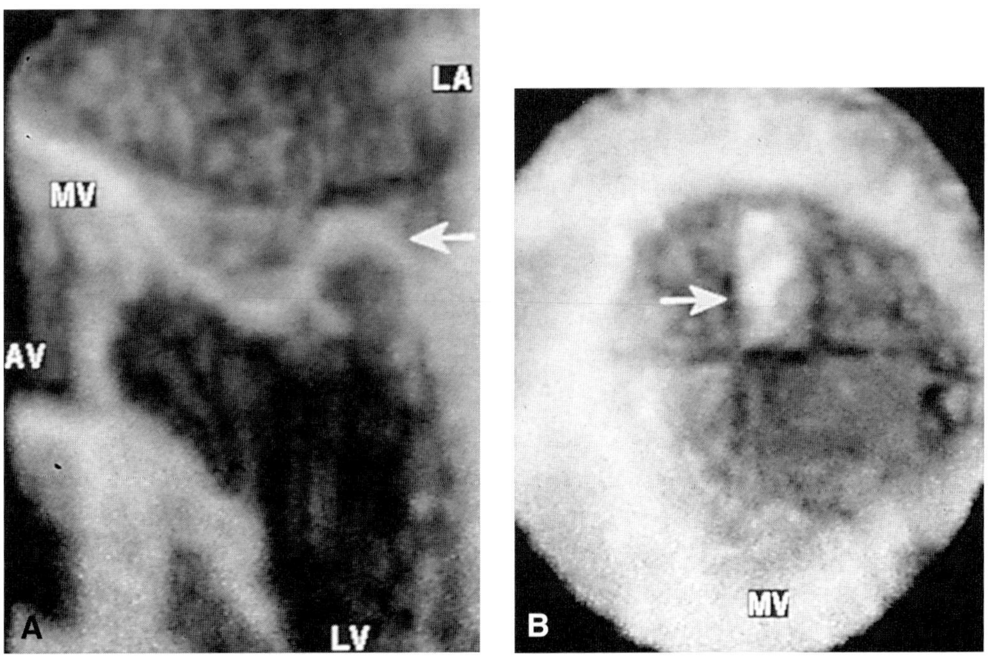

Figure 17. Transesophageal long-axis (**A**) and short-axis (**B**) orientation of the mitral and aortic valves in a patient with mitral valve prolapse of the posterior mitral valve leaflet (arrow). This view is very important to the surgeon performing mitral valve repair since it allows the exact intra-operative orientation to be selected and imaged in motion. This should allow the surgeon to most accurately and comprehensively prepare the most successful operation.

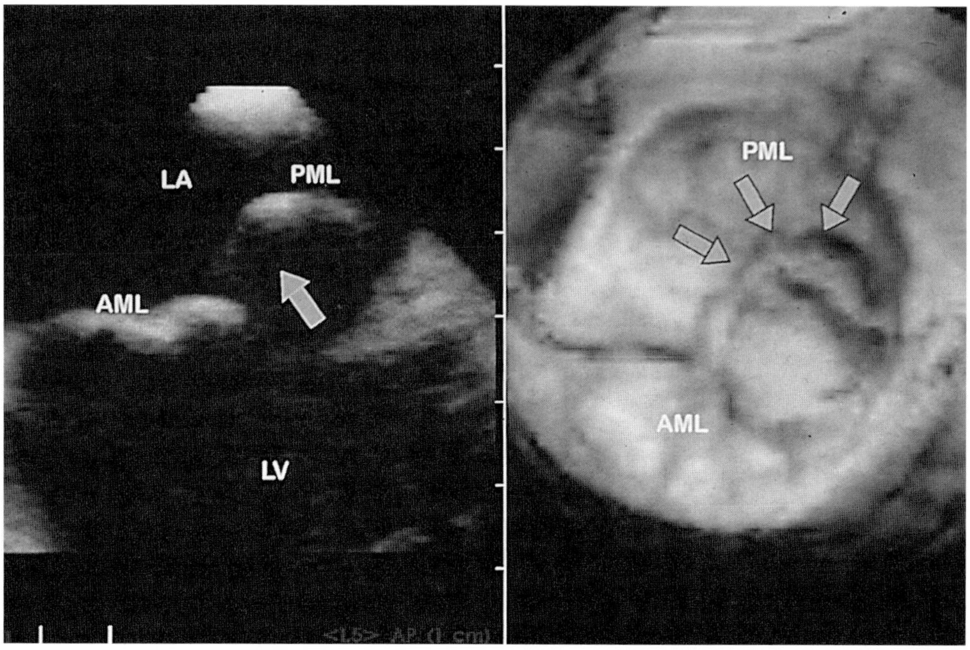

Figure 18. Left: A two-dimensional (2D) apical 4-chamber view of a 35-year-old male with myxomatous proliferation of the posterior mitral valve leaflet is shown. The entire extent of the prolapse cannot be determined from this 2D still frame. **Right:** A three-dimensional reconstruction of the mitral valve apparatus is appreciated from the perspective of the left atrium. Note the extent of the prolapse visualized more completely in this still frame image. From Annette Geibel, MD, Michael Handke, MD, Dietrich Markus Schäfer, MD, Anja Schöchlin, MA, and Helmut Wollschläger, MD.

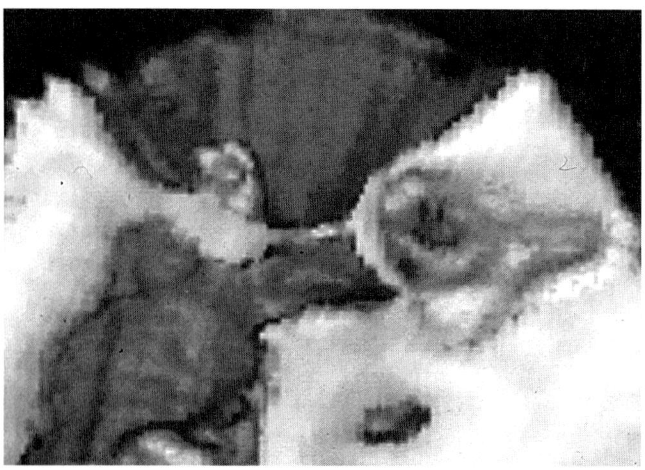

Figure 19. Oblique long-axis view of the left ventricle (**bottom**), left atrium (**top**) and outflow tract. The prolapse of the posterior leaflet has the shape of an aneurysm. From Cedric Vuille, MD and Rene Lerch, MD.

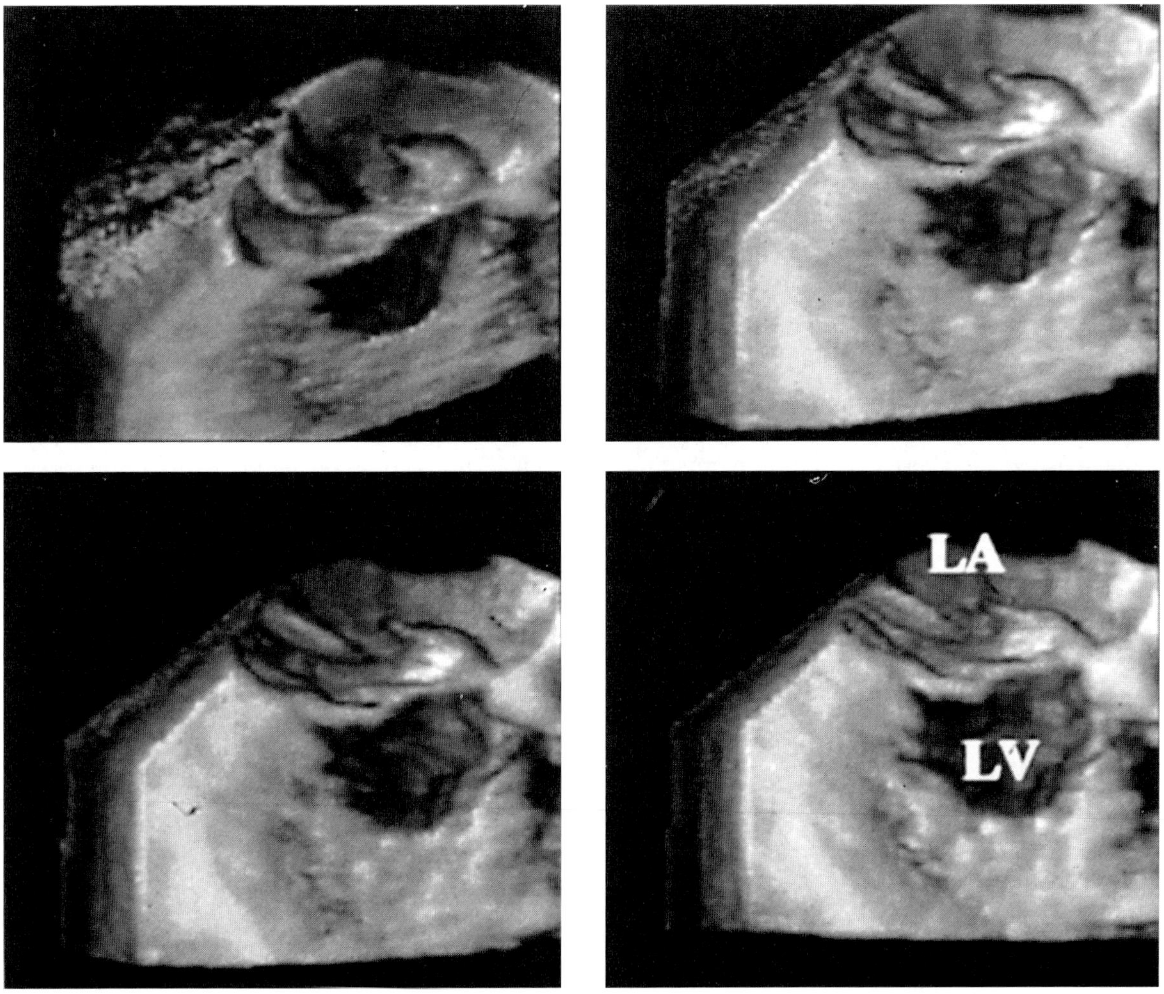

Figure 20. Mitral valve prolapse. Detailed anyplane views reconstructed from transesophageal acquisition of echo images. The prolapse of the anterior mitral leaflet is apparent at different points of view. From Jaroslaw Drozdz, MD and Jaroslaw D. Kasprzak, MD.

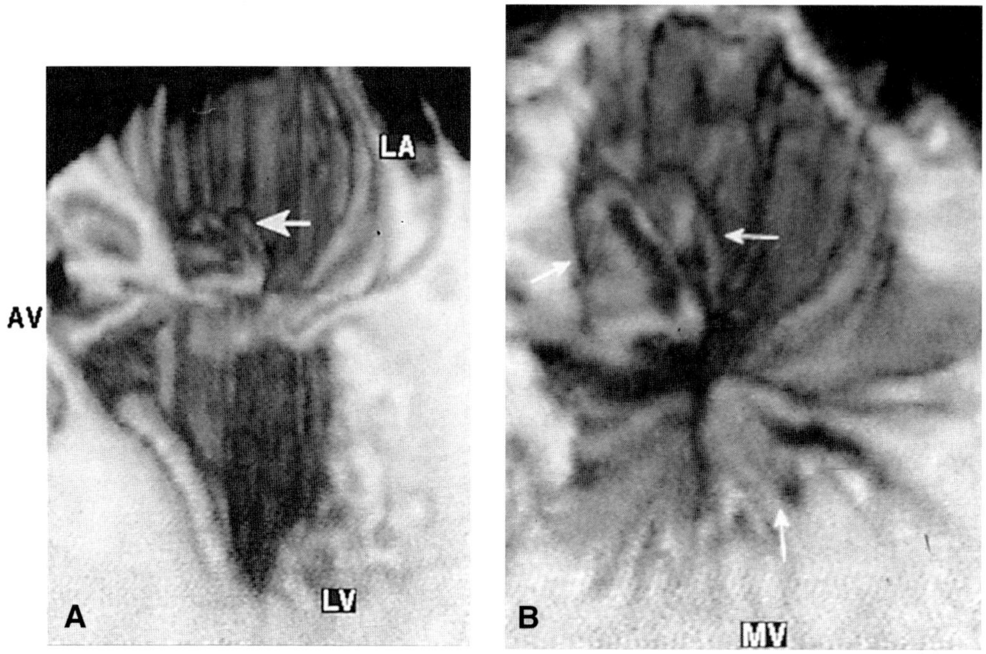

Figure 21. Long-axis (**A**) and short-axis (**B**) image from the mid-esophageal position in a patient with mitral valve prolapse of the anterior mitral valve leaflet (arrow). The extent of proliferative tissue is readily shown and allows the surgeon a more comprehensive assessment to plan surgery.

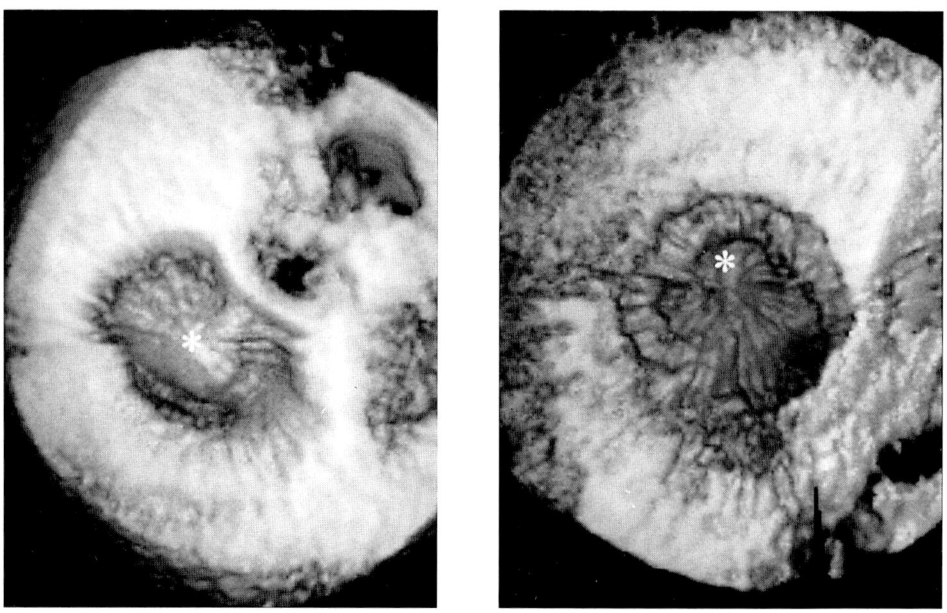

Figure 22. Anterior mitral leaflet prolapse: end systolic visualization from the left atrium (**left**) and the left ventricle (**right**). The prolapse of the whole leaflet is visualized (*) and the commissure is well defined on the left. From Albert A. Hagège, MD.

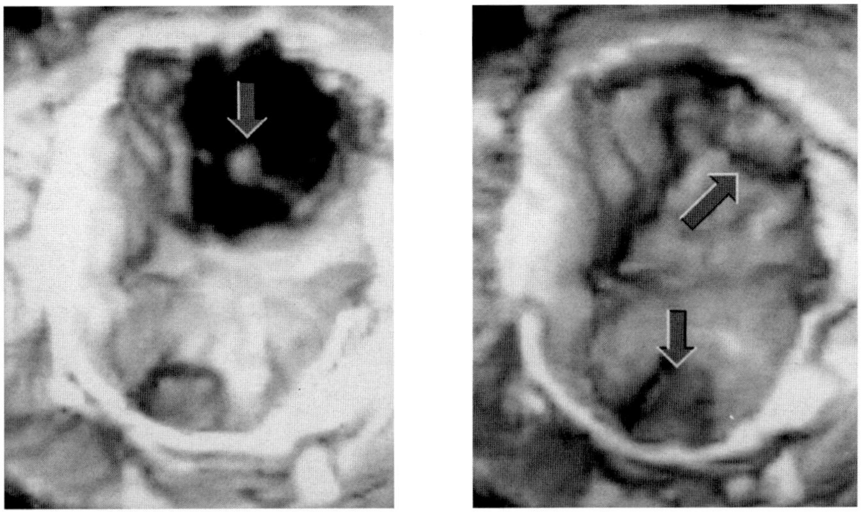

Figure 23. Posterior mitral valve prolapse (views from the left atrium). In diastole (**left**), the valve is open and the posterior papillary muscle is visualized with its main chordae (arrowhead). In systole (**right**), note the prolapse of the posterior scallop of the posterior leaflet (oblique arrow), its relationships with the annulus and the posterior commissure, and the left atrial appendage (vertical arrow). From Albert A. Hagège, MD.

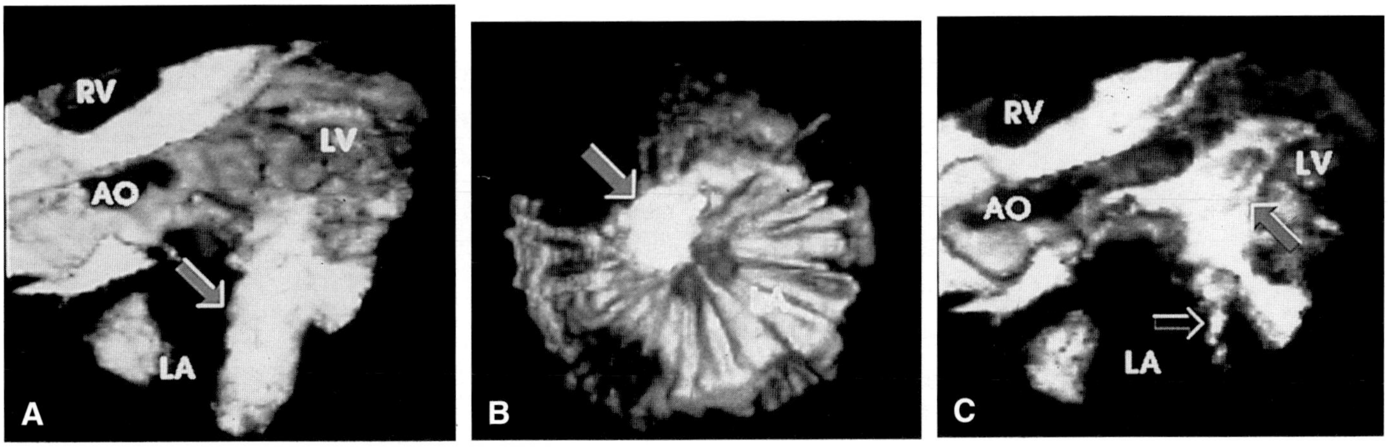

Figure 24. Dynamic three-dimensional images of mitral regurgitant jet. (**A**) Mitral regurgitant jet (arrow) shown in the left atrium (LA). (**B**) Cross sectional view of mitral regurgitant jet from the LA in the same patient as shown in A. (**C**) Diastolic mitral regurgitant jet (open arrow) visualized in the LA in another patient and diastolic mitral flow filling into the left ventricle (LV). AO = aorta; LVs = solid arrow; RA = right atrium; RV = right ventricle. Reproduced with permission from Li Z et al. Dynamic three-dimensional reconstruction of abnormal intracardiac blood flow. *Echocardiography* 1997;14:375–381.

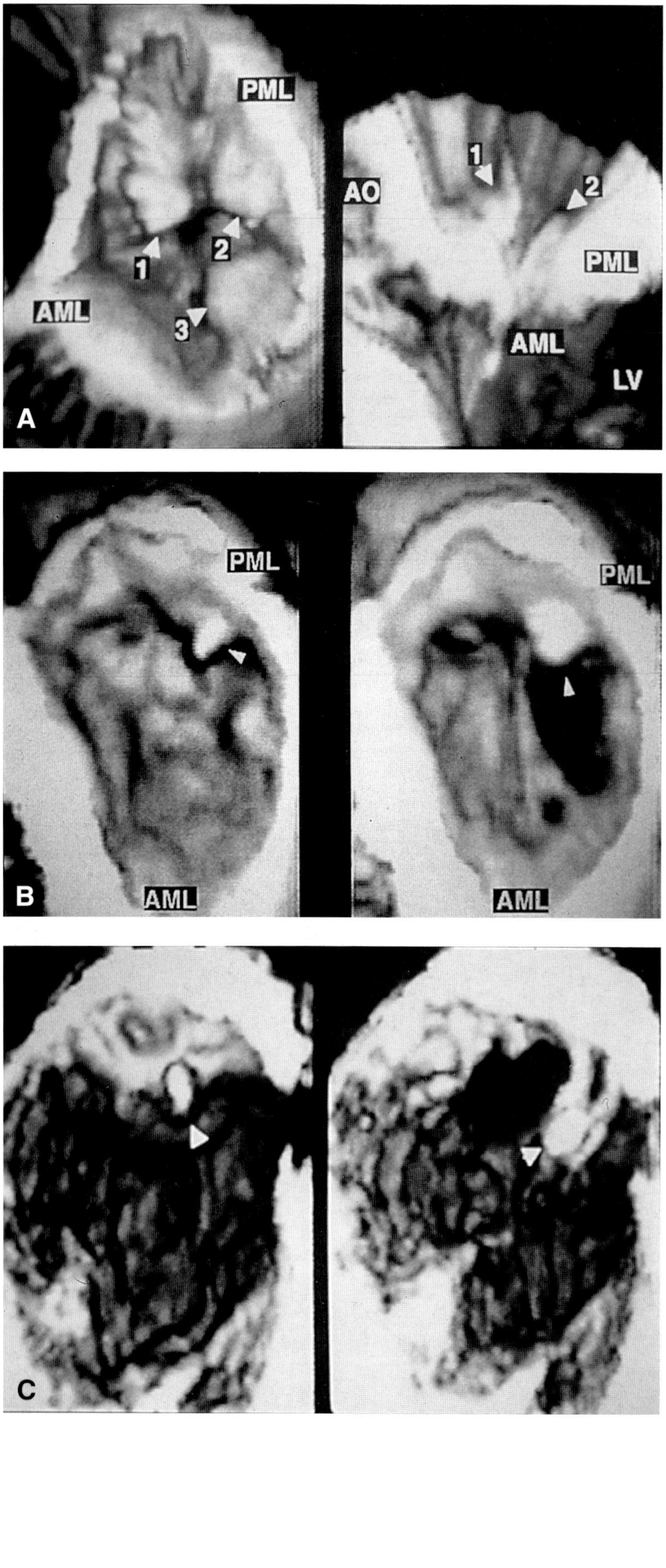

Figure 25. (**A**) Three-dimensional reconstructed short-axis and long-axis views of the mitral valve in a patient showing multiple vegetations (arrows). (**B, C**) Large vegetation (arrows in **B**) on the posterior mitral leaflet (PML) as well as a vegetation (arrows in **C**) on the mitral valve chordae tendinae. Portions of the left ventricular papillary muscles are also visualized in **C.** AML = anterior mitral leaflet; AO = aorta; LV = left ventricle. Reproduced with permission from Nanda NC et al. Incremental value of three-dimensional echocardiography over transesophageal multiplane two-dimensional echocardiography in qualitative and quantitative assessment of cardiac masses and defects. *Echocardiography* 1995; 12:619–628.

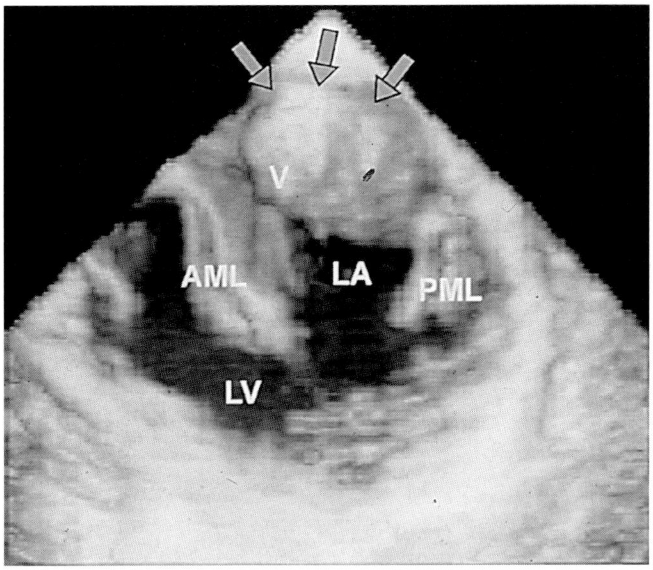

Figure 26. Three-dimensional view. Thirty-five-year-old patient with infective endocarditis. The vegetation (arrow) is located on the posterior mitral leaflet (PML). The patient was operated and the diagnosis was histologically confirmed. AML = anterior mitral leaflet; LA = left atrium; LV = left ventricle; V = vegetation. From Annette Geibel, MD, Michael Handke, MD, Dietrich Markus Schäfer, MD, Anja Schöchlin, MA, and Helmut Wollschläger, MD.

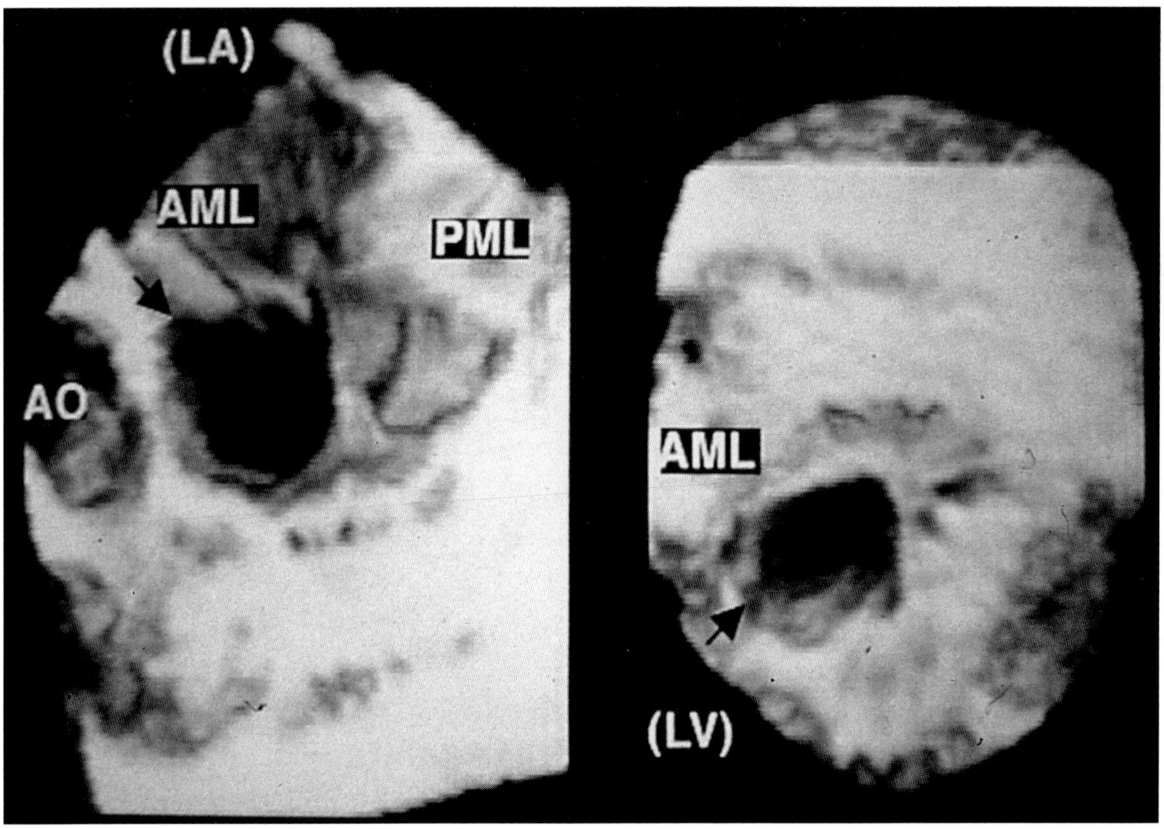

Figure 27. Large perforation (arrows) in the anterior mitral leaflet (AML). The patient had endocarditis. The posterior mitral leaflet (PML) was intact, and there were no vegetations. Thickening of the rim of the perforation was visualized when it was viewed from the ventricular side (**right**). No thickening of the rim was noted on the atrial aspect (**left**). Reproduced with permission from Nanda NC et al. Incremental value of three-dimensional echocardiography over transesophageal multiplane two-dimensional echocardiography in qualitative and quantitative assessment of cardiac masses and defects. *Echocardiography* 1995;12:619–628.

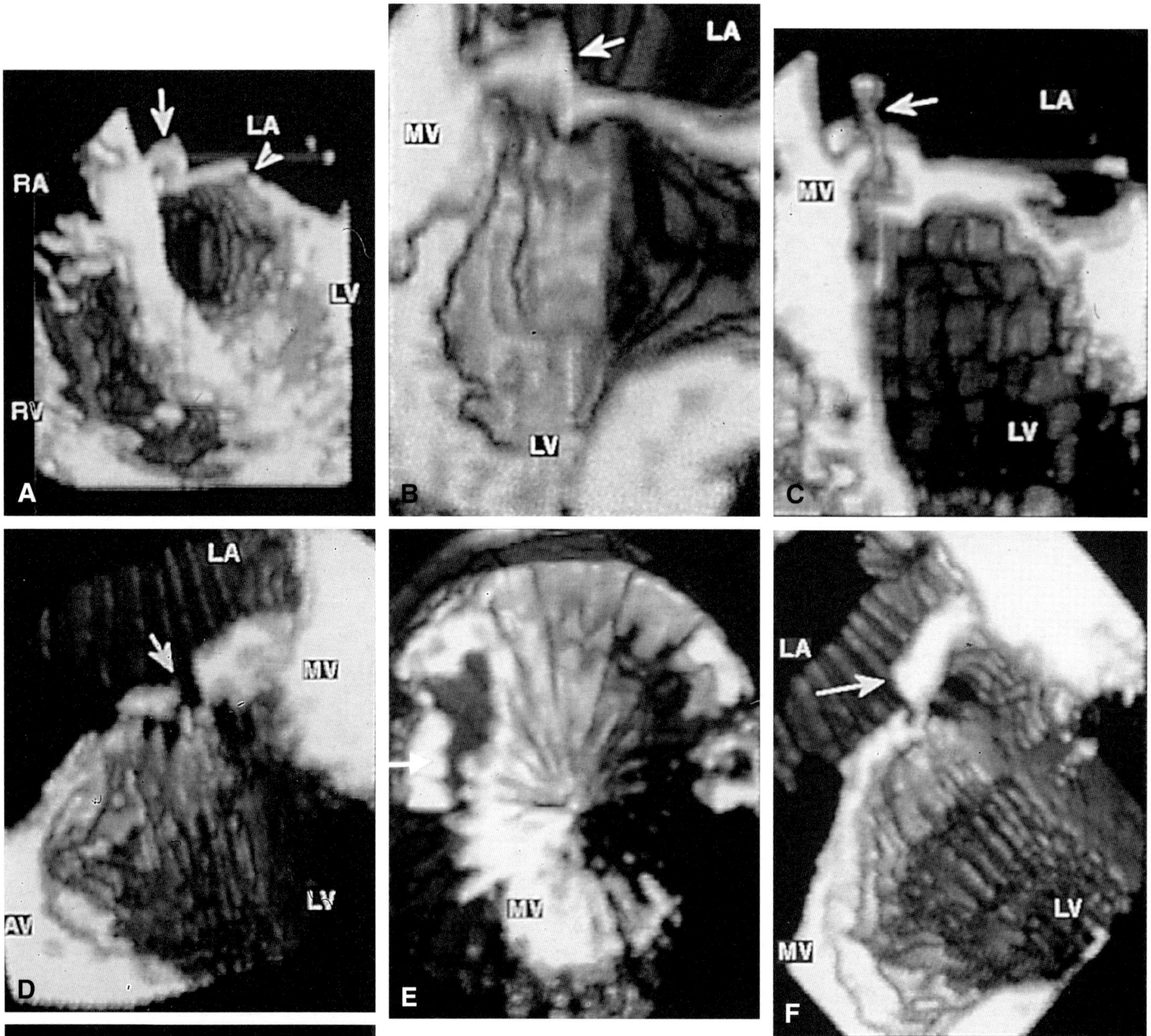

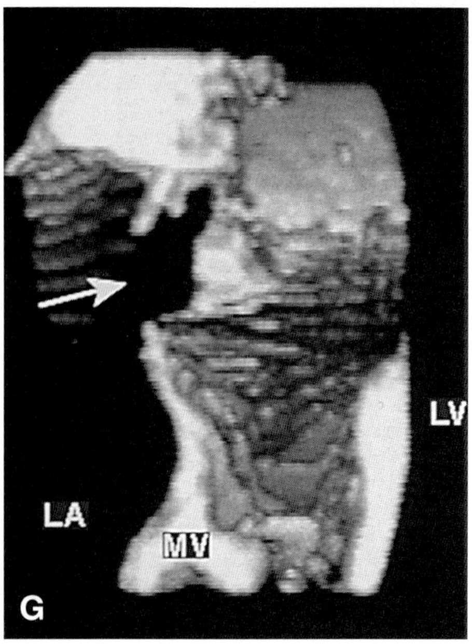

Figure 28. (**A**) Three-dimensional (3D) image of a patient with endocarditis (arrow) and mitral valve perforation (arrowhead) orientated in an apical 4-chamber view. Additional images allow further delineation of the pathology and a complete anatomic understanding of the surrounding tissues. (**B**) Apical long-axis image. (**C**) The exact location of the perforation is highlighted with color Doppler (displayed in gray). (**D**) Apical 2-chamber orientation (perforation = arrow). **E.** Long axis view that reveals the size and shape of the perforation. (**F, G**) Utilizing unusual perspectives (from the medial and lateral walls of the mitral valve annulus), additional information not available with standard 2D imaging may be obtained.

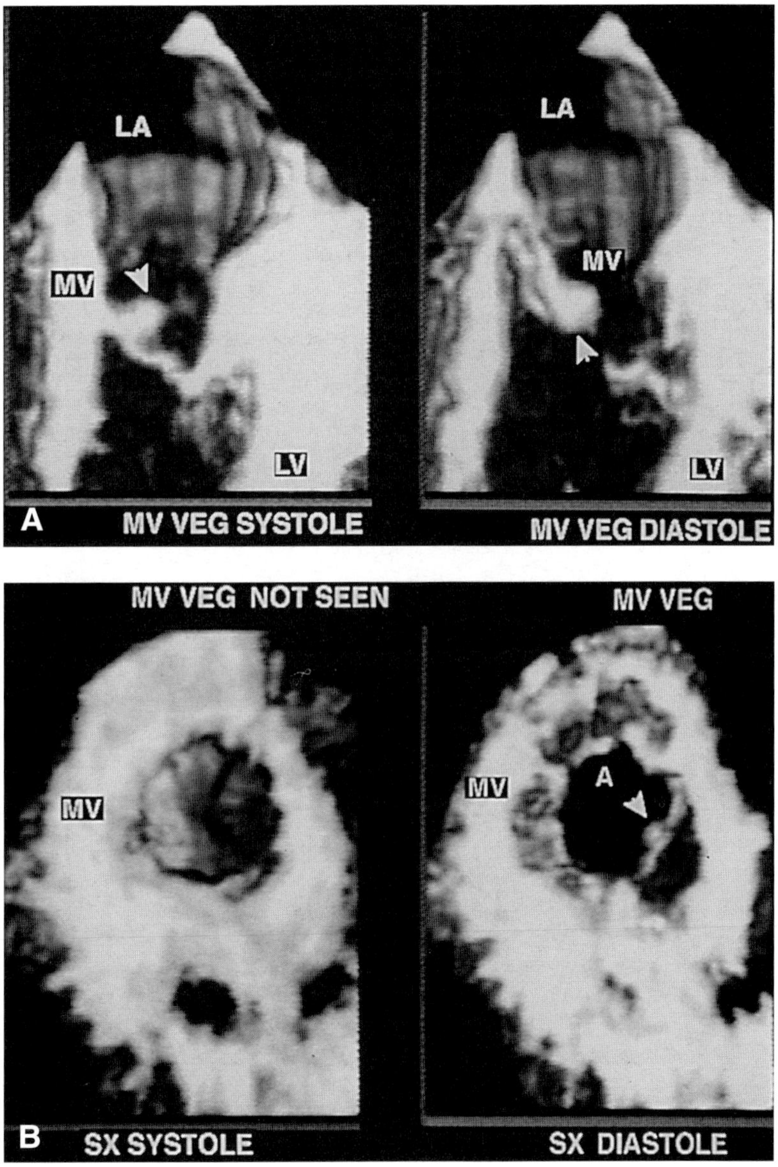

Figure 29. (**A**) transesophageal echo (TEE) long-axis image, apical 2-chamber orientation of a vegetation involving the anterior mitral valve leaflet (arrow) in systole (**left**) and diastole (**right**). (**B**) TEE short-axis image of the same patient as in the previous figure. Note the inability to visualize the vegetative lesion during systole (**left**) but enhanced visualization (arrowhead) during diastole (**right**).

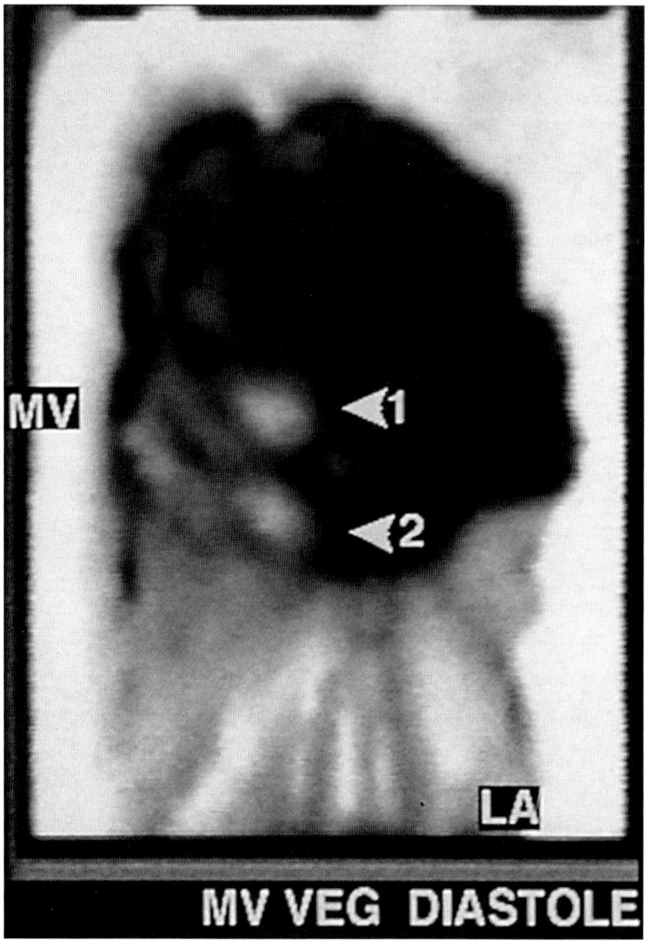

Figure 29. Continued. (**C**) Additional, focused interrogation with zoom imaging and anyplane orientation allows a more complete assessment of the mitral valve and identifies two vegetative lesions (arrows). This is the same patient as in the previous 2 figures.

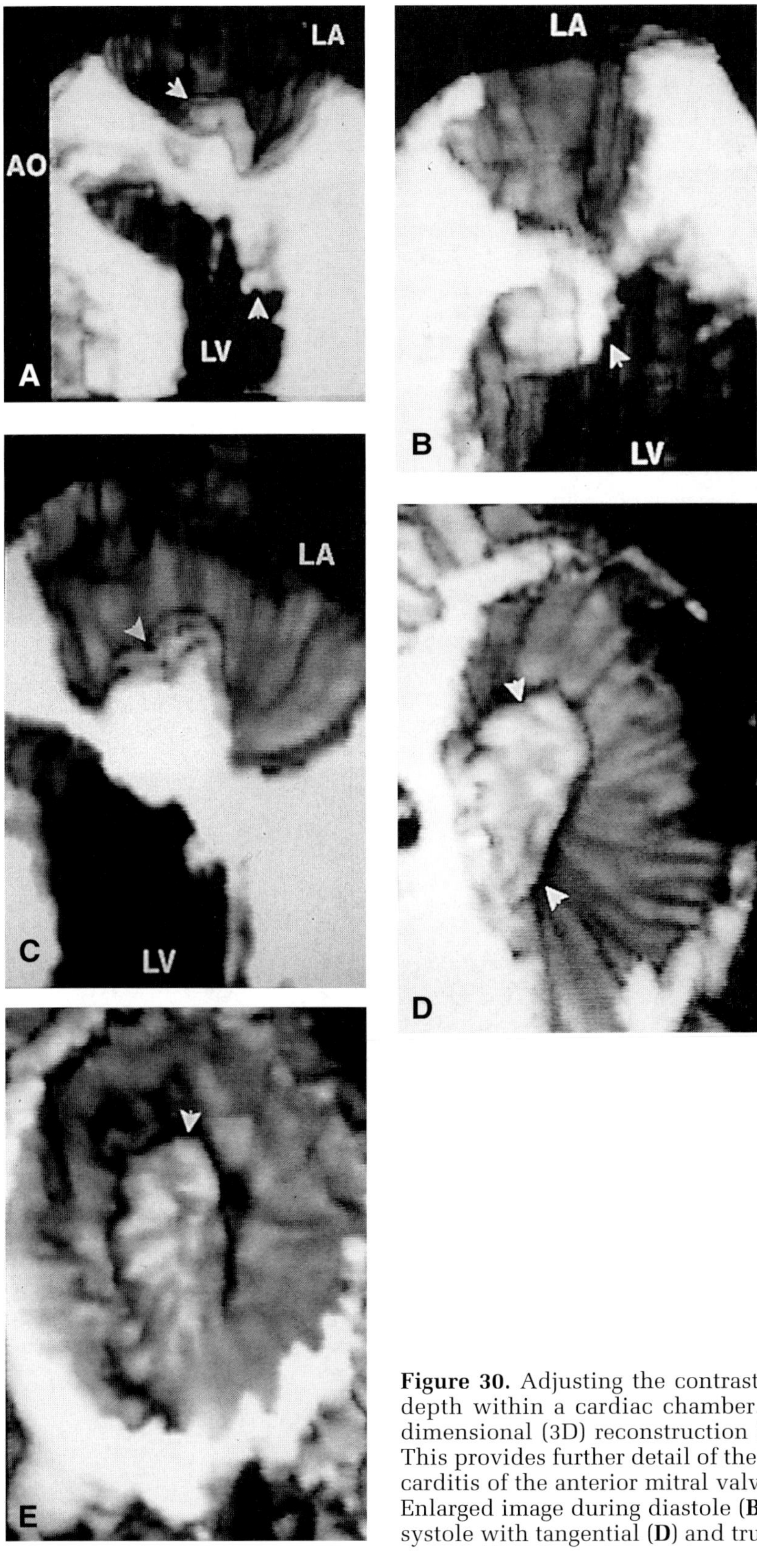

Figure 30. Adjusting the contrast and shadowing allows a greater appreciation of the depth within a cardiac chamber. Additionally, multiple off-axis imaging and three-dimensional (3D) reconstruction further enhances the detail of the desired pathology. This provides further detail of the size of the vegetative lesion in this patient with endocarditis of the anterior mitral valve leaflet. (**A**) Apical 5-chamber view in systole. (**B, C**) Enlarged image during diastole (**B**) and systole (**C**). (**D, E**) Focused 3D reconstruction in systole with tangential (**D**) and true *en-face* (**E**) views. arrows = vegetation.

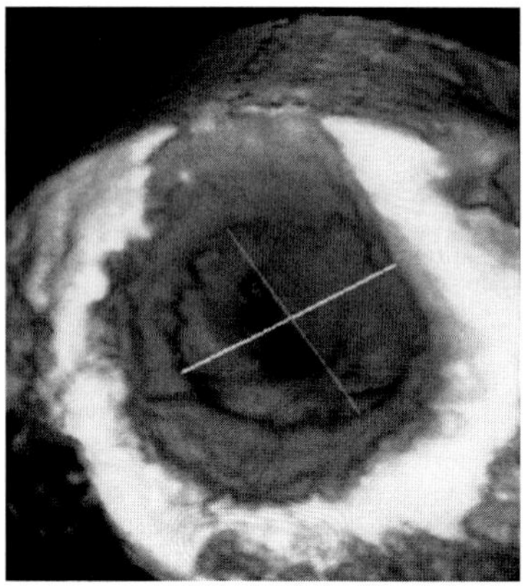

Figure 31. Direct assessment of longitudinal and transverse diameters of the mitral valve annulus. From Stefano De Castro, MD and Rachele Adorisio, MD.

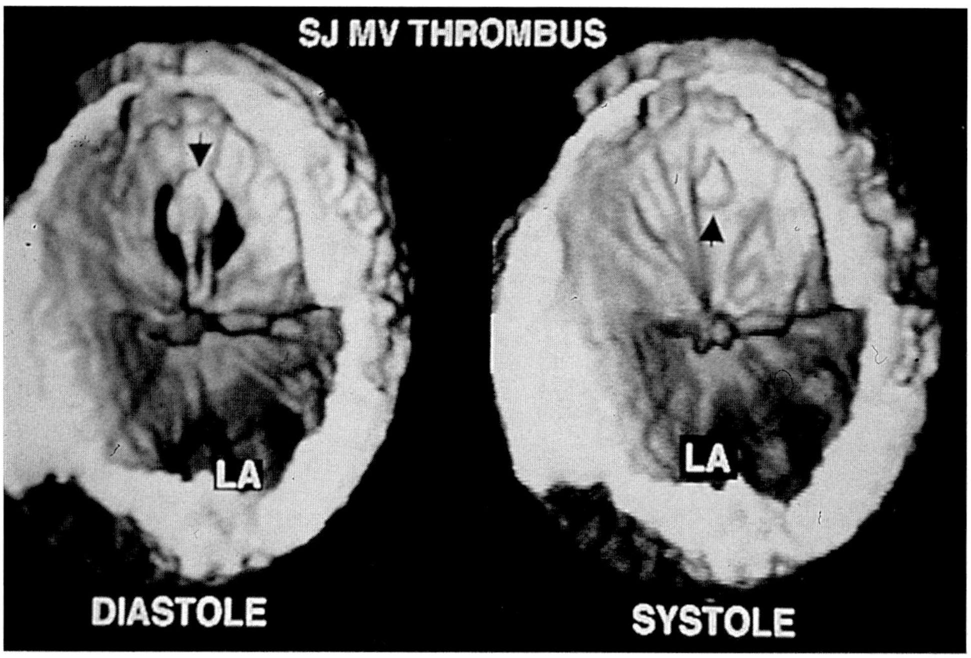

Figure 32. Thrombus (arrow) involving a St. Jude mitral valve (SJMV) (St. Jude, St. Paul, MN) prosthesis seen in the open (**left**) and closed positions (**right**). Reproduced with permission from Nanda NC et al. Incremental value of three-dimensional echocardiography over transesophageal multiplane two-dimensional echocardiography in qualitative and quantitative assessment of cardiac masses and defects. *Echocardiography* 1995;12:619–628.

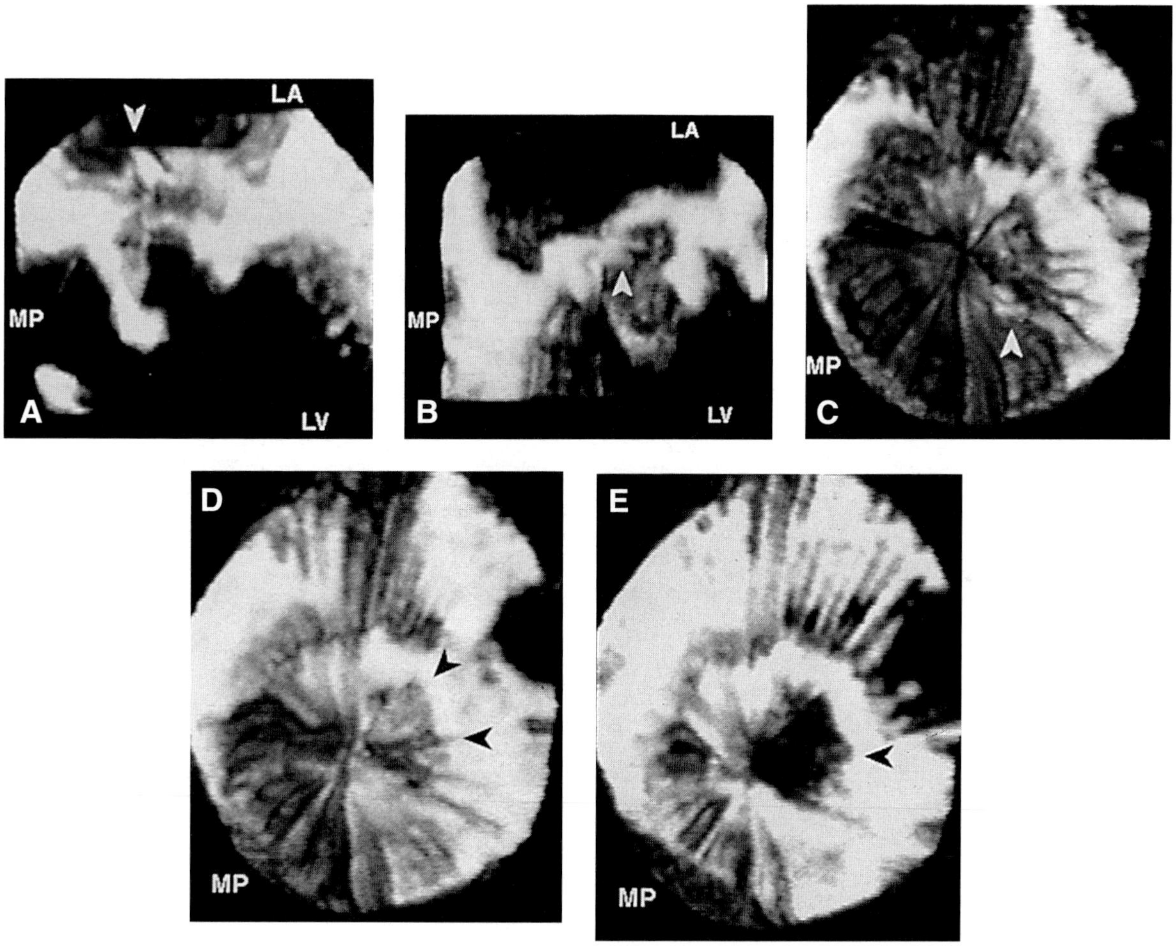

Figure 33. (**A, B**) Transesophageally (TEE)-obtained, long-axis image of the mitral valve in a patient status-post mitral valve replacement with a bioprosthetic valve. Note the small leaflet prolapse (arrow). (**C, D**) Short axis TEE images of the same patient as in the previous figures highlighting the prosthetic valve ring (arrows) in systole. (**E**) The full extent of the bioprosthesis is now shown in diastole.

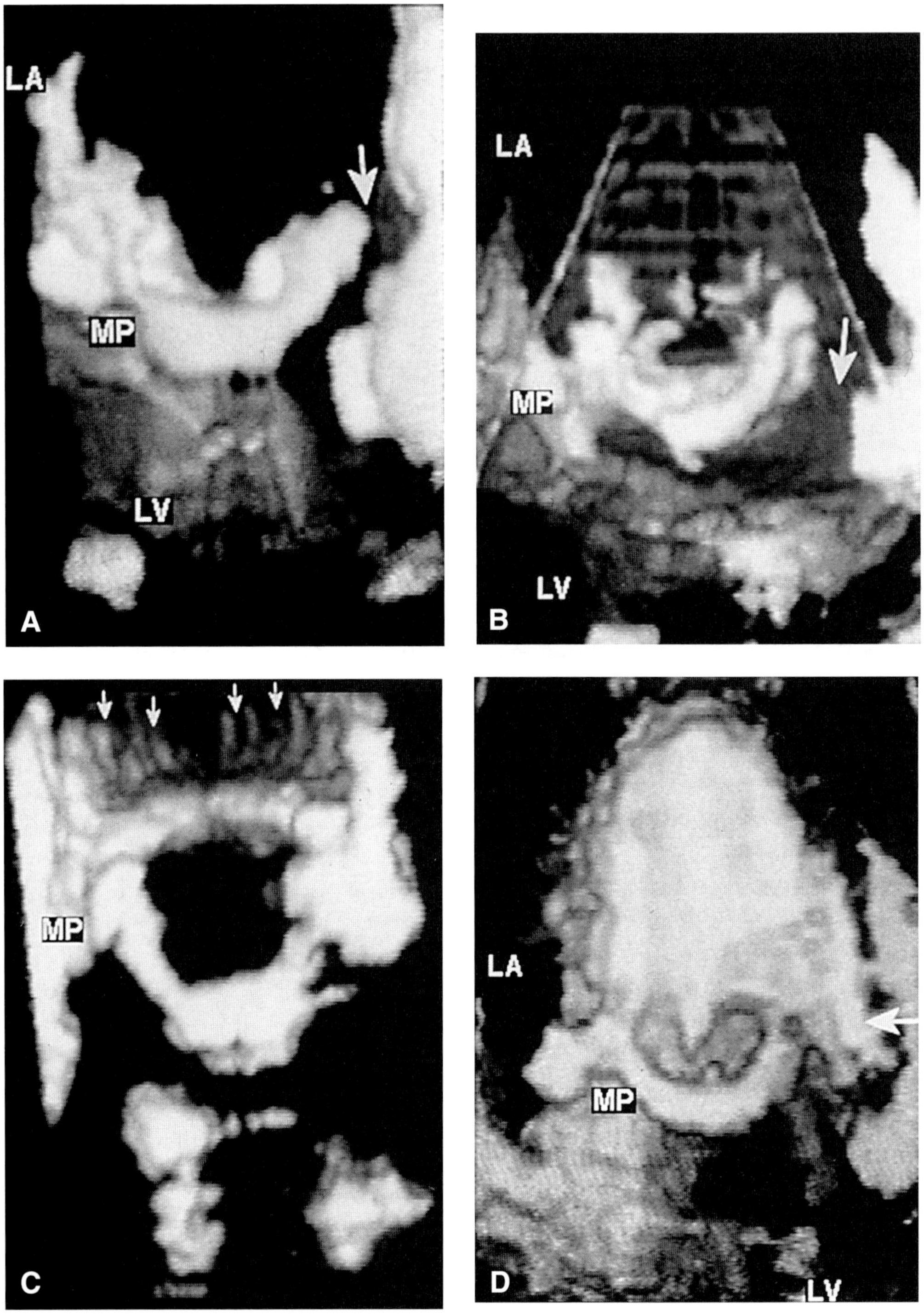

Figure 34. (**A**) Transesophageal long-axis image of a patient with a prosthetic valve and a peri-valvular area of dehiscence (arrow). Note the well-defined extent of the valve and the adjacent ventricular wall. (**B**) Same patient as in the previous figure. Off-axis imaging provides a greater understanding of the degree of dehiscence (arrow). MP = mitral prosthesis. (**C**) With color-flow Doppler (shown in gray), the regurgitant flow (arrows) is noted to arise outside of the valve lumen consistent with valvular dehiscence and paravalvular regurgitation. (**D**) Same patient as in the previous figure highlighting the color flow (gray) passing through the previously identified abnormal channel (arrow). Views such as these are not possible with two-dimensional echocardiography, and further enhance our understanding of prosthetic valve complications.

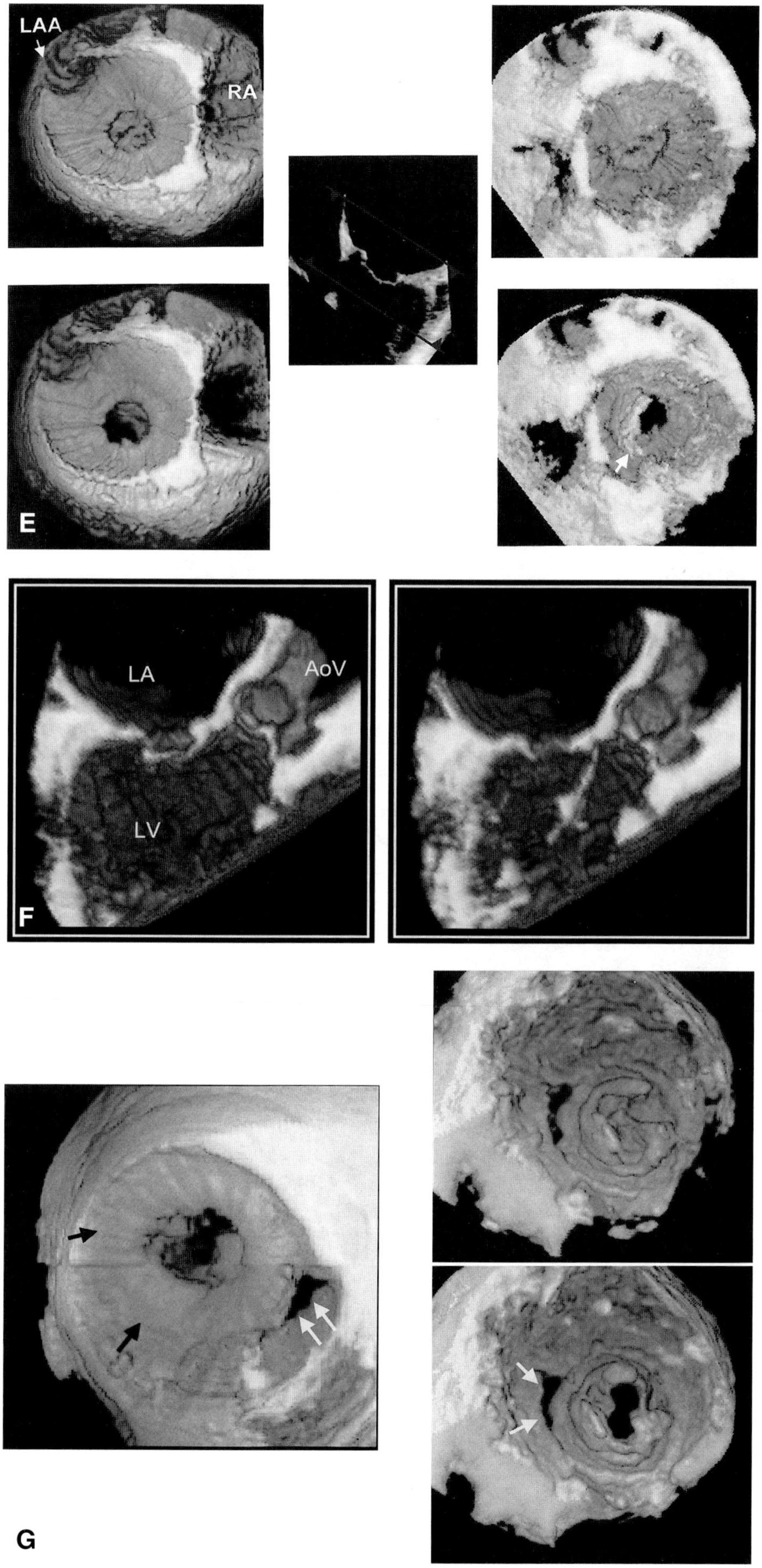

Figure 34. Continued. (**E**) Three-dimensional reconstructions of a bioprosthetic mitral valve are seen from the left atrium (**left**) and from the left ventricle (**right**) in systole (**top**) and diastole (**bottom**). The cutting planes are represented on the center image. From a left atrial orientation, the bioprosthetic valve is clearly defined in an enlarged left atrium. The reverse view from the left ventricle visualizes the large anterior leaflet (white arrow). (**F**) A long axis orientation of the bioprosthetic valve, looking anteriorly is seen in systole and diastole. The cusps of the aortic valve are distinctly seen. (**G**) **Left:** Evaluation of a patient with a bioprosthetic valve in the mitral position who had dyspnea, demonstrated the bioprosthesis viewed from the left atrium. The edge of the valve can be discerned entirely (black arrows). An area of dehiscence is noted (double white arrows) from above as well as from the ventricular aspect (upper and lower right). Three distinct struts and valvular leaflets are shown from a left ventricular view in systole (**upper right**) and diastole (**lower right**). **E, F,** and **G** are from Lissa Sugeng, MD, Ivan Godoy, MD, Kirk T. Spencer, MD, Jim Bednarz, BS, Lynn Weinert, BS, and Roberto M. Lang, MD.

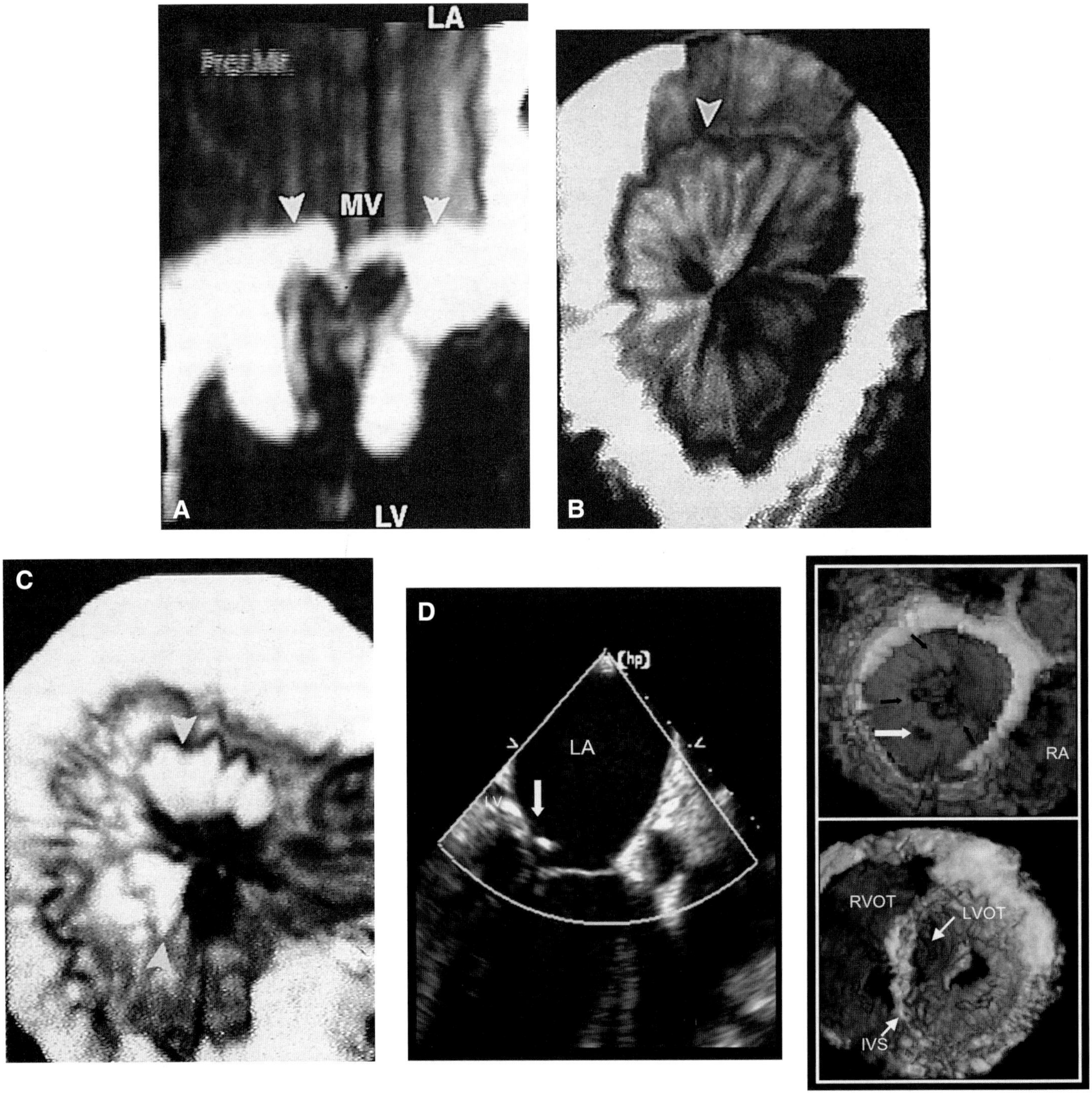

Figure 35. (**A**) Long axis transesophageal echo zoom image of a bioprosthetic mitral valve. The arrows point to the thickened, degenerative cusps. (**B, C**) The prosthetic valve is now seen from the perspective of the LA during systole (**B**) and the LV during diastole (**C**). Note the thickened cusps (arrows). MV = mitral valve; LA = left atrium; LV = left ventricle. (**D**) A patient with a mitral valve ring and paravalvular mitral regurgitation. On the 2-chamber view (**left**) a pledget is seen protruding inito the left atrium. A gray scale three-dimensional reconstruction was performed looking at the ring from the left atrium (**upper right**) (indicated by the black arrows). An area of dehiscence is observed on the posterior aspect of the ring (white arrow). From the left ventricle, the left ventricular outflow tract (LVOT) and mitral valve is seen opening in diastole (**lower right**). The area of dehiscence is not delineated from this orientation. 35**D** is from Lissa Sugeng, MD, Ivan Godoy, MD, Kirk T. Spencer, MD, Jim Bednarz, BS, Lynn Weinert, BS, and Roberto M. Lang, MD.

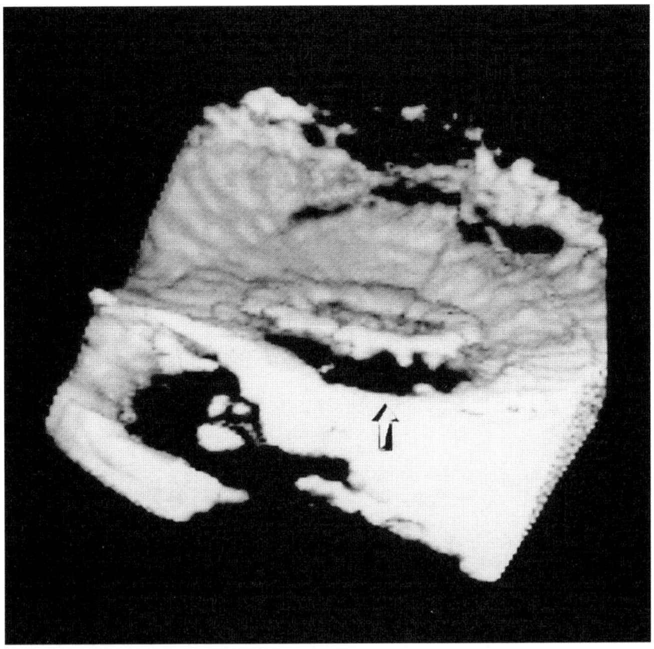

Figure 36. Dehiscence of a mitral Carpentier-Edwards prosthetic ring. The left atrium is up and the left ventricle is down. Note the large dehiscence of the prosthesis (arrowhead). From Albert A. Hagège, MD.

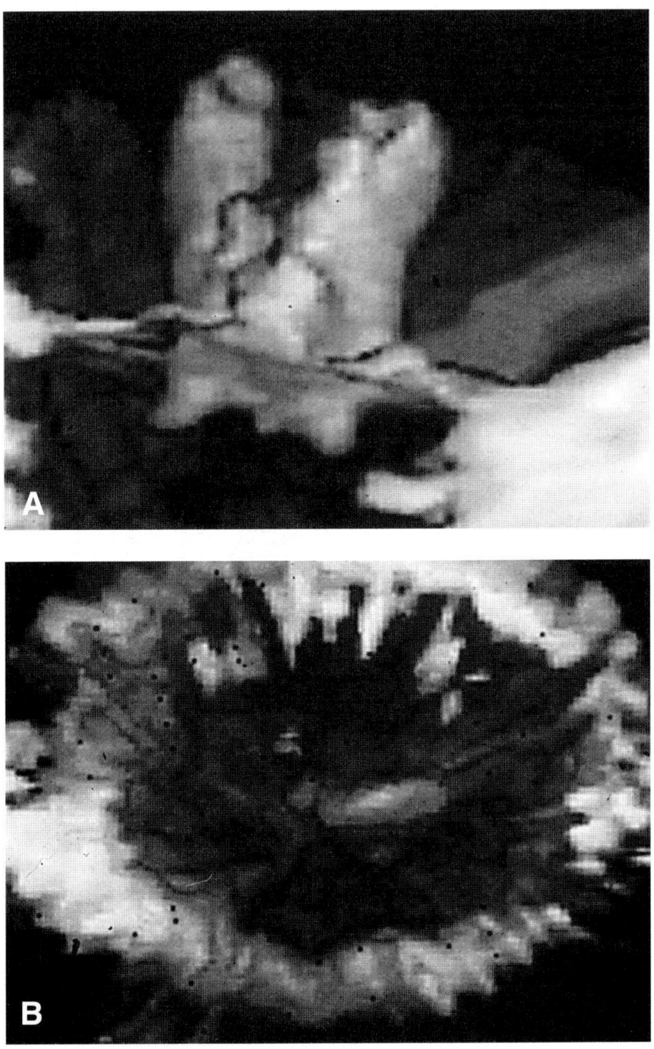

Figure 37. Mitral regurgitant jet (native valve). Black and white reconstruction from color-Doppler maps of a mitral regurgitation (MR) jet. (**A**) Cutplane through left atrium (**top**) and left ventricle (**bottom**) parallel to the closing line of the mitral valve. The large jet of MR is made of two diverging jets originating at each commissure, and of smaller cental jets. The flow converging toward the regurgitant orifice is seen on the ventricular side of the valve. (**B**) MR flow converging toward the regurgitant orifice. Short-axis view of the left ventricle with anterior wall at top. In systole, the flow converging toward the regurgitant orifice has an elongated shape, unlike the hemispheric shape required for the PISA method. (**C**) Images showing mitral valve prolapse along systolic phase. Such imaging may be of help in planning mitral valve repair through the precise assessment of the size and location of mitral prolapsing scallop as viewed by the surgeon *in situ*. (**D**) Abnormal regurgitant jet of a bileaflet mitral prosthesis. Side view of a mitral prosthesis, with left atrium at top. In addition to two normal small jets (converging in the shape of a triangle on the rear side of the prosthesis), a large jet extending into the left atrium is seen. **A, B, D** from Cedric Vuille, MD and Rene Lerch, MD; **C** from Stefano De Castro, MD and Rachele Adorisio, MD.

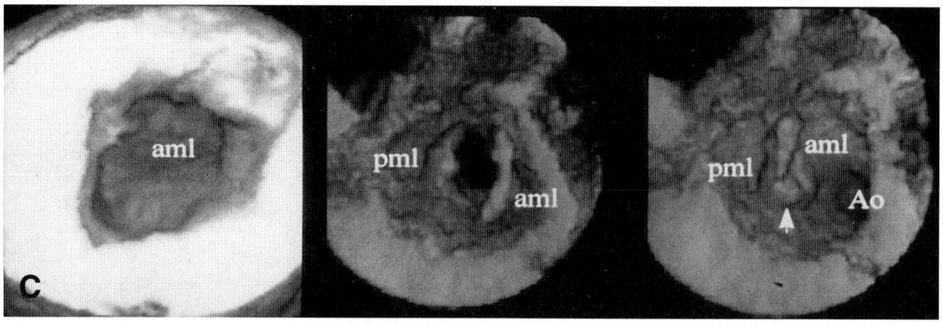

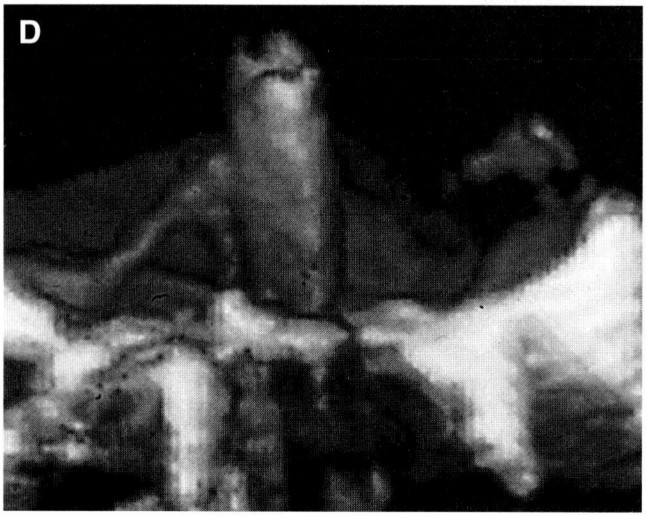

Figure 37. Continued. (**C**) Images showing mitral valve prolapse along systolic phase. Such imaging may be of help in planning mitral valve repair through the precise assessment of the size and location of mitral prolapsing scallop as viewed by the surgeon *in situ*. (**D**) Abnormal regurgitant jet of a bileaflet mitral prosthesis. Side view of a mitral prosthesis, with left atrium at top. In addition to two normal small jets (converging in the shape of a triangle on the rear side of the prosthesis), a large jet extending into the left atrium is seen. **A, B, D** from Cedric Vuille, MD and Rene Lerch, MD; **C** from Stefano De Castro, MD and Rachele Adorisio, MD.

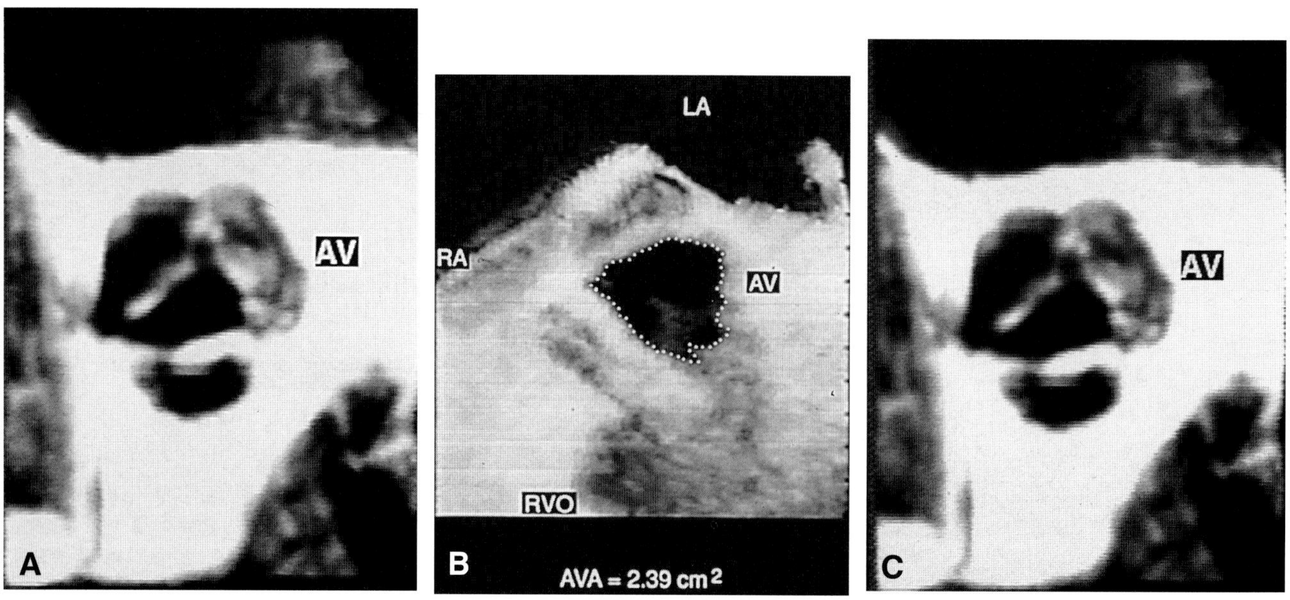

Figure 38. (**A**) Transesophageal (TEE), three-dimensionally reconstructed image of a normal aortic valve viewed from the left ventricular outflow tract during systole. (**B**) From the aortic viewpoint, the maximal systolic opening of the aortic valve can be easily planimetered to calculate the aortic valve area. The area in this patient is normal at 2.39 cm^2. All three leaflets can be seen well. RVO = right ventricular outflow tract. (**C**) TEE image of the aortic valve from the aortic position in a patient with mild aortic stenosis. Note how the maximal opening is reduced.

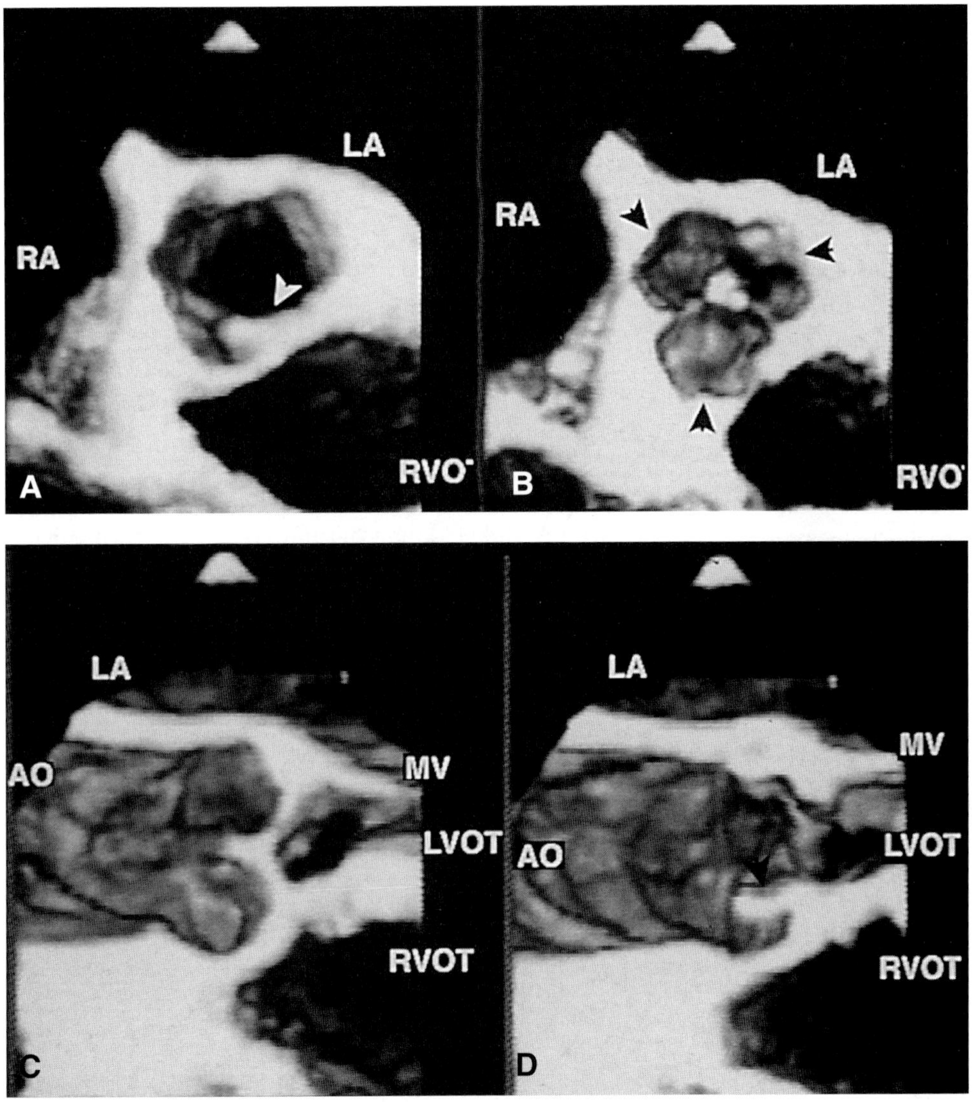

Figure 39. Transesophageal (TEE), three-dimensionally reconstruction short-axis image of the aortic valve during systole (**A**) and diastole (**B**) in a patient with mild aortic sclerosis and calcification of the right-coronary cusp (white arrowhead; left figure). (**C, D**) A TEE long-axis image of a mildly thickened aortic valve seen during systole (**C**) and diastole (**D**). Note the detail of the aortic lumen.

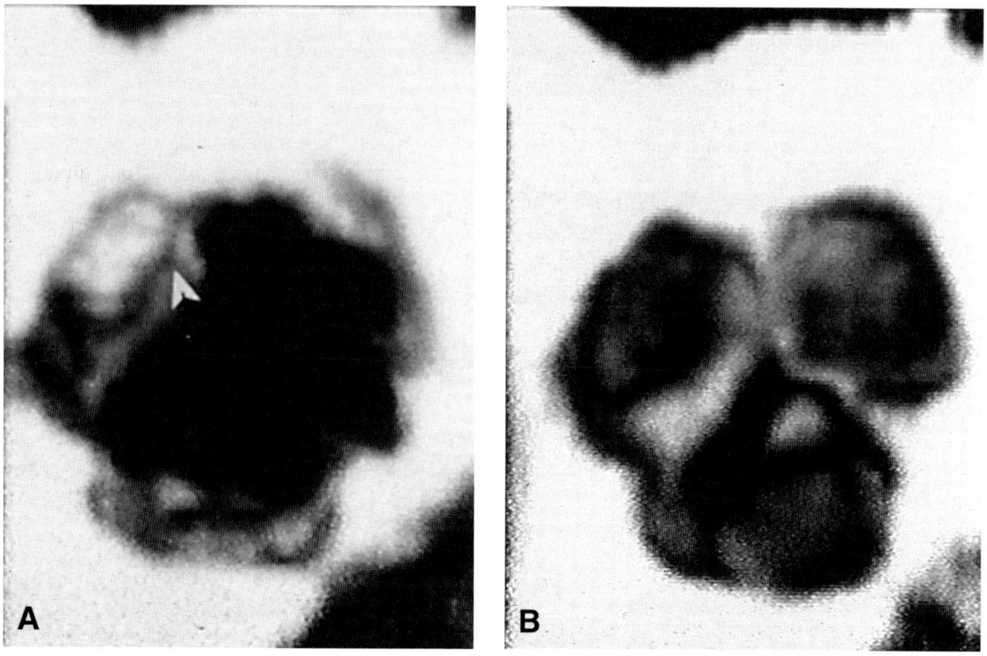

Figure 40. Transesophageal echo image of a mildly calcified aortic valve viewed from the aortic position. The noncoronary cusp has an area of focal calcification seen better during systole (**A**) than diastole (**B**). However, the details of the leaflets are best imaged during diastole.

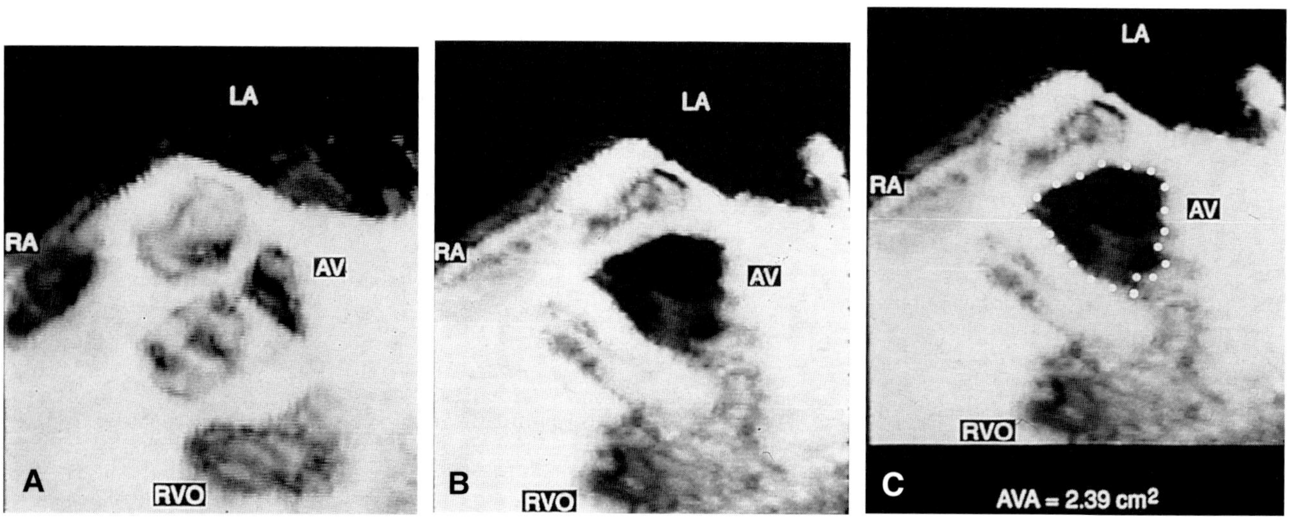

Figure 41. Transesophageal three-dimensional reconstruction of thickened aortic valve with no significant stenosis. The aortic valve leaflets show dense areas in both diastole (**A**) and systole (**B,C**) indicative of thickening and calcification. The aortic valve area obtained by planimetry (**C**) measured 2.39 cm^2. AV = aortic valve; B = moderator band in the right ventricle; LA = left atrium; LSPV = left superior pulmonary vein; LV = left ventricle; MV = mitral valve; RA = right atrium; RVO = right ventricular outflow tract; RSPV = right superior pulmonary vein; RV = right ventricle; VS = ventricular septum. Reproduced with permission from Nanda NC et al. Quantitative assessment of normal and stenotic aortic valve using transesophageal three-dimensional echocardiography. *Echocardiography* 1994;11:617–625.

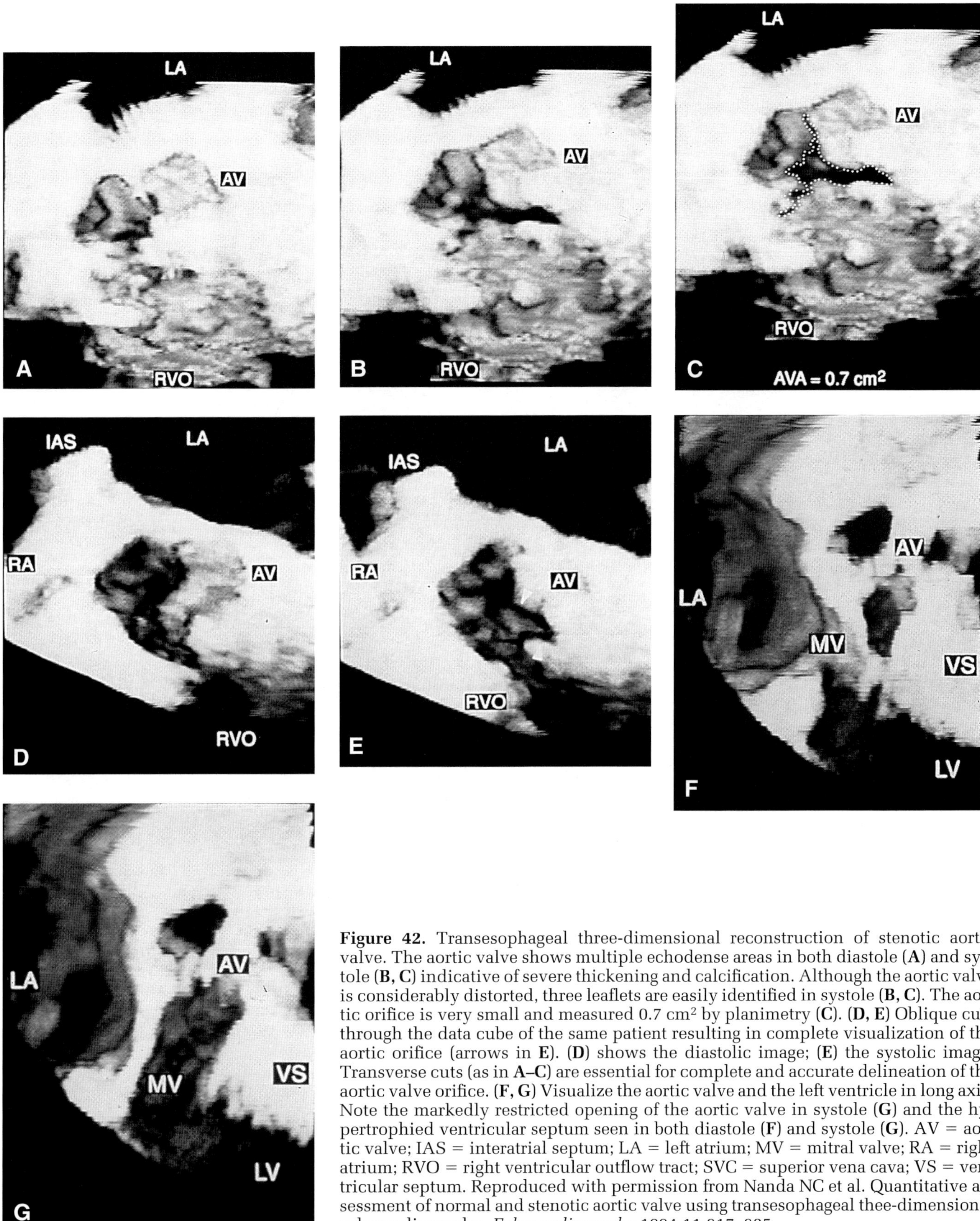

Figure 42. Transesophageal three-dimensional reconstruction of stenotic aortic valve. The aortic valve shows multiple echodense areas in both diastole (**A**) and systole (**B, C**) indicative of severe thickening and calcification. Although the aortic valve is considerably distorted, three leaflets are easily identified in systole (**B, C**). The aortic orifice is very small and measured 0.7 cm^2 by planimetry (**C**). (**D, E**) Oblique cuts through the data cube of the same patient resulting in complete visualization of the aortic orifice (arrows in **E**). (**D**) shows the diastolic image; (**E**) the systolic image. Transverse cuts (as in **A–C**) are essential for complete and accurate delineation of the aortic valve orifice. (**F, G**) Visualize the aortic valve and the left ventricle in long axis. Note the markedly restricted opening of the aortic valve in systole (**G**) and the hypertrophied ventricular septum seen in both diastole (**F**) and systole (**G**). AV = aortic valve; IAS = interatrial septum; LA = left atrium; MV = mitral valve; RA = right atrium; RVO = right ventricular outflow tract; SVC = superior vena cava; VS = ventricular septum. Reproduced with permission from Nanda NC et al. Quantitative assessment of normal and stenotic aortic valve using transesophageal thee-dimensional echocardiography. *Echocardiography* 1994;11:617–625.

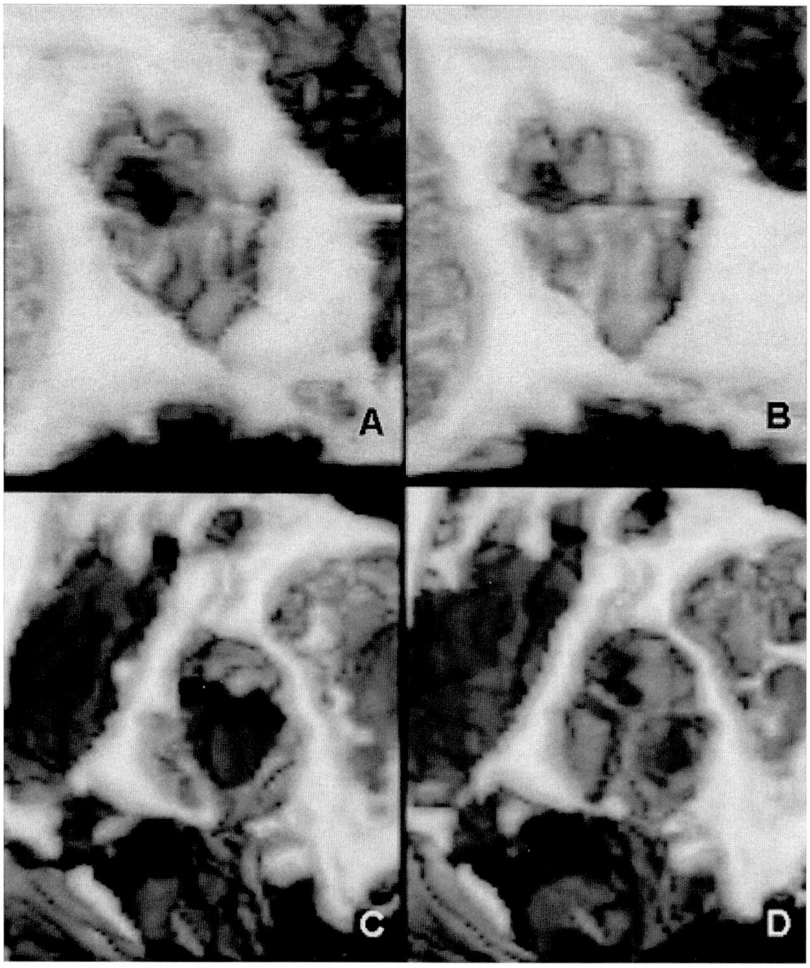

Figure 43. (**A–D**). A 65-year-old white male was admitted to the intensive care unit with chest pain. On auscultation a harsh diamond-shaped systolic murmur was heard and the electrocardiogram revealed marked left ventricular hypertrophy. A transthoracic two- and three-dimensional (2D, 3D) echocardiographic evaluation was performed. Top panels show a transthoracic 3D reconstruction of the aortic valve during systole (**A**) and diastole (**B**), visualized from the ascending aorta. 3D echocardiography revealed thickened and deformed commissures with a pinpoint valve orifice with a calculated valve area of 0.68 cm^2. Bottom panels show a transthoracic three-dimensional reconstruction of a normal aortic valve viewed from ascending aorta during systole (**C**) and diastole (**D**). The calculated valve area of this normal valve is 3.4 cm^2. Note the wide systolic opening of all three cusps compared with the stenotic valve. From Lissa Sugeng, MD, Ivan Godoy, MD, Kirk T. Spencer, MD, Jim Bednarz, BS, Lynn Weinert, BS, and Roberto M. Lang, MD.

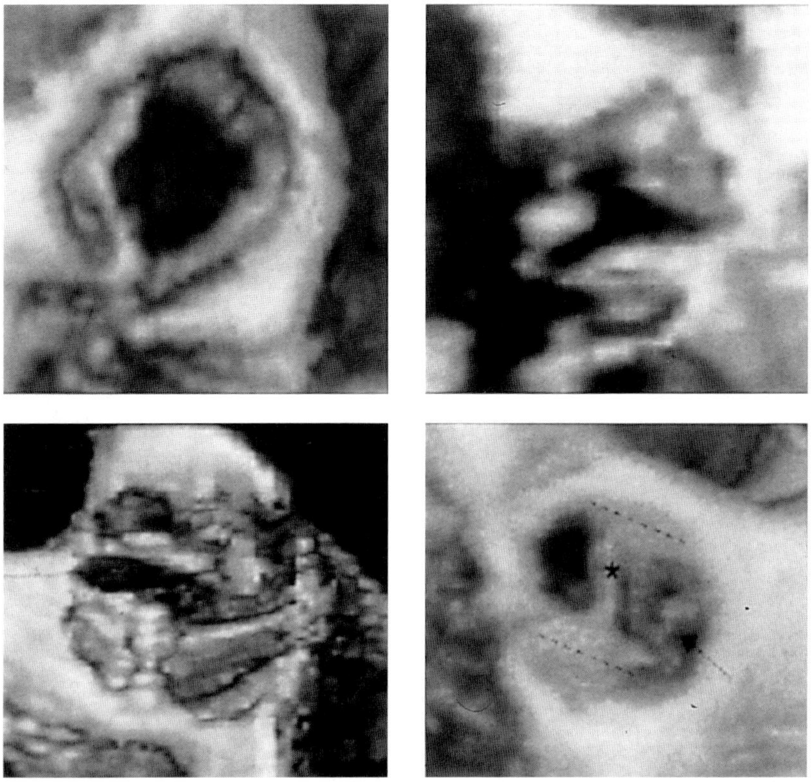

Figure 44. Volume rendering of aortic valve: normal triangular orifice (**upper left**), star-shaped orifice of a stenotic valve (**upper right**), bicuspid valve (**lower left**) and open St. Jude bileaflet prosthesis (St. Jude Medical, St. Paul, MN) (**lower right**). Note the open disks (dashed line), details of prosthesis framework (arrow) and an artifact (*). From Jaroslaw D. Kasprzak, MD and Jaroslaw Drozdz, MD.

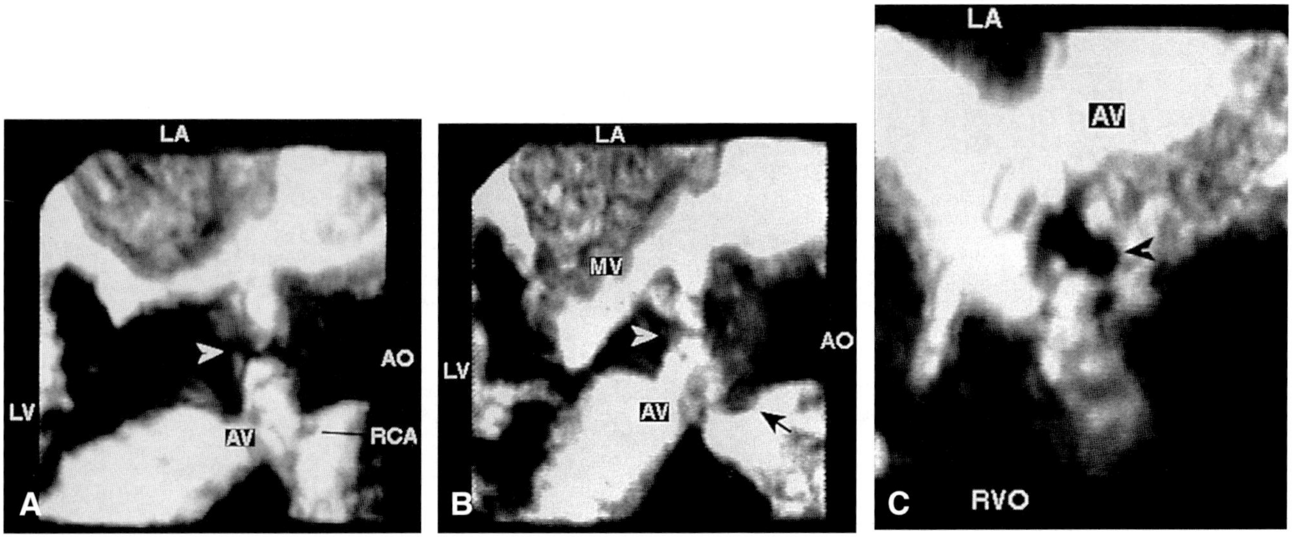

Figure 45. Long axis transesophageal echo (TEE) image of a very stenotic aortic valve in systole (**A**) and diastole (**B**). The proximal right coronary artery (RCA) is also visualized. (**C**) Short axis TEE image of the same aortic valve during systole showing the very small opening.

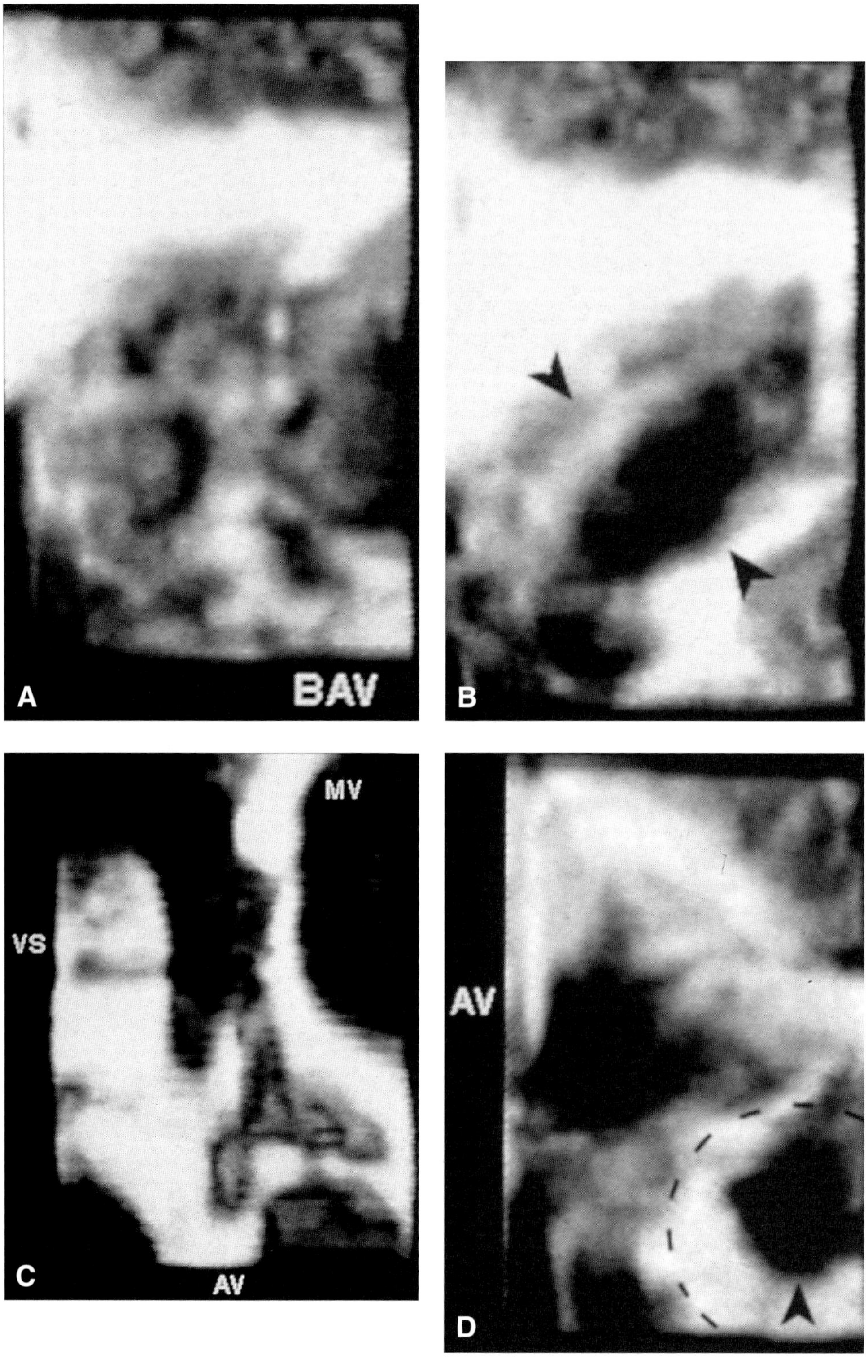

Figure 46. Short axis transesophageal echo (TEE) image of a bicuspid aortic valve with aortic stenosis visualized in diastole (**A**) and systole (**B**). Note the two, linear cusps (arrowheads). (**C**) TEE three-dimensional (3D) reconstruction, long-axis image of the bicuspid aortic valve with greater detail of the left ventricular outflow tract (LVOT) (a subaortic membrane is also seen arising from the ventricular septum). (**D**) TEE 3D short-axis image of the left and right ventricular outflow tracts (RVO; arrow) highlighting the anatomic relationship of these structures.

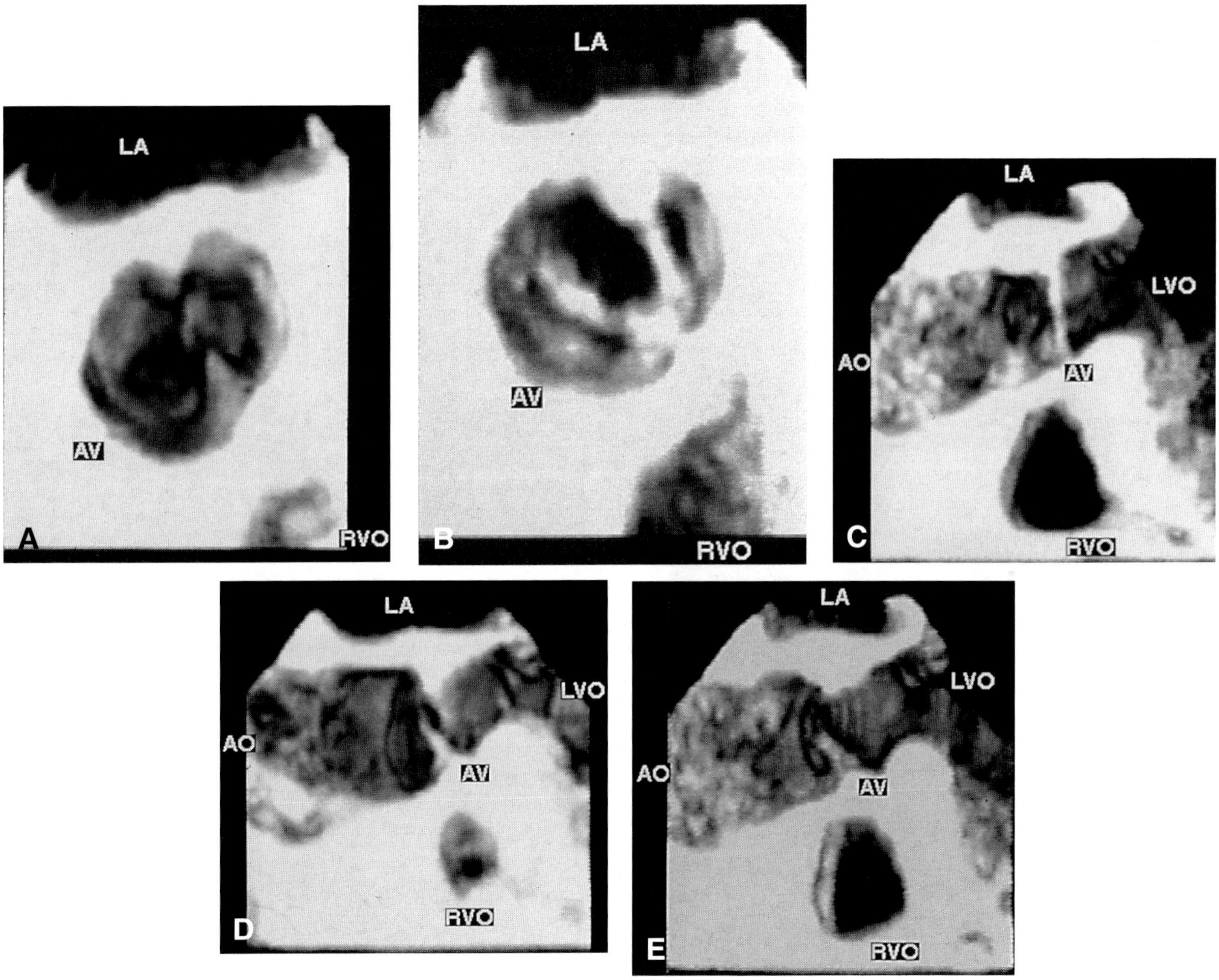

Figure 47. Transesophageal echo (TEE) short axis three-dimensional reconstruction of another bicuspid aortic valve during diastole (**A**) and systole (**B**). TEE long-axis reconstruction of the aortic valve during diastole (**C**), mid-systole (**D**) and systole (**E**) showing the thickened, calcified and restricted leaflets.

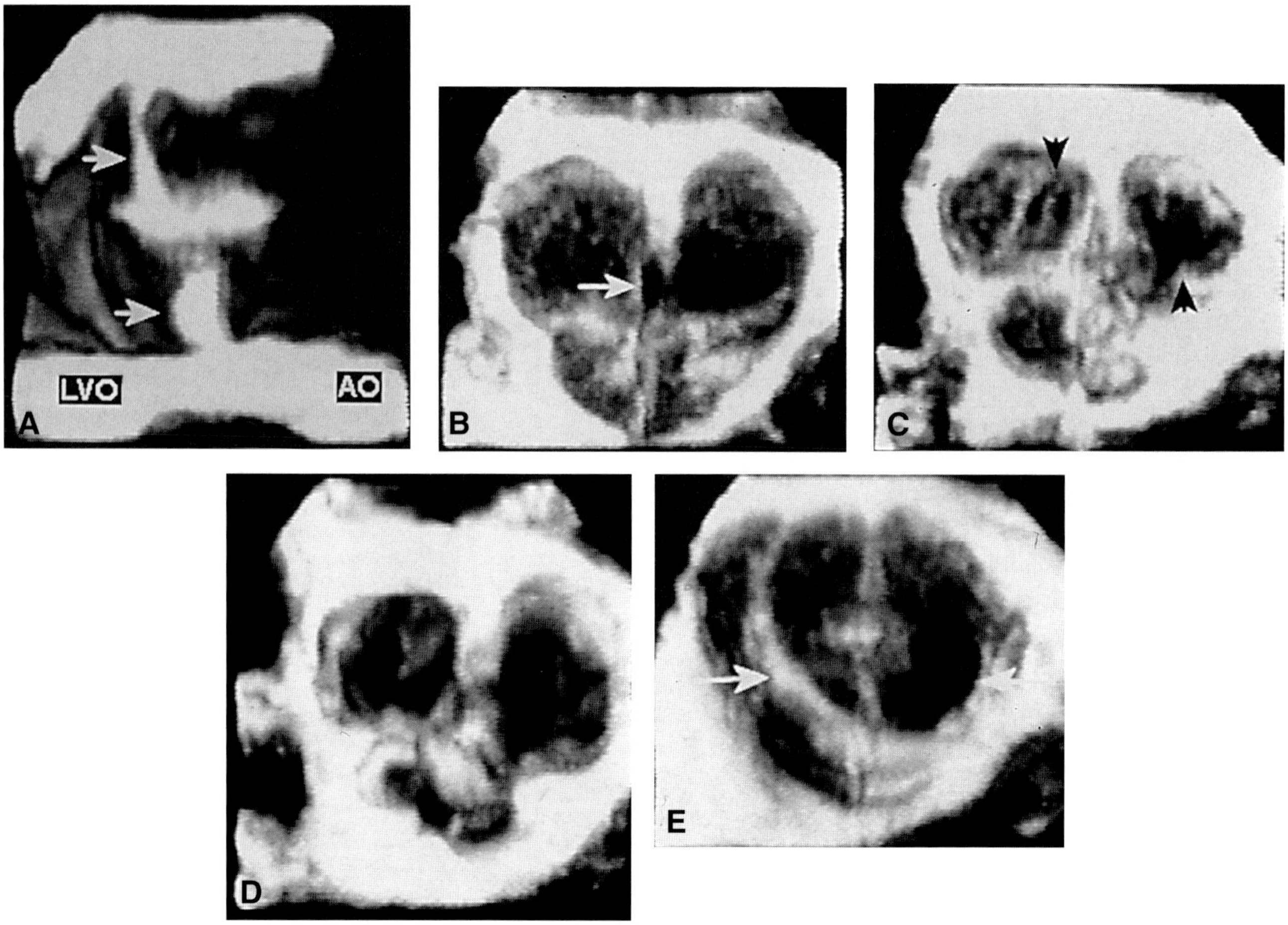

Figure 48. This series of three-dimensional (3D) images highlights the ability of 3D to choose cutplanes to illustrate various anatomic details. (**A**) Enlarged long-axis image of a bicuspid aortic valve. (**B**) Enlarged short-axis image of the bicuspid aortic valve illustrating malcoaptation of the leaflet tips (arrow) during diastole. (**C, D**) These two images were obtained during diastole and appear to represent a tri-leaflet valve. (**E**) This is the same image during systole clarifying the actual bicuspid valve and lack of significant aortic valve stenosis.

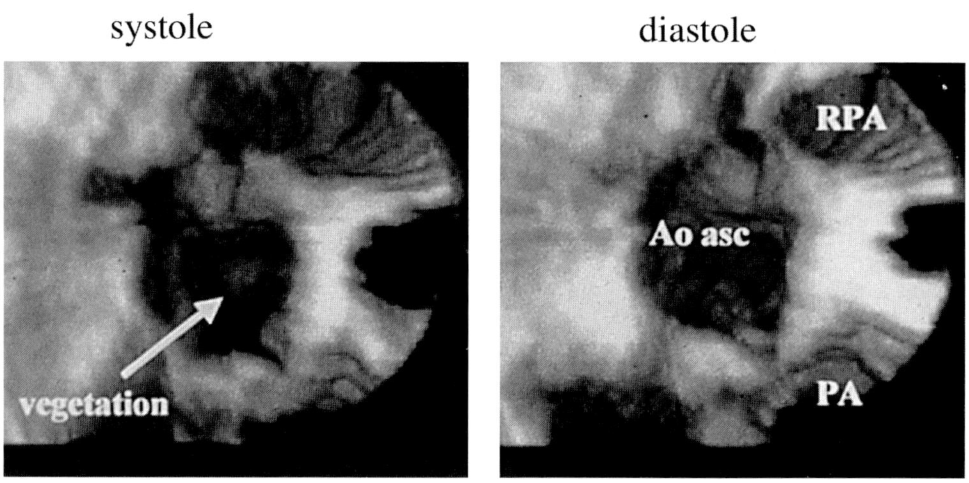

Figure 49. Bacterial endocarditis of the aortic valve—early stage. Anyplane reconstruction from a three-dimensional dataset shows the vegetation, localized on the right coronary cusp of the aortic valve, during systole (**left**) and diastole (**right**). The function of the aortic valve is preserved with complete opening and complete closure of the valve. From Jaroslaw Drozdz, MD and Jaroslaw D. Kasprzak, MD.

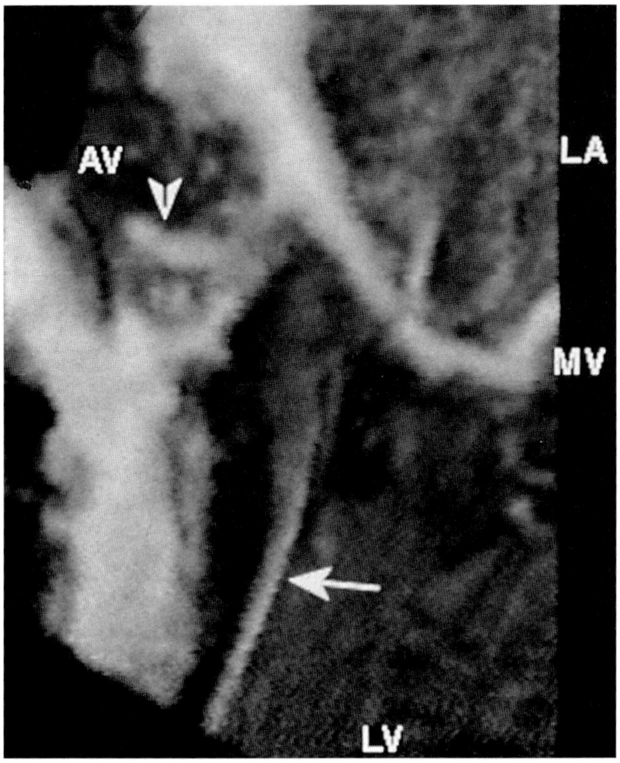

Figure 50. This is an apical 4-chamber, three-dimensional transesophageal zoom image of the aortic valve and left ventricular (LV) outflow tract area. There is an aortic valve vegetation (arrowhead) seen on the left coronary cusp. A linear structure is seen within the LV cavity and represents a reconstruction artifact (arrow).

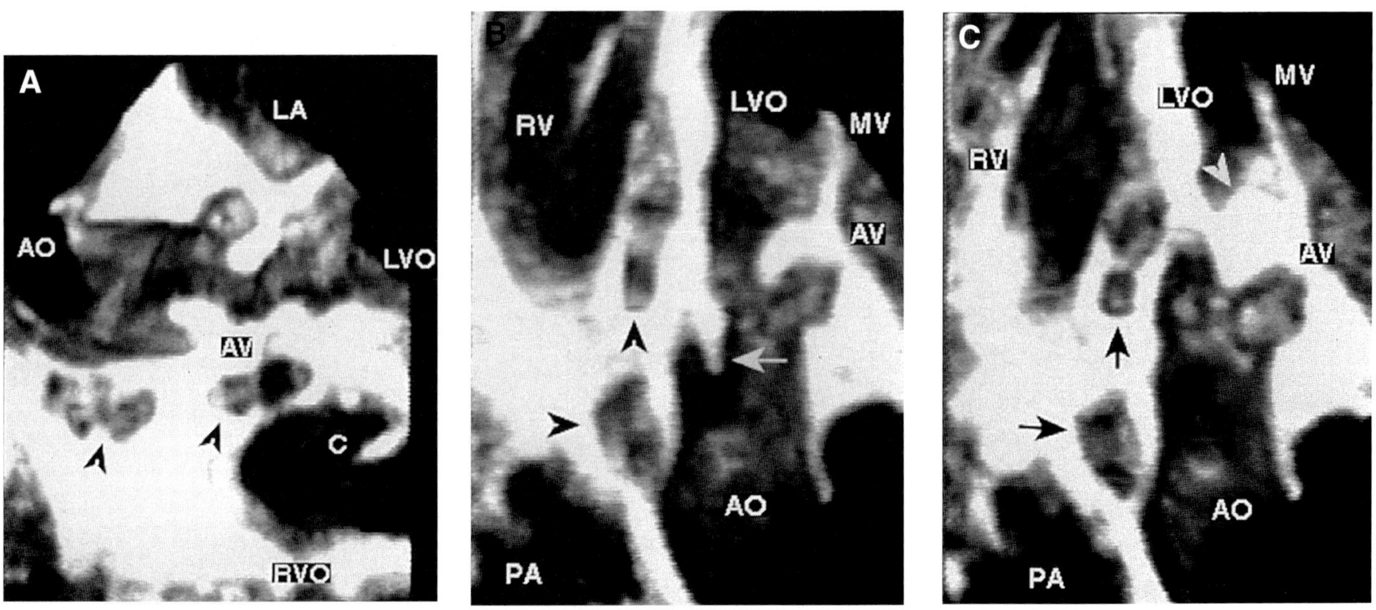

Figure 51. Series of images in another patient with endocarditis. (**A**) Transesophageal (TEE) horizontal long axis image showing multiple areas of perivalvular extension highly suggestive of abscesses (arrowheads). "C" = catheter. (**B, C**) TEE, vertical long-axis image showing the entire dimension of the abscess cavities (arrowheads) in systole (**B**) and diastole (**C**). The aortic valve vegetation is also noted (arrow).

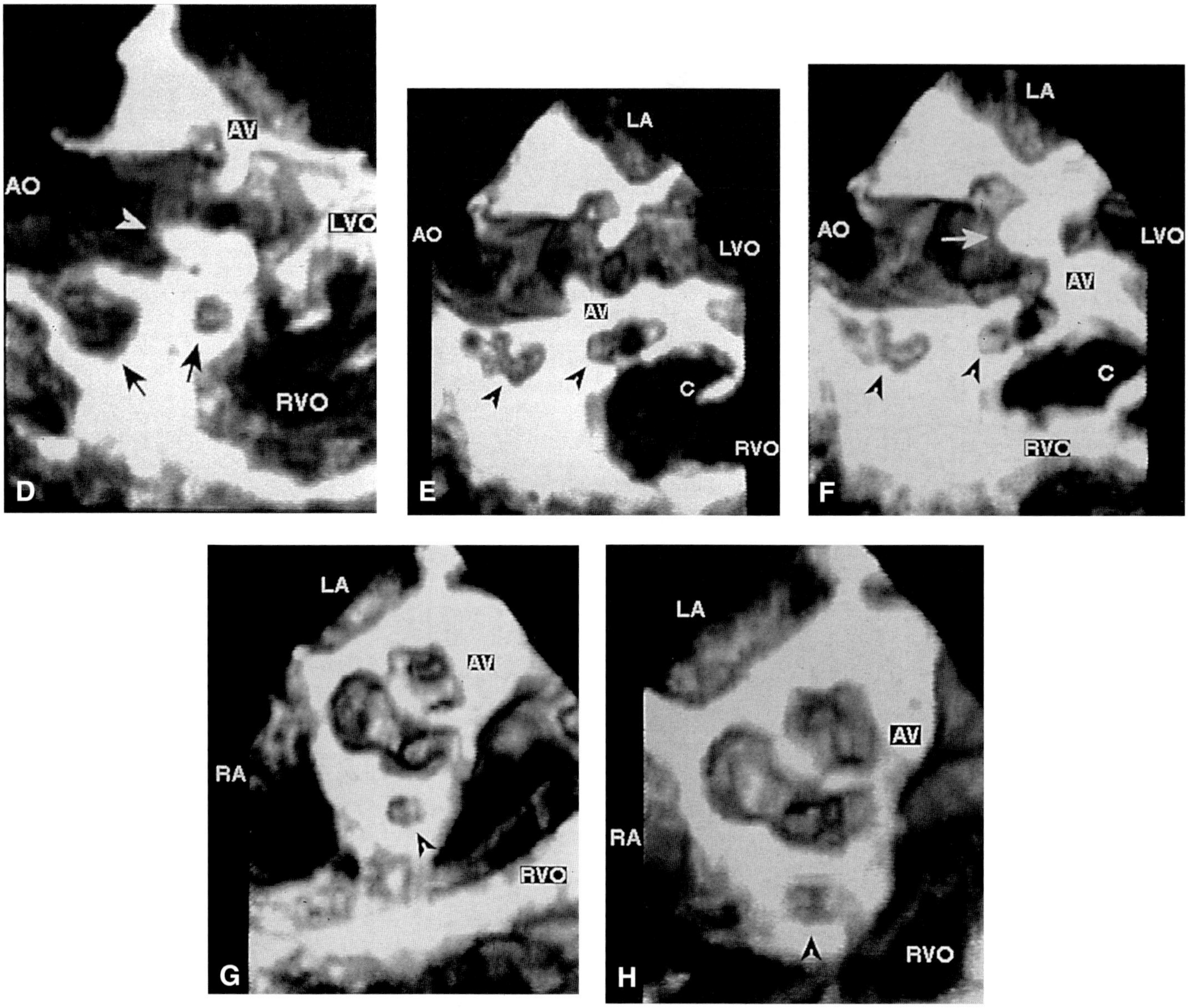

Figure 51. Continued. (**D, E, F**) TEE horizontal off-axis images showing the complex shape of these abscess cavities in systole (**D, E**) and diastole (**F**). Note the catheter tip better seen in the right ventricular outflow in **E.** (**G, H**) TEE, short-axis image of the same patient allowing the exact location and proximity to the right coronary cusp to be determined. (H = larger zoomed image) Arrowhead = abscess.

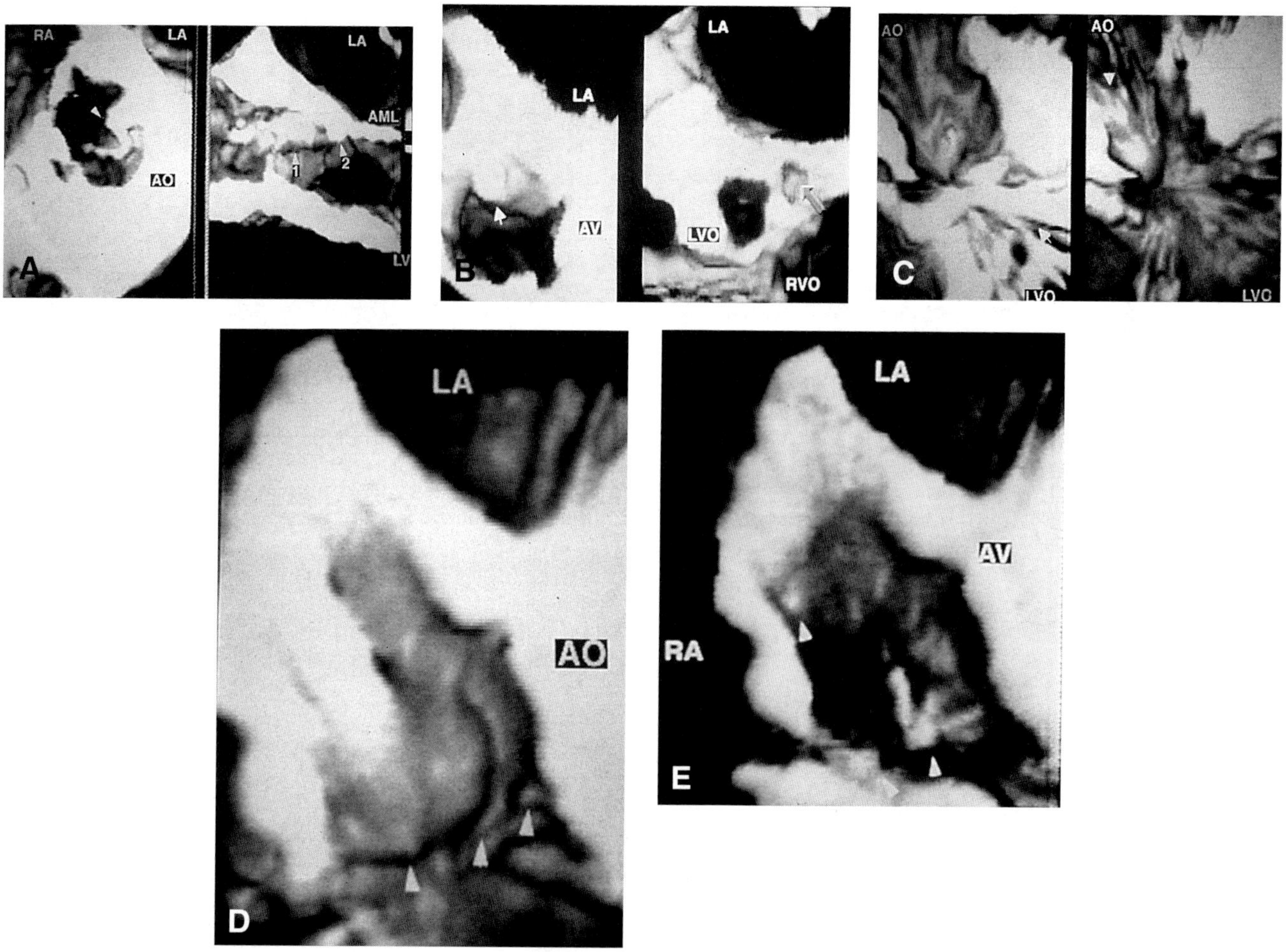

Figure 52. (**A**) Large vegetations (arrows, #1, #2) are seen involving the aortic valve reconstructed in short-axis (left) and long-axis (right) views. (**B**) A large vegetation (left, arrow) is noted on the aortic valve (AV) together with an abscess cavity (right, arrow) involving the itral-aortic intervalvular fibrosa. (**C–E**) "Peeling off of layers" of the aortic root and valve to delineate more clearly aortic valve vegetations (arrows). In **C**, both diastolic (left) and systsolic (right) frames are shown. AML = anterior mitral leaflet; AO = aorta; LA = left atrium; LV = left ventricle; LVO = left ventricular outflow tract; RA = right atrium; RVO = right ventricular outflow tract. Reproduced with permission from Nanda NC et al. Incremental value of three-dimensional echocardiography over transesophageal multiplane two-dimensional echocardiography in qualitative and quantitative assessment of cardiac masses and defects. *Echocardiography* 1995;12:619–628.

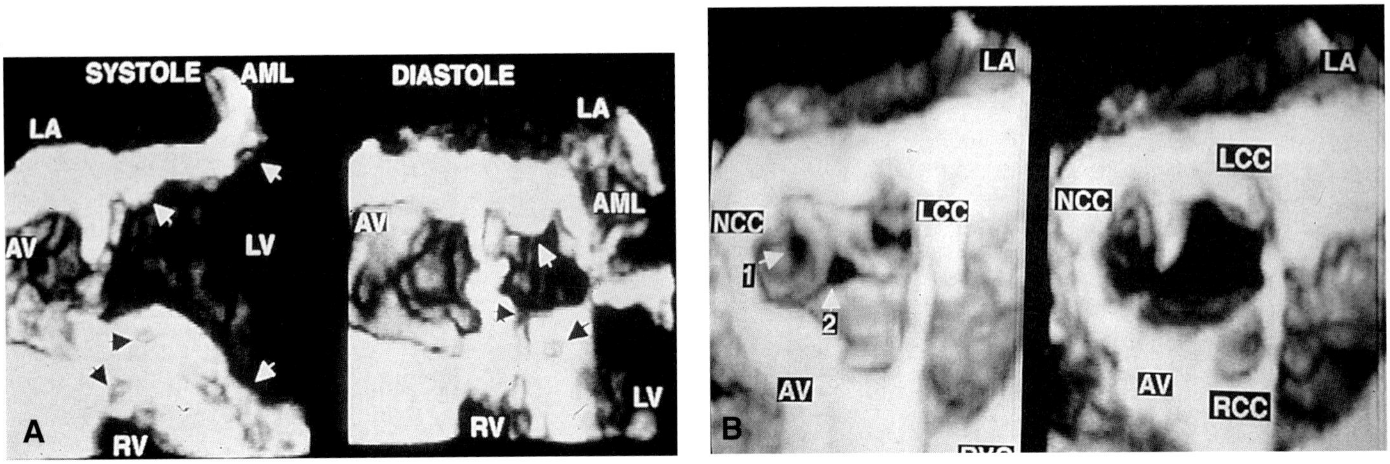

Figure 53. (**A**) Three-dimensionally reconstructed images of the aortic valve viewed in long axis showing multiple abscesses (arrows) involving the aortic root region, ventricular septum, mitral-aortic intervalvular fibrosa, and body of the anterior mitral leaflet. (**B**) Short-axis view in the same patient showing a large perforation (#1) in the two noncoronary cusps (NCC), extensive destruction of the left coronary cusp (LCC), and a large area of noncoaptation (#2) of aortic valve leaflets in diastole (left). The systolic frame is shown on the right. RCC = right coronary cusp; RV = right ventricle. Other abbreviations as in Figure 51. Reproduced with permission from Nanda NC et al. Incremental value of three-dimensional echocardiography over transesophageal multiplane two-dimensional echocardiography in qualitative and quantitative assessment of cardiac masses and defects. *Echocardiography* 1995;12:619–628.

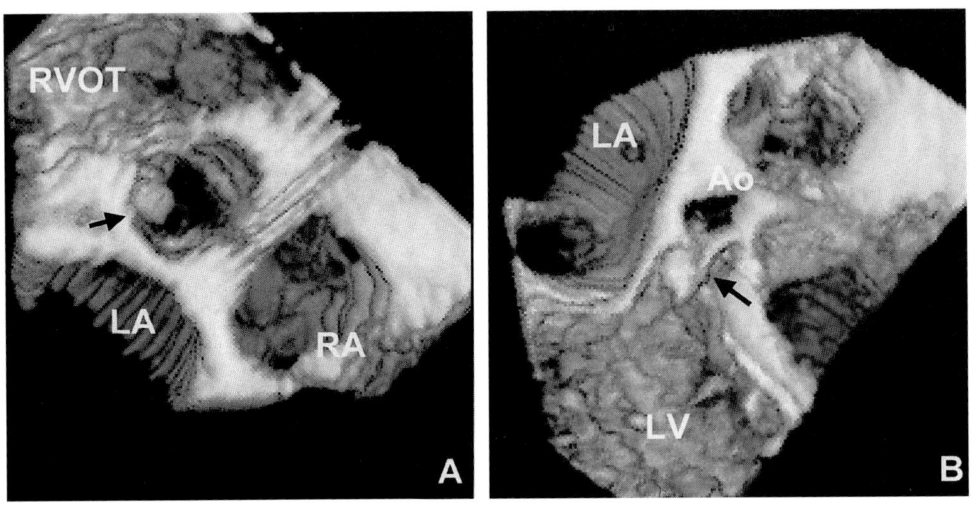

Figure 54. A transesophageal study performed on a middle aged male with a history of IV drug use demonstrating a vegetation o the left coronary cusp of the aortic valve viewed from the ascending aorta (**A**). A unique view of the vegetation (**B**) is demonstrated by a 3-chamber view looking towards the anterior aspects of the heart. During early diastole, the vegetation prolapses back into the left ventricle (black arrow). From Lissa Sugeng, MD, Ivan Godoy, MD, Kirk T. Spencer, MD, Jim Bednarz, BS, Lynn Weinert, BS, and Roberto M. Lang, MD

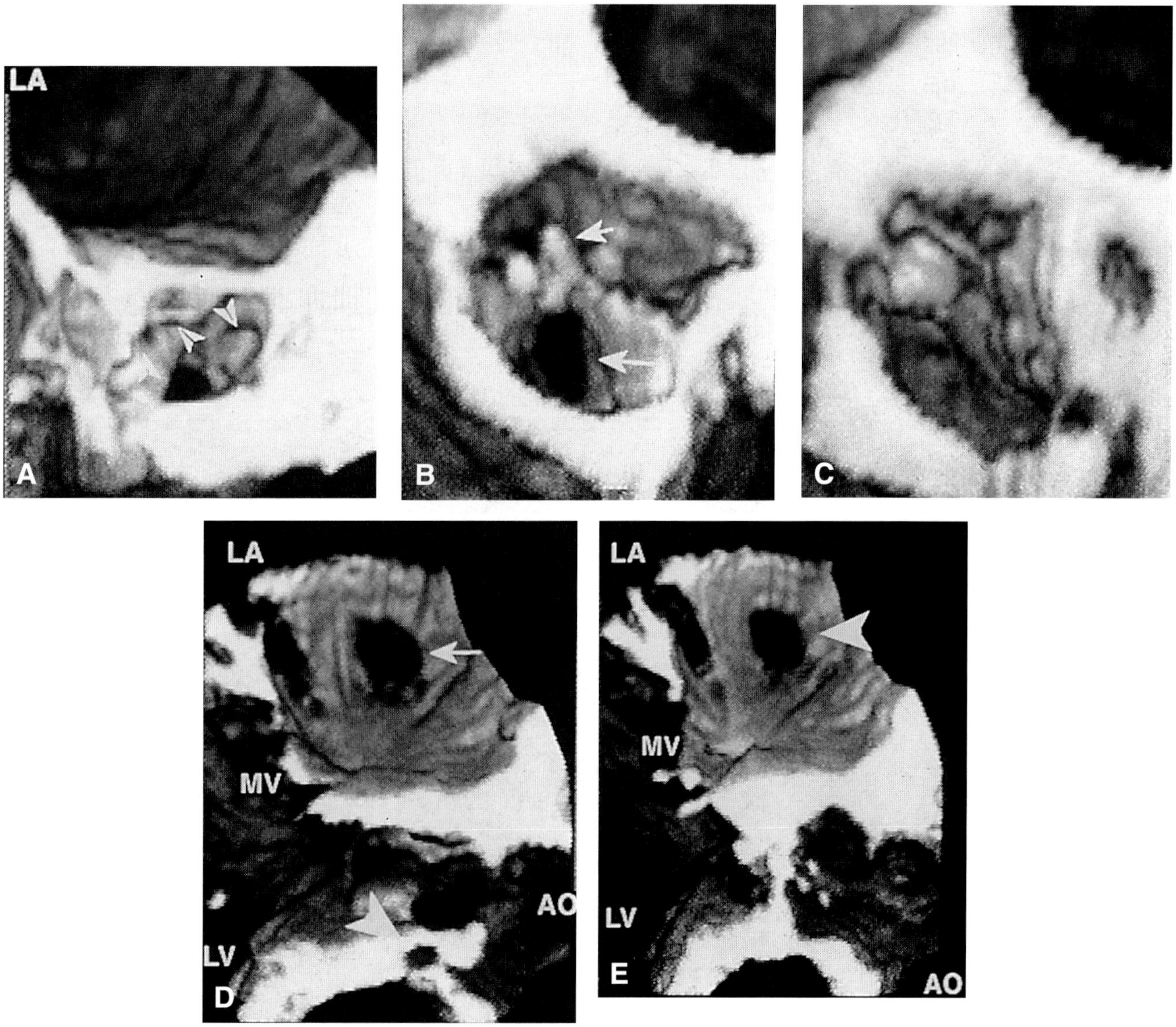

Figure 55. (**A**) Short-axis, anyplane transesophageal echo (TEE) image of the aortic valve in a patient with endocarditis (arrowheads) and a large perforation of the right coronary cusp. (**B**) TEE, short-axis, zoom image of the same patient with endocarditis (short arrow) and perforated leaflet (longer arrow). (**C**) With a slightly different orientation, the vegetative lesion on the aortic valve is seen more clearly, but the perforation is less apparent. (**D**) This is a vertical, long axis, TEE image of the left ventricular outflow tract, aorta, left ventricle, mitral valve, and left atrium. The pulmonary vein inlet is well visualized in systole (arrow). Also note the abscess cavity at the base of the aortic valve (arrowhead). (**E**) The same image is now reconstructed during diastole (note the closed aortic valve). The orifice of the pulmonary vein is noted to be smaller.

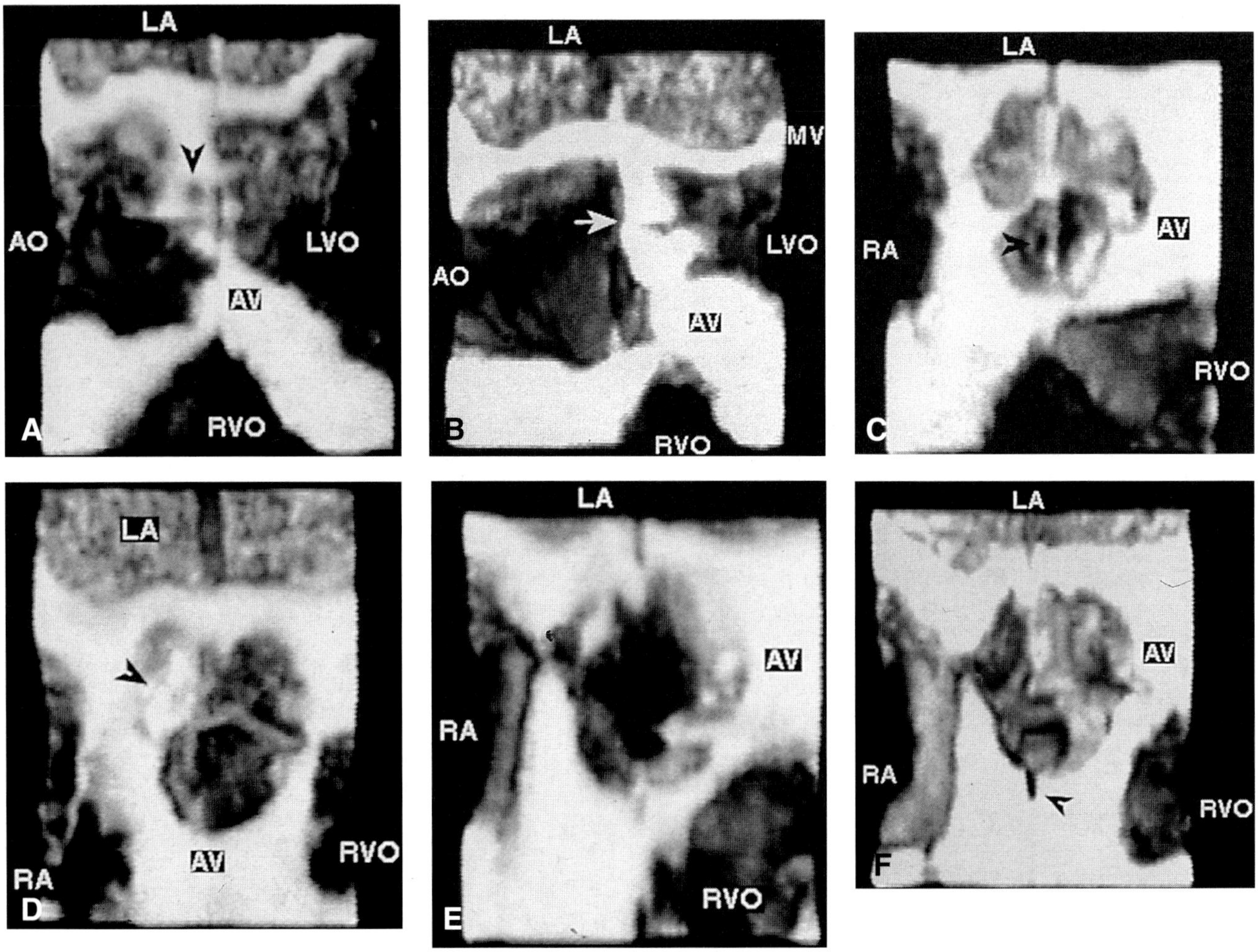

Figure 56. (**A, B**) Transesophageal echo (TEE) long-axis images in diastole in a patient with aortic valve endocarditis and a perforated right and noncoronary cusp (arrowhead). The slight differences in shading allow greater detail of the perforation (**A**) or the valve tissue (**B**). TEE short axis image from the aortic viewpoint showing the perforation in the right coronary cusp (arrowhead, **C**) and the vegetative lesion of the noncoronary cusp (arrowhead, **D**). (**E, F**) TEE three-dimensional short axis image of the same aortic valve in systole (**E**) and diastole (**F**).

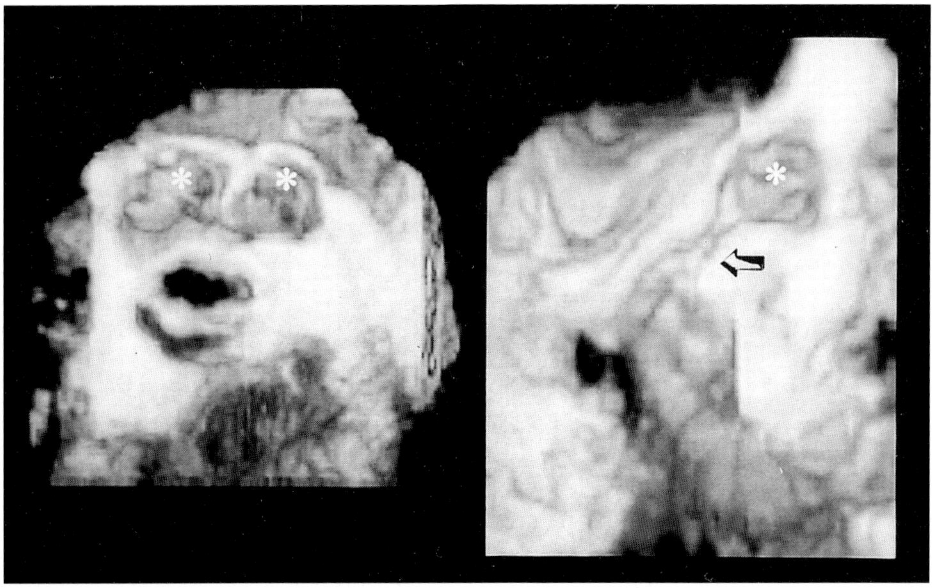

Figure 57. Endocarditis of the aortic valve with an adjacent ring abscess and left ventricular fistula. On a superior view (**left**), note the presence of 2 abscess cavities (*) in the aortic annulus, just behind the aortic valve. On a sagittal view (**right**), one of these cavities (*) communicates with the left ventricle through a tiny channel (arrowhead) which emerges just below the mitral valve. From Albert A. Hagège, MD.

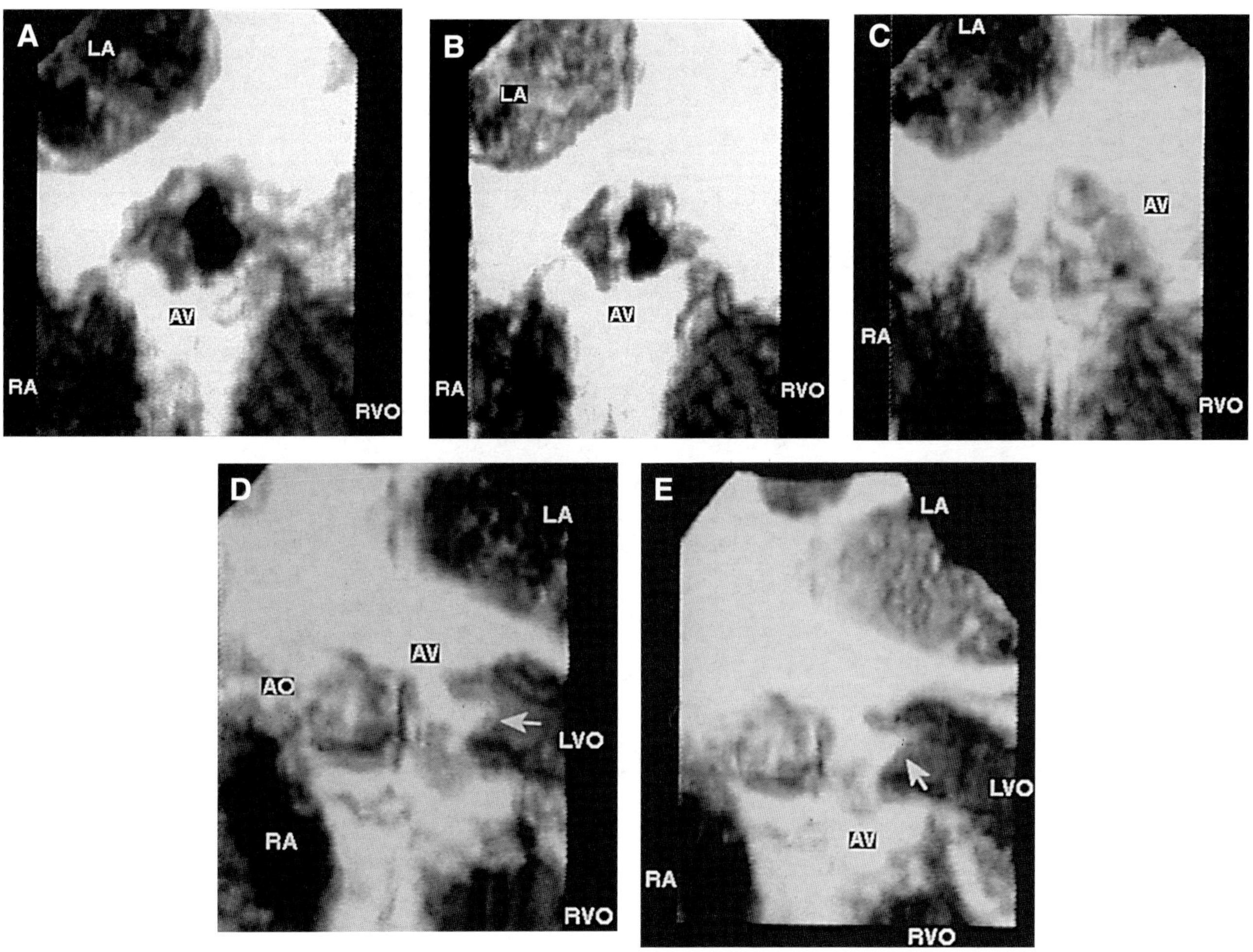

Figure 58. Transesophageal echo (TEE) three-dimensional (3D) short axis image of an aortic valve homograft in systole (**A**). In **A,** the contrast is slightly darker and the systolic phase is different than in **B,** giving a mild variation in the maximal opening and contour of this valve. (**C**) Same patient and general orientation of the aortic valve now in diastole. (**D**) TEE long-axis image of the AV homograft shown in the previous figures. Note the leaflet prolapse into the left ventricular outflow (arrow). In **E,** the image is displayed from a slightly different anyplane position and the contrast is also adjusted differently.

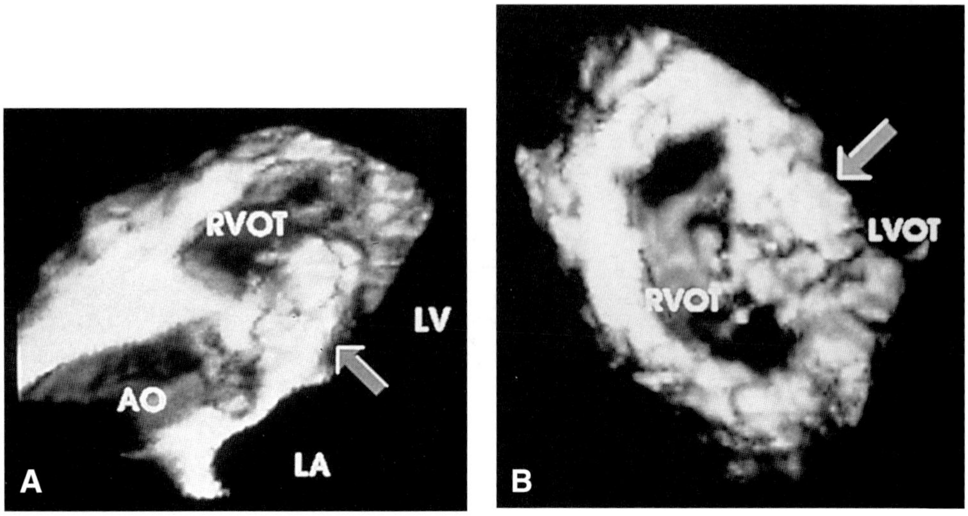

Figure 59. Dynamic three-dimensional images of aortic regurgitant jet. (**A**) Aortic (AO) regurgitant jet arrow displayed in the left ventricular outflow tract (LVOT). (**B**) Cross-sectional view of aortic regurgitant jet (arrow). LA = left atrium; LV = left ventricle; RVOT = right ventricular outflow tract. Reproduced with permission for Li Z et al. Dynamic three-dimensional reconstruction of abnormal intracardiac blood flow. *Echocardiography* 1997;14:375–381.

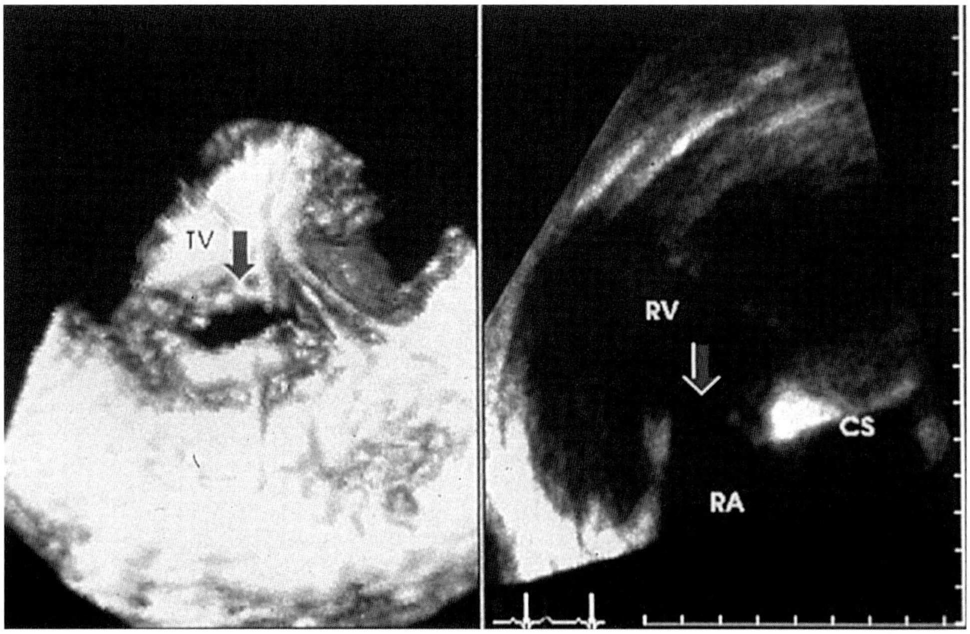

Figure 60. Tricuspid stenosis in a carcinoid disease. *En-face* view of the tricuspid valve in systole (**left**) clearly demonstrates a huge regurgitant orifice (++++ insufficiency). A long-axis anyplane view (**right**) confirms the lack of coaptation of rigid leaflets in systole (arrow). CS = coronary sinus; RA = right atrium; RV = right ventricle; TV = tricuspid valve. From Jaroslaw D. Kasprzak, MD and Jaroslaw Drozdz, MD.

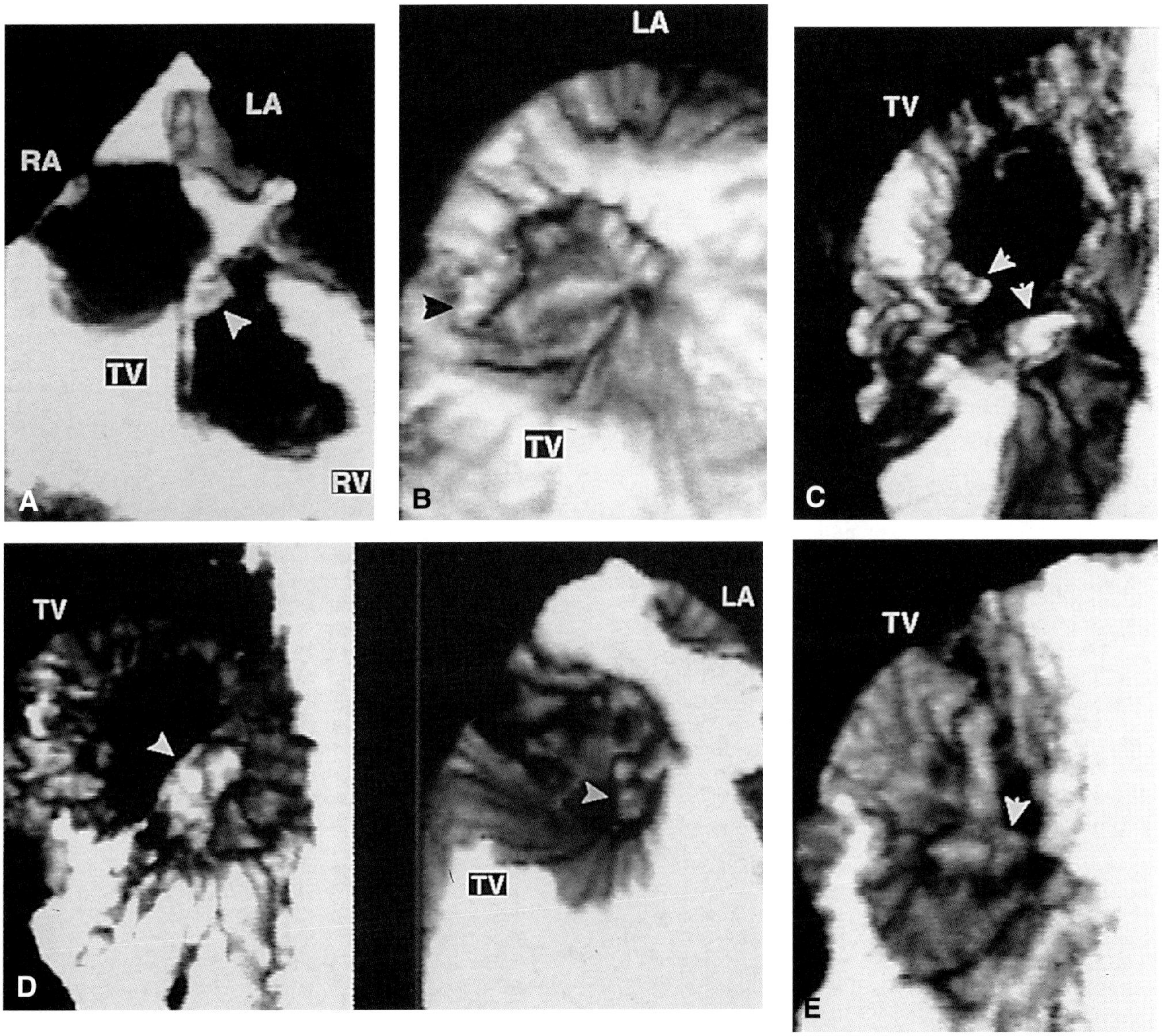

Figure 61. (**A**) Transesophageal echo (TEE) apical long-axis image highlighting the right atrium (RA) and right ventricle (RV). The tricuspid valve (TV) is abnormal with a small vegetation noted in systole (arrow). (**B**) TEE short-axis image of a closed (systolic) TV from the RA viewpoint. Note the vegetation (arrowhead). (**C**) RV viewpoint, TEE short-axis, diastolic image of the TV shown in the previous figures. From this viewpoint, at least two separate vegetative lesions can be seen (arrows). (**D**) These images represent a comparison of the previously shown abnormal TV with prominent vegetation (arrowheads) from the viewpoint of the RV (left) and RA (right). (**E**) By selecting a tangential plane through the TV annulus, additional images of the abnormal TV may be obtained. These orientations may provide the total extent of leaflet involvement and more fully reveal the size of the vegetation, as in this image. Vegetation = arrow.

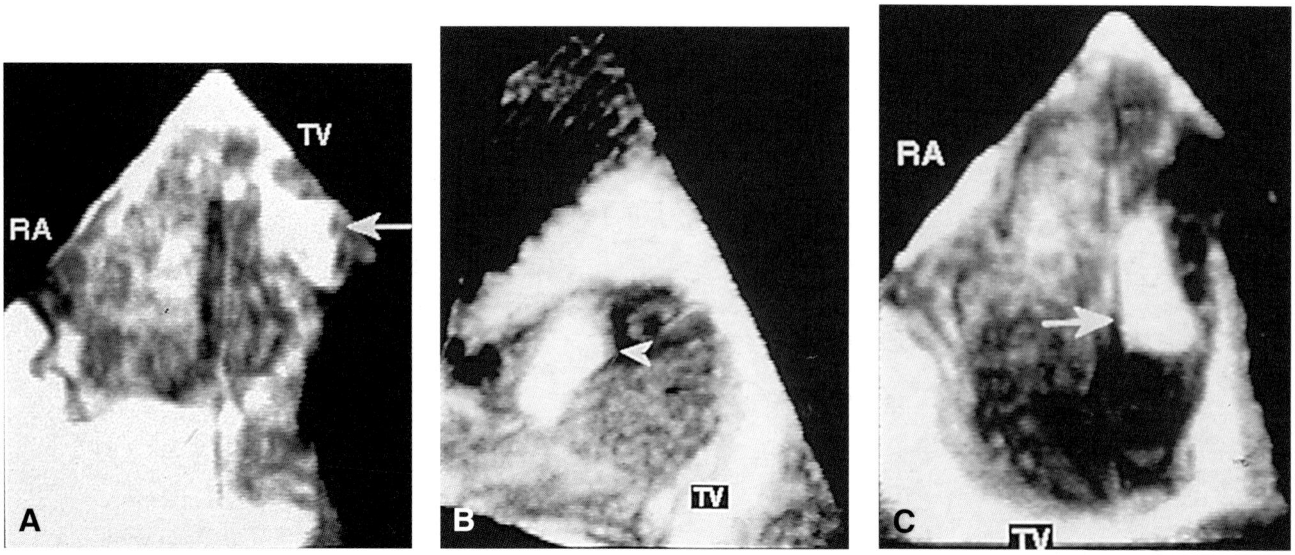

Figure 62. Transesophageal echo three-dimensional reconstruction of the right atrium and the tricuspid valve (TV). (**A**) Large vegetation is seen attached to the TV leaflet (arrow). (**B, C**) Additional off-axis orientations allow further clarification of the extent of the lesion and provide a complete interrogation of the size of the pathology.

Suggested Reading List

1. Nanda NC, Roychoudhury D, Chung SM, et al. Quantitative assessment of normal and stenotic aortic valve using transesophageal three-dimensional echocardiography. *Echocardiography* 1994;11:617–625.
2. Mikami T, Teranishi J, Saito N, et al. [Evaluation of valvular lesions by three-dimensional echocardiography]. [Japanese]. *J Cardiology* 1996;27 Suppl 2:39–43; discussion 44:39–43.
3. Laskari CV, Masani ND, Pandian NG. Three-dimensional echocardiography in mitral regurgitation. [Review] [19 refs]. *Coronary Artery Disease* 1996;7:206–210.
4. Abraham TP, Warner JGJ, Kon ND, et al. Feasibility, accuracy, and incremental value of intraoperative three-dimensional transesophageal echocardiography in valve surgery. *Am J Cardiology* 1997;80:1577–1582.
5. Chen Q, Nosir YF, Vletter WB, et al. Accurate assessment of mitral valve area in patients with mitral stenosis by three-dimensional echocardiography. *J Am Soc Echocardiography* 1997;10:133–140.
6. Ge S, Warner JGJ, Fowle KM, et al. Morphology and dynamic change of discrete subaortic stenosis can be imaged and quantified with three-dimensional transesophageal echocardiography. *J Am Soc Echocardiography* 1997;10:713–716.
7. Hozumi T, Yoshikawa J, Yoshida K, et al. Assessment of flail mitral leaflets by dynamic three-dimensional echocardiographic imaging. *Am J Cardiology* 1997;79:223–225.
8. Yamaura Y, Yoshida K, Hozumi T, et al Three-dimensional echocardiographic evaluation of configuration and dynamics of the mitral annulus in patients fitted with an annuloplasty ring. *J Heart Valve Dis* 1997;6:43–47.
9. Sugeng L, Cao QL, Delabays A, et al. Three-dimensional echocardiographic evaluation of aortic disorders with rotational multiplanar imaging: Experimental and clinical studies. *J Am Soc Echocardiography* 1997;10:120–132.
10. Vesely I, Fawzy HF, Fukamachi K, et al. Use of three-dimensional sonomicrometry to study the motion of the mitral valve. *ASAIO Journal* 1997;43:M465–M469.
11. Lange A, Walayat M, Turnbull CM, et al. Assessment of atrial septal defect morphology by transthoracic three dimensional echocardiography using standard grey scale and Doppler myocardial imaging techniques: Comparison with magnetic resonance imaging and intraoperative findings. *Heart* 1997;78:382–389.
12. Sezai A, Shiono M, Orime Y, et al. [Three-dimensional transesophageal echocardiographic assessment for prosthetic valves]. [Japanese]. *J Japanese Assoc Thoracic Surg* 1997;45:1084–1089.
13. Otsuji Y, Handschumacher MD, Schwammenthal E, et al. Insights from three-dimensional echocardiography into the mechanism of functional mitral regurgitation: Direct in vivo demonstration of altered leaflet tethering geometry. *Circulation* 1997;96:1999–2008.
14. Menzel T, Mohr-Kahaly S, Kolsch B, et al. Quantitative assessment of aortic stenosis by three-dimensional echocardiography. *J Am Soc Echocardiography* 1997;10:215–223.
15. Breburda CS, Griffin BP, Pu M, et al. Three-dimensional echocardiographic planimetry of maximal regurgitant orifice area in myxomatous mitral regurgitation: Intraoperative comparison with proximal flow convergence. *J Am Coll Cardiol* 1998;32:432–437.
16. Cheng TO. Assessment of mitral valve volume by quantitative three-dimensional echocardiography in patients with rheumatic mitral valve stenosis. [letter; comment]. *Clin Cardiol* 1998;21:869–870.
17. Dall'Agata A, Taams MA, Fioretti PM, et al. Cosgrove-Edwards mitral ring dynamics measured with transesophageal three-dimensional echocardiography. *Ann Thorac Surg* 1998;65:485–490.
18. El-Sayed AA, Nanda NC, Hassanein HA, et al. Value of three dimensional echo in the assessment of infective endocarditis: Quantification of volumes and weights of vegetations. (Abstract) *J Am Coll Cardiol* 1998;31:99C.
19. Ge S, Warner JGJ, Abraham TP, et al. Three-dimensional surface area of the aortic valve orifice by three-dimensional echocardiography: clinical validation of a novel index for assessment of aortic stenosis. *Am Heart J* 1998;136:1042–1050.

20. Godoy IE, Lang RM. Aortic stenosis. [see comments]. *Clin Cardiol* 1998;21:845.
21. Sadaniantz A, Burtt D, Nanda NC, et al. Three dimensional echocardiography of right heart pathology. *Echocardiography* 1998;15:795–806.
22. Yao J, Masani ND, Cao QL, et al. Clinical application of transthoracic volume-rendered three-dimensional echocardiography in the assessment of mitral regurgitation. *Am J Cardiol* 1998;82:189–196.
23. Yamaura Y, Yoshida K, Hozumi T, et al. Evaluation of the mitral annulus by extracted three-dimensional images in patients with an annuloplasty ring. *Am J Cardiol* 1998;82:534–536.
24. Kasprzak JD, Nosir YF, Dall'Agata A, Elhendy A, Taams M, Ten Cate FJ, Roelandt Jret al. Quantification of the aortic valve area in three-dimensional echocardiographic data sets: Analysis of orifice overestimation resulting from suboptimal cut-plane selection. *A Heart J* 1998;135:995–1003.
25. Menzel T, Mohr-Kahaly S, Wagner S, et al. Calculation of left ventricular outflow tract area using three-dimensional echocardiography. Influence on quantification of aortic valve stenosis. *Int J Cardiac Imaging* 1998;14:373–379.
26. Limbu YR, Shen X, Pan C, et al. Assessment of mitral valve volume by quantitative three-dimensional echocardiography in patients with rheumatic mitral valve stenosis. [see comments]. *Clin Cardiol* 1998;21:415–418.
27. Zhang GC, Tsukada T, Nakatani S, et al. Comparison of automatic boundary detection and manual tracing technique in echocardiographic determination of left atrial volume. *Japanese Circ J* 1998;62:755–759.
28. Acar P, Laskari C, Rhodes J, et al. Three-dimensional echocardiographic analysis of valve anatomy as a determinant of mitral regurgitation after surgery for atrioventricular septal defects. *Am J Cardiol* 1999;83:745–749.
29. Acar P, Jones M, Shiota T, et al. Quantitative assessment of chronic aortic regurgitation with 3-dimensional echocardiographic reconstruction: comparison with electromagnetic flowmeter measurements. *J Am Soc Echocardiography* 1999;12:138–148.
30. Anayiotos AS, Smith BK, Kolda M, et al. Morphological evaluation of a regurgitant orifice by 3-D echocardiography: Applications in the quantification of valvular regurgitation. *Ultrasound Med Biology* 1999;25:209–223.
31. De Simone R, Glombitza G, Vahl CF, et al. Three-dimensional color Doppler: a clinical study in patients with mitral regurgitation. *J Am Coll Cardiol* 1999; 33:1646–1654.
32. De Simone R, Glombitza G, Vahl CF, et al. Three-dimensional color Doppler: A new approach for quantitative assessment of mitral regurgitant jets. *J Am Soc Echocardiography* 1999;12:173–185.
33. Kanzaki Y, Yoshida K, Hozumi T, et al. [Evaluation of mitral valve lesions in patients with infective endocarditis by three-dimensional echocardiography]. [Japanese]. *J Cardiology* 1999;33:7–11.
34. Samal AK, Nanda NC, Thakur AC, et al. Three-dimensional echocardiographic assessment of Lambl's excrescences on the aortic valve. *Echocardiography* 1999;16:437–441.
35. Vogel M, Ho SY, Anderson RH, et al. Transthoracic 3-dimensional echocardiography in the assessment of subaortic stenosis due to a restrictive ventricular septal defect in double inlet left ventricle with discordant ventriculoarterial connections. *Cardiol in the Young* 1999;9:549–555.
36. Shandas R, Kwon J, Valdes-Cruz L. Real-time 3-dimensional volumetric ultrasound imaging of the vena contracta for stenotic valves with the use of echocardiographic contrast imaging: In vitro pulsatile flow studies. *J Am Soc Echocardiography* 1999;12:541–550.
37. Ratanasopa S, Bolson EL, Sheehan FH, et al. Performance of a Fourier-based program for three-dimensional reconstruction of the mitral annulus on application to sparse, noisy data. *Int J Cardiac Imaging* 1999;15:301–307.
38. Kuhl HP, Franke A, Hoffmann R, et al. [The value of echocardiography for the assessment of chronic mitral valve insufficiency]. [see comments]. [Review] [56 refs] [German]. *Deutsche Medizinische Wochenschrift.* 1999;124: 1281–1289.
39. Maeno Y, Tananari Y, Ishii M, et al. [Assessment of the interatrial septum using three-dimensional transesophageal echocardiography]. [Japanese]. *J Cardiology* 1999;34: 159–161.
40. Ansingkar K, Nanda NC, Aaluri SR, et al. Transesophageal three dimensional color Doppler echocardiographic assessment of valvular and paravalvular mitral prosthetic regurgitation. *Echocardiography* 2000;17:579–583.
41. Binder TM, Rosenhek R, Porenta G, et al. Improved assessment of mitral valve stenosis by volumetric real-time three-dimensional echocardiography. [see comments]. *J Am Coll Cardiology* 2000;36(4):1355–1361.
42. Buck T, Mucci RA, Guerrero JL, et al. The power-velocity integral at the vena contracta: A new method for direct quantification of regurgitant volume flow. *Circulation* 2000;102(9):1053–1061.
43. Chauvel C, Bogino E, Clerc P, Fernandez G, Vernhet JC, Becat A, Dehant P: Usefulness of three-dimensional echocardiography for the evaluation of mitral valve prolapse: An intraoperative study. *J Heart Valve Disease* 2000;9(3):341–349.
44. Flachskampf FA, Chandra S, Gaddipatti A, et al. Analysis of shape and motion of the mitral annulus in subjects with and without cardiomyopathy by echocardiographic 3-dimensional reconstruction. *J Am Soc Echocardiography* 2000;13(4):277–287.
45. Huang WY, Nanda NC, Miller A, et al. Fibrotic aortic stenosis in a patient with dwarfism. *Echocardiography* 2000;17(7):701–704.
46. Zabalgoitia M. Echocardiographic assessment of prosthetic heart valves. [Review] [154 refs]. *Curr Prob Cardiol* 2000;25(3):157–218.
47. Vogel M, Ho SY, Lincoln C, et al. Transthoracic three-dimensional echocardiography for the assessment of straddling tricuspid or mitral valves. *Cardiol in theYoung* 2000;10(6):603–609.
48. Kaplan SR, Bashein G, Sheehan FH, et al. Three-dimensional echocardiographic assessment of annular shape changes in the normal and regurgitant mitral valve. *Am Heart J* 2000;139(3):378–387.
49. Sutaria N, Northridge D, Masani N, et al. Three dimensional echocardiography for the assessment of mitral valve disease. [Review] [20 refs]. *Heart* 2000;84(Suppl.2):II7–10.
50. Lassige TA, Benkeser PJ, Fyfe D, et al. Comparison of septal defects in 2D and 3D echocardiography using active contour models. *Comp Medical Imag Graphics* 2000;24(6):377–388.
51. Liel-Cohen N, Guerrero JL, Otsuji Y, et al. Design of a new surgical approach for ventricular remodeling to relieve ischemic mitral regurgitation: Insights from 3-dimensional echocardiography. *Circulation* 2000;101(23):2756–2763.
52. Martin RP: The fish mouth and three-dimensional echocardiography: New technology catches an old problem. [letter; comment]. [Review] [6 refs]. *J Am Coll Cardiol* 2000;36(4):1362–1364.
53. Otsuji Y, Handschumacher MD, Liel-Cohen N, et al.

Mechanism of ischemic mitral regurgitation with segmental left ventricular dysfunction: Three-dimensional echocardiographic studies in models of acute and chronic progressive regurgitation. *J Am Coll Cardiol* 2001;37(2):641–648.

54. Izumi C, Himura Y, Iga K, et al. Relationship between papillary muscle size and benefit to cardiac function in mitral valve replacement with chordal preservation. *J Heart Valve Disease* 2001;10(1):57–64.
55. Horton Jr. CJ, Nanda NC, Nekkanti R, et al. Prosthetic aortic valve abscess producing total right coronary artery occlusion: Diagnosis by transesophageal three-dimensional echocardiography. *Echocardiography* (In press, August 2002).

Chapter 4

Aortic Pathology

Navin C. Nanda, MD and Vincent L. Sorrell, MD

Owing to its proximal location to the esophagus, no other diagnostic modality (invasive or noninvasive) exists that is capable of such high resolution images of the aorta as three-dimensional transesophageal echo (3D TEE). Furthermore, cardiac magnetic resonance imaging (MRI) and computed tomography (CT) do not image in real-time, additionally limiting the detection of mobile atherosclerotic debris. It has been our anecdotal experience that this finding is one of the most common pathologies identified in patients with unexplained strokes and without cardiovascular symptoms. Three-dimensionally acquired data sets allow complete visualization of these complexly shaped lesions and often improve the traditional knowledge obtained with conventional two-dimensional (2D) data.

Aortic dissections are life threatening and require rapid diagnosis and emergent surgery if they involve the ascending or transverse aorta (Stanford Type A). It has been reported that patients will experience a 1% per hour mortality rate for the first 48 hours. The extent of the dissection, as well as the involvement of the aortic valve, coronary arteries, pericardium or great vessels, is vitally important to the surgeon performing the operation. The great vessels are occasionally difficult to visualize even with experienced TEE operators, and this extended field of vision is the one clear advantage of CT and MRI. With 3D imaging, which requires the desired object to be placed in the middle of the region of interest, the great vessels are even more difficult to interrogate. However, the tradeoff for this small limitation is worthwhile. With TEE, as opposed to MRI or CT imaging, the information is obtained in the patient's room, preventing the need to transport the often clinically ill patient. Information is interpreted immediately. The left ventricular (LV) size and function, aortic valve competence, pericardium, pleural space, proximal coronary arteries, as well as an extensive search for other cardiac causes of the patient's symptoms are also rapidly noted.

Importantly, 3D imaging enhances the interpreter's confidence by more clearly interrogating the intimal flap. With 2D imaging, this flap is seen as a thin, linear, mobile intra-aortic echo, and is occasionally difficult to differentiate from reverberation artifacts. This fact has been previously reported in the literature in erroneous, false-positive case reports. This is less common with experienced TEE performers who use multiple imaging planes and combine 2D with Doppler data, but is likely nonexistent with 3D imaging, since the intimal flap has a distinct appearance. With 3D imaging, the flap is seen as a membrane or a sheet, and the surface of the dissected aortic intima in no way appears as a linear artifact. This fact should further enhance the advantage of TEE imaging for a suspected aortic dissection.

This chapter provides multiple examples of aortic aneurysms, uncomplicated and complicated dissections, and aortic atherosclerotic debris. Readers should also see the images in the following chapters: Aortic abscess (Valvular Heart Diseases); Coarctation of the aorta and right sided aortic arch (Congenital Heart Diseases).

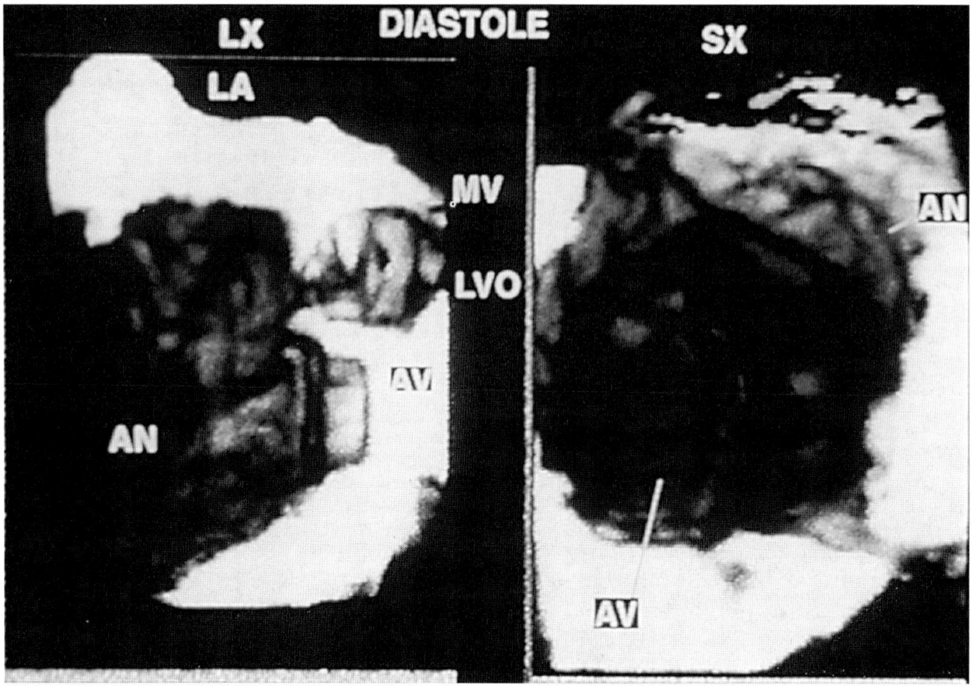

Figure 1. Transesophageal three-dimensional echocardiographic reconstruction in aortic aneurysm without dissection. Note the absence of a dissection flap. AN = aortic aneurysm; AV = aortic valve; LA = left atrium; MV = mitral valve; LX = long axis; SX = short axis. Reproduced with permission from Nanda NC et al. Three-dimensional echocardiographic assessment of aortic dissection. *Echocardiography* 1998;15:745–754.

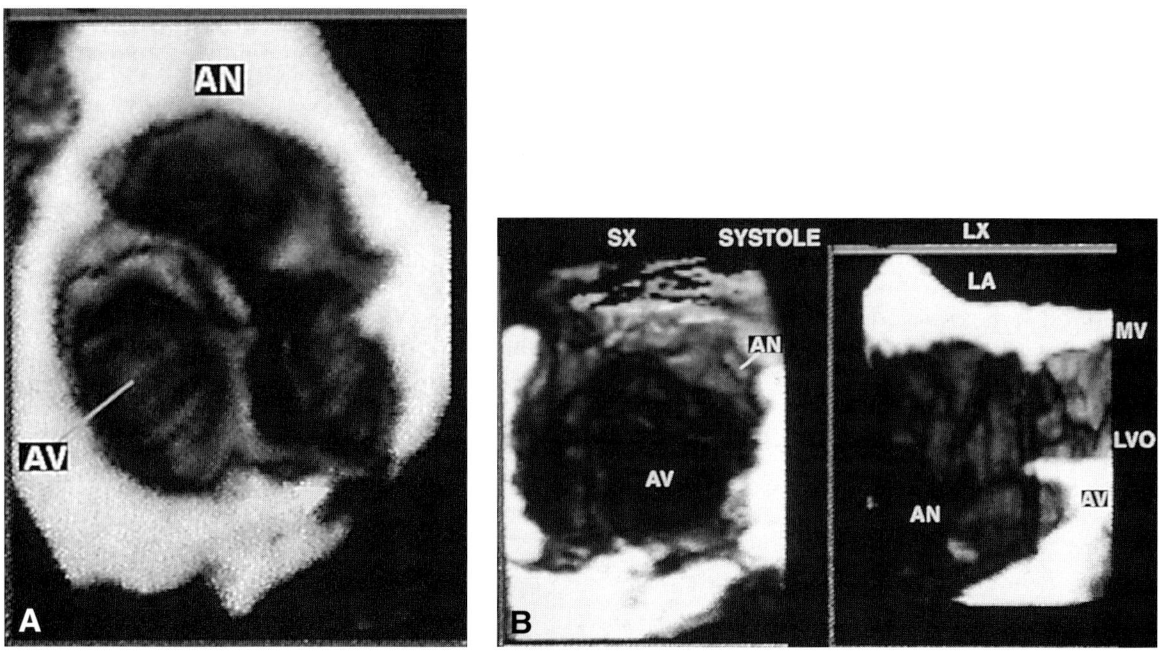

Figure 2. (**A**) Transesophageal short-axis, upper esophageal image of the aortic valve (AV) in a patient with an aortic aneurysm (AN). Arrow = left main coronary artery ostium. (**B**) Same patient as in the previous figure. The AN is seen in short axis (left) and long axis (right). LA = left atrium; LVO = left ventricular outflow tract; MV = mitral valve.

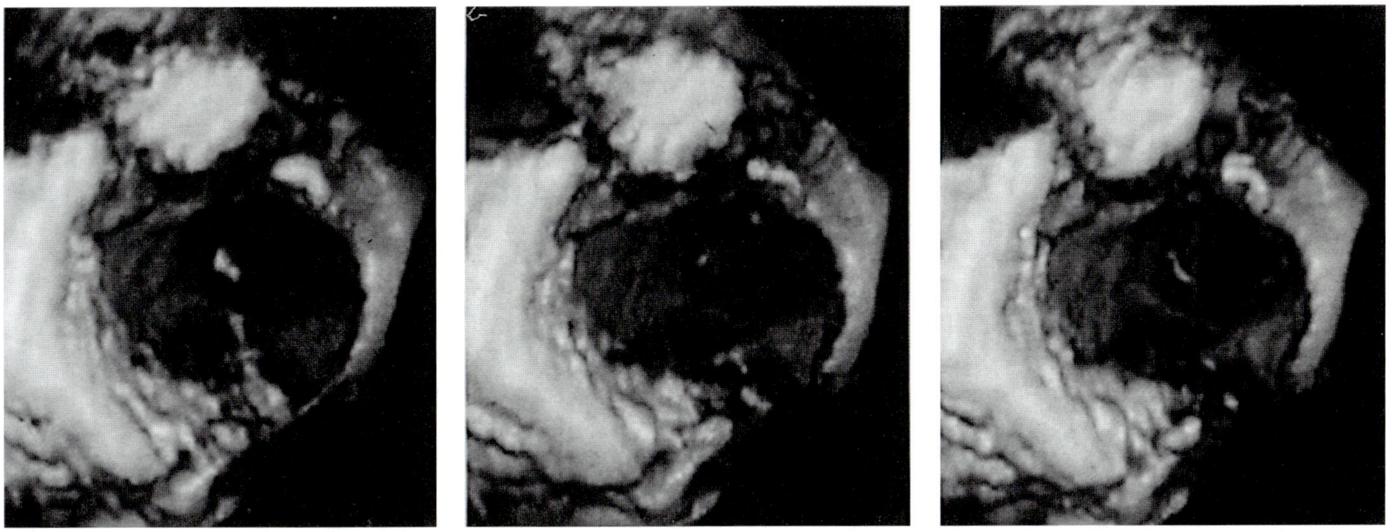

Figure 3. Aneurysm of the ascending aorta with aortic regurgitation. Three-dimensional reconstruction of spatial structure of the aorta. The maximal dimension of the aorta ascendens is 8.4 cm. Aortic annulus is involved in the aortic dilation, which is the key mechanism of the aortic regurgitation. Spontaneous echo contrast in the aorta is reconstructed and presented as a solid structure inside the aortic lumen. From Jaroslaw Drozdz, MD, and Jaroslaw D. Kasprzak, MD.

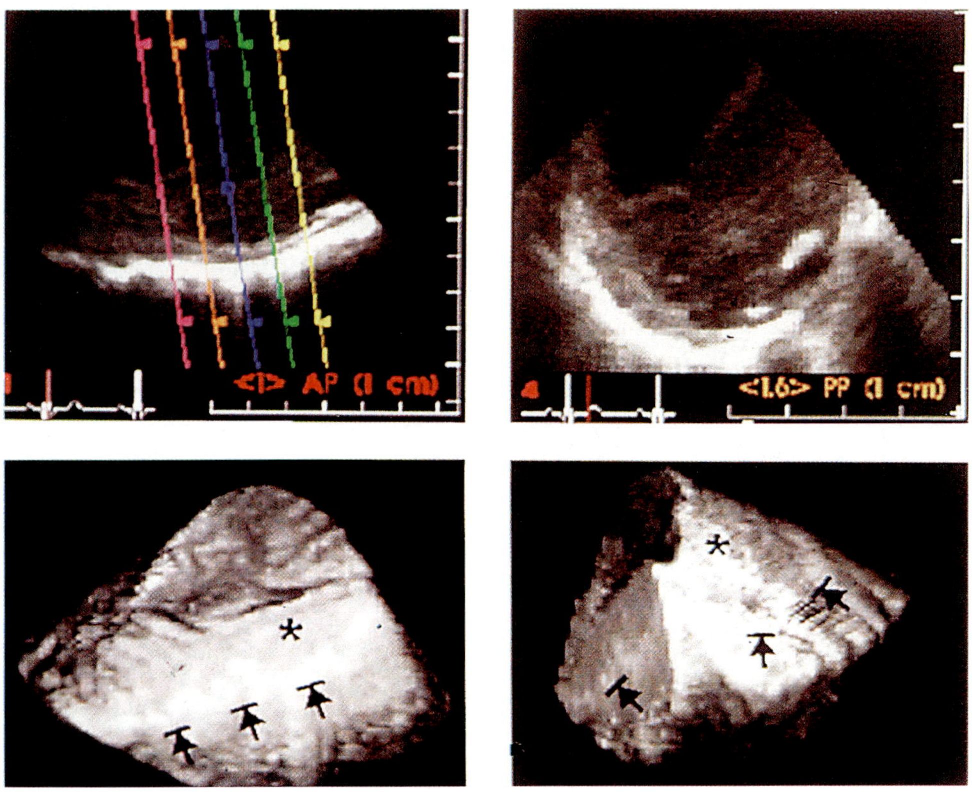

Figure 4. Three-dimensional echocardiogram of an aneurysmal segment of the descending aorta with a large mural thrombus (*). Upper panels are anyplane reconstructed views of the lesion: in aortic long and short axis. In volume-rendered views (bottom panels) the appropriate use of shading allows to display the borders of thrombus and the aortic wall contour (arrows). The aortic segment is visualized from different viewpoints to improve the perception of depth. From Jaroslaw D. Kasprzak, MD.

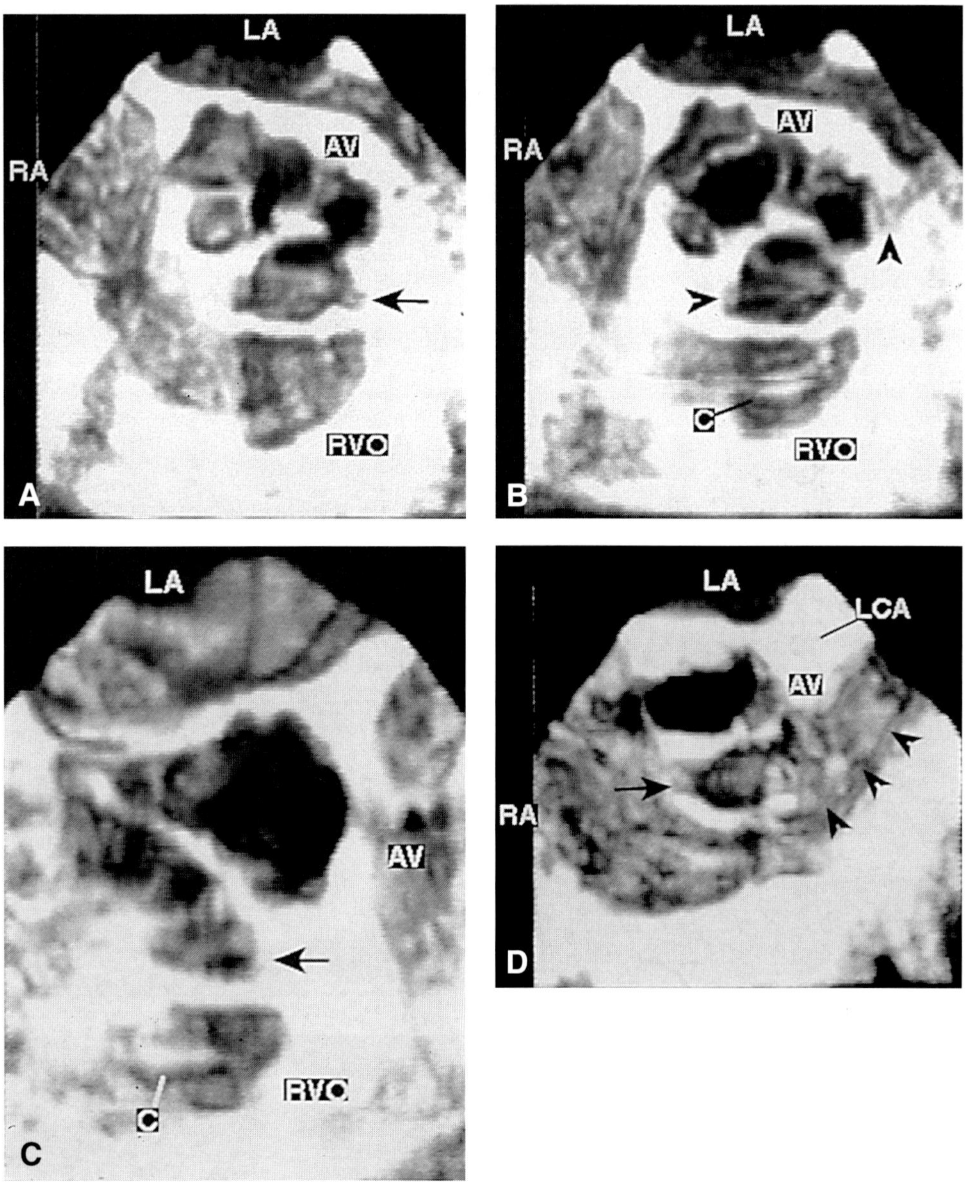

Figure 5. (**A**) Transesophageal echocardiographic short axis image of the aortic valve in a patient with endocarditis and extension of infection into the aortic wall creating an aortic abscess. (**B**) The arrowheads point to multiple abscess cavities. (**C**) A catheter "C" is seen in the right ventricular outflow tract. (**D**) Additional adjustment of the imaging perspective allows the three-dimensional dataset to be displayed for optimal clarification of the extent of these abscesses (arrows). AV = aortic valve; LA = left atrium; LCA = left coronary artery; RA = right atrium.

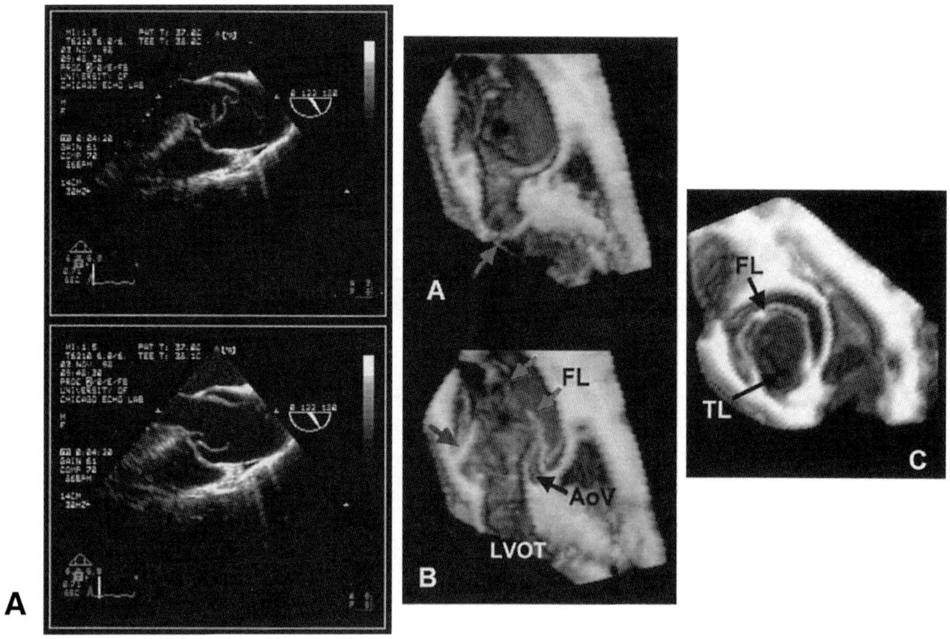

Figure 6A. Two-dimensional echo images of a Type A aortic dissection are shown on the left. (**A**) Three-dimensional reconstructions of the dissection flap (FL) in a long-axis orientation was observed prolapsing into the left ventricular outflow tract indicated by the red arrow. (**B**) In systole, the aortic valve was better observed with the dissection flap arising above the aortic valve and followed for a small portion of the ascending aorta. (**C**) A cross-sectional view of the flap viewed cranially towards the ascending aorta demonstrating the true lumen and the intimal flap.

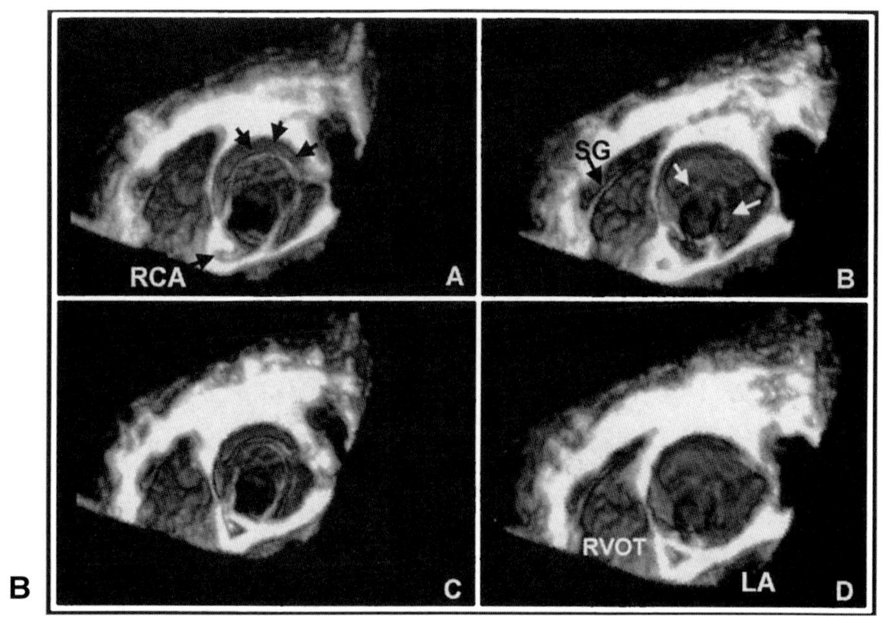

Figure 6B. In the same patient with a type A dissection, several short axis cuts were performed to define coronary artery involvement. All views are from the ascending aorta looking down towards the aortic valve. (**A**) The dissection flap can be followed around (black arrows) from the ostia of the right coronary artery. Through this dissection flap, which is the true lumen, the tips of the aortic valve leaflets and left ventricular outflow tract are observed. During diastole (**B**), the dissection flap prolapses through the aortic valve into the left ventricular outflow tract. The flap covers the aortic valve leaflets shown by the white arrows. A Swan-Ganz (SG) catheter is seen in the right ventricular outflow tract. In panels **C** and **D,** the cutplane is set above the sinotubular junction. From Lissa Sugeng, MD, Ivan Godoy, MD, Kirk T. Spencer, MD, Jim Bednarz, BS, Lynn Weinert, BS, and Roberto M. Lang, MD.

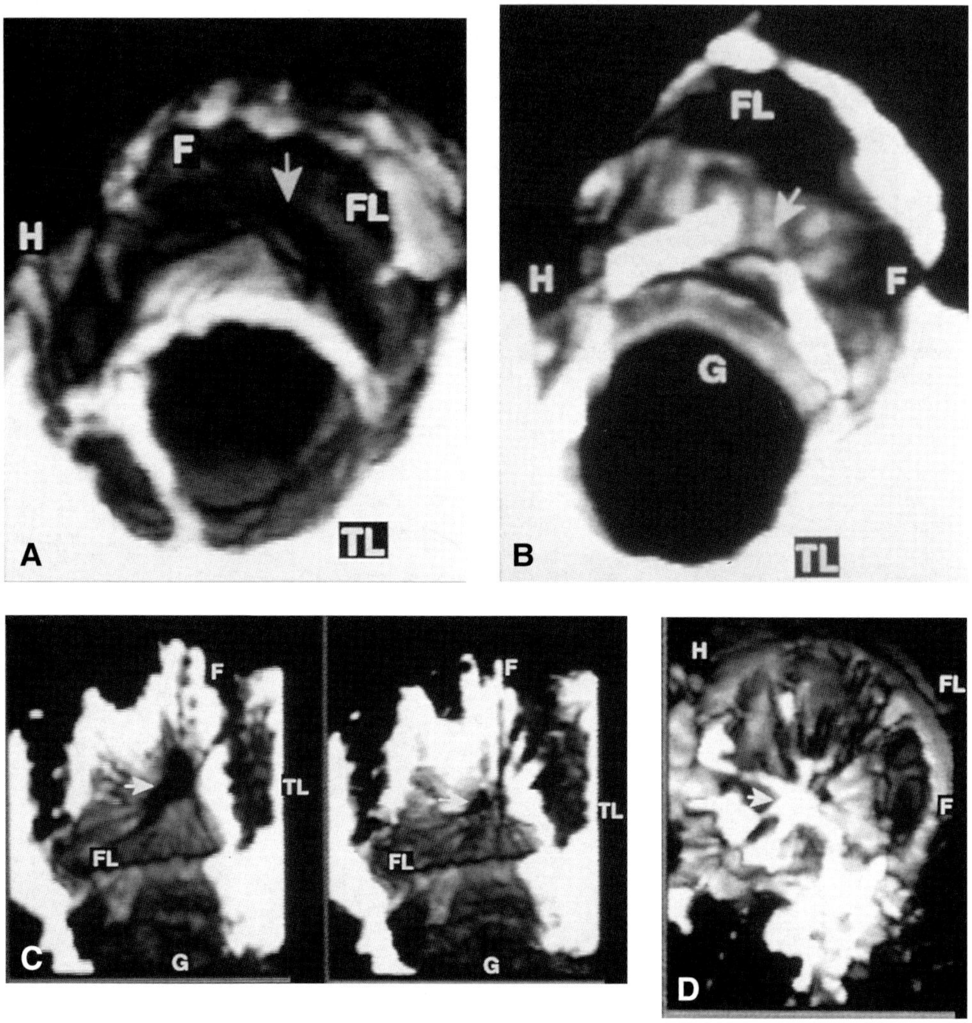

Figure 7. (**A**) A posteriorly directed transesophageal echocardiographic short axis image of the descending aorta in a patient with a surgically repaired, large, chronic type B dissection. (**B**) At a slightly different depth, the actual entry site into the subintimal space is readily visualized (arrow). (**C**) The comprehensive, three-dimensional data set allows the orientation to be chosen, as seen in this image of the patient in the previous figures. Here, the entry site is visualized in an *en face* view and noted to be larger in systole (**left**) than diastole (**right**). (**D**) The Doppler flow can also be reconstructed and can be seen entering (arrow) into this entry site noted in the previous few figures. FL = false lumen; TL = true lumen; H = hematoma; arrow = entry site; G= graft from surgical repair; F = intimal flap.

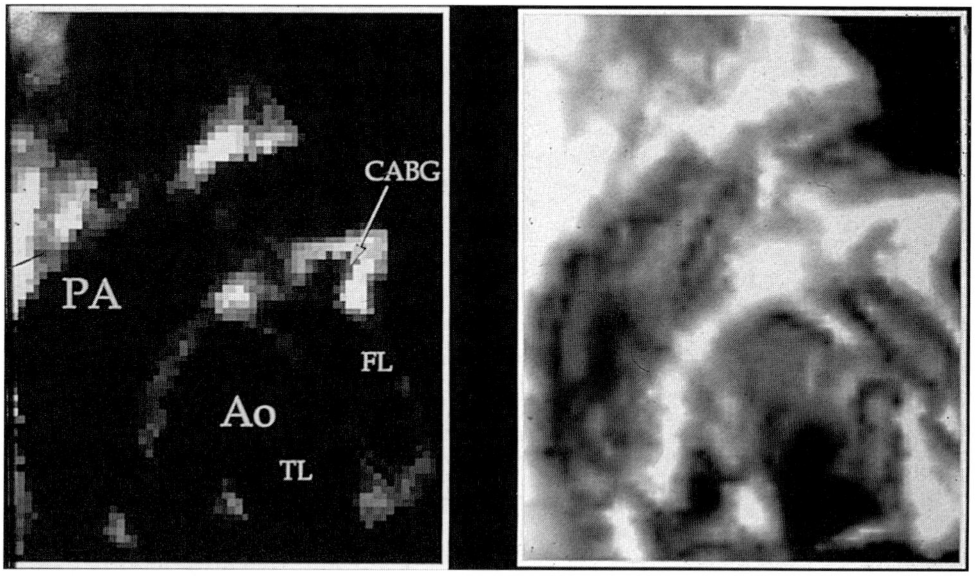

Figure 8. Aortic dissection. **Right:** Three-dimensional reconstruction showing a flap in the ascending aorta, the true lumen and the false lumen. Ostium of a coronary artery bypass graft is seen arising from the false lumen, and was not identified in the original two-dimensional images. **Left:** corresponding slice through the reconstructed volume with legends. Ao = aorta; CABG = coronary artery bypass graft; FL = false lumen; PA = pulmonary artery; TL = true lumen. From Cedric Vuille, MD and Rene Lerch, MD.

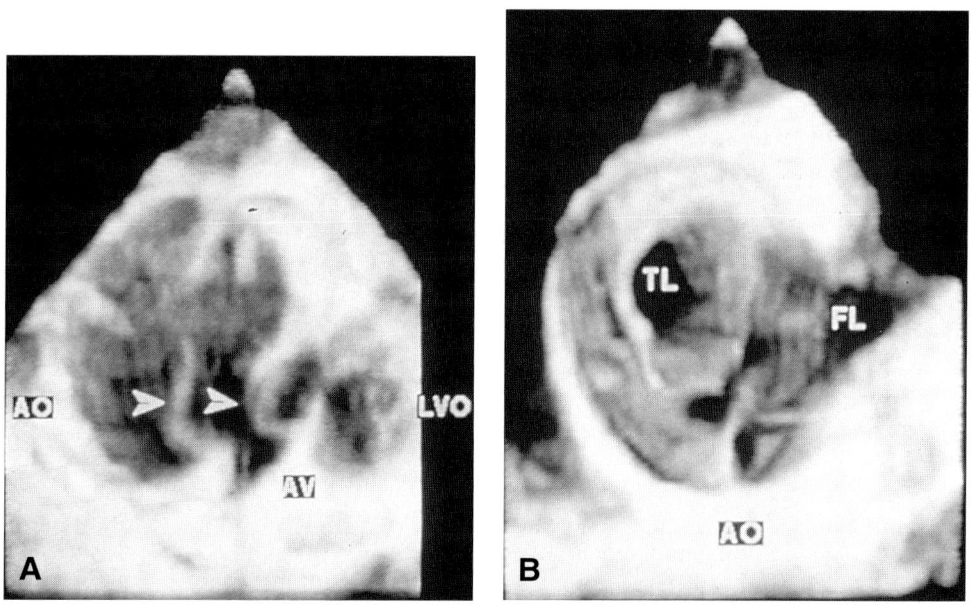

Figure 9. (**A,B**) Transesophageal three-dimensional echocardiographic reconstruction in aortic dissection. The dissection flap (arrowheads in **A**) is shown impinging on the aortic valve (AV). AO = aorta; FL = false lumen; LVO = left ventricular outflow tract; TL = true lumen. Reproduced with permission from Nanda NC et al. Three-dimensional echocardiographic assessment of aortic dissection. *Echocardiography:* 1998;15:745–754.

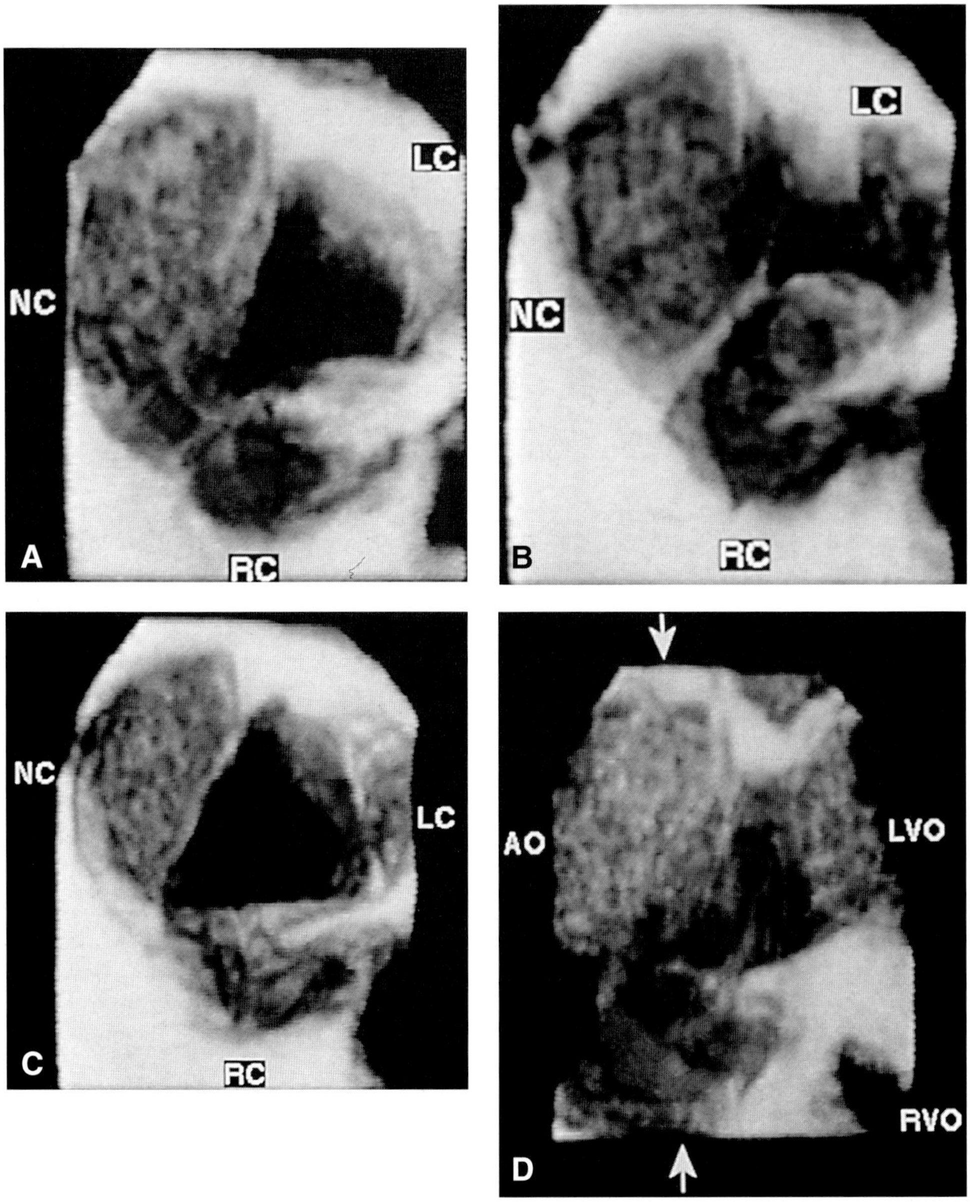

Figure 10. (**A**) Transesophageal echo zoom, short-axis image of an aortic valve in a patient with dilatation of the sinuses of Valsalva. Note the greatest dilatation of the noncoronary region (NC). LC = left coronary cusp; RC = right coronary cusp. (**B, C**) Additional images may be displayed to provide further insight into the complete anatomic relationships. (**D**) Longitudinal aortic root image that displays the characterization of the sinuses of Valsalva and their relationship to the left and right ventricular outflow tracts.

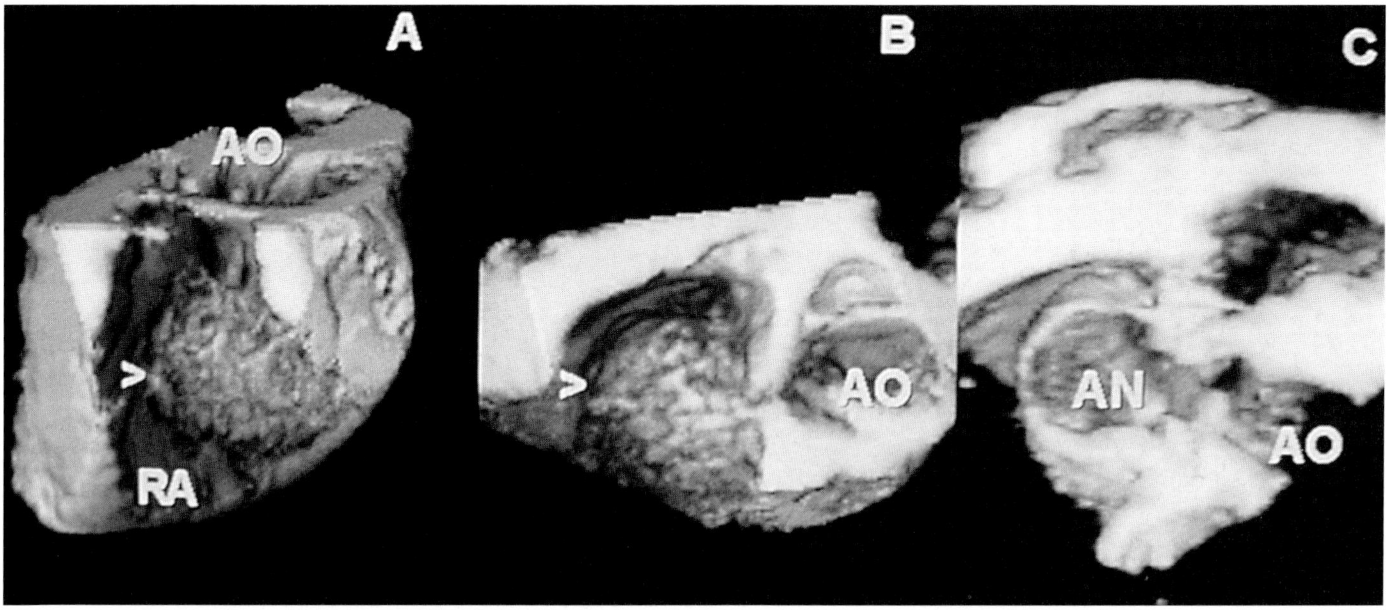

Figure 11. Aneurysm of sinus of Valsalva. In this patient, the aneurysm originated in the noncoronary sinus and entered into the right atrium. (**A, B**) The wall of the aneurysm in the right atrium was adjacent to the aorta. (**C**) After cutting the aneurysm and removing the anterior wall, a hole located between the aneurysm and the aortic root could be seen. From Xin-Fang Wang, MD. Adapted from Wang XF, Li ZA, Cheng TO, et al: Four-dimensional echocardiography: Methods and clinical application. *Am Heart J* 1996;132:682.

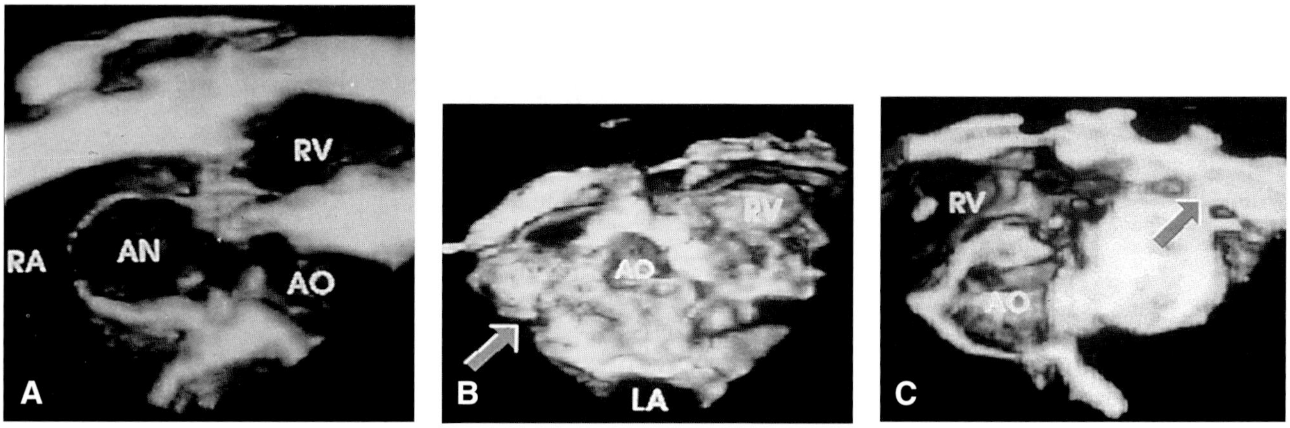

Figure 12. Dynamic three-dimensional images of shunt flow in ruptured aneurysm of sinus of Valsalva. (**A**) Stereoscopic aneurysm body (AN) protruding into the right atrium (RA). (**B**) Shunt flow originating from the aorta (AO) and moving into the aneurysm and the RA (arrow) in the same patient. (**C**) Shunt flow (arrow) originating from the AO and moving into the aneurysm and the right ventricle (RV) in another patient. LA = left atrium. Reproduced with permission from Li Z et al. Dynamic three-dimensional reconstruction of abnormal intracardiac blood flow. *Echocardiography* 1997;14:375–381.

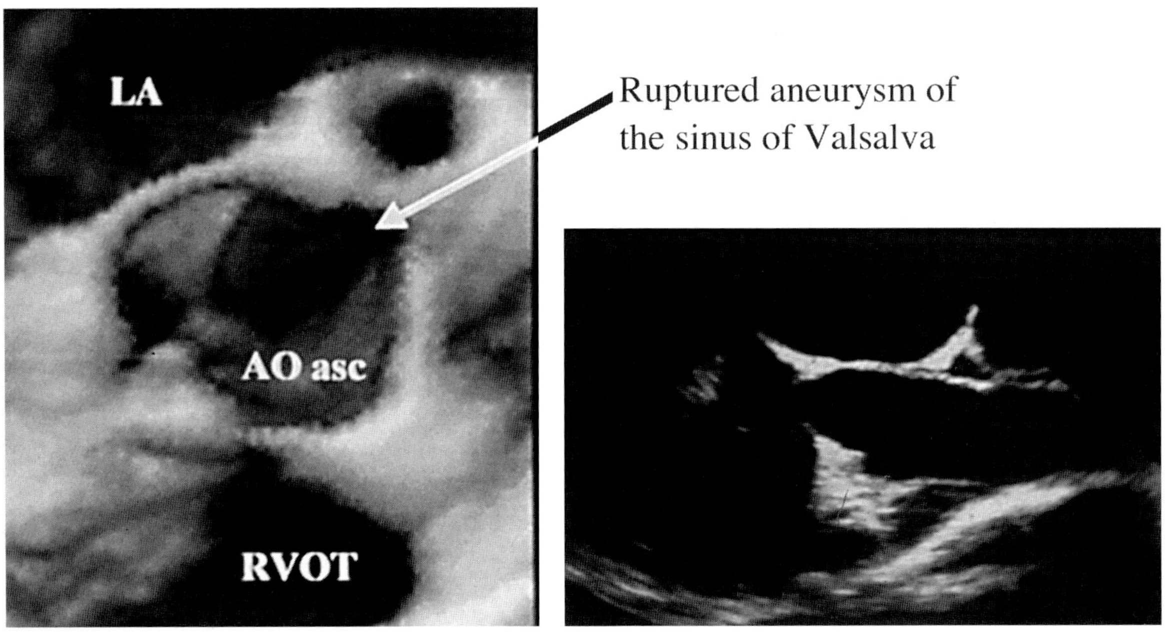

Figure 13. Ruptured Valsalva sinus aneurysm. A 46-year-old male with clinical picture of progressive congestive heart failure. Two-dimensional transesophageal echo view reveals Valsalva sinus ruptured into the right atrium (**right**). Detailed anatomical perspective from the aorta is obtained in volume-rendered three-dimensional (3D) view of the rupture (**left**). The optimal cutplane and angulation, enabled by anyplane 3D echocardiography, enabled the measurement of the orifice of the rupture of 0.97 cm^2. From Jaroslaw Drozdz, MD and Jaroslaw D. Kasprzak, MD.

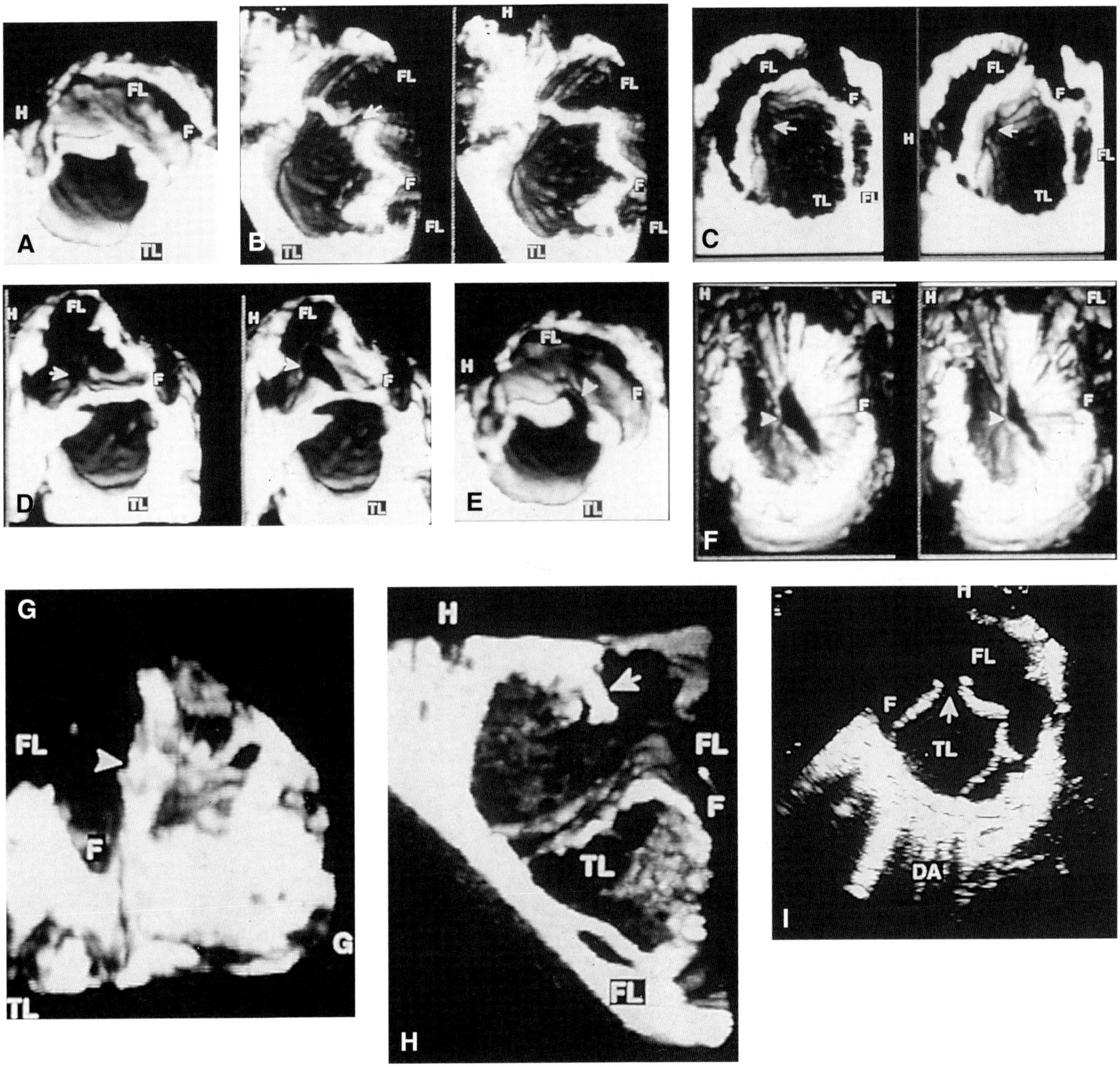

Figure 14. Transesophageal three-dimensional echocardiographic reconstruction in aortic dissection. (**A–I**) The descending thoracic aorta was examined using multiple cut sections and various viewing angles. Both the true (TL) and the false (FL) lumens are well visualized, and the dissection flap (F) presents as a sheet-like structure along the aortic length. The communication (arrows) between the true and false lumens is viewed from within the true (**C**) and false lumens (**D–F**) as well as *en face* (**F**) using a transverse section. As would be expected, the communication is larger in systole than in diastole (**D** and **F**). The arrowhead in **G** shows color Doppler flow signals moving from the true lumen into the false lumen. In **H,** the arrow points to a linear echo density attached to the wall of the false lumen adjacent to a mediastinal hematoma (H), which resulted from rupture of the dissection. This echo density is consistent with a fibrin plug. (**I**) represents a two-dimensional image shown for comparison. Note that the dissection flap (F) in the descending aorta (DSA) appears only as a linear structure, which has been difficult to differentiate from an artifact in some patients. Reproduced with permission from Nanda NC et al. Three-dimensional echocardiographic assessment of aortic dissection. *Echocardiography* 1998;15:745–754.

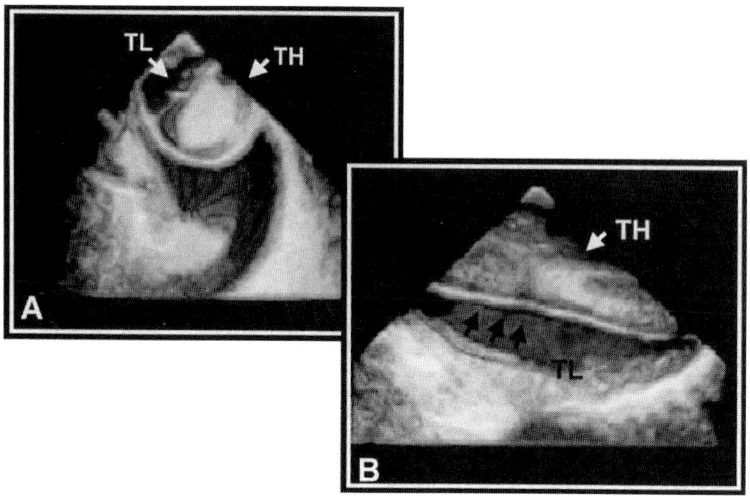

Figure 15. A three-dimensional study of a patient with a type B aortic dissection. The true lumen (TL) and false lumen filled with thrombus (TH) can be observed in a cross sectional view (**A**) and longitudinal cut (**B**). The length of the dissection flap is noted by the black arrows. From Lissa Sugeng, MD, Ivan Godoy, MD, Kirk T. Spencer, MD, Jim Bednarz, BS, Lynn Weinert, BS, and Roberto M. Lang, MD.

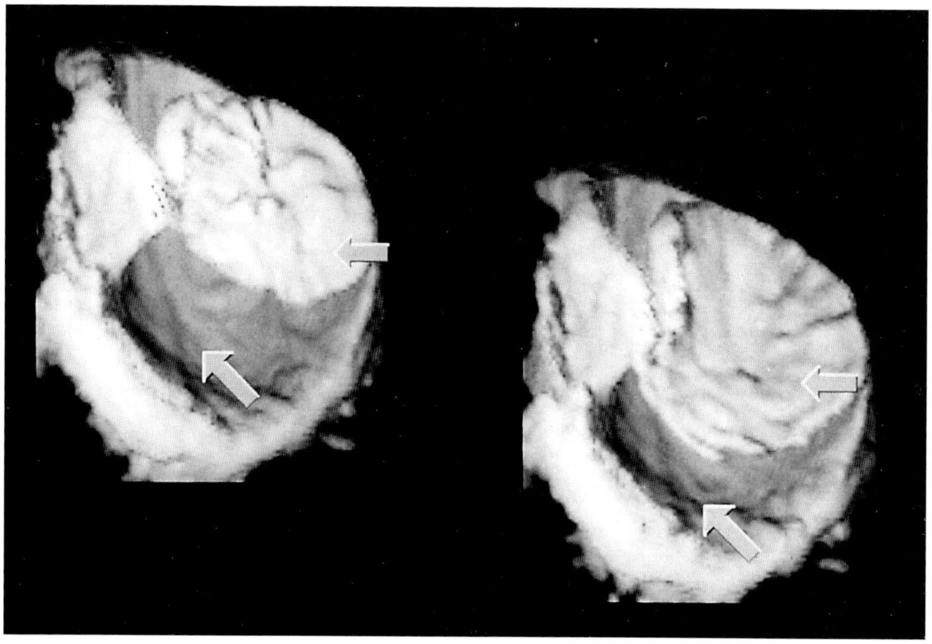

Figure 16. Dissection of the thoracic aorta. The flap (horizontal arrow) is moving during the cardiac cycle and the false channel is well displayed (oblique arrow). From Albert A. Hagège, MD.

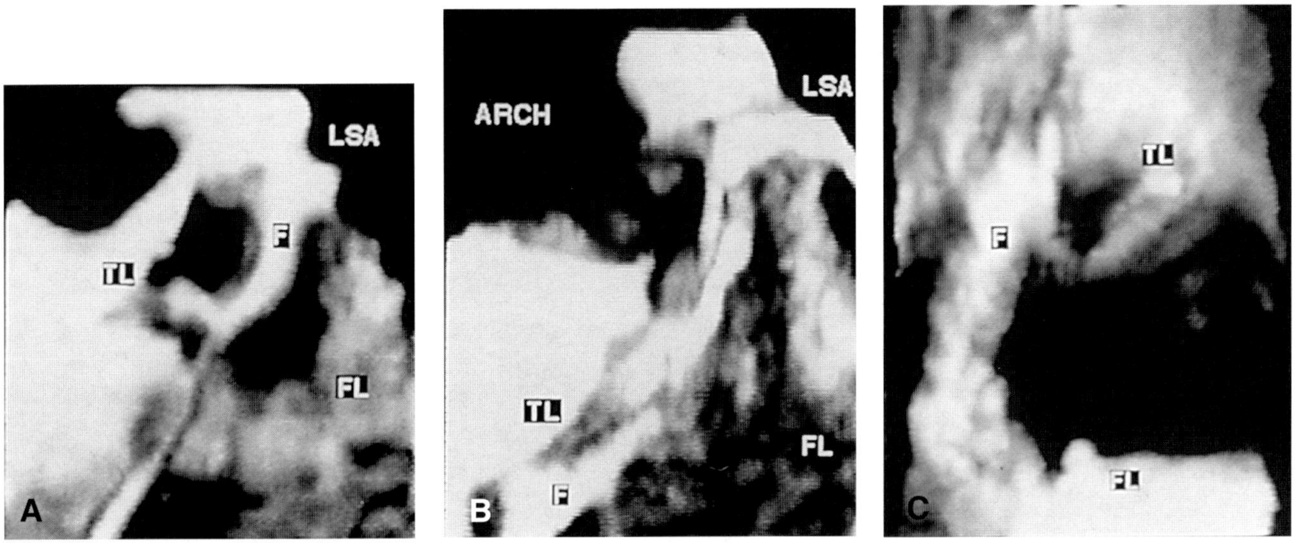

Figure 17. Transthoracic three-dimensional reconstruction in aortic dissection. (**A** and **B**) The dissection flap (F) presents as a sheet-like structure in the descending thoracic aorta. The left subclavian artery (LSA) is uninvolved. (**C**) The dissected abdominal aorta is viewed in three-dimensions. FL = false lumen; TL = true lumen. Reproduced with permission from Nanda NC et al. Three-dimensional echocardiographic assessment of aortic dissection. *Echocardiography* 1998;15:745–754.

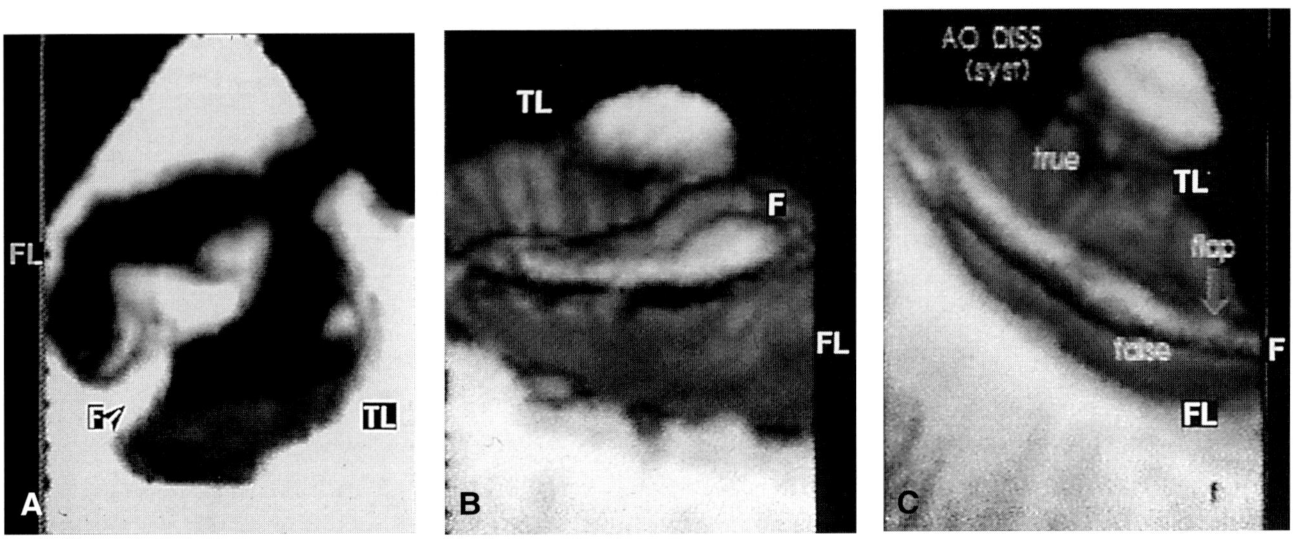

Figure 18A-C. Transesophageal short-axis image of the descending aorta in a patient with a dissection. (**A**) The communication between the true lumen (TL) and the false lumen (FL) is readily identified. The intimal "flap" is well seen (F). (**B**) Long-axis orientation of the same patient. Note the inequality of the thickness of the intimal flap, not possible with conventional two-dimensional imaging. (**C**) With a slightly different cutplane, an additional horizontal long-axis image is obtained and reveals even greater anatomic detail and a greater extent of the "flap."

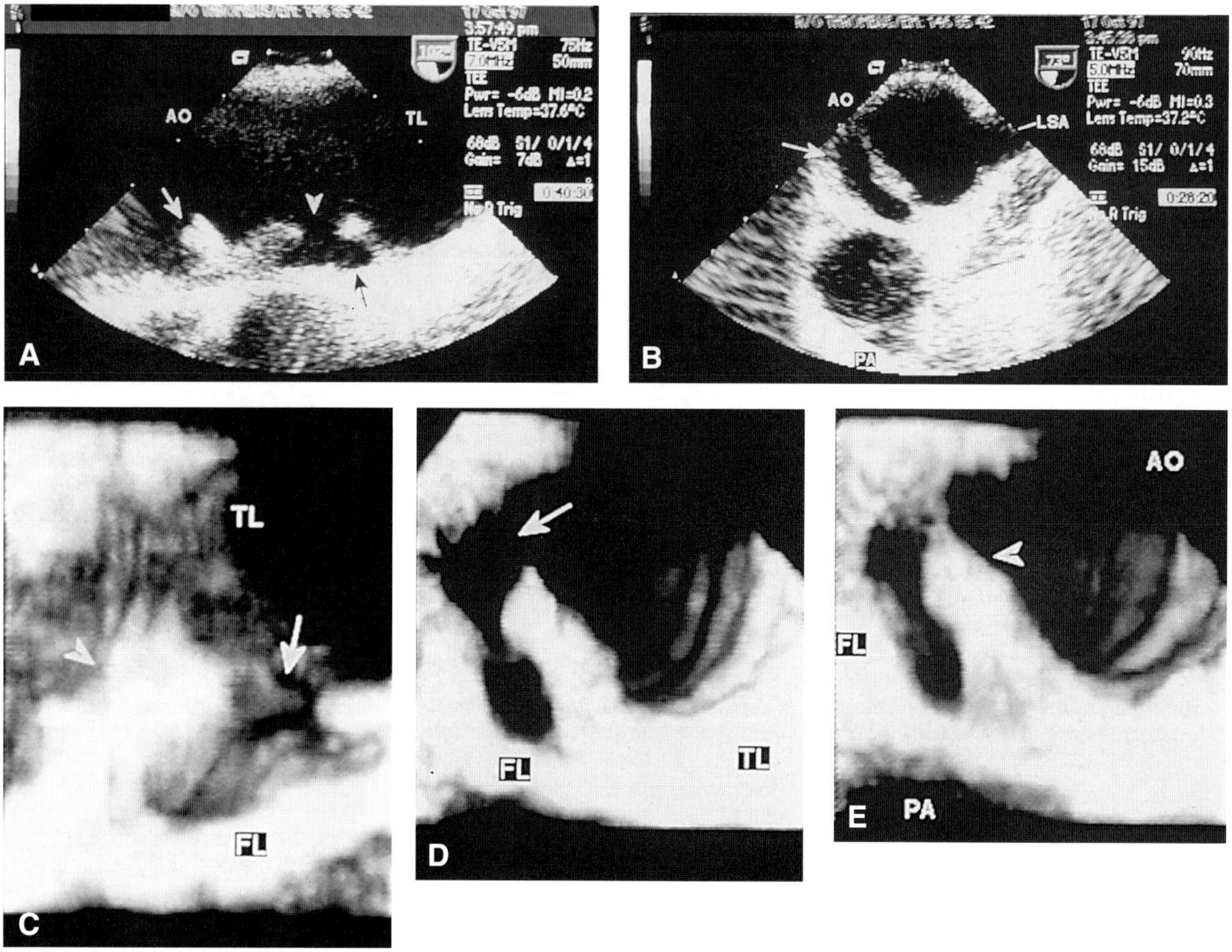

Figure 19. Traumatic rupture of atherosclerotic plaque-producing aortic isthmus dissection. Multiplane transesophageal echocardiographic examination. (**A**) The arrowhead indicates the site of rupture in the atherosclerotic plaque (yellow arrow). Black arrow shows resulting dissection. The site of rupture is at the junction of a relatively less calcified and heavily calcified area of the plaque. (**B**) Circumferential extent of aortic dissection (arrow). (**C–E**) Three-dimensionally reconstructed transesophageal echocardiographic images graphically demonstrate the site of rupture (arrows in **C** and **D**) in the atherosclerotic plaque (arrowheads in **C** and **E**). AO = aorta; FL = false lumen; LSA = left subclavian artery; PA = pulmonary artery; TL = true lumen. Reproduced with permission from Samal AK et al. Traumatic rupture of atherosclerotic plaque producing aortic isthmus dissection. *Echocardiography* 1998;15:695–702.

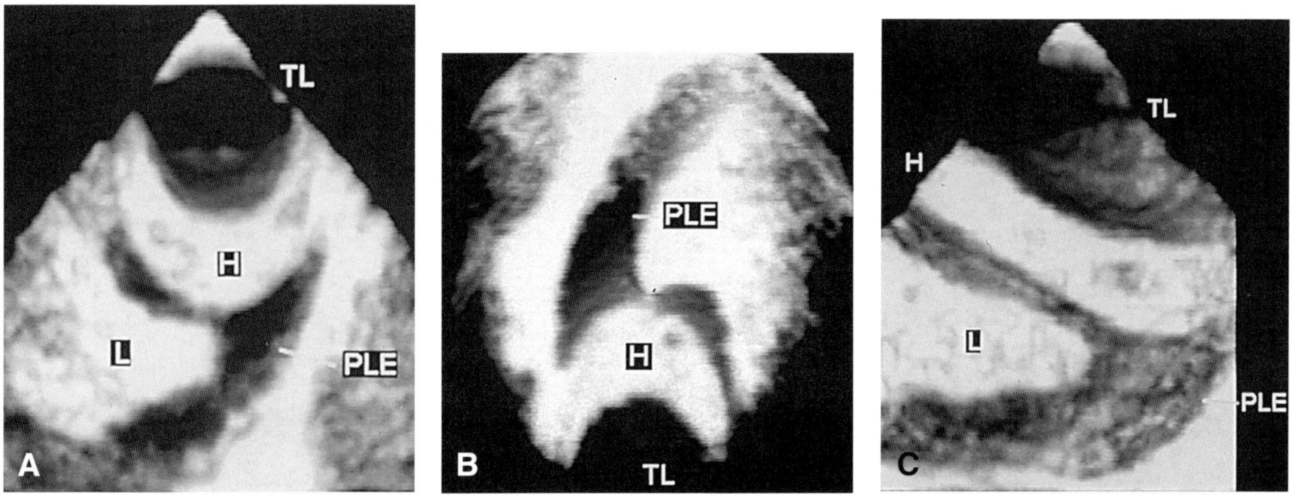

Figure 20. (**A**) In this patient, an aortic dissection is not visible, but a hematoma (H) and pleural effusion (PLE) can be seen near the lung (L). (**B**) By inverting the image, some readers may be more adjusted to interpreting certain pathologies from specific orientations. This is the same image as the previous slide. Because of the slightly tilted imaging perspective, the aortic lumen is visualized to a greater extent than in the previous image, but the aortic wall is less well clarified. (**C**) This is the same patient now shown in a long-axis orientation. Note the excellent definition of the internal aortic wall. TL = aortic lumen.

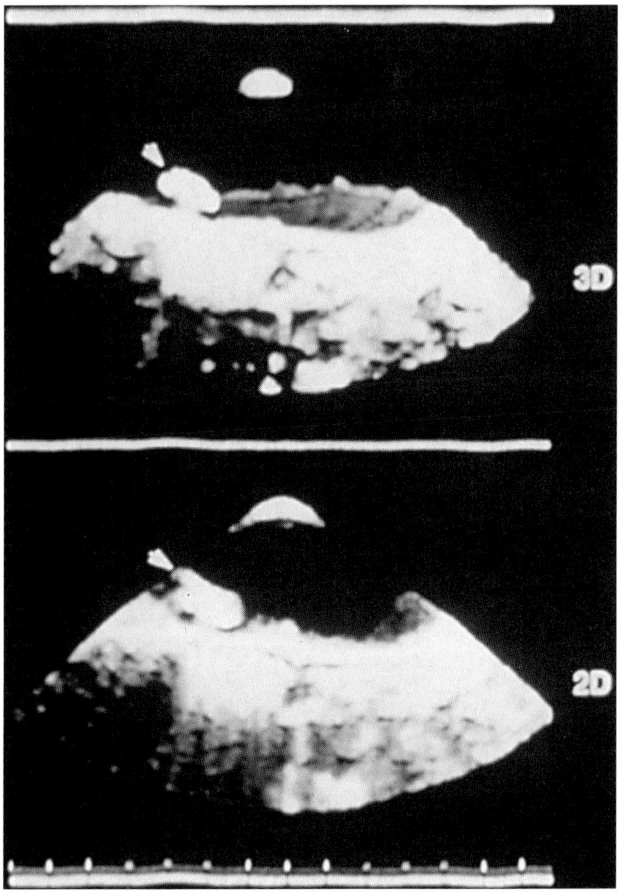

Figure 21. Atheromatous plaque (arrow) in the aortic arch seen in three dimensions (3D) (**top**). The two-dimensional (2D) image is shown (**bottom**) for comparison. Reproduced with permission from Nanda NC et al. Incremental value of three-dimensional echocardiography over transeosphageal multiplane two-dimensional echocardiography in qualitative and quantitative assessment of cardiac masses and defects. *Echocardiography* 1995;12:619–628

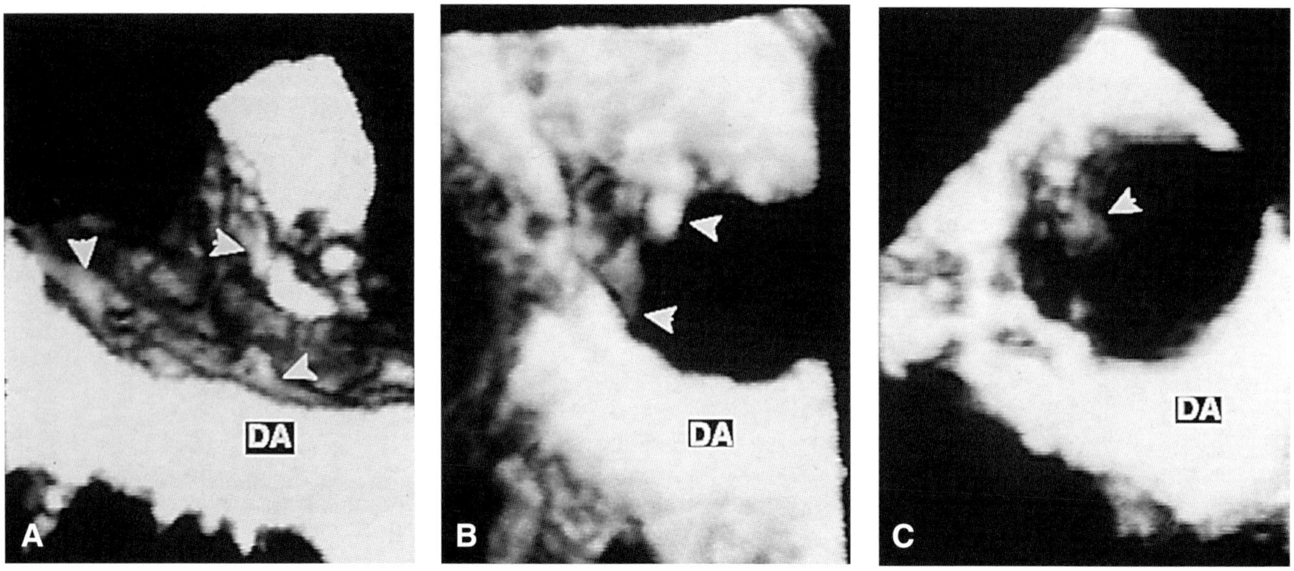

Figure 22A-C. (**A**) Transesophageal (TEE), long-axis image of the descending aorta in a patient with atheromatous debris (arrows). A zoom tangential (**B**) and short axis (**C**) of the TEE three-dimensional echo images shown in the previous figure. Arrow (s) = atheroma.

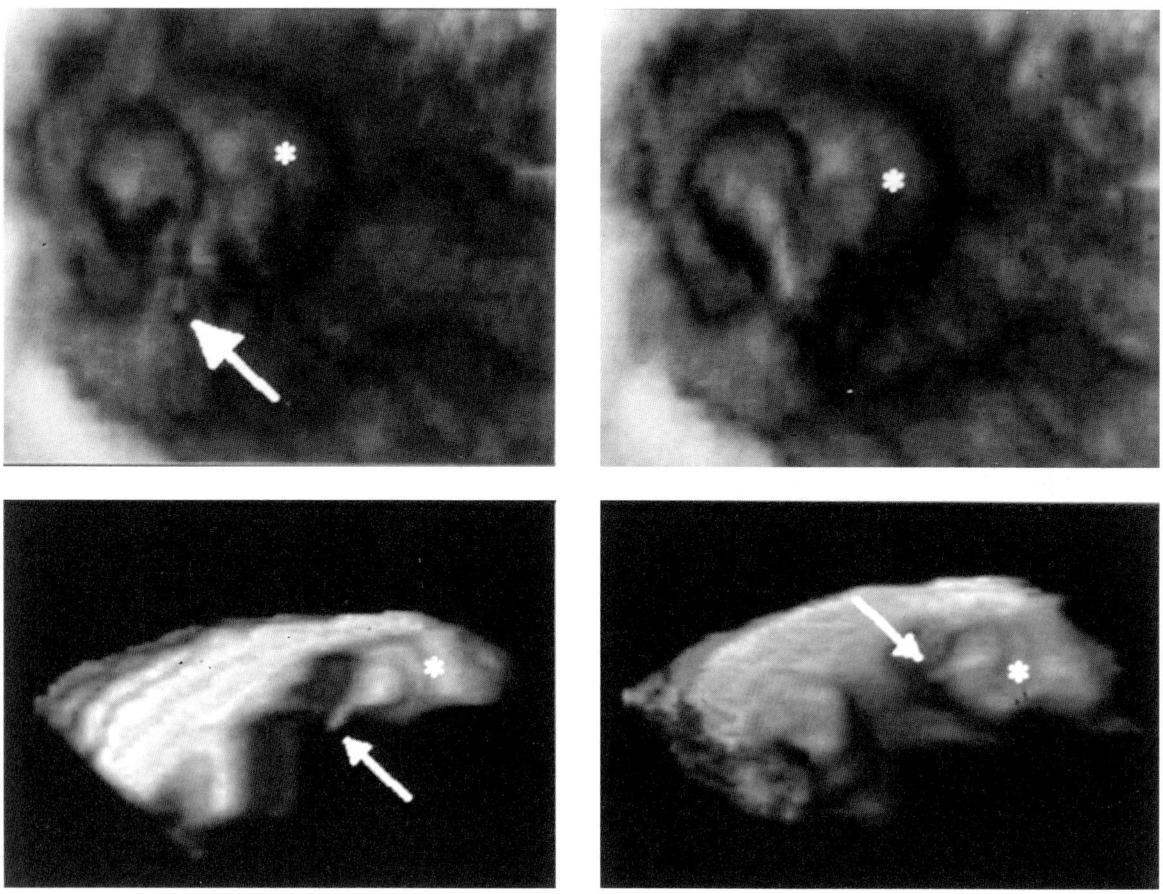

Figure 23. Volume-rendered reconstruction of an atherosclerotic lesion (*) in the aortic arch with an attached mobile thrombus (arrows). **Upper panels** are taken from a dynamic clip representing different phases of cardiac cycle, thus displaying a waving motion in the stream of blood. **Lower panels** represent electronically dissected segment of the aortic wall with the atheroma, visualized from different angles. From Jaroslaw D. Kasprzak, MD.

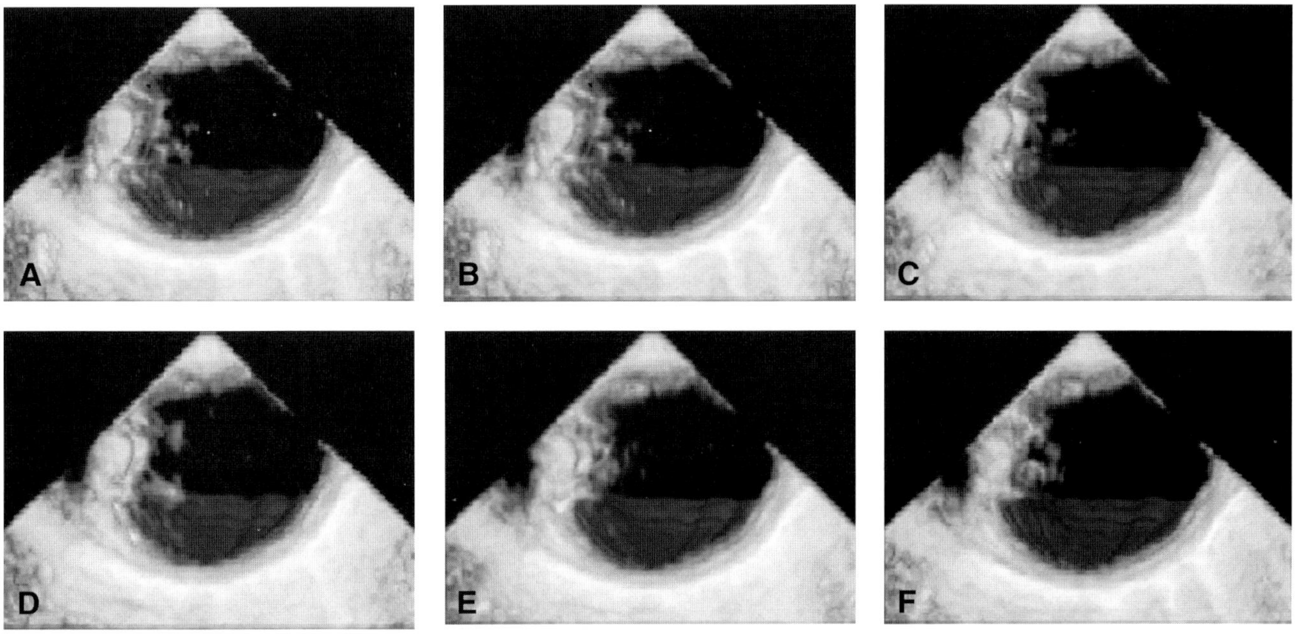

Figure 24. Aortic Atherosclerotic Debris. (**A–F**) Transesophageal echo (TEE) three-dimensional short axis image of the thoracic aorta. This series of images was obtained in a patient referred for TEE to evaluate a potential cardiac source of embolism after an unexplained stroke. Multiple frond-like structures were noted within the medial wall of the proximal descending aorta and protruding more than 1 cm into the aortic lumen. These were highly mobile and are displayed in sequence at different portions of the cardiac cycle. From Vincent L. Sorrell, MD.

Suggested Reading List

1. Khatri GK, Abd El-Rahman S, Fuisz AR, et al. Incremental value of 3-D echo over multiplane 2-D echo in aortic dissection and aortic rupture. (Abstract) *Circulation* 1996;94:117–176.
2. Nanda NC, Khatri GK, Samal A, et al. Three-dimensional echocardiographic assessment of aortic dissection. *Echocardiography* 1998;15:745–754.
3. Samal A, Nanda NC, Biederman RWW, et al. Traumatic rupture of atherosclerotic plaque producing aortic isthmus dissection. *Echocardiography* 1998;15:695–701.
4. Nanda NC, Samal AK, Bakir S, et al. Transesophageal echocardiographic diagnosis of right sided aortic arch. *Echocardiography* 1998;15:409–417.
5. Aaluri SR, Miller A, Nanda NC, et al. Transesophageal three dimensional color Doppler echocardiographic findings in traumatic aortic isthmus pseudoaneurysm. *Am J Geriatric Cardiol* 2000;9:286–288.
6. Ansingkar KG, Aaluri SR, Nanda NC. Three dimensional transesophageal echocardiographic demonstration of aortic dissection flap extending into right coronary artery ostium. *Am J Geriatric Cardiol* 2000;9:344–345.
7. Ansingkar KG, Nanda NC, Nekkanti Ret al. Transesophageal three dimensional color Doppler echocardiographic reconstruction of the left vertebral artery. *Echocardiography* (In press, October 2001).
8. Miller AP, Aaluri SR, Mukhtar OM, et al. Three-dimensional color Doppler transpharyngeal echocardiographic reconstruction of the left common, internal and external carotid arteries. *Echocardiography* (In press, May 2002).

Chapter 5

Coronary Artery Disease

Navin C. Nanda, MD and Vincent L. Sorrell, MD

Coronary artery disease remains the greatest killer in the United States and is soon to become the number one killer in the world. Traditional echocardiography is frequently used in these patients to evaluate the left ventricular (LV) function as well as the presence and size of myocardial aneurysms or intracavitary thrombi. More recently, direct visualization of the coronary arteries with transesophageal echocardiography (TEE) has provided clinically useful information.

In addition to the above common uses that are enhanced with three-dimensional (3D) imaging techniques, postinfarction complications (LV pseudoaneurysm; ventricular septal aneurysm; ruptured papillary muscle) are more clearly delineated with 3D and offer the surgeon clinically useful, incremental data above that obtained with two-dimensional (2D) echo. Imaging the coronary arteries highlights another important advantage of 3D data acquisition. Since these are extremely tortuous, they may not be interrogated within a single 2D imaging plane. However, since they remain within the 3D data set, they can be displayed to a greater extent. See also the chapter on Normal Anatomy, Normal Variants and Artifacts (anomalous coronary artery).

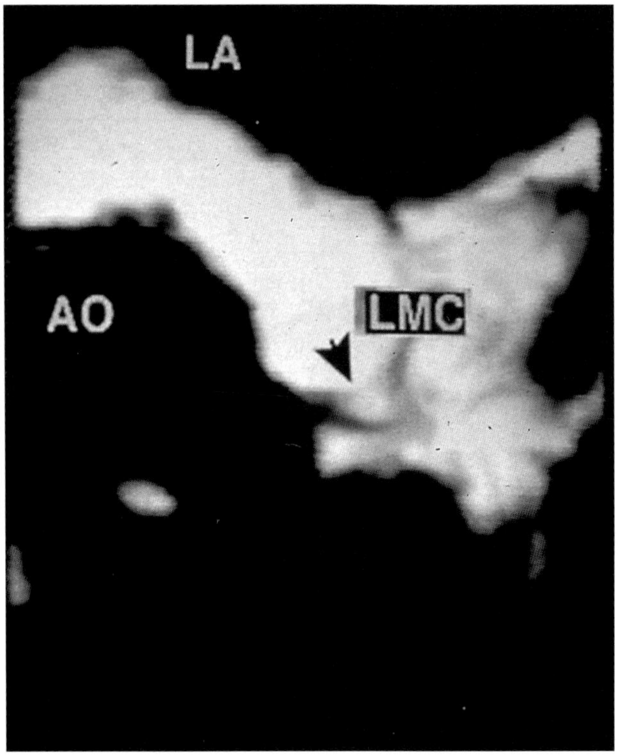

Figure 1. Transesophageal three-dimensional echocardiographic examination of coronary arteries. There is significant discrete narrowing (arrow) of the left main coronary artery (LMC). AO = aortic root; LA = left atrium. Reproduced with permission from Abd El-Rahman SM et al. Transesophageal three-dimensional echocardiographic assessment of normal and stenosed coronary arteries. *Echocardiography* 1996;13:503–510.

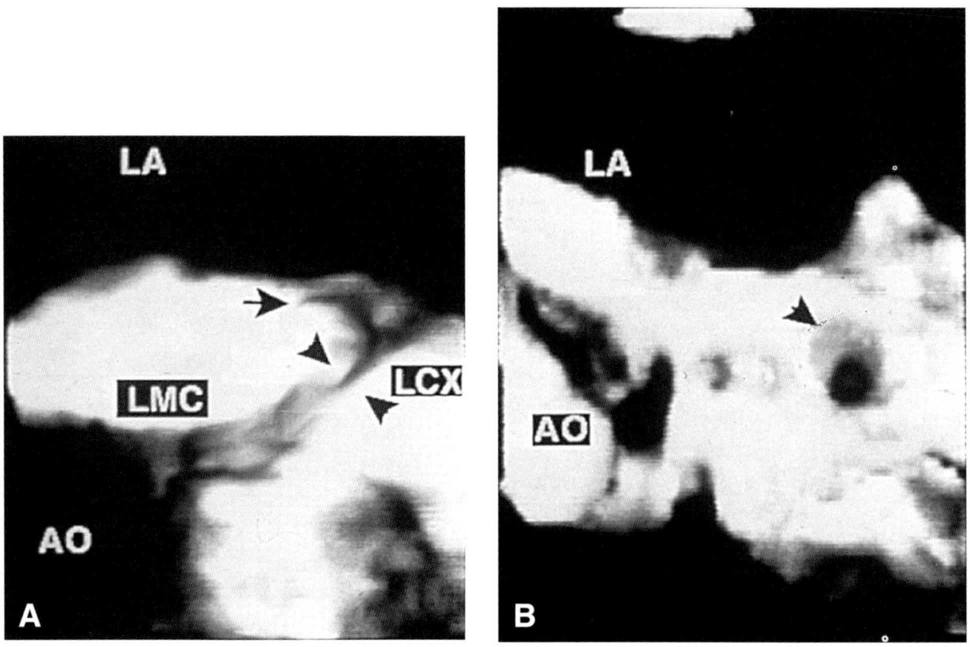

Figure 2. Transesophageal three-dimensional echocardiographic examination of coronary arteries. There is tight stenosis (arrowheads) of the circumflex coronary artery (LCX) imaged in both long—(**A**) and short axis (**B**) views in three dimensions. The arrow points to an atrial branch. Other abbreviations as in Figure 1. Reproduced with permission from Abd El-Rahman SM et al. Transesophageal three-dimensional echocardiographic assessment of normal and stenosed coronary arteries. *Echocardiography* 1996;13:503–510.

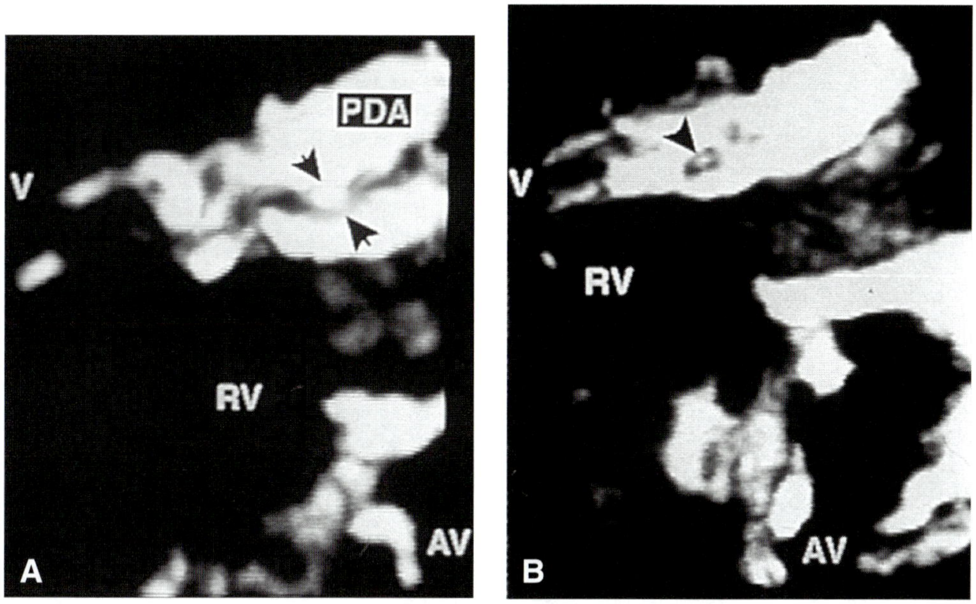

Figure 3. Transgasteric three-dimensional echocardiographic examination of posterior descending coronary artery. Severe stenosis (arrows) is noted in the mid portion of the posterior descending branch of the right coronary artery (PDA) imaged in both long- (**A**) and short-axis (**B**) views. AV = aortic valve; RV = right ventricle; V = small cardiac vein. Reproduced with permission from Abd El-Rahman SM et al. Transesophageal three-dimensional echocardiographic assessment of normal and stenosed coronary arteries. *Echocardiography* 1996;13:503–510.

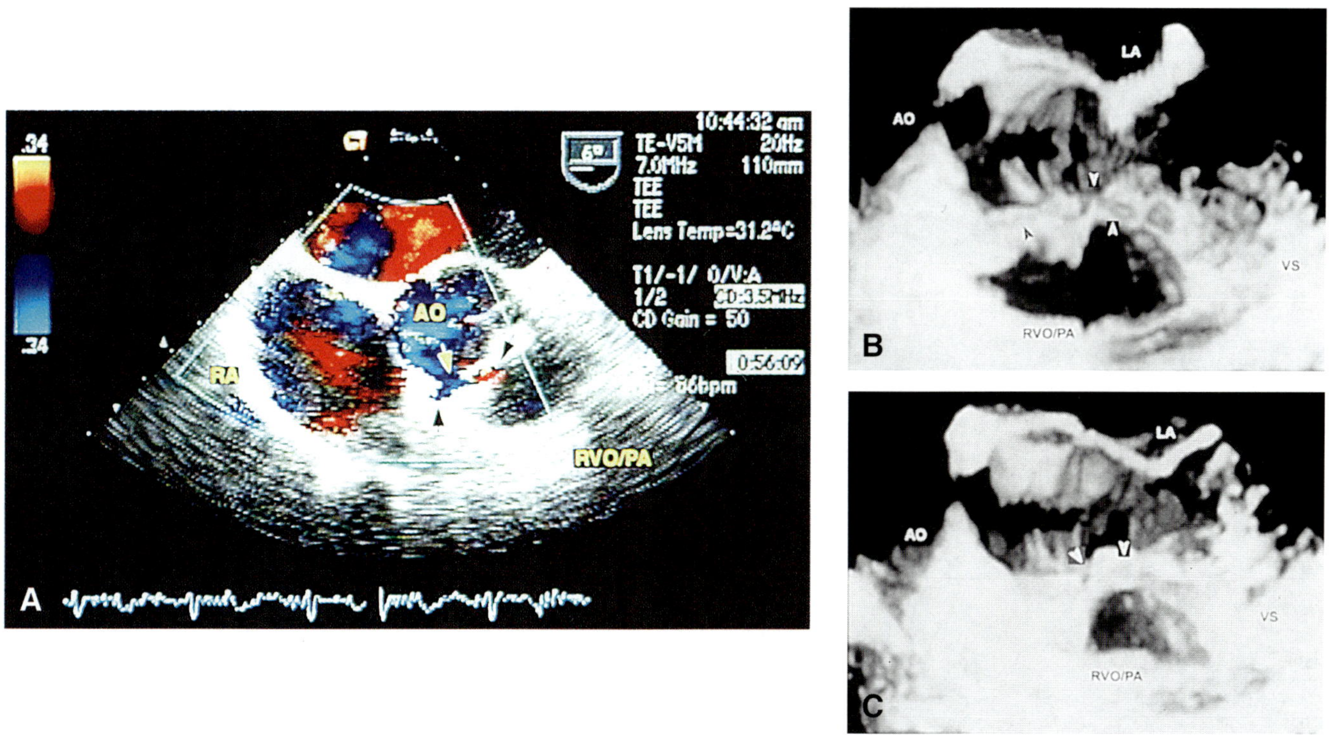

Figure 4. Transesophageal two- and three-dimensional echocardiography in an adult with anomalous coronary artery. **A–C.** Both left main and right coronary arteries (black arrows in **A**, lower arrowheads in **B**) arise from a common ostium (yellow arrow in **A**, upper arrowhead in **B**, left arrowhead in **C**) in the right sinus of Valsalva. The left main coronary artery courses between the aorta (A) and the right ventricular outflow tract/pulmonary artery (RVO/PA). The right arrowhead in (**C**) points to the left main coronary artery. LA = left atrium; RA = right atrium; VS = ventricular septum. Reproduced with permission from Nanda NC et al. Transesophageal three-dimensional echocardiographic assessment of anomalous coronary arteries. *Echocardiography* 2000;17:53–60.

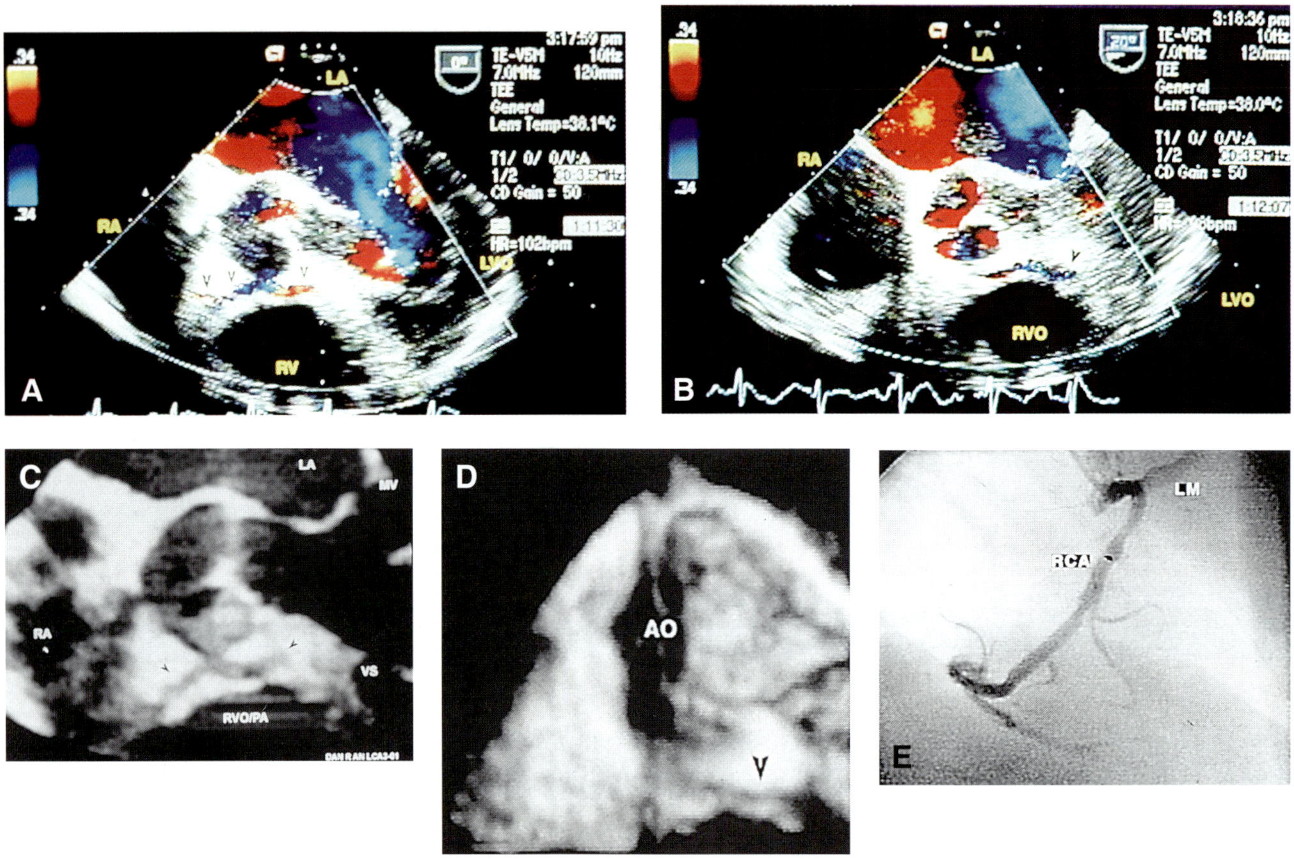

Figure 5. Transesophageal two- and three-dimensional echocardiography in another adult patient with anomalous coronary artery. (**A–D**) In this patient, both left main and right coronary arteries (arrowheads) arise from a common ostium in the right sinus with the left main coursing between AO and RVO/PA. In (**B**), the arrowhead points to intramyocardial course of the LAD coronary artery within the ventricular septum. (**E**) Coronary angiogram showing the common origin of the left main (LM) and right coronary (RCA) arteries. LVO = left ventricular outflow tract; MV = mitral valve; RV = right ventricle; other abbreviations as in Figure 4. Reproduced with permission from Nanda NC et al. Transesophageal three-dimensional echocardiographic assessment of anomalous coronary arteries. *Echocardiography* 2000;17:53–60

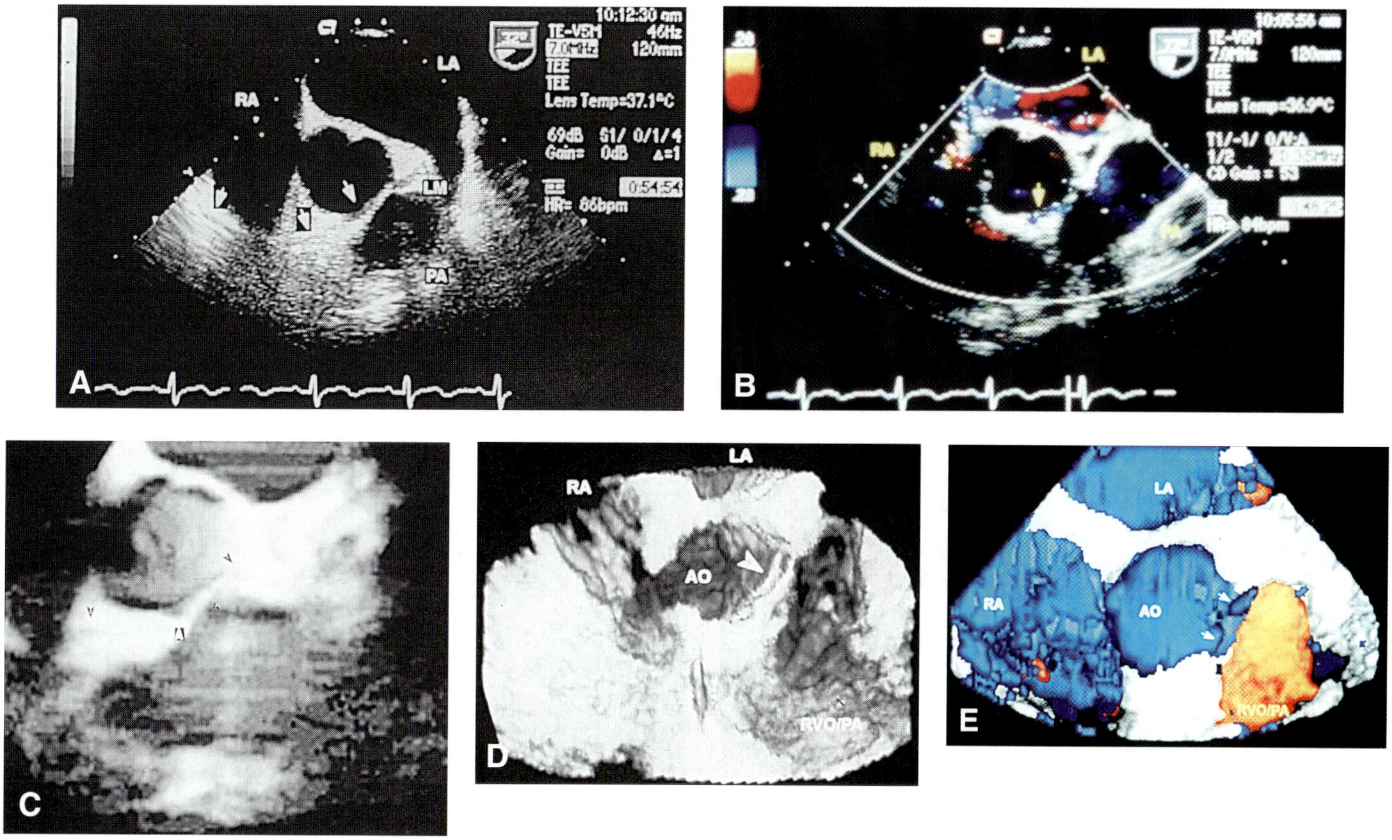

Figure 6. Transesophageal two- and three-dimensional echocardiography in a 50-year-old patient with anomalous coronary artery. (**A–E**) The arrows demonstrate the anomalous RCA arising from the left sinus, coursing within the aortic wall between the AO and the PA toward the right sinus and then following its usual course. (**E**). Represents color Doppler 3-D reconstruction. Abbreviations as in Figures 4 and 5. Reproduced with permission from Nanda NC et al. Transesophageal three-dimensional echocardiographic assessment of anomalous coronary arteries. *Echocardiography* 2000;17:53–60.

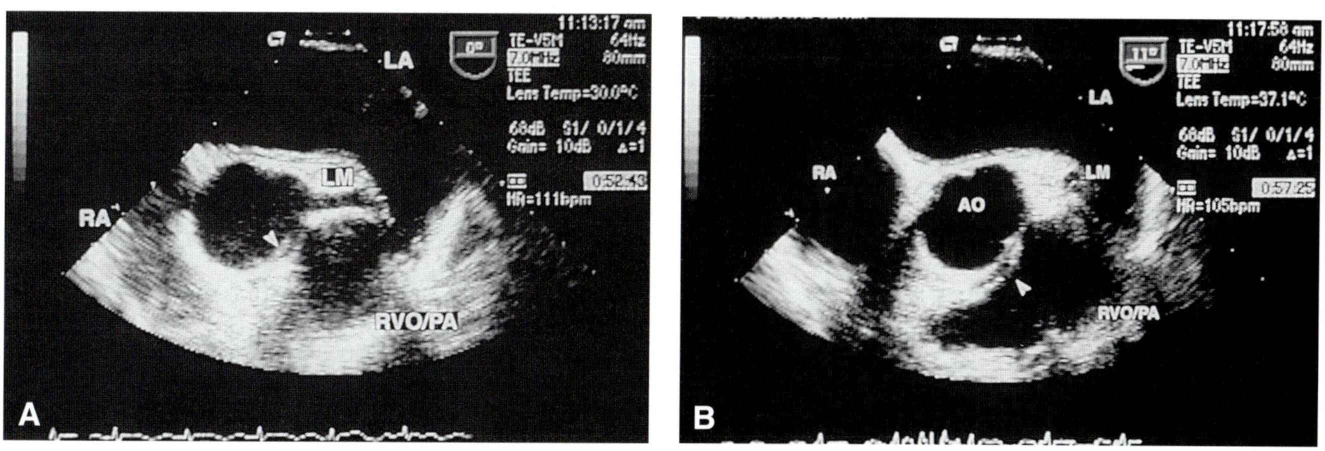

Figure 7. Transesophageal two- and three-dimensional echocardiography in a 59-year-old patient with anomalous coronary artery. (**A–F**) The arrowheads point to an anomalous right coronary artery (RCA) arising from the left sinus very close to the origin of the left main coronary artery (LM). This anomalous RCA also courses within the aortic wall between the aorta (AO) and right ventricular outflow tract/pulmonary artery (RVO/PA) toward the right sinus and then follows its usual course.

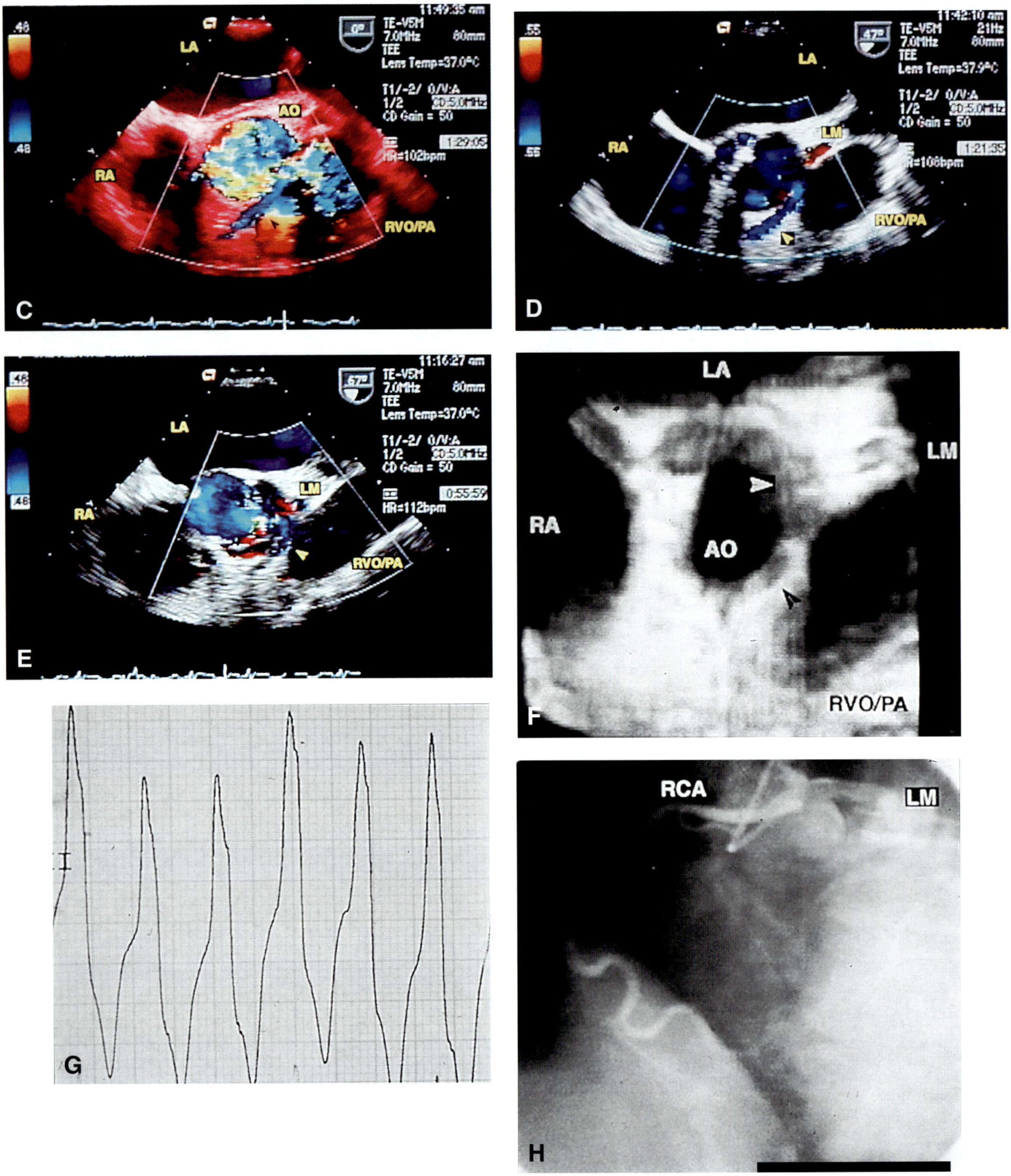

Figure 7. Continued. Transesophageal two- and three-dimensional echocardiography in a 59-year-old patient with anomalous coronary artery. (**A–F**) The arrowheads point to an anomalous right coronary artery (RCA) arising from the left sinus very close to the origin of the left main coronary artery (LM). This anomalous RCA also courses within the aortic wall between the aorta (AO) and right ventricular outflow tract/pulmonary artery (RVO/PA) toward the right sinus and then follows its usual course. The upper arrowhead in (**F**) points to the origin of the anomalous RCA. (**G**) ECG demonstrating ventricular tachycardia which developed 2 minutes and 24 seconds into treadmill exercise. (**H**) Coronary angiogram showing the anomalous RCA. Abbreviation as in Figures 4–6. Reproduced with permission from Nanda NC et al. Transesophageal three-dimensional echocardiographic assessment of anomalous coronary arteries. *Echocardiography* 2000;17:53–60.

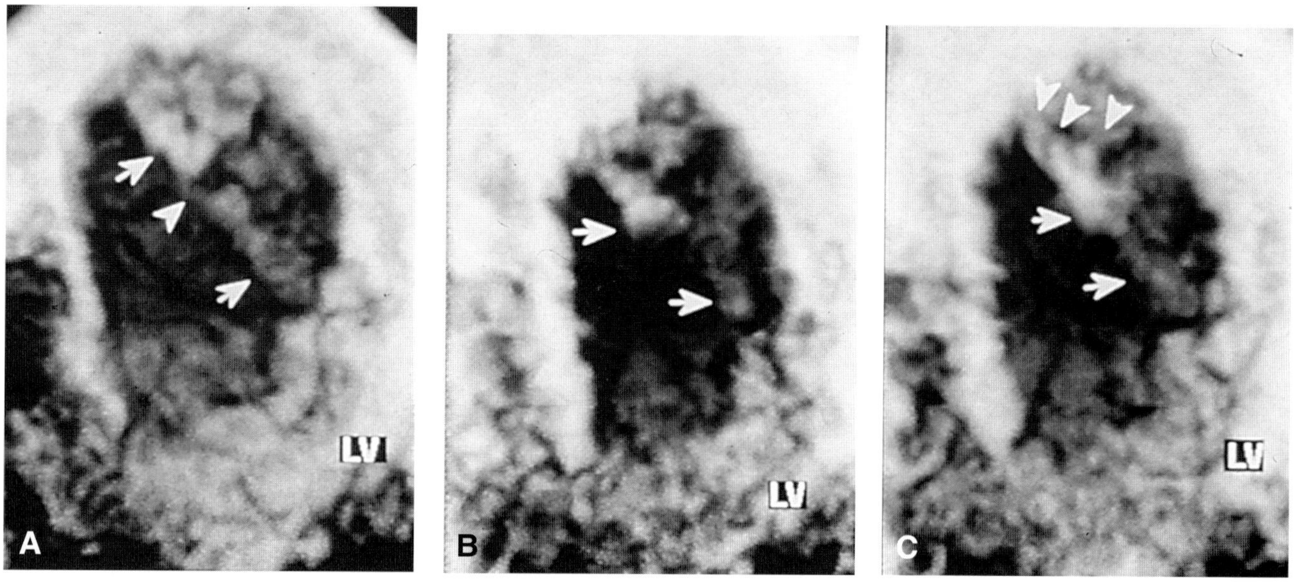

Figure 8. Transesophageal three-dimensional reconstruction in papillary muscle rupture. (**A, B**) Both the ruptured head (top arrow) and the portion of the papillary muscle still attached to the left ventricular wall (bottom arrow) are shown. The site of rupture is indicated by an arrowhead. (**C**) The arrowheads point to the chordae attached to the ruptured head. The finding of complete papillary muscle rupture was confirmed at surgery. The patient underwent excision of the mitral valve with replacement by a Carbomedics prosthesis (Carbomedics, Austin, TX). Reproduced with permission from Malhotra S et al. Transesophageal three-dimensional echocardiography in papillary muscle rupture. *Echocardiography* 1998;15:603–604.

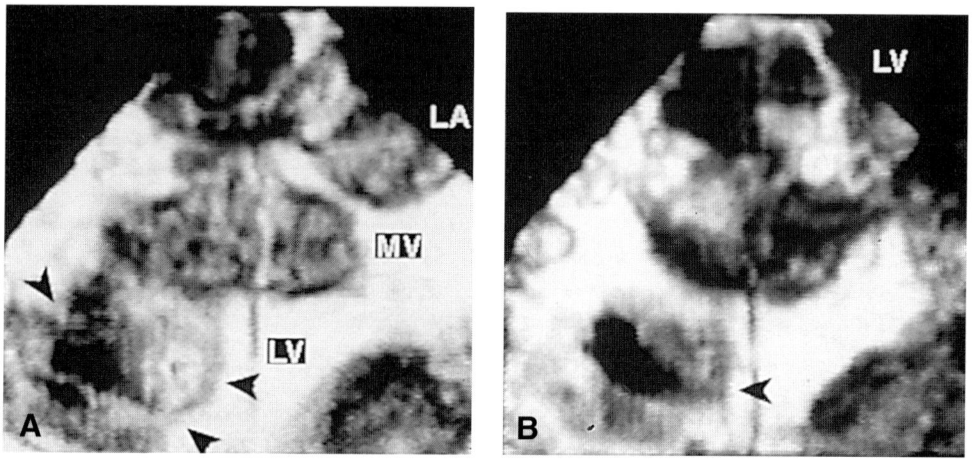

Figure 9. (**A**) Transesophageal echo (TEE), long-axis image of an apical 2-chamber view showing a left ventricular (LV) aneurysm (arrowheads). (**B**) TEE, tangential view of the previous figure. Note the appearance of the LV aneurysm in short axis (arrowhead).

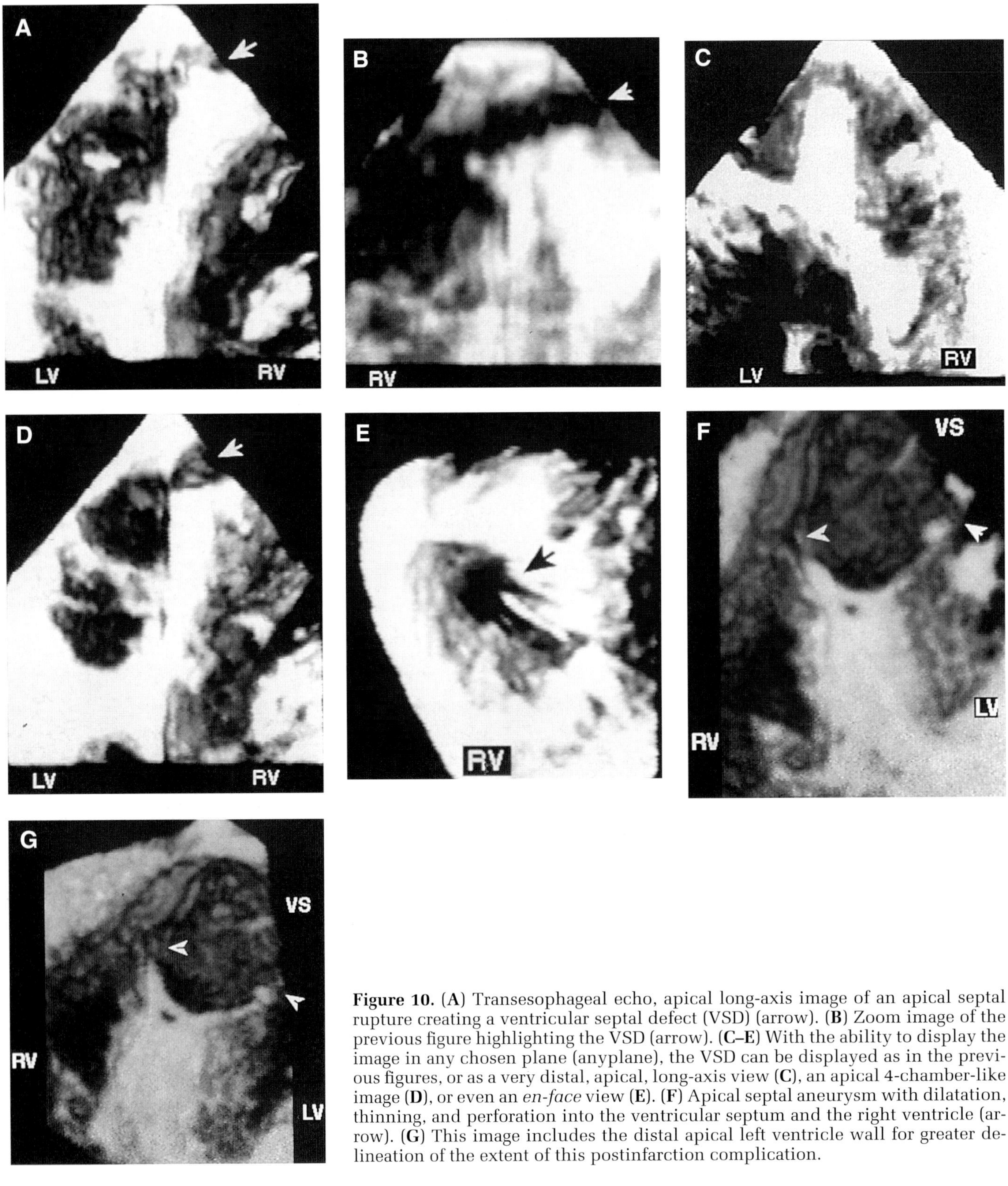

Figure 10. (**A**) Transesophageal echo, apical long-axis image of an apical septal rupture creating a ventricular septal defect (VSD) (arrow). (**B**) Zoom image of the previous figure highlighting the VSD (arrow). (**C–E**) With the ability to display the image in any chosen plane (anyplane), the VSD can be displayed as in the previous figures, or as a very distal, apical, long-axis view (**C**), an apical 4-chamber-like image (**D**), or even an *en-face* view (**E**). (**F**) Apical septal aneurysm with dilatation, thinning, and perforation into the ventricular septum and the right ventricle (arrow). (**G**) This image includes the distal apical left ventricle wall for greater delineation of the extent of this postinfarction complication.

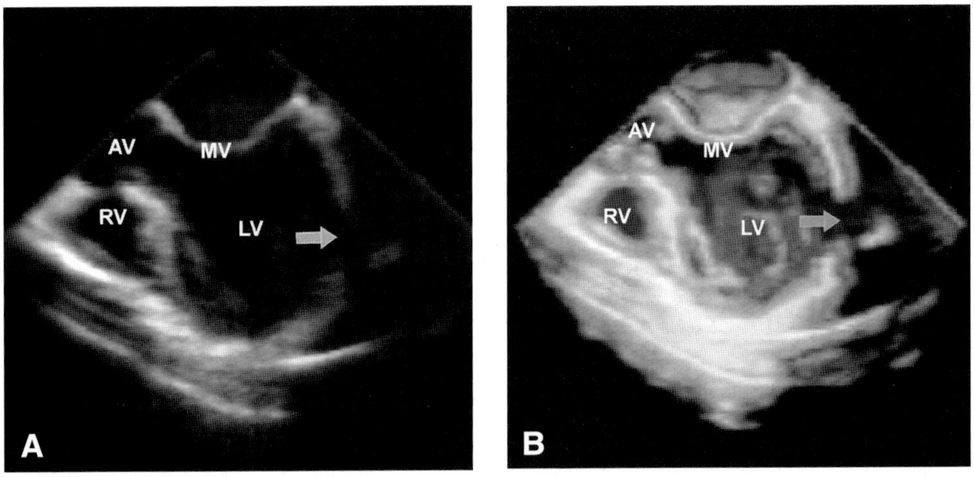

Figure 11. (**A**) Two-dimensional echocardiogram. A 59-year-old patient with myocardial rupture after acute myocardial infarction (arrow). (**B**) Three-dimensional view. A 59-year-old patient with myocardial rupture after acute myocardial infarction (arrow). AV = aortic valve; LV = left ventricle; MV = mitral valve; RV = right ventricle. From Annette Geibel, MD, Michael Handke, MD, Dietrich Markus Schäfer, MD, Anja Schöchlin, MA, and Helmut Wollschläger, MD.

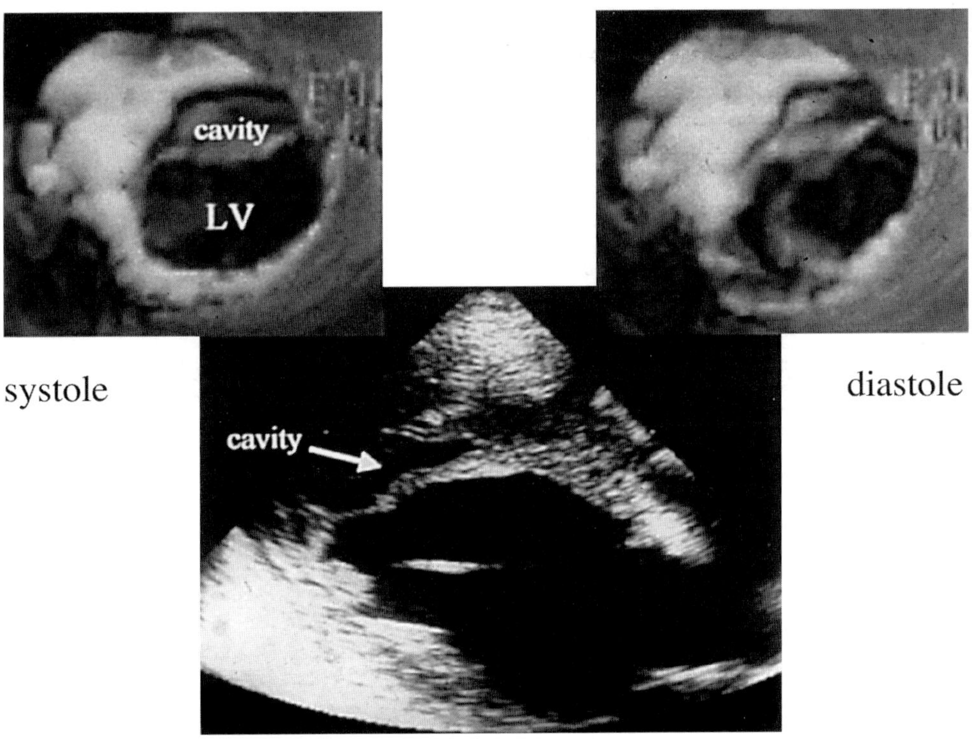

Figure 12. Left ventricular intramyocardial dissection. A 54-year-old male in stable clinical status referred for coronography 6 months after myocardial infarction. Transthoracic echocardiogram revealed depressed left ventricular function with apical aneurysm and an ejection fraction of 24%. A cavity within apical region of the left ventricle was also apparent (bottom panel). Three-dimensional reconstruction showed constant volume of the cavity of 4.5 mL with no systolic-diastolic difference (without communication with left ventricle). Repeated three-dimensional studies revealed gradual decrease of the volume of the cavity with its subsequent total thrombosis and closure. From Jaroslaw Drozdz, MD and Jaroslaw D. Kasprzak, MD.

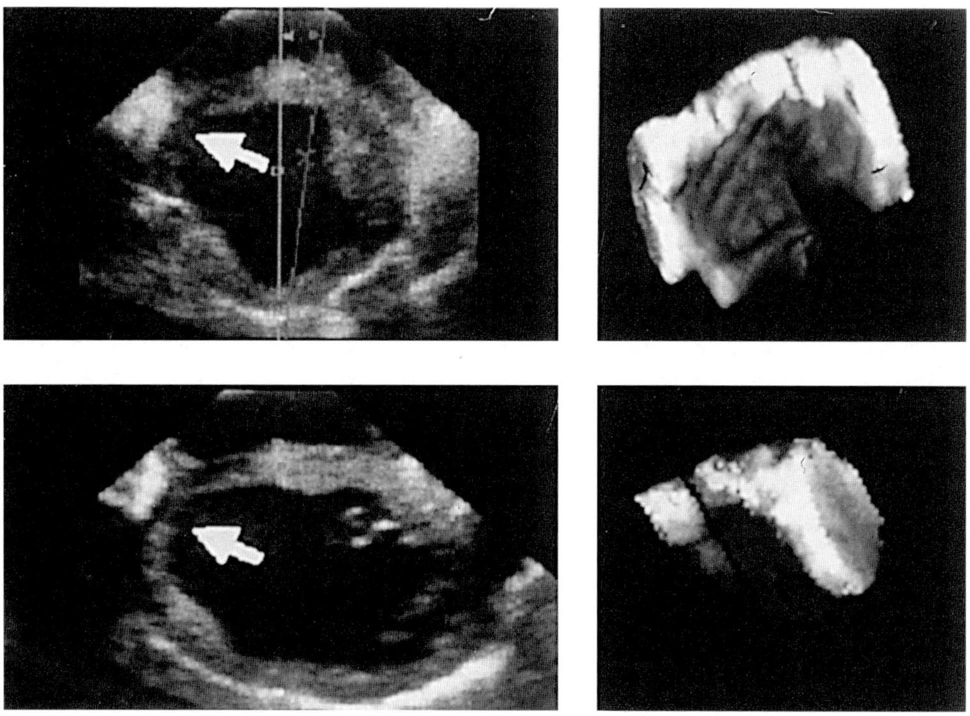

Figure 13. Three-dimensional contrast echocardiography. The data set reliably retains regional differences in myocardial opacification. Perfusion defect (arrow) can be displayed in orthogonal reconstructed cutplanes and used for volume-rendering (**right panels**). The use of different viewing points allows to improve the perception of three-dimensional geometry of irregular myocardial segment. From Jaroslaw D. Kasprzak, MD.

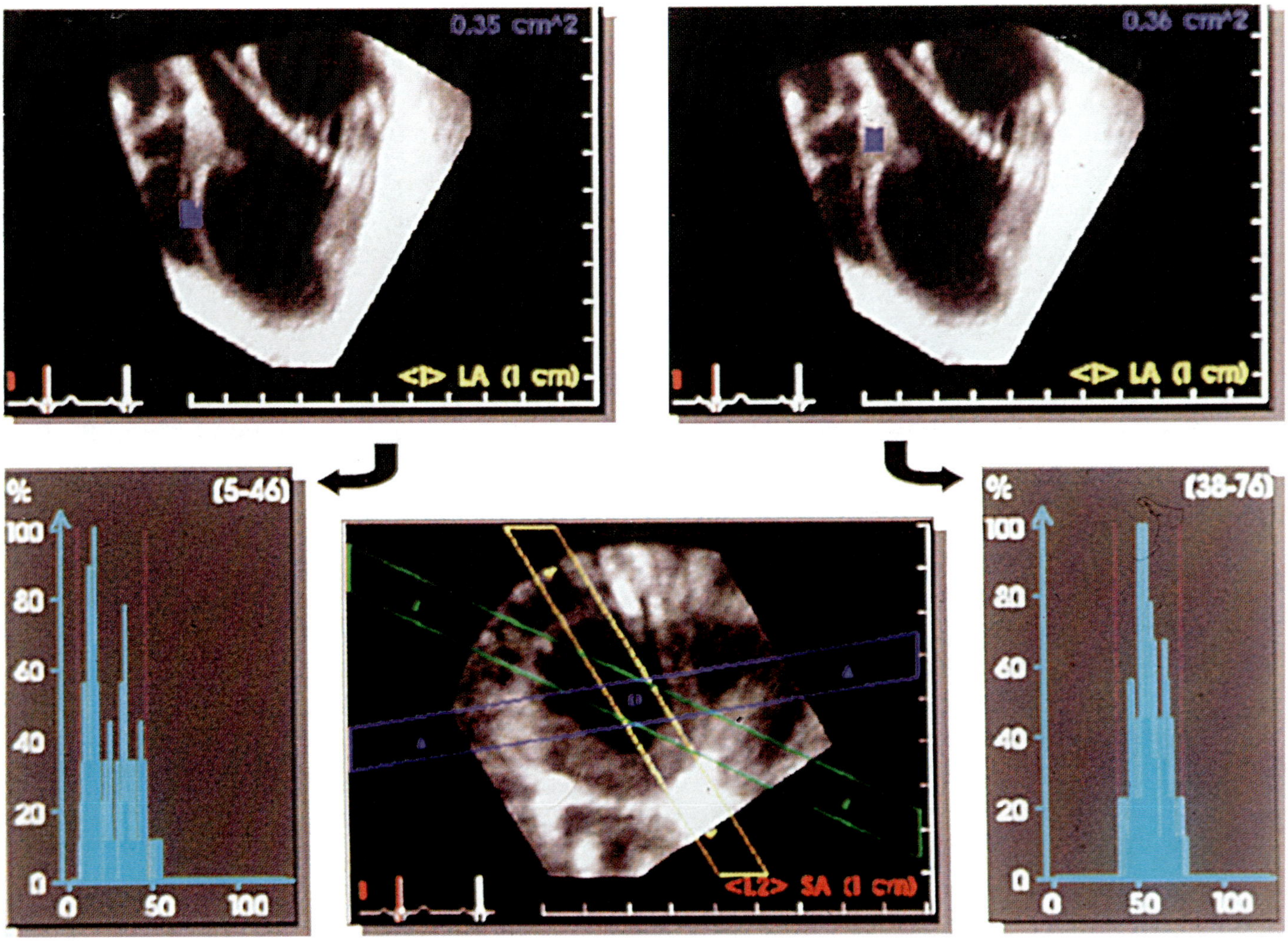

Figure 14. Intensity quantification in a three-dimensional contrast echocardiographic study. Data sets were acquired after a deposit contrast injection in a pig with an occluded left anterior descending artery. Rectangular masks mark the regions of interests (**upper panels**), from which voxel intensity histograms were derived as shown below. A corresponding orthogonal view (**center bottom**) illustrates the concept of spatial region of interest and definition of the third dimension—the thickness of a slice, corresponding with the rectangular masks. From Jaroslaw D. Kasprzak, MD.

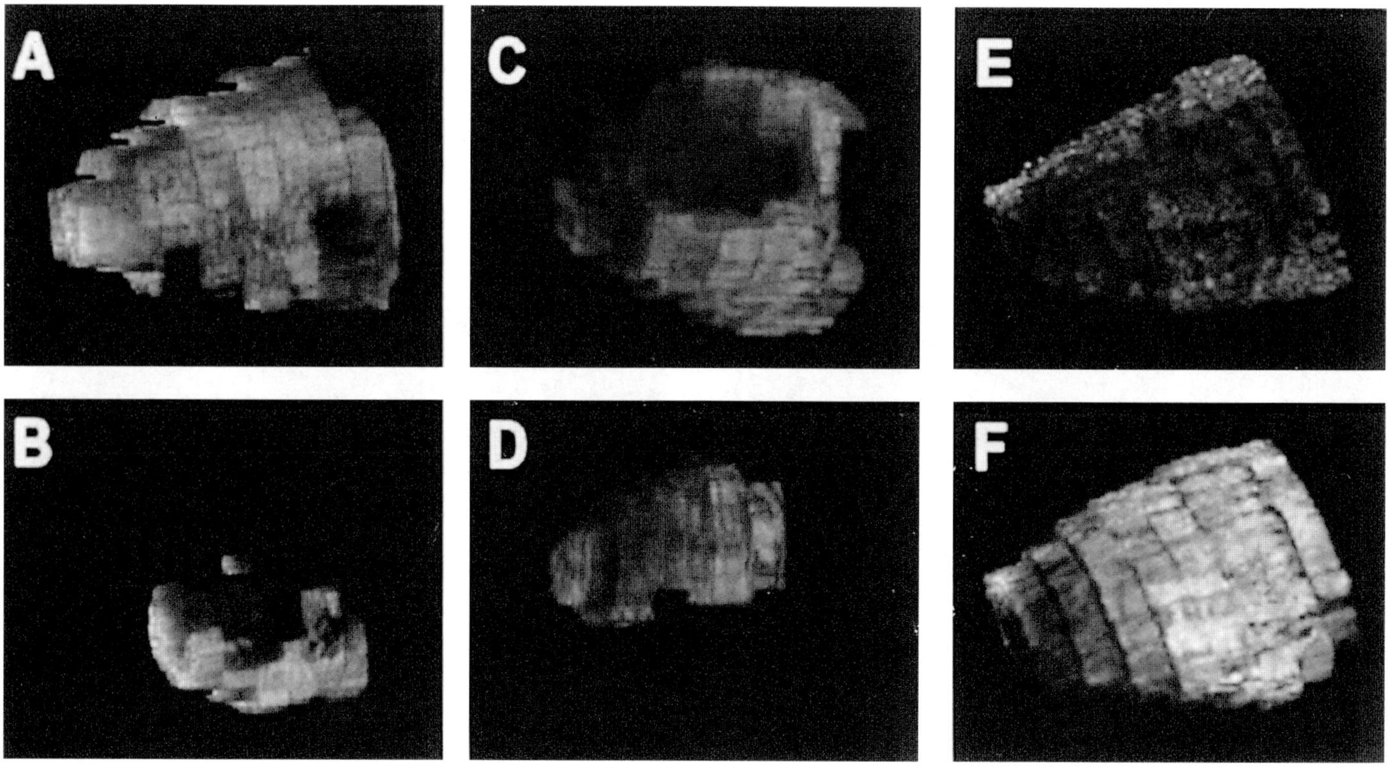

Figure 15. Three-dimensional imaging of left ventricular perfusion maps. Perfused myocardial regions (**A, C**) were separated from nonperfused myocardium (**B, D**) based upon the intensity difference and displayed separately. Data sets were collected after an injection of a deposit contrast agent during the occlusion of the circumflex artery (**A, B**) and the left anterior descending artery (**C, D**). Volume-rendered presentation of the entire myocardium is helpful for the recognition of local wall thickening (in a semitransparent presentation, **E**) and global contraction pattern (**F**). From Jaroslaw D. Kasprzak, MD.

Suggested Reading List

1. Abd El-Rahman SM, Khatri G, Nanda N, et al. Transesophageal three-dimensional assessment of normal and stenosed coronary arteries. *Echocardiography* 1996;13:503–510.
2. Azevedo J, Garcia-Fernandez MA, Puerta P, et al. [Three-dimensional echocardiography reconstruction of the left ventricle using 3 different myocardial encoding techniques with Doppler tissue imaging]. [Portuguese]. *Revista Portuguesa Cardiologia* 1996;15:841–846.
3. Azevedo J, Coucelo J, Jacques AK, et al. [Relation of left ventricular mass, volume and systolic function in three-dimensional transesophageal echocardiography. Multifactorial linear regression analysis]. [Portuguese]. *Revista Portuguesa Cardiologia.* 1996;15:819–824.
4. Bjornstad K, Maehle J, Aakhus S, et al. Evaluation of reference systems for quantitative wall motion analysis from three-dimensional endocardial surface reconstruction: an echocardiographic study in subjects with and without myocardial infarction. *Am J Cardiac Imaging* 1996;10:244–253.
5. Legget ME, Bashein G. Automatic border detection and three-dimensional reconstruction with echocardiography. [Review] [101 refs]. *Critical Care Clinics* 1996;12:471–496.
6. Muller S, Bartel T, Baumann G, et al. Preliminary report: evaluation of three-dimensional echocardiographic volumetry by simultaneous thermal dilution in coronary heart disease. *Cardiology* 1996;87:552–559.
7. Nicosia A, von Birgelen C, Di Mario C, et al. 3-dimensional reconstruction in intracoronary echocardiography: the advantages, limits and future prospects. [Review] [84 refs] [Italian]. *Cardiologia* 1996;41:1165–1174.
8. Qiang M, Que X, Sun P. [Three-dimensional echocardiography in evaluation of left ventricular systolic function after mitral valve replacement for chronic mitral diseases with preservation of mitral apparatus]. [Chinese]. *Chinese Medical Journal* 1996;76:516–518.
9. Azevedo J, Garcia-Fernandez MA, Puerta P, et al. [Dynamic tridimensional echocardiography and evaluation of functional alterations in acute ischemia]. [Portuguese]. *Revista Portuguesa Cardiologia* 1997;16:913–917.
10. Azevedo J, Garcia-Fernandez MA, Puerta P, et al. [Left ventricular mass identified with tridimensional echocardiography and myocardial tissue Doppler]. [Portuguese]. *Revista Portuguesa Cardiologia* 1997;16:907–911.
11. Gopal AS, Schnellbaecher MJ, Shen Z, et al. Freehand three-dimensional echocardiography for measurement of left ventricular mass: In vivo anatomic validation using explanted human hearts. *J Am Coll Cardiol* 1997;30:802–810.
12. Iwase M, Kondo T, Hasegawa K, et al. Three-dimensional echocardiography by semi-automatic border detection in assessment of left ventricular volume and ejection fraction: comparison with magnetic resonance imaging. *J Cardiol* 1997;30:97–105.
13. Jamil F, Nanda NC, Thakur AC, et al. Echocardiographic detection of intramyocardial coronary obstruction produced by pericardial hydatid cyst. *Echocardiography* 1997;14:631–635.

14. Kuhl HP, Franke A, Frielingsdorf J, et al. Determination of left ventricular mass and circumferential wall thickness by three-dimensional reconstruction: In vitro validation of a new method that uses a multiplane transesophageal transducer. *J Am Soc Echocardiography* 1997;10:107–119.
15. Linka AZ, Ates G, Wei K, et al. Three-dimensional myocardial contrast echocardiography: Validation of in vivo risk and infarct volumes. *J Am Coll Cardiol* 1997;30:1892–1899.
16. Nakazato M, Yoshida K, Hozumi T, et al. [Measurement of plaque volume using three-dimensional intravascular ultrasound: in vitro study]. [Japanese]. *J Cardiology* 1997; 30:227–230.
17. Pini R, Giannazzo G, Di Bari M, et al. Transthoracic three-dimensional echocardiographic reconstruction of left and right ventricles: In vitro validation and comparison with magnetic resonance imaging. *Am Heart J* 1997;133:221–229.
18. Prati F, Gil R, Di Mario C, et al. Is quantitative angiography sufficient to guide stent implantation? A comparison with three-dimensional reconstruction of intracoronary ultrasound images. *Giornale Italiano Cardiologia* 1997; 27:328–336.
19. Prati F, Di Mario C, Gil R, et al. On-line three-dimensional intracoronary ultrasound for guidance of catheter based interventions. [Review] [40 refs]. *Giornale Italiano Cardiologia* 1997;27:123–132.
20. Rodevand O, Bjornerheim R, Kolbjornsen O, et al. Left ventricular mass assessed by three-dimensional echocardiography using rotational acquisition. *Clin Cardiol* 1997;20:957–962.
21. Vogel M, Gutberlet M, Dittrich S, et al. Comparison of transthoracic three dimensional echocardiography with magnetic resonance imaging in the assessment of right ventricular volume and mass. *Heart* 1997;78:127–130.
22. Yao J, Cao QL, Masani N, et al. Three-dimensional echocardiographic estimation of infarct mass based on quantification of dysfunctional left ventricular mass. *Circulation* 1997;96:1660–1666.
23. Azevedo J, Coucelo J, Jacques AK, et al. [Variation in the calculation of the left ventricular mass using three-dimensional echocardiography]. [Portuguese]. *Revista Portuguesa Cardiologia* 1998;17:81–84.
24. Danias PG, Chuang ML, Parker RA, et al. Relation between the number of image planes and the accuracy of three-dimensional echocardiography for measuring left ventricular volumes and ejection fraction. *Am J Cardiol* 1998;82:1431–1434, A9.
25. De Castro S, Yao J, Fedele F, et al. Three-dimensional echocardiography in ischemic heart disease. [Review] [35 refs]. *Coronary Artery Disease* 1998;9:427–434.
26. De Castro S, Yao J, Magni G, et al. Three-dimensional echocardiographic assessment of the extension of dysfunctional mass in patients with coronary artery disease. *Am J Cardiol* 1998;81:103G–106G.
27. Frielingsdorf J, Franke A, Kuhl HP, et al. Evaluation of regional systolic function in hypertrophic cardiomyopathy and hypertensive heart disease: A three-dimensional echocardiographic study. *J Am Soc Echocardiography* 1998;11:778–786.
28. Fujimoto S, Mizuno R, Nakagawa Y, Dohi K, Nakano H: Estimation of the right ventricular volume and ejection fraction by transthoracic three-dimensional echocardiography. A validation study using magnetic resonance imaging. *Int J Cardiac Imaging* 1998;14:385–390.
29. Kasprzak JD, Vletter WB, Nosir YF, et al. Improved quantification of myocardial mass by three-dimensional echocardiography using a deposit contrast agent. *Ultrasound Med & Biol* 1998;24:647–653.
30. Kasprzak JD, Vletter WB, Roelandt JR, et al. Visualization and quantification of myocardial mass at risk using three-dimensional contrast echocardiography. *Cardiovasc Research* 1998;40:314–321.
31. Legget ME, Leotta DF, Bolson EL, et al. System for quantitative three-dimensional echocardiography of the left ventricle based on a magnetic-field position and orientation sensing system. *IEEE Transact Biomed Engineer* 1998;45:494–504.
32. Malhotra S, Nanda NC, McElderry HT, et al. Transesophageal three-dimensional echocardiography in papillary muscle rupture. *Echocardiography* 1998;15:603–604.
33. Maxted WCJ, Swanson ST, Huntley M, et al. Location of stents in the left anterior descending coronary artery using three dimensionally acquired, two dimensionally displayed transthoracic echocardiography. *Am J Cardiol* 1998;82:1434–1436.
34. Mele D, Maehle J, Pedini I, et al. Three-dimensional echocardiographic reconstruction: Description and applications of a simplified technique for quantitative assessment of left ventricular size and function. [Review] [31 refs]. *Am J Cardiol* 1998;81:107G–110G.
35. Munt BI, Leotta DF, Bolson EL, et al. Left ventricular shape analysis from three-dimensional echocardiograms. *J Am Soc Echocardiography* 1998;11:761–769.
36. Nosir YF, Lequin MH, Kasprzak JD, et al. Measurements and day-to-day variabilities of left ventricular volumes and ejection fraction by three-dimensional echocardiography and comparison with magnetic resonance imaging. *Am J Cardiol* 1998;82:209–214.
37. Nosir YF, Salustri A, Kasprzak JD, et al. Left ventricular ejection fraction in patients with normal and distorted left ventricular shape by three-dimensional echocardiographic methods: A comparison with radionuclide angiography. *J Am Soc Echocardiography* 1998;11:620–630.
38. Prati F, Mallus MT, Lioy E. Three-dimensional reconstruction techniques applied to intracoronary images. [Review] [27 refs]. *Giornale Italiano Cardiologia* 1998;28:460–467.
39. Rodevand O, Bjornerheim R, Aakhus S, et al. Left ventricular volumes assessed by different new three-dimensional echocardiographic methods and ordinary biplane technique. *Int J Cardiac Imaging* 1998;14:55–63.
40. Shiota T, Jones M, Chikada M, et al. Real-time three-dimensional echocardiography for determining right ventricular stroke volume in an animal model of chronic right ventricular volume overload. *Circulation* 1998;97: 1897–1900.
41. Chuang ML, Beaudin RA, Riley MF, et al. Impact of on-line endocardial border detection on determination of left ventricular volume and ejection fraction by transthoracic 3-dimensional echocardiography. *J Am Soc Echocardiography* 1999;12:551–558.
42. Chuang ML, Parker RA, Riley MF, et al. Three-dimensional echocardiography improves accuracy and compensates for sonographer inexperience in assessment of left ventricular ejection fraction. *J Am Soc Echocardiography* 1999;12:290–299.
43. Collins M, Hsieh A, Ohazama CJ, et al. Assessment of regional wall motion abnormalities with real-time 3-dimensional echocardiography. *J Am Soc Echocardiography* 1999;12:7–14.
44. Duann JR, Chiang SH, Lin SB, et al. Assessment of left ventricular cardiac shape by the use of volumetric cur-

vature analysis from 3D echocardiography. *Comp Medical Imaging & Graphics* 1999;23:89–101.
45. Geil S, Rao L, Menzel T, et al. [Determination of left ventricular mass by transthoracic three-dimensional echocardiography in patients with dilated cardiomyopathy]. [German]. *Zeitschrift Kardiologie* 1999;88:922–931.
46. Heusch A, Koch JA, Krogmann ON, et al. Volumetric analysis of the right and left ventricle in a porcine heart model: Comparison of three-dimensional echocardiography, magnetic resonance imaging and angiocardiography. *Eur J Ultrasound* 1999;9:245–255.
47. Nosir YF, Stoker J, Kasprzak JD, et al. Paraplane analysis from precordial three-dimensional echocardiographic data sets for rapid and accurate quantification of left ventricular volume and function: a comparison with magnetic resonance imaging. *Am Heart J.* 1999;137:134–143.
48. Rodevan O, Bjornerheim R, Ljosland M, et al. Left atrial volumes assessed by three- and two-dimensional echocardiography compared to MRI estimates. *Int J Cardiac Imaging* 1999;15:397–410.
49. Yao J, Kasprzak JD, Nosir YF, et al. Appropriate 3-dimensional echocardiography data acquisition interval for left ventricular volume quantification: Implications for clinical application. *J Am Soc Echocardiography* 1999;12:1053–1057.
50. Yao J, Taams MA, Kasprzak Jdet al. Usefulness of three-dimensional transesophageal echocardiographic imaging for evaluating narrowing in the coronary arteries. *Am J Cardiol* 1999;84:41–44.
51. Zwas DR, Takuma S, Mullis-Jansson S, et al. Feasibility of real-time 3-dimensional treadmill stress echocardiography. *J Am Soc Echocardiography* 1999;12:285–289.
52. Ansingkar KG, Aaluri SR, Nanda NC. Three dimensional transesophageal echocardiographic demonstration of aortic dissection flap extending into right coronary artery ostium. *Am J Geriatric Cardiol* 2000;9:344–345.
53. Arbeille P, Eder V, Casset D, et al. Real-time 3-D ultrasound acquisition and display for cardiac volume and ejection fraction evaluation. *Ultrasound Medicine & Biology* 2000;26(2):201–208.
54. Chuang ML, Beaudin RA, Riley MF, et al. Three-dimensional echocardiographic measurement of left ventricular mass: comparison with magnetic resonance imaging and two-dimensional echocardiographic determinations in man. *Int J Cardiac Imaging* 2000;16(5):347–357.
55. Chuang ML, Hibberd MG, Salton CJ, et al. Importance of imaging method over imaging modality in noninvasive determination of left ventricular volumes and ejection fraction: Assessment by two- and three-dimensional echocardiography and magnetic resonance imaging. *J Am Coll Cardiol* 2000;35(2):477–484.
56. Eder V, Herault S, Hudelo C, et al. Evaluation of left ventricular systolic function by 3D echocardiography: a comparative study with X-ray angiography and radionuclide angiography. *Eur J Ultrasound* 2000;11(2):105–115.
57. Hibberd MG, Chuang ML, Beaudin RA, et al. Accuracy of three-dimensional echocardiography with unrestricted selection of imaging planes for measurement of left ventricular volumes and ejection fraction. *Am Heart J* 2000;140(3.:469–475.
58. Keller AM. Positional localization: Three-dimensional transthoracic echocardiographic techniques for the measurement of cardiac mass, volume, and function. [Review] [20 refs]. *Echocardiography* 2000;17(8):745–748.
59. Kim WY, Terp KA, Nyengaard JR, et al. Unbiased and efficient estimation of left ventricular volumes by three-dimensional echocardiography with coaxial sections. Validation with magnetic resonance imaging. *Heart & Vessels* 2000;15(1):35–43.
60. Kuhl HP, Bucker A, Franke A, et al. Transesophageal 3-dimensional echocardiography: In vivo determination of left ventricular mass in comparison with magnetic resonance imaging. *J Am Soc Echocardiography* 2000;13(3):205–215.
61. Marcus EN, Munoz RA, Palacio G, et al. A new quantitative method for the diagnosis of right ventricular hypertensive disorders in 3 dimensions. *J Am Soc Echocardiography* 2000;13(3):186–193.
62. Mele D, Levine RA. Quantitation of ventricular size and function: principles and accuracy of transthoracic rotational scanning. [Review] [33 refs]. *Echocardiography* 2000;17(8):749–755.
63. Munoz R, Marcus E, Palacio G, et al. Reconstruction of 3-dimensional right ventricular shape and volume from 3 orthogonal planes. *J Am Soc Echocardiography* 2000;13(3):177–185.
64. Nadkarni SK, Boughner DR, Drangova M, et al. Three-dimensional echocardiography: Assessment of inter- and intra-operator variability and accuracy in the measurement of left ventricular cavity volume and myocardial mass. *Phys Med Biol* 2000;45(5):1255–1273.
65. Nanda NC, Bhambore MM, Jindal A, et al. Transesophageal three-dimensional echocardiographic assessment of anomalous coronary arteries. *Echocardiography* 2000;17(1):53–60.
66. Qin JX, Shiota T, McCarthy PM, et al. Real-time three-dimensional echocardiographic study of left ventricular function after infarct exclusion surgery for ischemic cardiomyopathy. *Circulation* 2000;102(Suppl.3):III101–106.
67. Qin JX, Shiota T, Thomas JD. Determination of left ventricular volume, ejection fraction, and myocardial mass by real-time three-dimensional echocardiography. [Review] [34 refs]. *Echocardiography* 2000;17(8):781–786.
68. Qin JX, Jones M, Shiota T, et al.Validation of real-time three-dimensional echocardiography for quantifying left ventricular volumes in the presence of a left ventricular aneurysm: In vitro and in vivo studies. *J Am Coll Cardiol* 2000;36(3):900–907.
69. Rusk RA, Mori Y, Davies CH, et al. Comparison of ventricular volume and mass measurements from B- and C-scan images with the use of real-time 3-dimensional echocardiography: studies in an in vitro model. *J Am Soc Echocardiography* 2000;13(10):910–917.
70. Suguta M, Nakamura T, Kurabayashi M, et al. [Prognostic significance of quantification of left ventricular mass in hypertensive patients]. [Review] [13 refs] [Japanese]. *Japanese J Clin Med* 2000;58(Suppl.1):740–743.
71. Yalcin F, Shiota T, Odabashian J, et al. Comparison by real-time three-dimensional echocardiography of left ventricular geometry in hypertrophic cardiomyopathy versus secondary left ventricular hypertrophy. *Am J Cardiol* 2000;85(8):1035–1038.
72. Yao J, Teupe C, Takeuchi M, et al. Quantitative 3-dimensional contrast echocardiographic determination of myocardial mass at risk and residual infarct mass after reperfusion: Experimental canine studies with intravenous contrast agent NC100100. *J Am Soc Echocardiography* 2000;13(6):570–581.
73. Ahmad M, Xie T, McCulloch M, et al. Real-time three-dimensional dobutamine stress echocardiography in assessment stress echocardiography in assessment of ischemia: Comparison with two-dimensional dobutamine stress echocardiography. *J Am Coll Cardiol* 2001;37(5):1303–1309.

74. Bauer F, Shiota T, Qin JX, et al. [Measurement of left atrial and ventricular volumes in real-time 3D echocardiography. Validation by nuclear magnetic resonance]. [French]. *Arch Mal Coeur et Vaisseaux* 2001;94(1):31–38.
75. Belohlavek M, Tanabe K, Jakrapanichakul D, et al. Rapid three-dimensional echocardiography: Clinically feasible alternative for precise and accurate measurement of left ventricular volumes. *Circulation* 2001;103:2882–2884
76. Corsi C, Borsari M, Consegnati F, Sarti A, Lamberti C, Travaglini A, Shiota T, Thomas JD: Left ventricular endocardial surface detection based on real-time 3D echocardiographic data. *Eur J Ultrasound* 2001;13(1):41–51.
77. Kim WY, Sogaard P, Mortensen PT, et al. Three dimensional echocardiography documents haemodynamic improvement by biventricular pacing in patients with severe heart failure. *Heart* 2001;85(5):514–520.
78. Kim WY, Sogaard P, Egeblad H, et al. Three-dimensional echocardiography with tissue harmonic imaging shows excellent reproducibility in assessment of left ventricular volumes. *J Am Soc Echocardiography* 2001;14(6):612–617.
79. Kim WY, Sogaard P, Kristensen BO, et al. Measurement of left ventricular volumes by 3-dimensional echocardiography with tissue harmonic imaging: A comparison with magnetic resonance imaging. *J Am Soc Echocardiography* 2001;14(3):169–179.
80. Papademetris X, Sinusas AJ, Dione DP, et al. Estimation of 3D left ventricular deformation from echocardiography. *Medical Image Analysis* 2001;5(1):17–28.
81. Takuma S, Ota T, Muro T, et al. Assessment of left ventricular function by real-time 3-dimensional echocardiography compared with conventional noninvasive methods. *J Am Soc Echocardiography* 2001;14(4): 275–284.
82. Zotz RJ, Zirlik A, Raeder T, et al. Three-dimensional visualization of coronary arteries in excised hearts. *J Am Soc Echocardiography* 2001;14:11–19.
83. Nekkanti R, Nanda NC, Ansingkar KG, et al. Transesophageal three dimensional echocardiographic assessment of left ventricular pseudoaneurysm. *Echocardiography* (In press, February 2002).
84. Nekkanti R, Nanda NC, Zoghbi GJ, et al. Transesophageal two and three dimensional echocardiographic diagnosis of combined left ventricular pseudoaneurysm and ventricular septal rupture. *Echocardiography* (In press, July 2002).
85. Horton Jr. CJ, Nanda NC, Nekkanti R, et al. Prosthetic aortic valve abscess producing total right coronary artery occlusion: Diagnosis by transesophageal three-dimensional echocardiography. *Echocardiography* (In press, August 2002).

Chapter 6

Congenital Heart Disease

Navin C. Nanda, MD and Vincent L. Sorrell, MD

Congenital heart diseases include many extraordinary echocardiographic features not familiar to even the most experienced adult echocardiographer. Even pediatric echocardiographers, who are most accustomed to the various nuances of congenital aberrations, may have difficulty in optimally displaying the pathology. Three-dimensional (3D) echocardiography provides the greatest spatial resolution and anatomic understanding and should therefore significantly help to optimally diagnose the patient with congenital heart disease.

However, since many congenital heart disease patients become symptomatic while still very young or in infancy, the transthoracic ultrasound imaging probe provides exquisite details and transesophageal echocardiography (TEE) is much less commonly required. The TEE procedure is also more difficult in small weight children and babies. Therefore, until a more developed 3D transthoracic echocardiographic (TTE) probe is available, many of the potential advantages of 3D data sets in these individuals will not be known.

The adult with congenital heart disease is often studied with TEE and many examples have been included in this atlas. The most common congenital abnormality seen by adult echocardiographers is a bicuspid aortic valve. Atrial septal defects are also commonly seen and 3D imaging allows novel *en face* displays to directly assess the size of the defect (which, we have now learned with 3D knowledge, changes in systole and diastole). Other not infrequent congenital abnormalities seen in adults and best understood with 3D echo include: ventricular septal defects; subaortic membranes; left-sided superior vena cava; right-sided aortic arch; anomalous pulmonary venous drainage; patent ductus arteriosus; cor triatriatum; coarctation of the aorta; and Ebstein's anomaly.

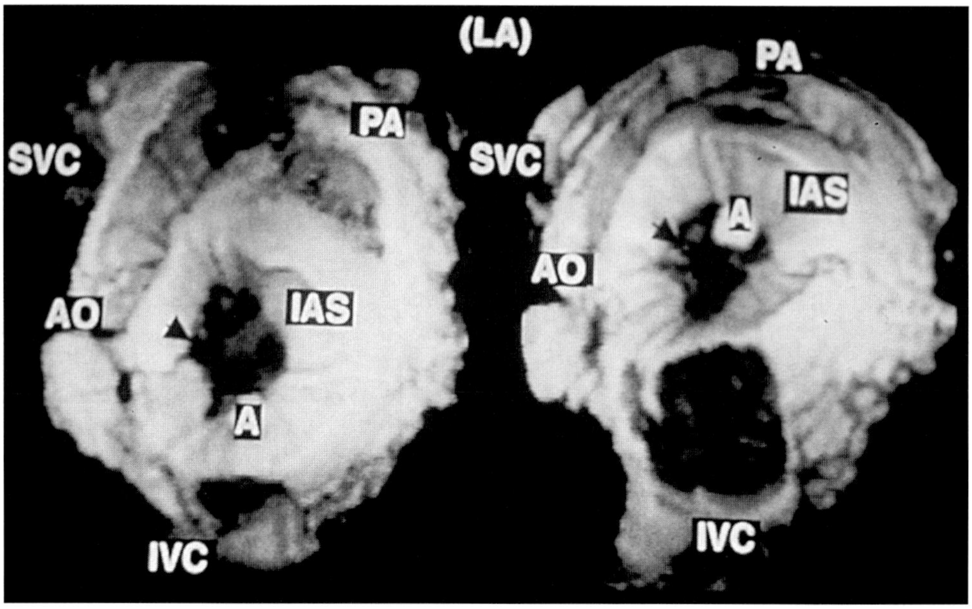

Figure 1. Three-dimensional image with a secundum atrial septal defect (arrows) viewed from the right atrium (RA) in systole and diastole. The image on the left has been rotated supero-inferiorly to demonstrate the great vessels more clearly. "A" represents a technical artifact. AO = aorta; IAS = interatrial septum; IVC = inferior vena cava; LA = left atrium; PA = pulmonary artery; SVC = superior vena cava. Reproduced with permission from Nanda NC et al. Incremental value of three-dimensional echocardiography over transesophageal multiplane two-dimensional echocardiography in qualitative and quantitative assessment of cardiac masses and defects. *Echocardiography* 1995;12:619–628.

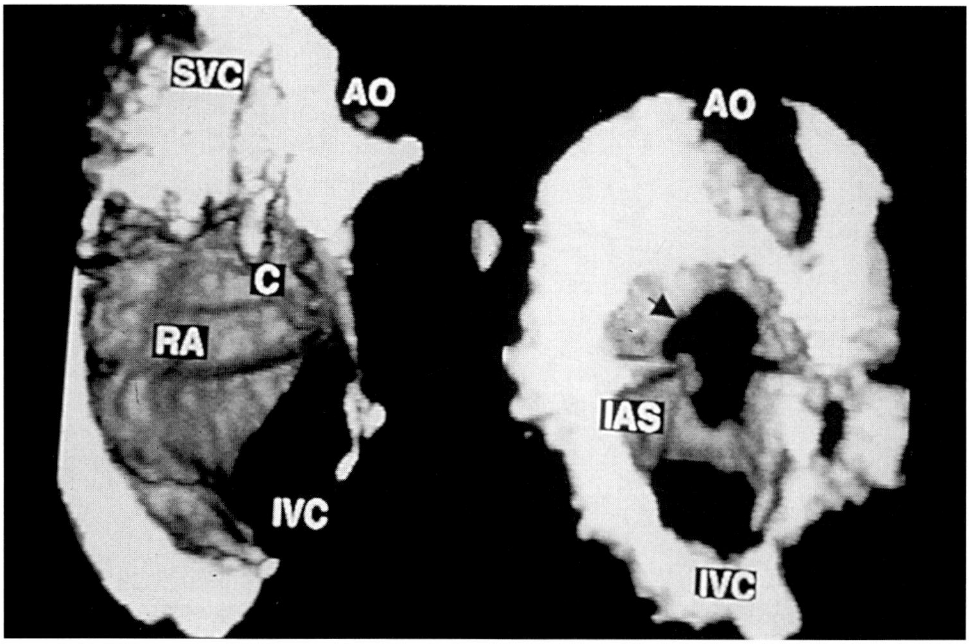

Figure 2. Atrial septal defect (arrow) viewed from the right side (**right**). The image on the **left** shows a catheter (C) in the right atrium. Abbreviations same as in 1. Reproduced with permission from Nanda NC et al. Incremental value of three-dimensional echocardiography over transesophageal multiplane two-dimensional echocardiography in qualitative and quantitative assessment of cardiac masses and defects. *Echocardiography* 1995;12:619–628.

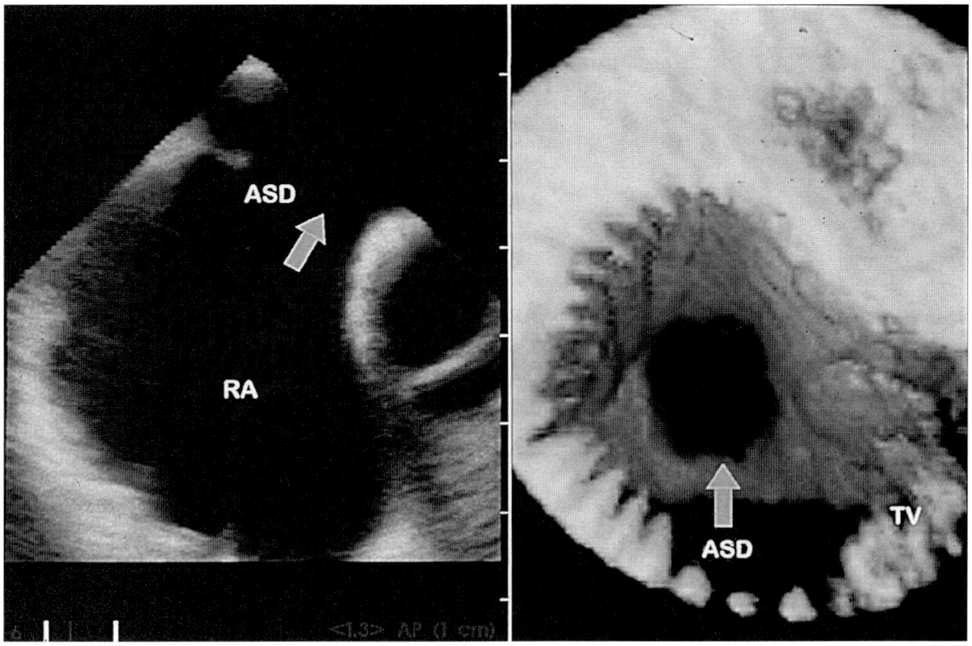

Figure 3. Left: A conventional two-dimensional image showing a large, secundum type atrial septal defect (arrow). **Right:** A three-dimensional reconstruction from the perspective of the left atrium showing the circumferential extent of this defect. From Annette Geibel, MD, Michael Handke, MD, Dietrich Markus Schäfer, MD, Anja Schöchlin, MA, and Helmut Wollschläger, MD.

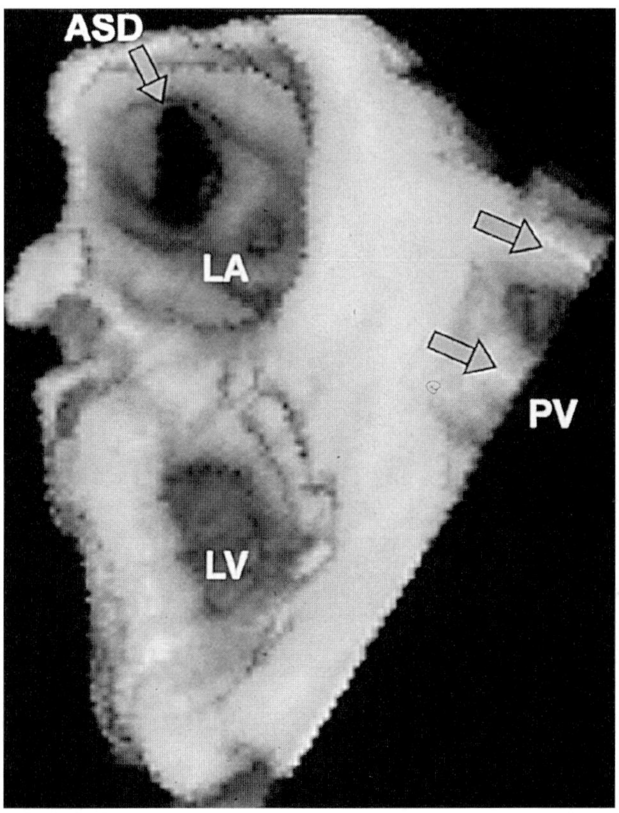

Figure 4. This is an expanded view of a patient with a secundum atrial septal defect that provides the complete interrogation of the atrial and ventricular septum, as well as the atrioventricular groove. The pulmonary veins (PV) are also well seen. From Annette Geibel, MD, Michael Handke, MD, Dietrich Markus Schäfer, MD, Anja Schöchlin, MA, and Helmut Wollschläger, MD.

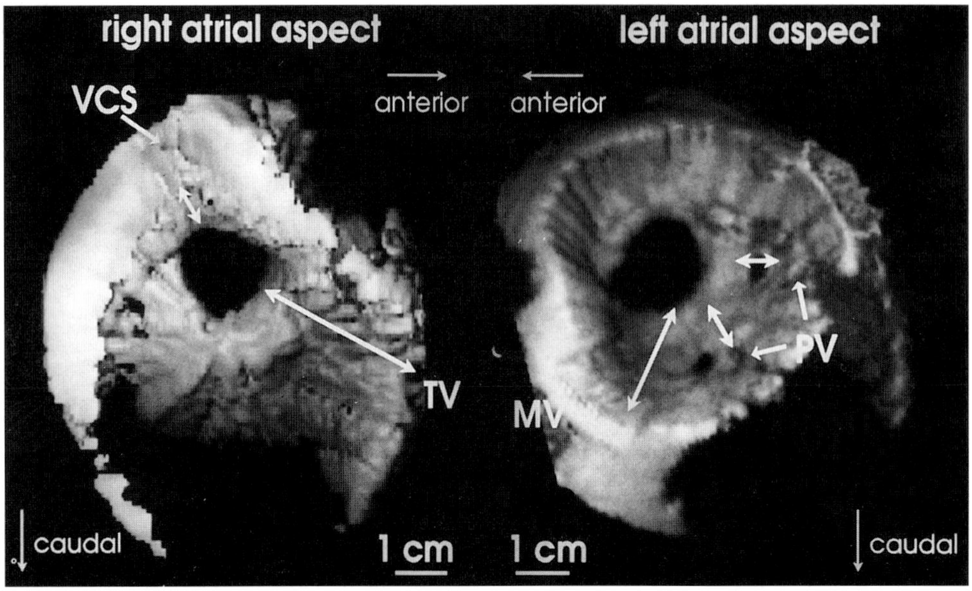

Figure 5. *En-face* view of a secundum-type atrial septal defect (ASD). Measurements of spatial distances from the defect to adjacent cardiac structures within the voxel-reconstructed three-dimensional image. Systolic stop frame images of a large ASD in a 40-year-old woman with a left-to-right shunt of 65%. **Left:** Right atrial aspect with upper caval vein (VCS) and parts of the tricuspid valve (TV). **Right:** Aspect from the left atrium with the distances to the mitral valve ring (MV) and the pulmonary veins (PV) marked by arrows. From Andreas Franke, MD, Harald P. Kühl, MD, and Peter Hanrath, MD. Reprinted with permission from Frank A. et al, Quantitative analysis of the morphology of secundum-type atrial septal defects and their dynamic change using transesophageal three-dimensional echocardiography. *Circulation* 1997;96(Suppl):II-323–327.

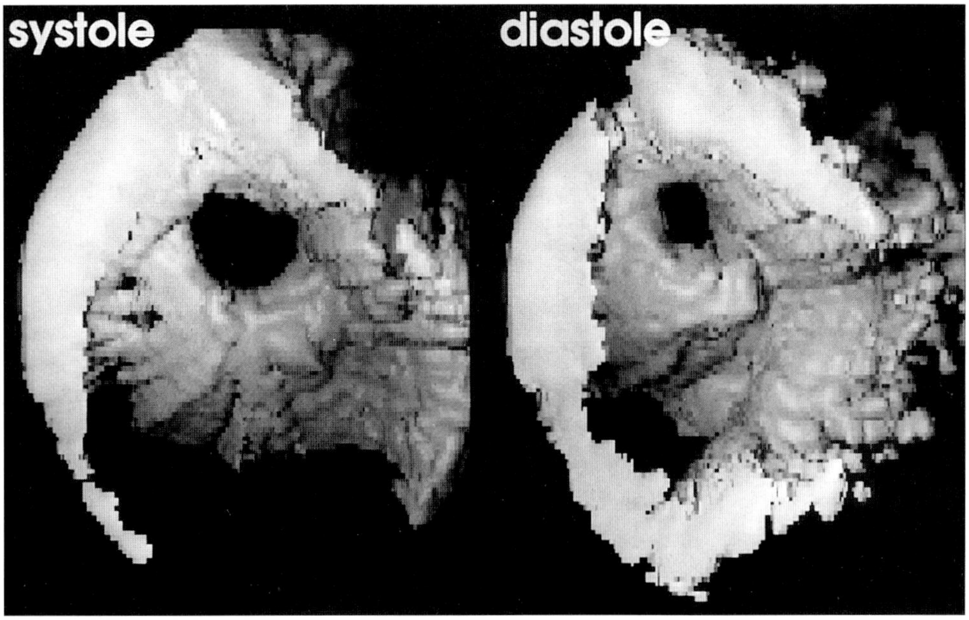

Figure 6. Area changes of a secundum-type atrial septal defect (ASD). **Left:** End-systolic three-dimensional stop-frame image with maximal ASD area viewed from the right atrium. Orientation is as in Figure 5. **Right:** End-diastolic stop-frame image with minimal area. From Andreas Franke, MD, Harald P. Kühl, MD, and Peter Hanrath, MD. Reprinted with permission from Frank A. et al. Quantitative analysis of the morphology of secundum-type atrial septal defects and their dynamic change using transesophageal three-dimensional echocardiography. *Circulation* 1997;96(Suppl):II-323–327.

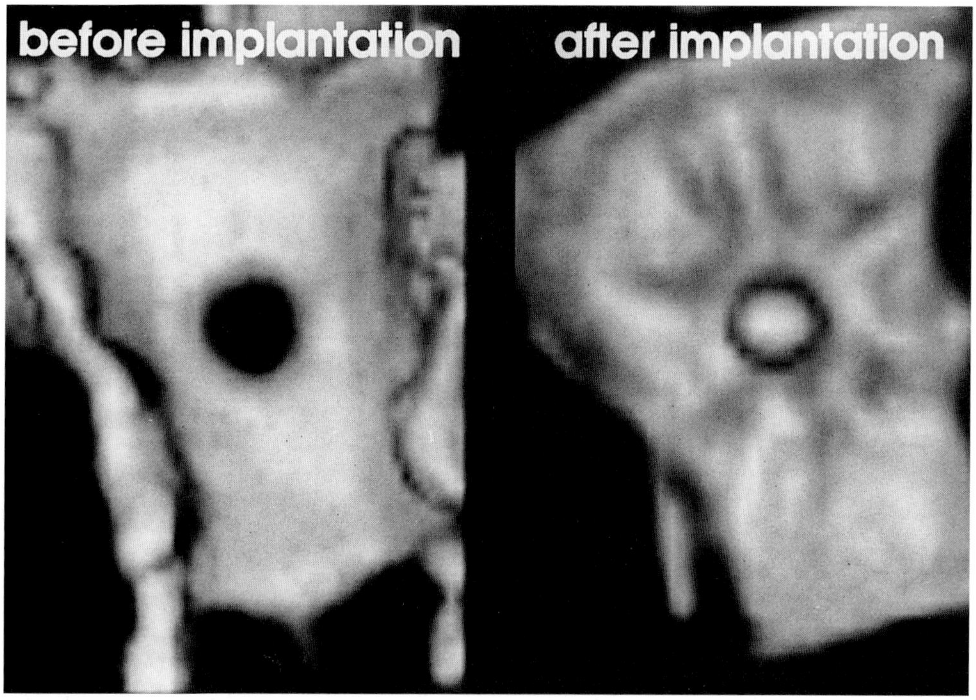

Figure 7. In vitro three-dimensional reconstruction of a simulated atrial septal defect before and after closure with an umbrella device (ASDOS device, Sulzer Osypka). From Andreas Franke, MD, Harald P. Kühl, MD, and Peter Hanrath, MD. Reprinted with permission from Frank A. et al, Quantitative analysis of the morphology of secundum-type atrial septal defects and their dynamic change using transesophageal three-dimensional echocardiography. *Circulation* 1997;96(Suppl):II-323–327.

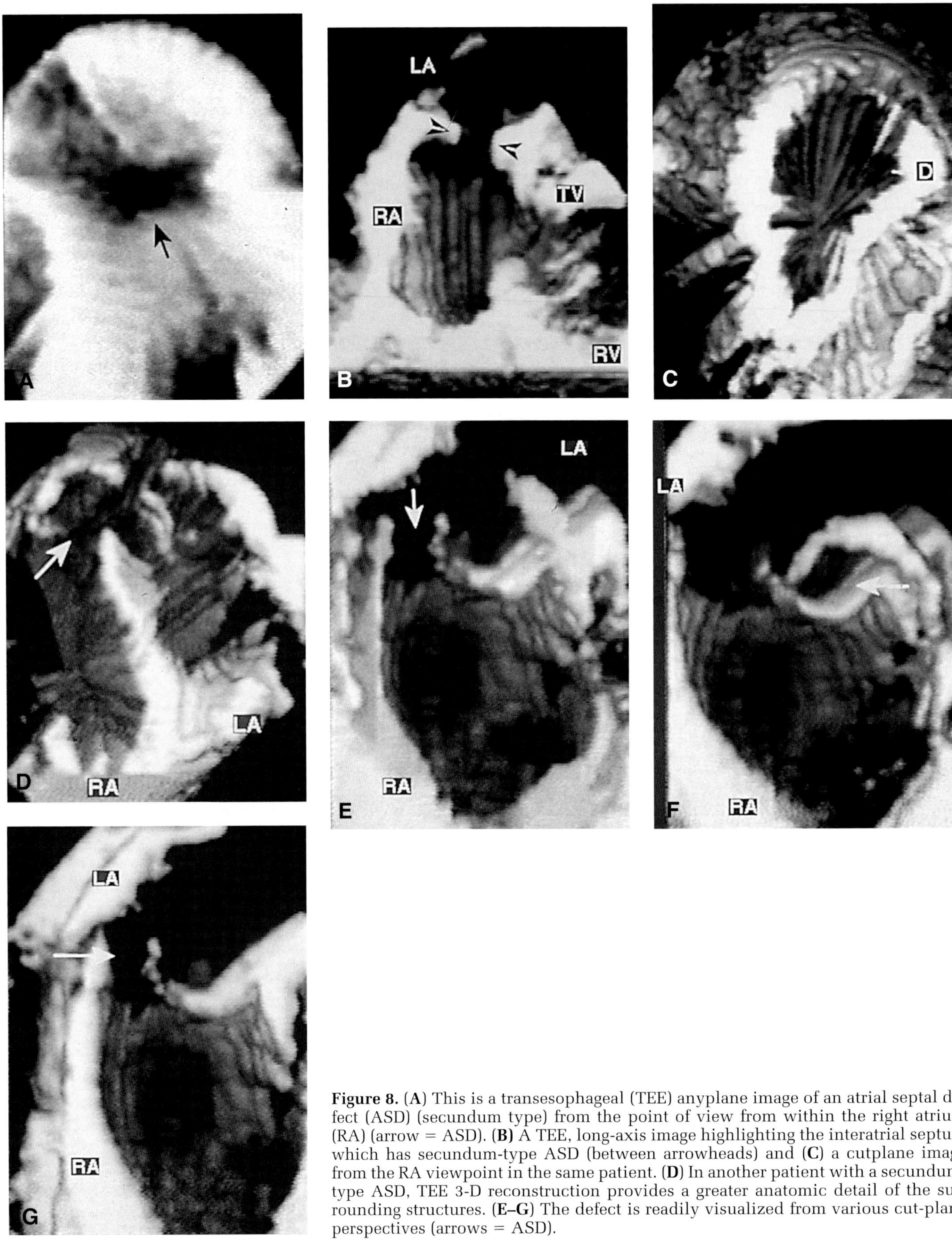

Figure 8. (**A**) This is a transesophageal (TEE) anyplane image of an atrial septal defect (ASD) (secundum type) from the point of view from within the right atrium (RA) (arrow = ASD). (**B**) A TEE, long-axis image highlighting the interatrial septum which has secundum-type ASD (between arrowheads) and (**C**) a cutplane image from the RA viewpoint in the same patient. (**D**) In another patient with a secundum-type ASD, TEE 3-D reconstruction provides a greater anatomic detail of the surrounding structures. (**E–G**) The defect is readily visualized from various cut-plane perspectives (arrows = ASD).

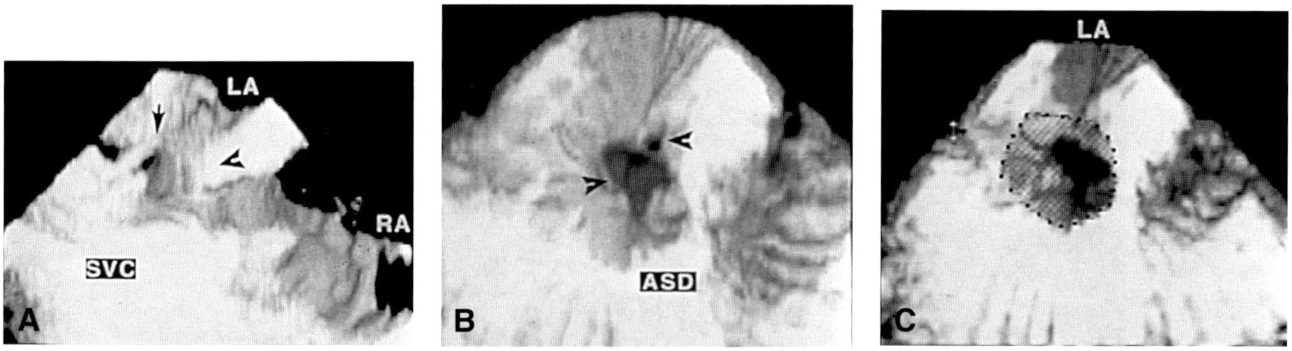

Figure 9. Multiplane transesophageal three-dimensional reconstruction of sinus venosus ASD. (**A**) The arrowhead points to the large defect in the superior portion of the atrial septum. The arrow shows the right superior pulmonary vein (PV) entering the SVC-atrial junction at the site of the defect. (**B, C**) Orthogonal views demonstrating the size of the defect, which measured 3.69cm^2 in area. The maximal dimension of the defect was 2.5 cm, which corresponded to the diameter of 2 cm measured at surgery. The top arrowhead in **B** points to the right superior PV, and the bottom arrowhead points to the defect. ASD=atrial septal defect; LA=left atrium; RA=right atrium; SVC=superior vena cava. Reproduced with permission from Nanda NC et al. Transesophageal three–dimensional echo assessment of sinus venosus atrial septal defect. *Echocardiography* 1999;16:835–837.

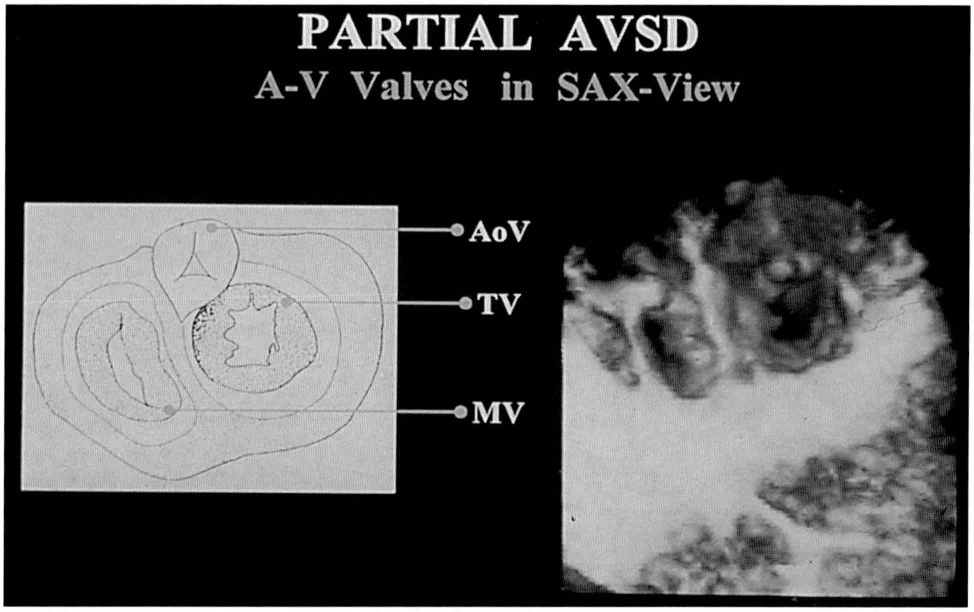

Figure 10. Partial atrial ventricular septal defect. Transthoracic three-dimensional reconstruction of a partial atrioventricular septal defect with an *en face* view of the atrioventricular junction directed from the atrial perspective (**right**) with corresponding schematic diagram (**left**). AoV = aortic valve; MV = mitral valve; TV = tricuspid valve. From Aleksandra Lange, MD.

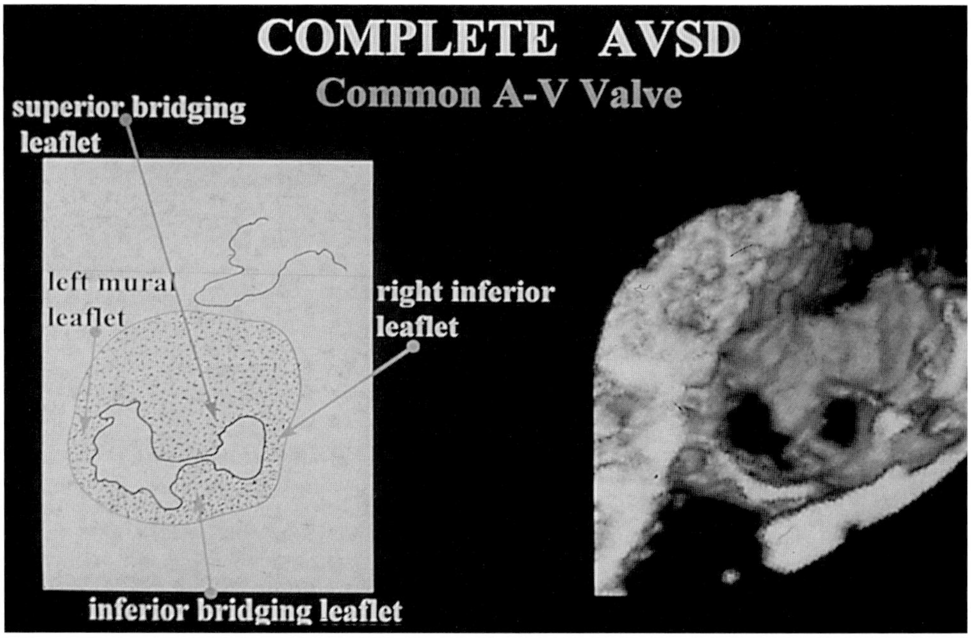

Figure 11. Complete atrial ventricular septal defect. Transthoracic three-dimensional reconstruction of a common atrioventricular valve *en face* from left ventricular perspective (**right**) with a corresponding schematic diagram taken at surgery (**left**). From Aleksandra Lange, MD.

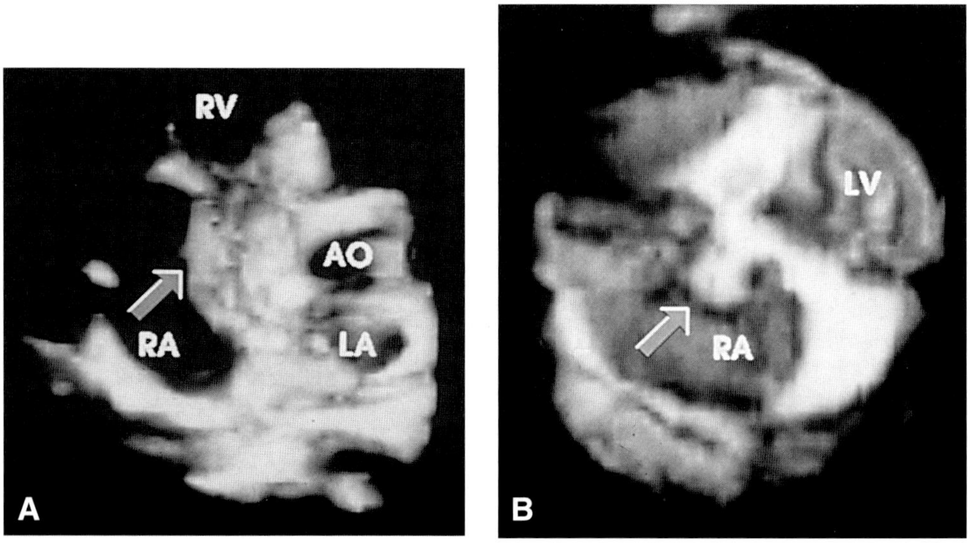

Figure 12. Dynamic three-dimensional images of intracardiac shunt. (**A**) Shunt jet (arrow) from the left atrium (LA) to the right atrium (RA) and then through the tricuspid valve into the right ventricle (RV) in atrial septal defect. (**B**) Cross-sectional view of shunt jet (arrow) from the RA in the same patient.. Reproduced with permission for Li Z et al. Dynamic three-dimensional reconstruction of abnormal intracardiac blood flow. *Echocardiography* 1997;14:375–381.

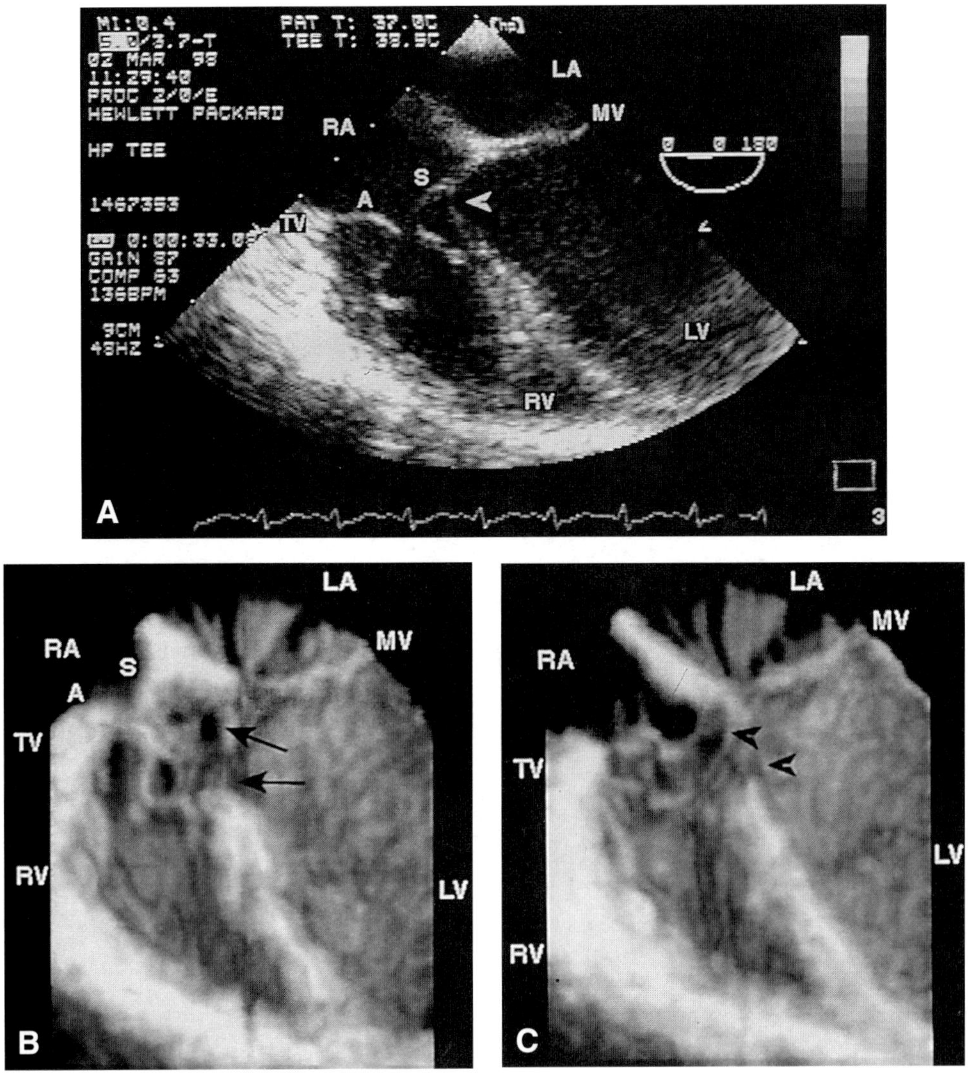

Figure 13. Transesophageal echo (TEE) two-dimensional image (**A**) from the mid-esophageal level showing an apical 4-chamber view of a patient with a basal membranous ventricular septal defect (VSD), compared directly with a similar cut-plane, 3-D reconstruction image of the same patient (**B**). Arrowheads = defect. The defect is noted to enter the right atrium in a manner consistent with a Gerbode defect. (**C**) Slightly different TEE, long-axis perspective of the VSD (arrows) in the previous figure. A= anterior TV leaflet; S = septal TV leaflet.

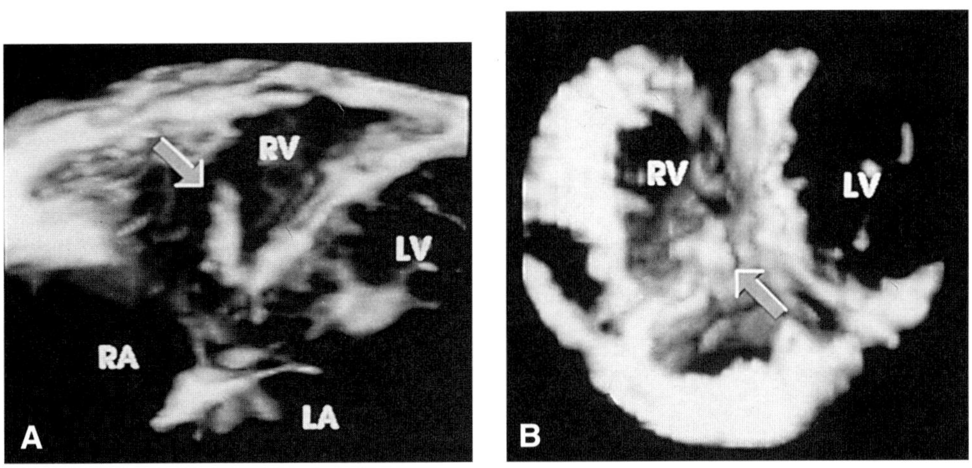

Figure 14. (**A**) Shunt jet (arrow) from the left ventricle (LV) to right ventricle (RV) with a ventricular septal defect. (**B**) Cross-sectional view of shunt jet (arrow) from the RV in the same patient. AO = aorta. Reproduced with permission for Li Z et al. Dynamic three-dimensional reconstruction of abnormal intracardiac blood flow. *Echocardiography* 1997;14:375–381.

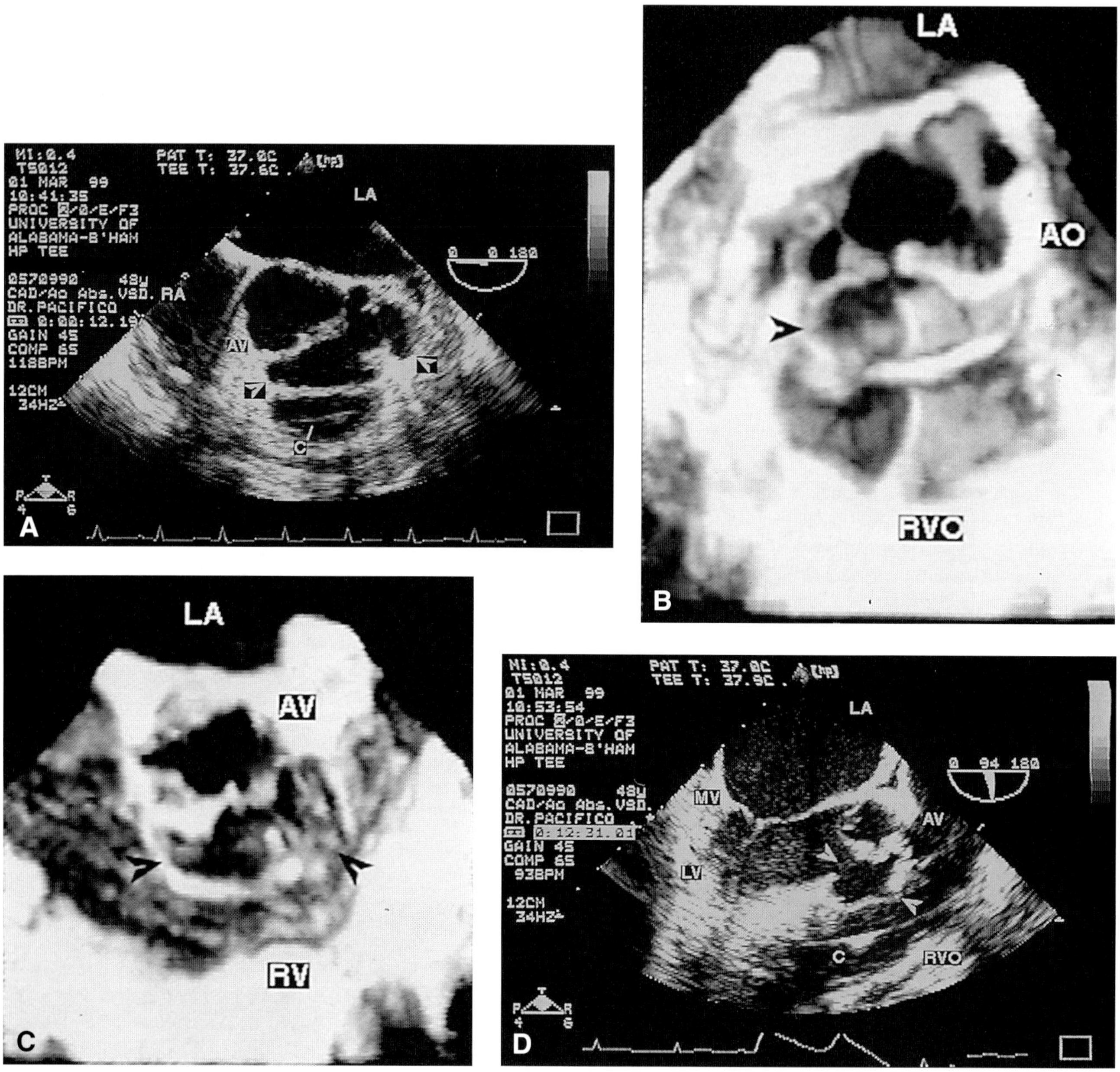

Figure 15. (**A**) Two-dimensional, transesophageal echo (2D TEE), short axis, upper esophageal view of the aortic valve showing a large perivalvular extension of infection (abscess = arrowheads) in a typical location for a patient with ventricular septal defect. C = catheter in the right ventricular outflow tract. (**B**) A similarly chosen orientation, three-dimensional (3D) image is shown for comparison. (**C**) Slight adjustment in the image orientation of the previous figure allows optimal interrogation of this abscess (arrowheads). (**D**) 2D TEE image, upper-mid esophageal view highlighting the left ventricular outflow tract further illustrates the relationship of this abscess to the surrounding structures.

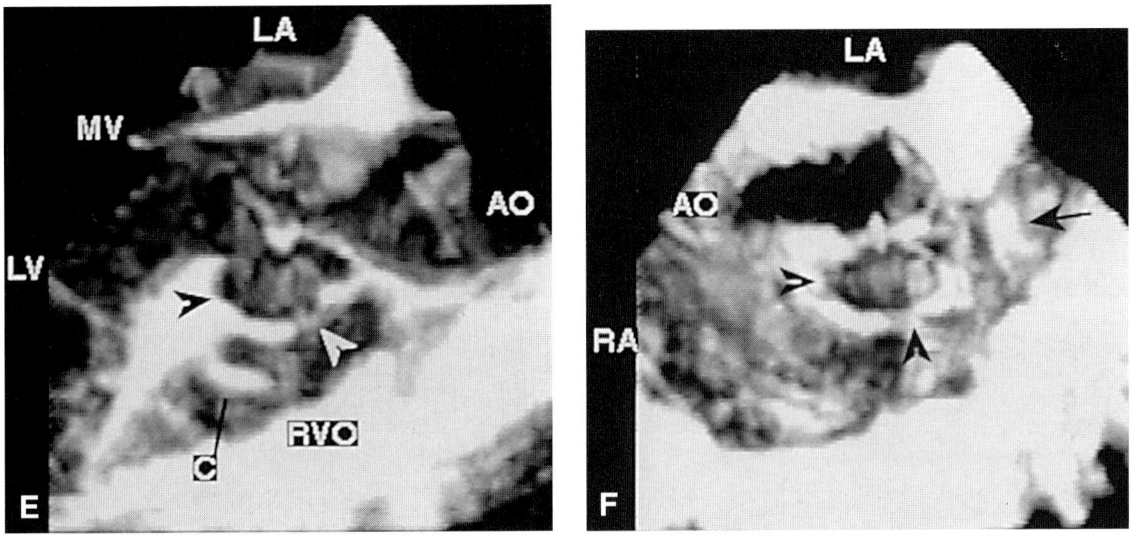

Figure 15. Continued. (**E**) A 3D reconstruction, zoom image of a very similar orientation as the 2D image. The extent of the abscess is appreciated to a much greater degree in the 3D image. (**F**) Short axis orientation providing another still-frame image of the abscess. It allows the reader to begin to obtain a better understanding of the image in motion (or 4D echo).

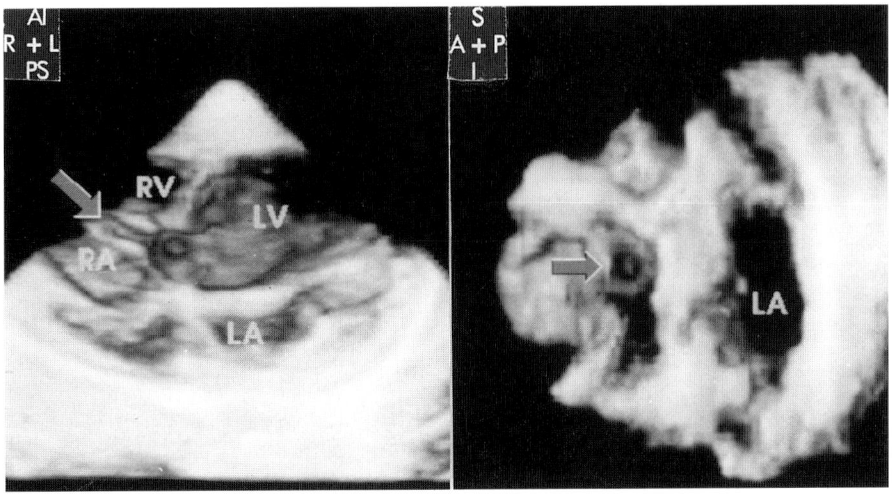

Figure 16. Interventricular septal defect examined by transthoracic echocardiography. **Left:** In four-chamber view, defect appears as a tunnel (arrow) between left and right ventricles. **Right:** By sectioning heart along septum and observing septum from perpendicular direction, defect appears as a circle (arrow). Reproduced with permission from Wang XF. Four-dimensional echocardiography; Methods and clinical application. *Am Heart J* 1996;132:678.

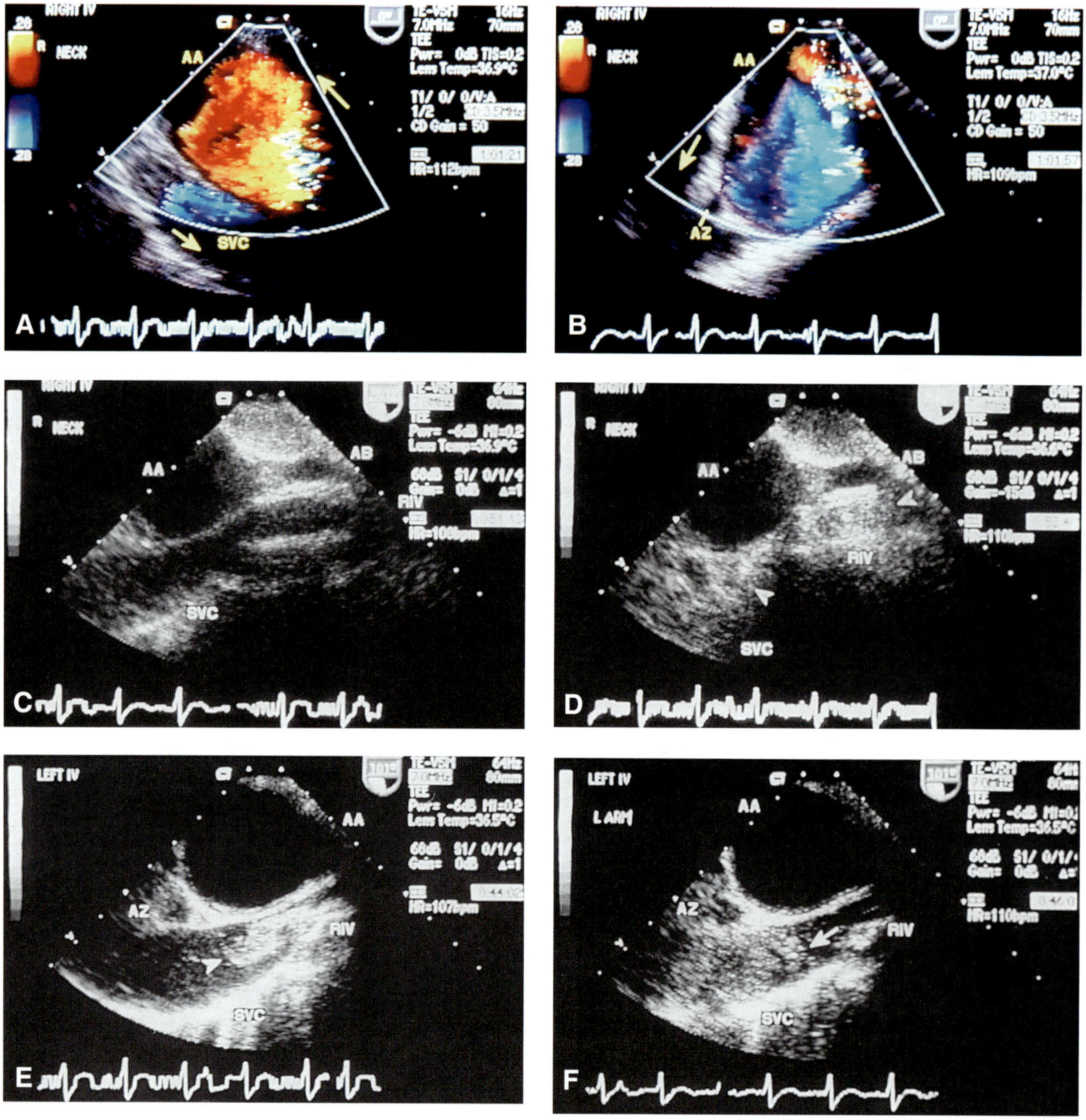

Figure 17. Transesophageal echocardiography in right-sided aortic arch without dissection. (**A**) Color Doppler examination shows the proximal aortic arch (AA) oriented in a left-to-right and anteroposterior direction. The superior vena cava (SVC) is imaged anterior to AA. Imaging of a large vascular structure such as the SVC next to the AA may mimic aortic dissection. (**B**) Slight advancement and rotation of the probe from the position used to image the proximal AA brings into view the distal portion of the AA, which is identified by posteroanterior direction of blood flow. Both **A** and **B** were imaged at a plane angulation of 0°. AZ = azygos vein. (**C-F**) The right innominate vein (RIV) is seen joining the SVC. The arch branch (AB) adjacent to RIV is the right subclavian artery. Saline contrast injections through a catheter placed in the right external jugular vein demonstrated contrast signals entering the SVC from RIV (arrowheads in **D** and **E**). On the other hand, saline contrast injections through a peripheral left arm vein fills the SVC (arrow in **F**) without any opacification of the RIV.

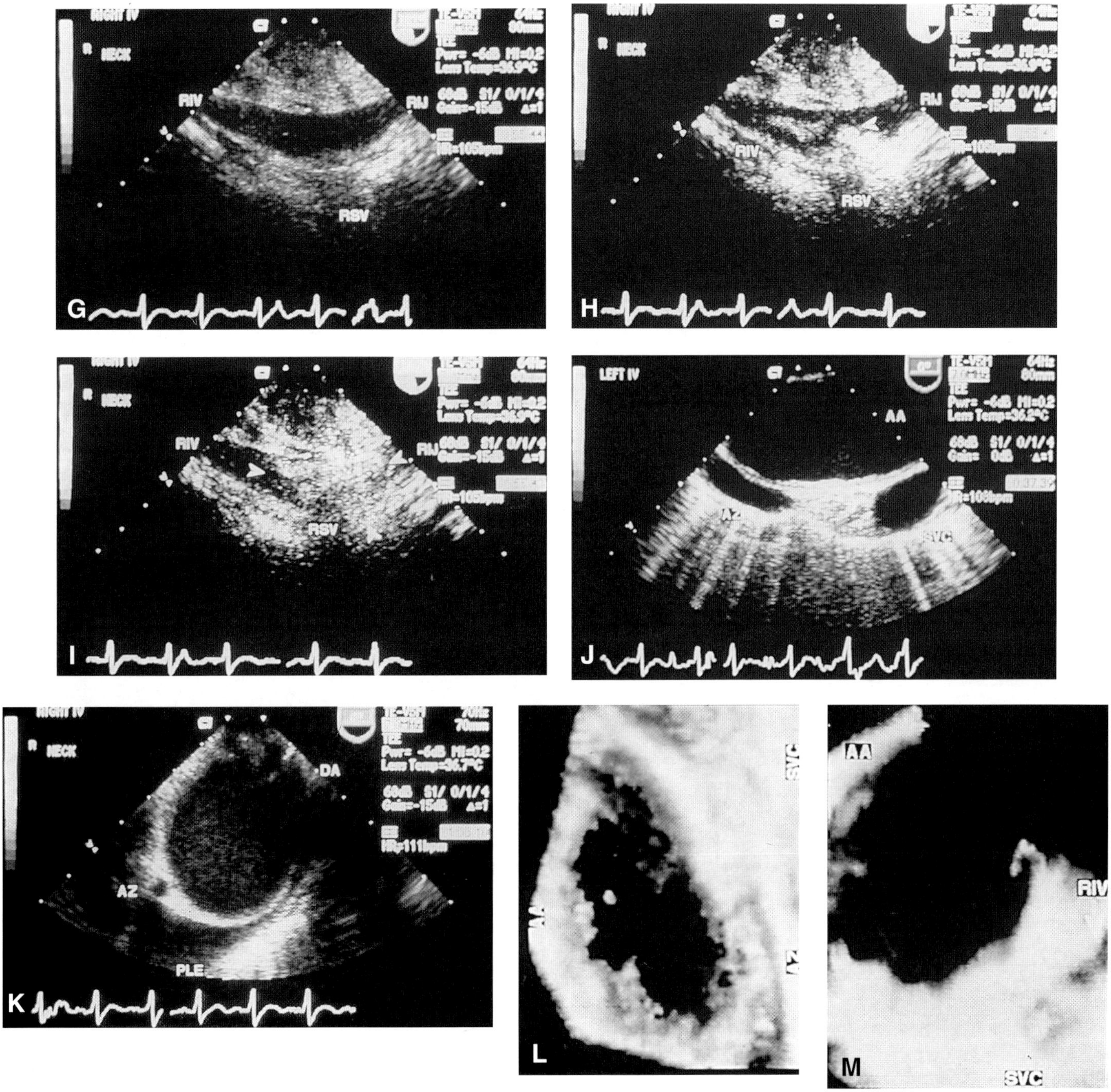

Figure 17. Continued. (**G–I**) Withdrawal of the probe from this position demonstrates the right subclavian (RSV) and the right internal jugular (RIJ) veins joining to form the RIV. Intravenous saline contrast injections through the right external jugular vein demonstrate contrast echoes (arrowheads) moving from the RSV into the RIV with some reflux into RIJ. (**J–K**) The azygos vein is also imaged anterior to AA and adjacent to SVC. (**J**) By advancing the probe from this position, it could be followed down to the level of the proximal descending thoracic aorta (DA). (**K**) Intravenous saline contrast injections from the right neck and from the left arm did not show any contrast echoes in the AX vein. PLE = left pleural effusion. (**L, M**) Three-dimensionally reconstructed images of the AA, SVC, AZ vein and RIV. Reproduced with permission from Nanda NC et al. Transesophageal echocardiographic diagnosis of right-sided aortic arch. *Echocardiography* 1998;409–417.

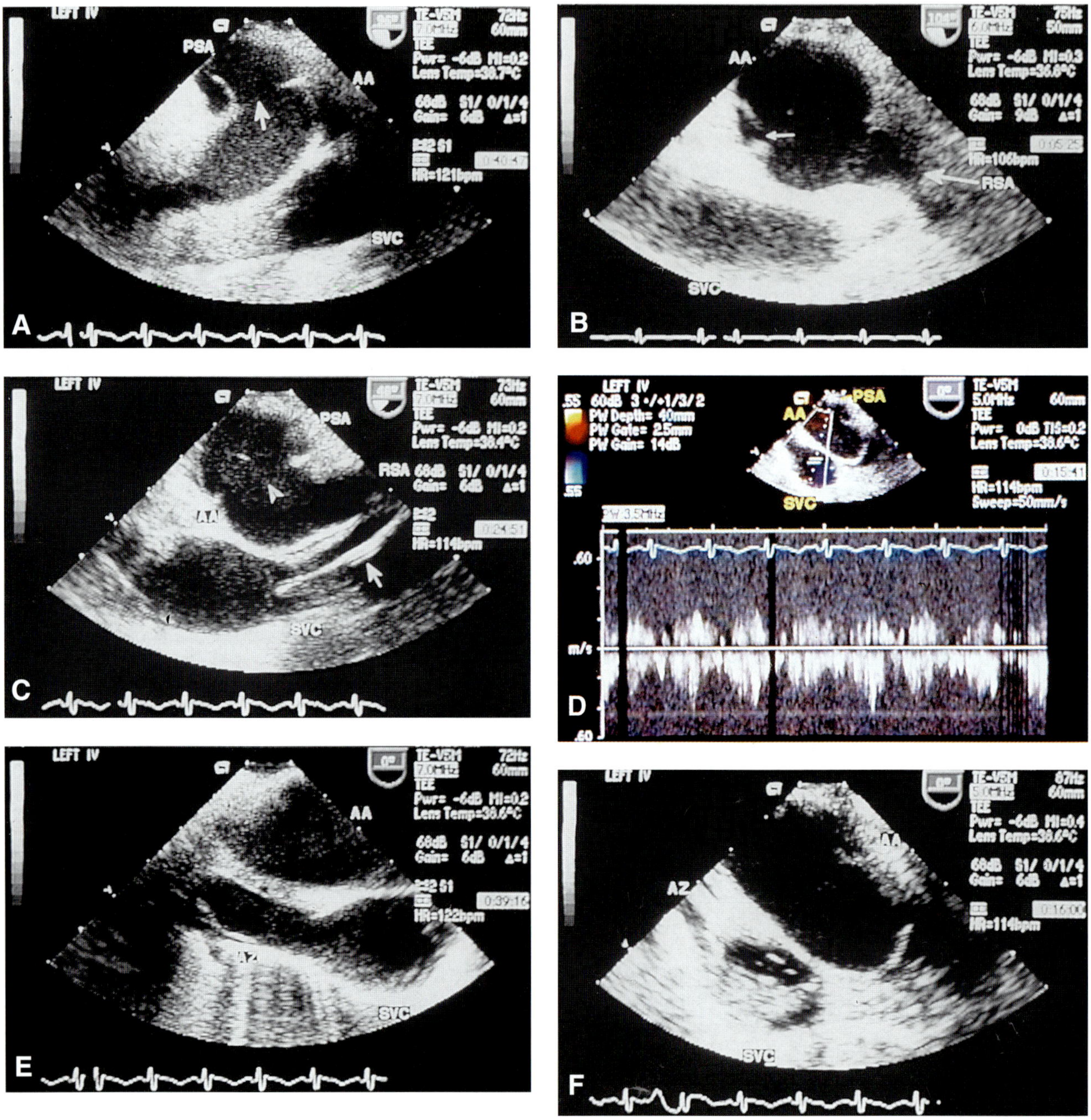

Figure 18. Transesophageal echocardiography in right-sided aortic arch with traumatic aortic injury (dissection). (**A**) The dissection flap as well as the communication (arrow) from the aortic arch (AA) into the pseudoaneurysm (PSA) are clearly shown. The superior vena cava (SVC) is imaged anterior to AA. (**B**) Shows the origin of the right subclavian artery (RSA) from the AA. The small arrow points to the dissection flap. (**C**) The arrow points to a catheter in the SVC. The arrowhead denotes the communication into the PSA. (**D**) Pulse Doppler interrogation of SVC demonstrates prominent flow signals throughout the cardiac cycle indicative of venous flow. (**E**) A prominent azygos (A) vein is connected to the SVC. (**F**) With left-sided intravenous saline contrast injections, contrast echoes first appeared in the SVC and then refluxed into the AZ vein.

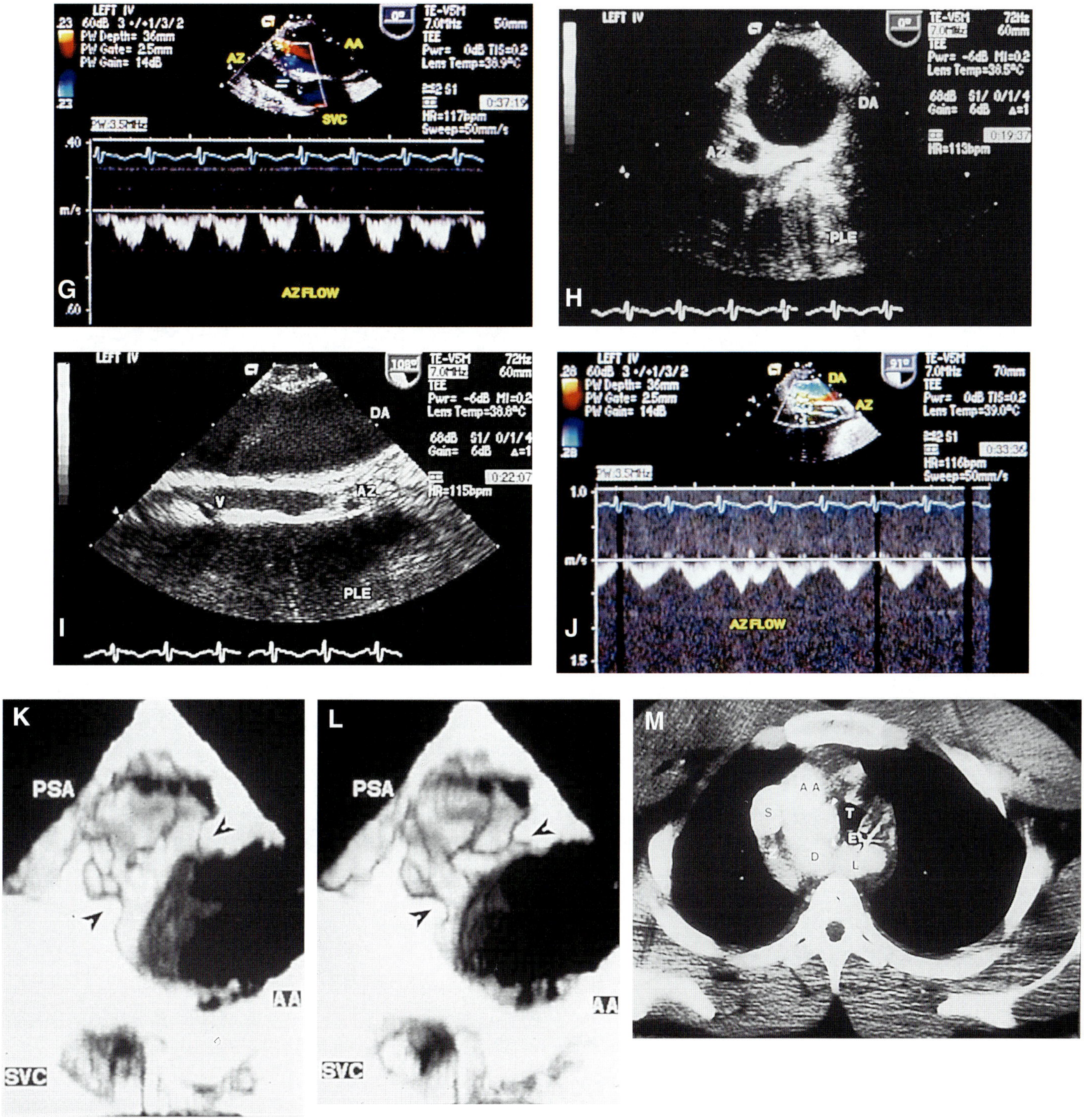

Figure 18. Continued. (**G**) Pulse Doppler interrogation of AZ vein also shows prominent flow signals throughout the cardiac cycle typical of venous flow. (**H**) Advancement of the probe from the arch position (keeping the same plane angulation of 0°) demonstrates both the proximal descending thoracic aorta (DA) and the AZ vein in short axis. Movement of the probe up and down the esophagus served to confirm the identity of the venous structure joining the SVC from the right side as the AZ vein. (**I**) AZ vein viewed in long axis next to the DA. V represents a venous valve at the junction of a tributary. (**J**) Pulse Doppler interrogation of the AZ vein shows typical venous type of flow. (**K, L**) Three-dimensionally reconstructed images showing the SVC, AA, PSA and the communication (arrowheads). (**M**) CT scan. The superior vena cava (S) and the azygos vein (Z) are imaged adjacent to the aortic arch (AA). The arrowheads point to possible pseudoaneurysm. D = descending thoracic aorta; E = esophagus; L = left subclavian artery; T = trachea. Reproduced with permission from Nanda NC et al. Transesophageal echocardiographic diagnosis of right-sided aortic arch. *Echocardiography* 1998;409–417.

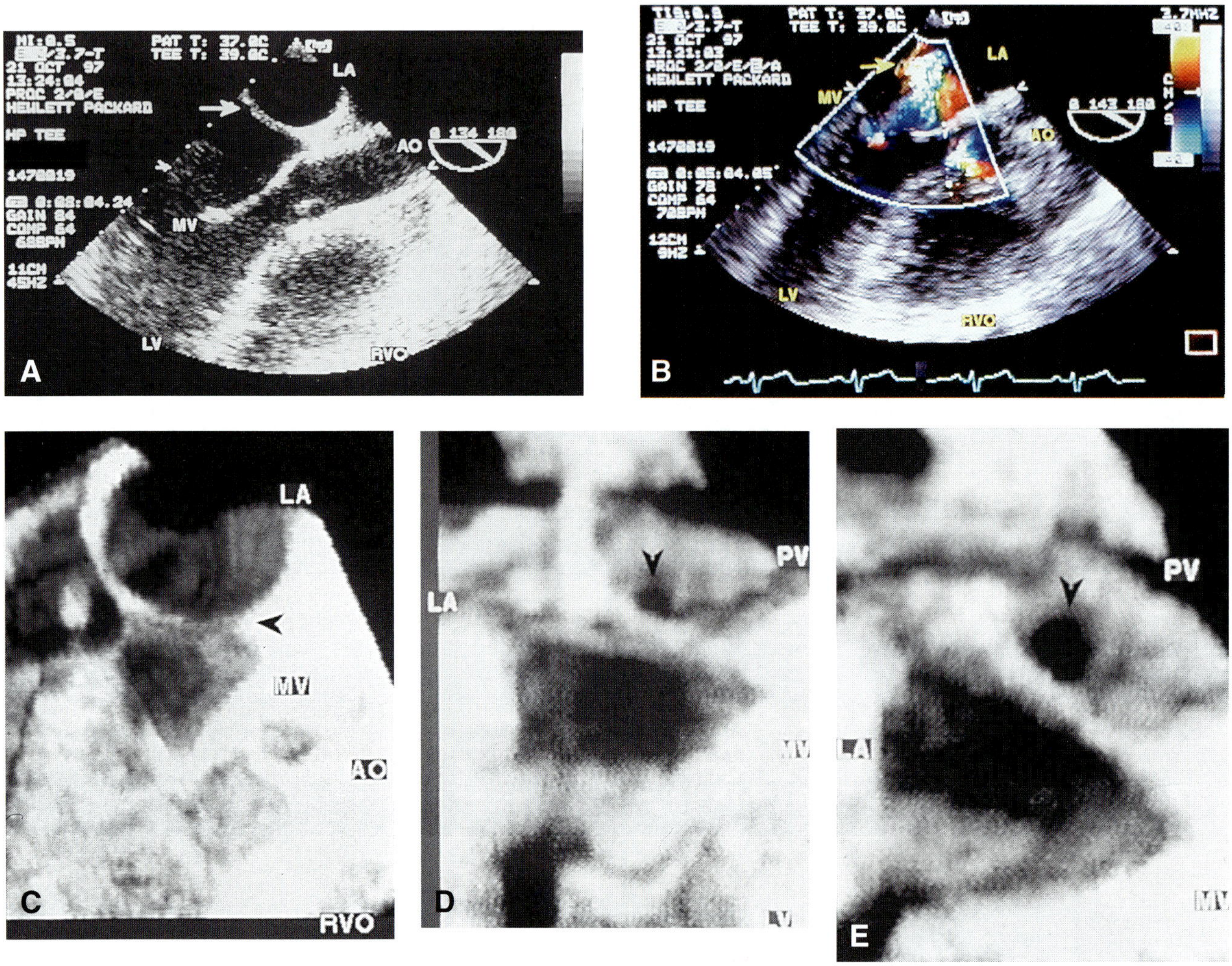

Figure 19. (**A, B**) Transesophageal (TEE) two-dimensional study showing a membrane (arrow in **A**) dividing the left atrium (cor triatriatum). The arrow in **B** points to turbulent flow across the membrane, indicative of obstruction. (**C–E**) TEE three-dimensionally reconstructed images. The arrowhead in **C** points to the membrane. The arrowheads in **D** and **E** demonstrate the opening in the membrane. (**E**) Tilting of the image resulted in optimal visualization of the opening. AO = aorta; AV = aortic valve; LA = left atrium; LV = left ventricle; MV = mitral valve; PV = pulmonary vein; RVO = right ventricular outflow tract. Reproduced with permission from Samal AK et al. Three-dimensional echocardiographic reconstruction of atrial membranes. *Echocardiography* 1998;15:605–610.

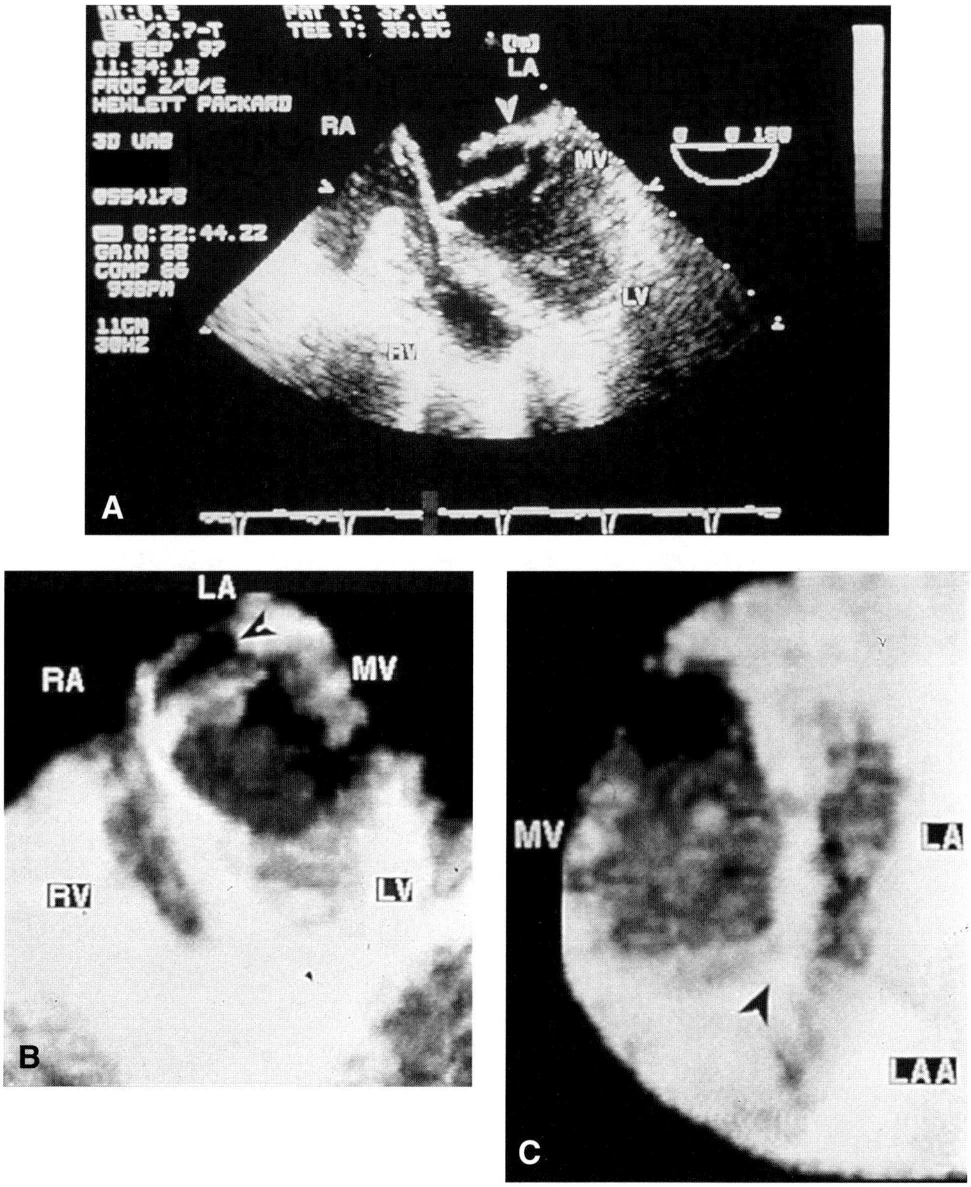

Figure 20. Mitral supravalvular membrane. (**A**) Transesophageal two-dimensional study. The arrowhead points to a membrane in the left atrium located just above the mitral valve (MV). (**B, C**) Transesophageal three-dimensionally reconstructed images. The arrowhead in **B** shows the opening in the membrane. (**C**) Membrane located inferior to the left atrial appendage (LAA); this finding serves to differentiate it from cor triatriatum sinister (sinistrum). RA = right atrium; RV = right ventricle. Other abbreviations as in Figure 18. Reproduced with permission from Samal AK et al. Three-dimensional echocardiographic reconstruction of atrial membranes. *Echocardiography* 1998;15:605–610.

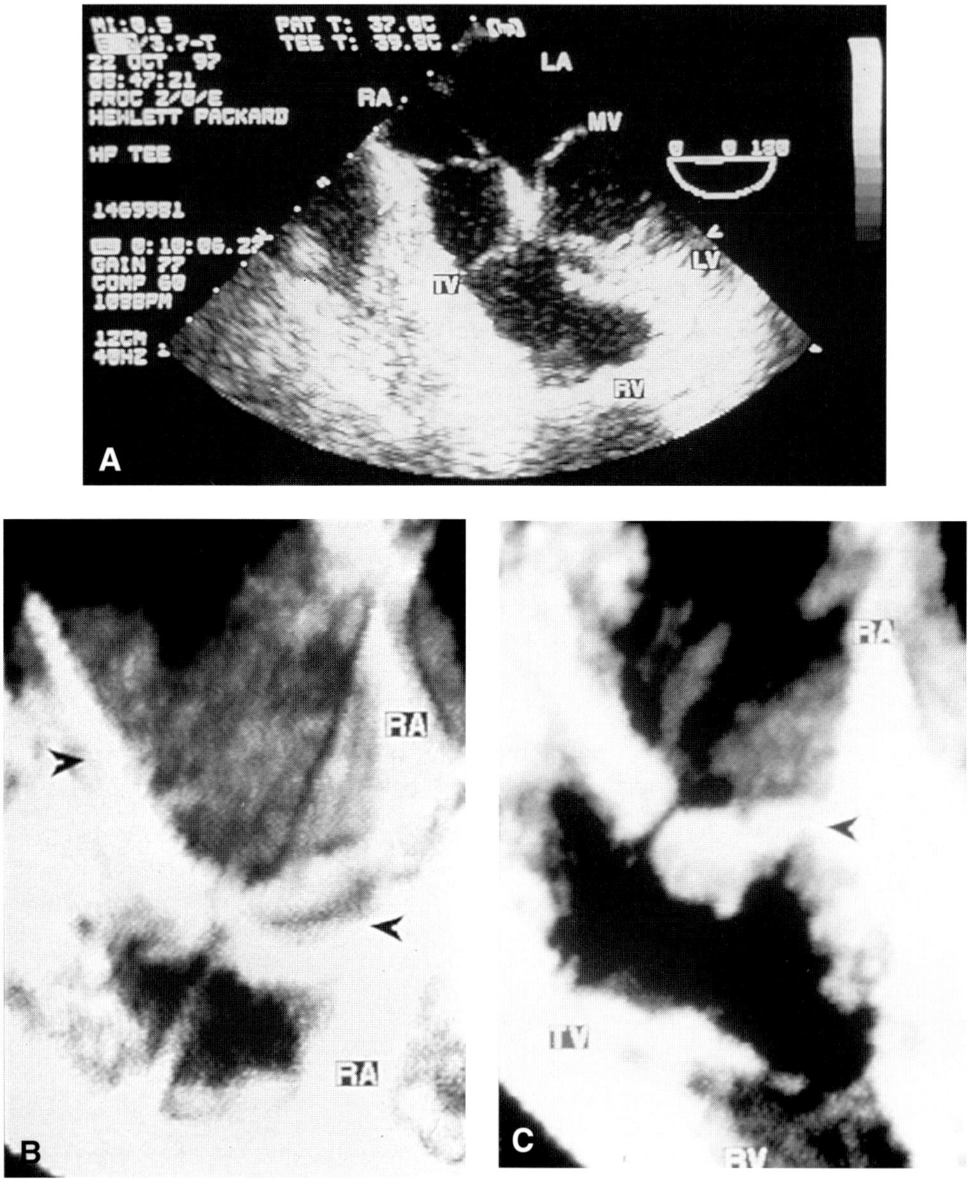

Figure 21. Cor triatriatum dexter. (**A**) Transesophageal two-dimensional image. The arrow points to the membrane in the right atrium (RA). (**B, C**) Transesophageal three-dimensional reconstructed images. The arrowheads demonstrate the membrane. TV = tricuspid valve. Other abbreviations as in Figures 18 and 19. Reproduced with permission from Samal AK et al. Three-dimensional echocardiographic reconstruction of atrial membranes. *Echocardiography* 1998;15:605–610.

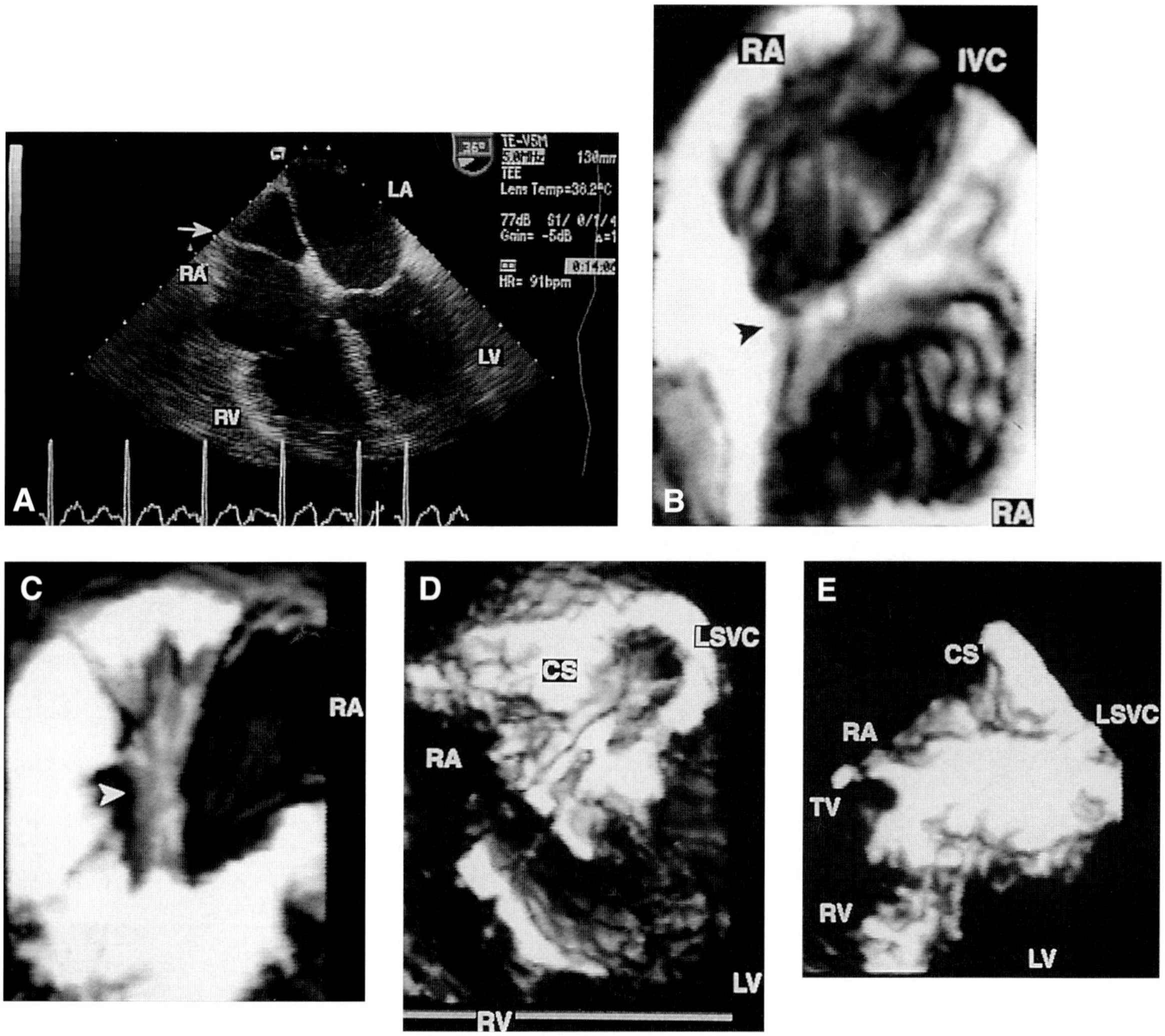

Figure 22. Cor Triatriatum Dexter with persistent left superior vena cava (LSVC) series. (**A**) Two-dimensional apical 4-chamber image of a patient with a cor triatriatum dexter (arrow) for comparison to the three-dimensional (3D) images that follow. (**B, C**) 3D reconstructed transesophageal echo (TEE) *en-face* images of the right atrium highlighting the membrane (arrow) separating the RA (cor triatriatum dexter). (**D, E**) TEE study, long-axis view, lower esophageal position, highlighting the ostium of the coronary sinus (CS) which was dilated due to a LSVC. The persistent LSVC can be displayed in short-axis (**D**) or long axis (**E**).

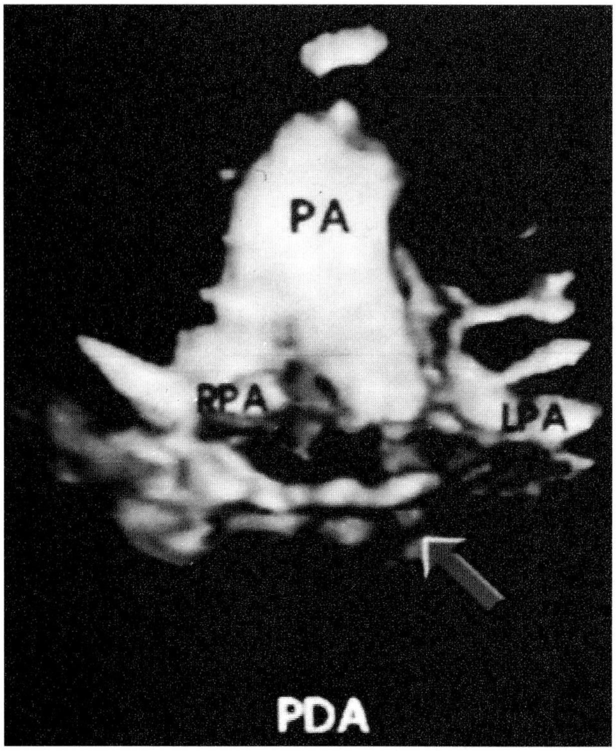

Figure 23. Obtained from patient with patent ductus arteriosus by transthoracic echo in diastole, showing main pulmonary artery (PA) and right and left pulmonary arteries; there was another stream of blood flow representing patent ductus arteriosus (PDA) (arrow) and joining left pulmonary artery. Reproduced with permission from Wang XF. Four-dimensional echocardiography: Methods and clinical application. *Am Heart J* 1996;132:672–684.

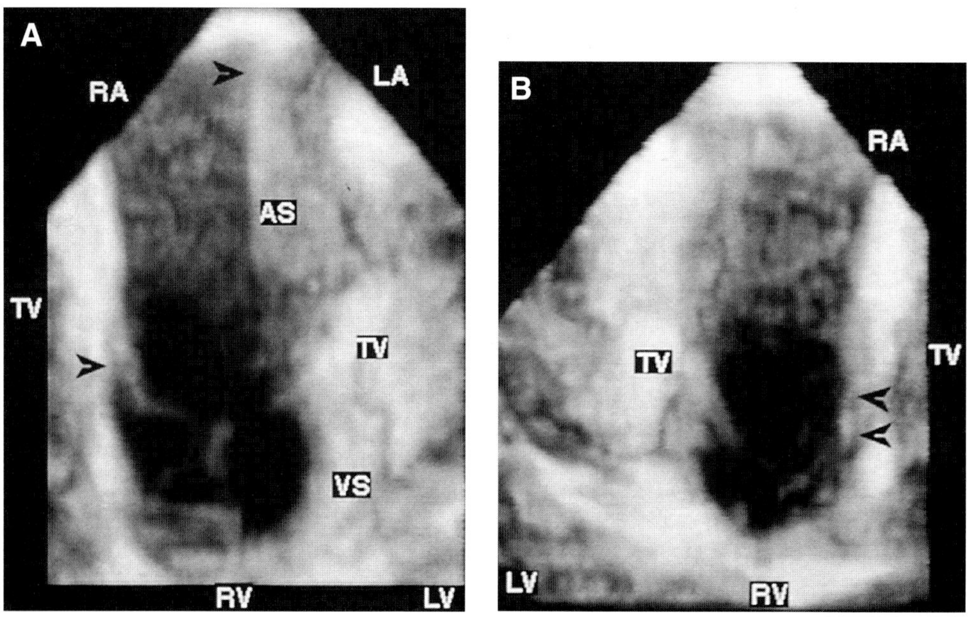

Figure 24. (**A**) Transesophageal echo, three-dimensional (TEE 3D) reconstruction image of a patient with an Ebstein's anomaly. Note the apically displaced tricuspid valve (TV) (lower arrowhead) shown in systole. An atrial septal defect is also noted (upper arrow) in the basal portion of the atrial septum (AS). (**B**) This TEE 3D reconstruction of the same patient with Ebstein's anomaly was chosen to illustrate to a greater degree the anterior TV leaflet in diastole. arrowheads = TV leaflets with tethering to the right ventricular free wall.

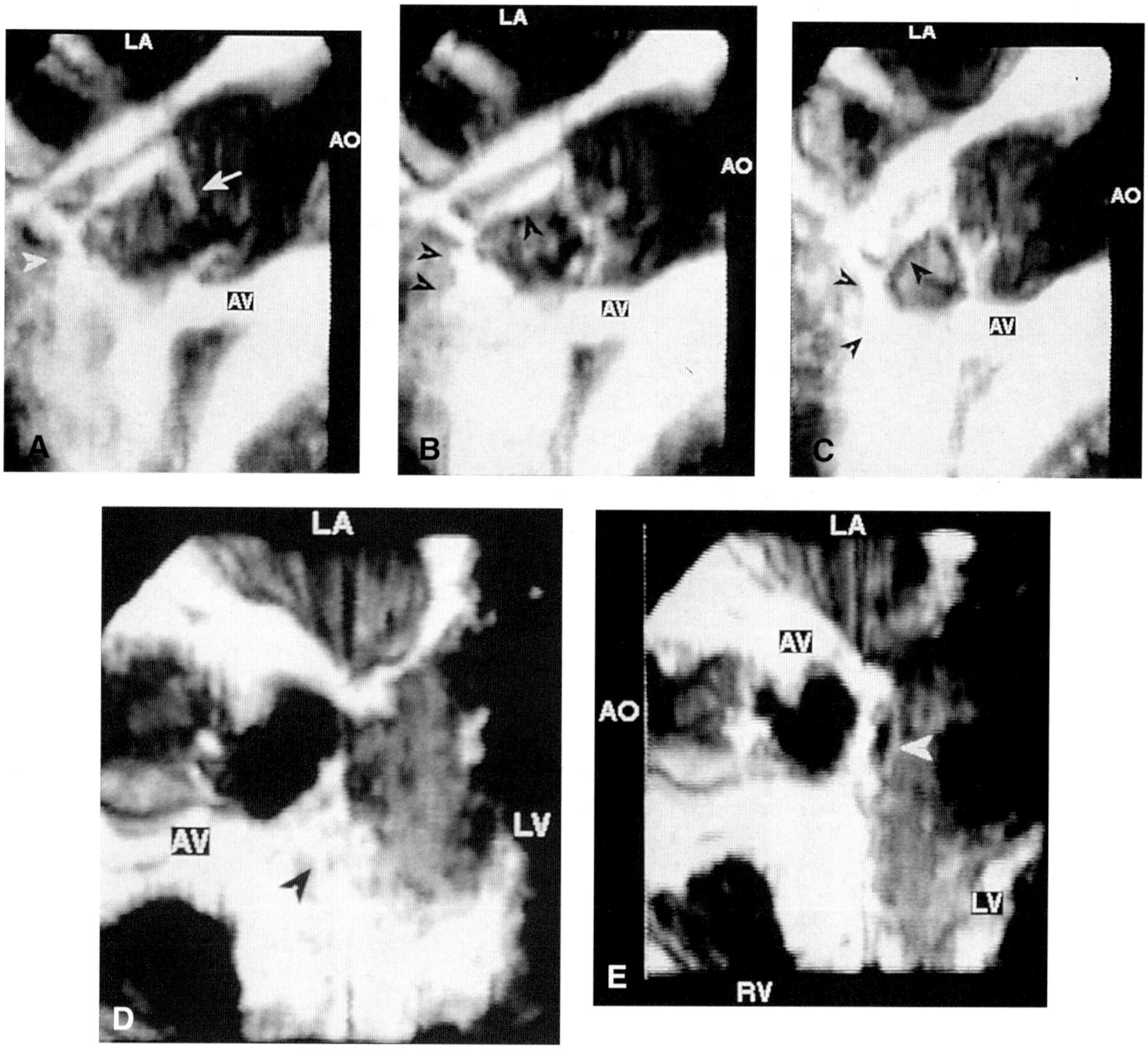

Figure 25. Subaortic membrane series. (**A, B**) Transesophageal echo (TEE), long-axis, zoom image of the left ventricular outflow tract (LVO) and aorta (AO) in a patient with a stenotic subaortic membrane (arrowheads left figure) shown in systole (**A**) and diastole (**B**). The aortic valve is mildly thickened and noted to characteristically close early (arrow in **A**). Calcification of the LVO is common and noted in **B**. (**C**) With a slightly different cutplane orientation, the extent of the membrane seen in the previous figures is more clearly delineated (arrowheads) and noted to completely encircle the LVO. (**D**) TEE, midesophageal, 3D apical 5-chamber equivalent image of the patient in the previous figures highlighting the LVO and the abnormal subaortic membrane (arrowhead). (**E**) By "opening" the LV further with a slightly varied cut-plane orientation, the membrane is noted to span the LVO (arrowhead). These types of post-acquisition, anyplane images provide an infinite number of views and often incrementally add to the final, limited baseline knowledge available with only 2D TEE.

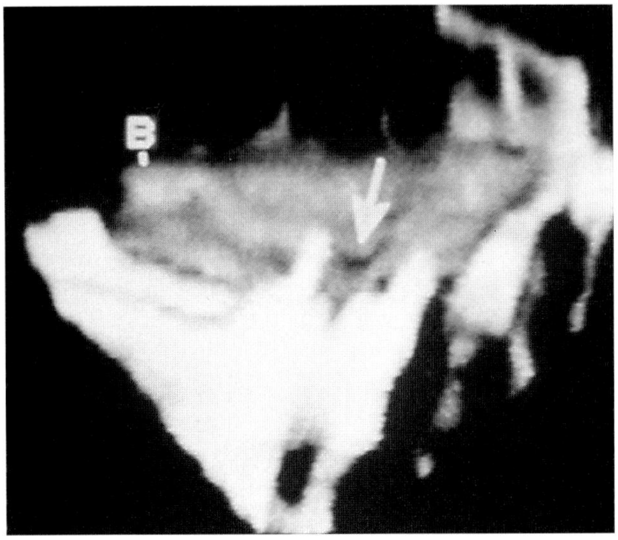

Figure 26. Atrial baffle (status post-Senning procedure). Transthoracic three-dimensionally reconstructed image. The arrow points to a small defect in the baffle (B). Reproduced with permission from Samal AK et al. Three-dimensional echocardiographic reconstruction of atrial membranes. *Echocardiography* 1998;15:605–610.

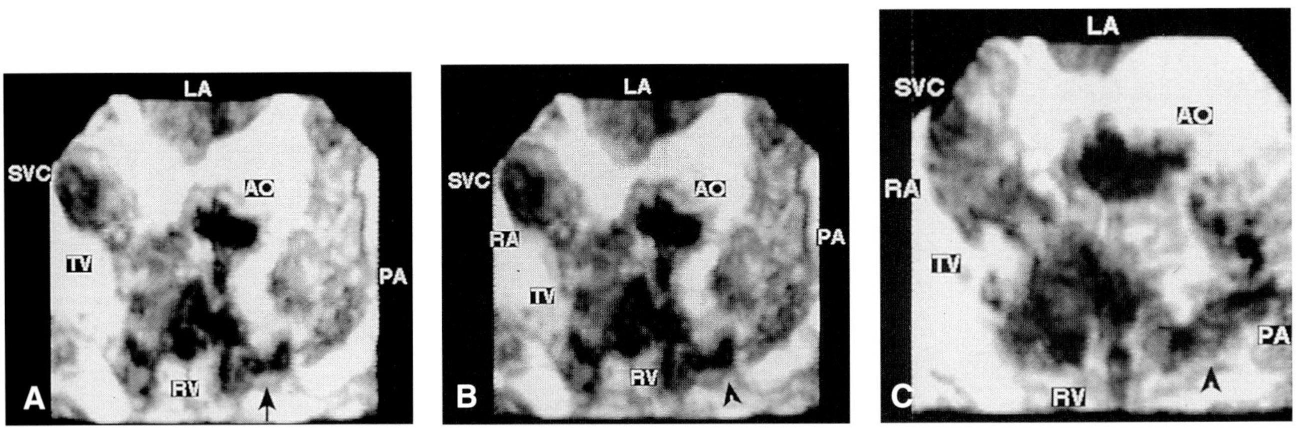

Figure 27. Subpulmonic stenosis series. (**A**) TEE oblique cutplane image of the right ventricular outflow tract (RVO) and main pulmonary artery (PA) in a patient with subpulmonic stenosis (arrow). (**B**) Less contrast and more shading may assist in imaging the desired structure as in this patient in which the subpulmonic stenosis (arrow) is better defined. (**C**) Additional cutplane views can be displayed to improve the anatomic relationships or the appearance in other cardiac cycles (systole).

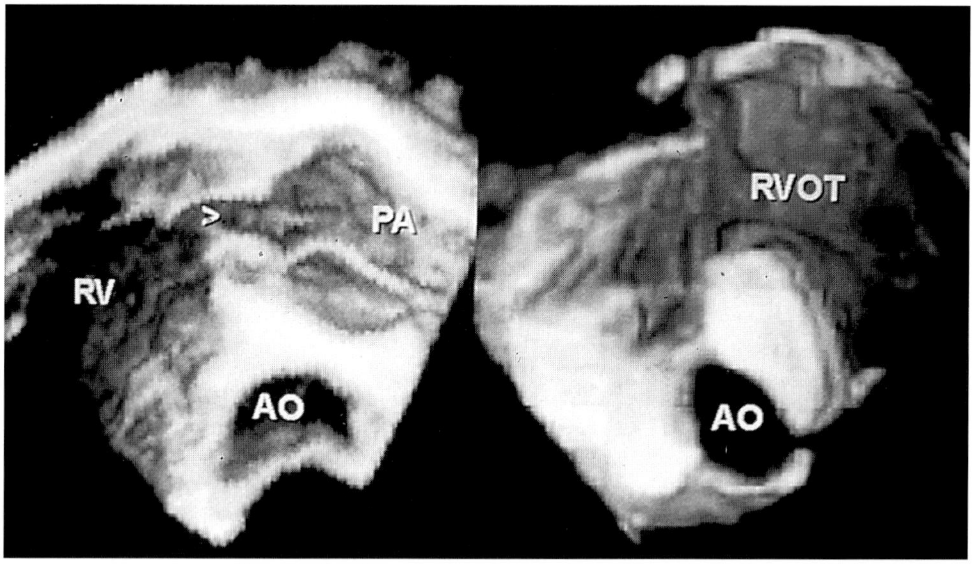

Figure 28. Dynamic three-dimensional image of patient with tetralogy of Fallot. **Left:** Preoperative long-axis view of the right ventricular outflow tract (RVOT). The right ventricle (RV), RVOT, and pulmonary artery (PA) were simultaneously observed; the RVOT had tube-like narrowing (arrow). **Right:** During operation, the RV anterior wall was repaired with a piece of pericardium and the RVOT was obviously extended (arrow). Reproduced with permission from Wang XF. Four-dimensional echocardiography: Methods and clinical application. *Am Heart J* 1996;132:672–684.

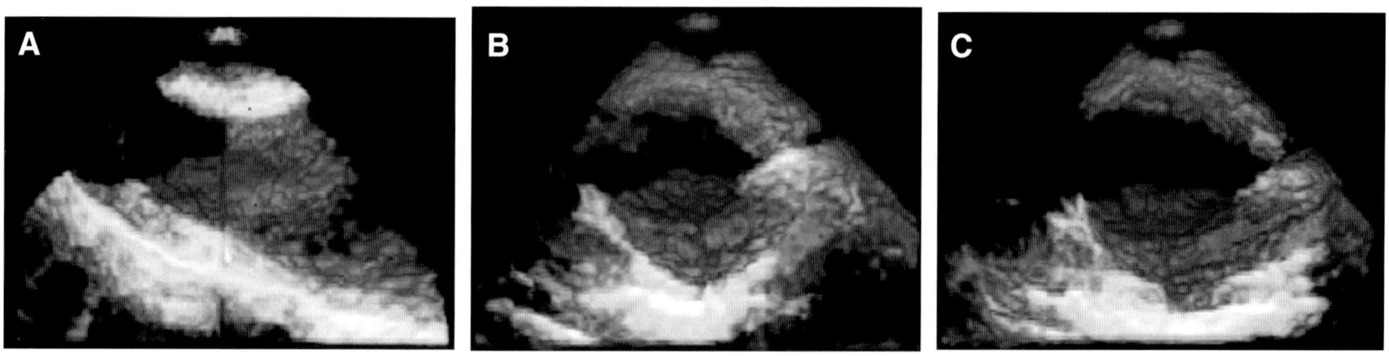

Figure 29. Coarctation of the aorta. (**A**) Transesophageal echo (TEE) three-dimensional (3D) display of the thoracic aorta. This data set was acquired in a young male with difficult to control hypertension, decreased lower extremity pulses and a loud, extensive systolic murmur. Note the much larger proximal aortic lumen (on right) compared with the relatively narrow coarctation (left). The perpendicular middle line represents a reconstruction artifact obtained from slight probe motion during data acquisition. Additional artifact is noted within the aortic lumen and a drop-out artifact is displayed on the left. (**B, C**) In this short-axis display, the coarctation is visualized from the perspective of the proximal, normal aorta, in diastole (**B**) and systole (**C**). Note that even with the marked artifact within this image, important anatomic detail was obtained concerning the circumferential nature of the coarctation that was confirmed at surgery. From Vincent L. Sorrell, MD.

Suggested Reading List

1. Li Z, Wang X, Nanda NC, et al. Three-dimensional reconstruction of transesophageal echocardiographic longitudinal images. *Echocardiography* 1995;12:367–375.
2. Nanda NC, Abd-El Rahman SM, Khatri G, et al. Incremental value of three-dimensional echocardiography over transesophageal multiplane two-dimensional echocardiography in qualitative and quantitative assessment of cardiac masses and defects. *Echocardiography* 1995; 12:619–628.
3. Deng J, Gardener JE, Rodeck CH, et al. Fetal echocardiography in three and four dimensions. *Ultrasound Med & Biol* 1996;22:979–986.
4. Meyer-Wittkopf M, Cook A, McLennan A, et al. Evaluation of three-dimensional ultrasonography and magnetic resonance imaging in assessment of congenital heart anomalies in fetal cardiac specimens. *Ultrasound Obstetr & Gynecol* 1996;8:303–308.
5. Vitarelli A. [Tridimensional echocardiography: general principles and clinical applications (with special reference to congenital heart diseases)]. [Italian]. *Minerva Cardioangiologica* 1996;44:545–554.
6. Altmann K, Shen Z, Boxt LM, et al. Comparison of three-dimensional echocardiographic assessment of volume,

mass, and function in children with functionally single left ventricles with two-dimensional echocardiography and magnetic resonance imaging. *Am J Cardiology* 1997; 80:1060–1065
7. Liang RI, Huang SE, Chang FM. Prenatal diagnosis of ectopia cordis at 10 weeks of gestation using two-dimensional and three-dimensional ultrasonography. [Review] [10 refs]. *Ultrasound Obstetr & Gynecol* 1997;10:137–139.
8. Nascimento R, Pereira D, Freitas A, et al. Comparison of left ventricular ejection fraction in congenital heart disease by visual versus algorithmic determination. *Am J Cardiol* 1997;80:1331–1335.
9. Acar P, Maunoury C, Antonietti T, et al. Left ventricular ejection fraction in children measured by three-dimensional echocardiography using a new transthoracic integrated 3D-probe. A comparison with equilibrium radionuclide angiography. *Eur Heart J* 1998;19:1583–1588.
10. Acar P, Piechaud JF, Bonhoeffer P, et al. [Anatomic evaluation of ostium secundum atrial septal defects by tridimensional echocardiography]. [French]. *Arch Mal Coeur et Vaisseaux* 1998;91:543–550.
11. Kardon RE, Cao QL, Masani N, et al. New insights and observations in three-dimensional echocardiographic visualization of ventricular septal defects: Experimental and clinical studies. *Circulation* 1998;98:1307–1314.
12. Levental M, Pretorius DH, Sklansky MS, et al. Three-dimensional ultrasonography of normal fetal heart: Comparison with two-dimensional imaging. *J Ultrasound Med* 1998;17:341–348.
13. Nanda NC, Samal AK, Bakir S, et al. Transesophageal echocardiographic diagnosis of right sided aortic arch. *Echocardiography* 1998;15:409–417.
14. Papavassiliou DP, Parks WJ, Hopkins KL, et al. Three-dimensional echocardiographic measurement of right ventricular volume in children with congenital heart disease validated by magnetic resonance imaging. *J Am Soc Echocardiography* 1998;11:770–777.
15. Sadaniantz A, Burtt D, Nanda NC, et al. Three dimensional echocardiography of right heart pathology. *Echocardiography* 1998;15:795–806.
16. Samal AK, Nanda NC, Thakur AC, et al. Three-dimensional echocardiographic reconstruction of atrial membranes. *Echocardiography* 1998;15:605–610.
17. Schneider M, Schneider I, Neu H. [Feasibility of sonography in the diagnosis of congenital heart diseases in dogs]. [Review] [23 refs] [German]. *Tierarztliche Praxis Ausgabe K , Kleintiere /Heimtiere* 1998;26:170–179.
18. Sklansky MS, Nelson TR, Pretorius DH. Three-dimensional fetal echocardiography: Gated versus nongated techniques. *J Ultrasound Med* 1998;17:451–457.
19. Tantibhedhyangkul W, Godoy I, Karp R, et al. Cor triatriatum in a 70-year-old woman: Role of transesophageal echocardiography and dynamic three-dimensional echocardiography in diagnostic assessment. *J Am Soc Echocardiography* 1998;11:837–840.
20. Acar P, Saliba Z, Aggoun Y, et al. [A new anatomical approach to congenital valve diseases by three-dimensional echocardiography]. [French]. *Arch Mal Coeur Vaisseaux* 1999;92:583–590.
21. Acar P, Aggoun Y, Saliba Z, et al. Effect of balloon dilatation on aortic stenosis assessed by 3-dimensional echocardiographic reconstruction. *Circulation* 1999;99: 2598–2599.
22. Dall'Agata A, Cromme-Dijkhuis AH, Meijboom F, et al. Use of three-dimensional echocardiography for analysis of outflow obstruction in congenital heart disease. *Am J Cardiol* 1999;83:921–925.
23. Dall'Agata A, McGhie J, Taams MA, et al. Secundum atrial septal defect is a dynamic three-dimensional entity. [see comments]. *Am Heart J* 1999;137:1075–1081.
24. Heusch A, Rubo J, Krogmann ON, et al. Volume measurement of the left ventricle in children with congenital heart defects: 3-dimensional echocardiography versus angiocardiography. *Cardiology* 1999;92:45–52.
25. Heusch A, Rubo J, Krogmann ON, et al. Volumetric analysis of the right ventricle in children with congenital heart defects: comparison of biplane angiography and transthoracic 3-dimensional echocardiography. *Cardiol in the.Young* 1999;9:577–584.
26. Li J, Sanders SP. Three-dimensional echocardiography in congenital heart disease. [Review] [29 refs]. *Curr Opin Cardiol* 1999;14:53–59.
27. Mizelle KM, Rice MJ, Sahn DJ. Practical application of three-dimensional echocardiography in evaluation of atrial septal defects. [letter; comment]. *Am Heart J* 1999;137:1000–1001.
28. Nanda NC, Ansingkar K, Espinal M, et al. Transesophageal three-dimensional echo assessment of sinus venosus atrial septal defect. *Echocardiography* 1999;16:835–837.
29. Sklansky MS, Nelson T, Strachan M, et al. Real-time three-dimensional fetal echocardiography: initial feasibility study. *J Ultrasound Med* 1999;18:745–752.
30. Alabdulkarim N, Knudson OA, Shaffer E, et al. Three-dimensional imaging of aortic arch anomalies in infants and children with intravascular ultrasound catheters from a transesophageal approach. *J Am Soc Echocardiography* 2000;13:924–931.
31. Balestrini L, Fleishman C, Lanzoni L, et al. Real-time 3-dimensional echocardiography evaluation of congenital heart disease. *J Am Soc Echocardiography* 2000;13: 171–176.
32. Blaas HG, Eik-Nes SH, Berg S. Three-dimensional fetal ultrasound. [Review] [69 refs]. *Best Practice & Research Clinical Obstetr Gynaecol* 2000;14(4):611–627.
33. Deng J, Ruff CF, Linney AD, et al. Simultaneous use of two ultrasound scanners for motion-gated three-dimensional fetal echocardiography. *Ultrasound Med & Biol* 2000; 26(6):1021–1032.
34. Ito H, Tamura H, Ito Y. Images in cardiology: coronary sinus ostial atresia with persistent left superior vena cava connected with atrial septal defect. *Heart* 2000;84(3):289.
35. Lange A, Mankad P, Walayat M, et al. Transthoracic three-dimensional echocardiography in the preoperative assessment of atrioventricular septal defect morphology. *Am J Cardiol* 2000;85(5):630–635.
36. Meyer-Wittkopf M, Rappe N, Sierra F, et al. Three-dimensional (3-D) ultrasonography for obtaining the four and five-chamber view: comparison with cross-sectional (2-D) fetal sonographic screening. *Ultrasound Obstetr & Gynecol* 2000;15(5):397–402.
37. Mizelle KM, Rice MJ, Sahn DJ. Clinical use of Real-time three-dimensional echocardiography in pediatric cardiology. [Review] [12 refs]. *Echocardiography* 2000;17(8): 787–790.
38. Nanda NC, Bhambore MM, Jindal A, et al. Transesophageal three dimensional echocardiographic assessment of anomalous coronary arteries. *Echocardiography* 2000;17:53–60.
39. Poutanen T, Ikonen A, Vainio P, et al. Left atrial volume assessed by transthoracic three dimensional echocardiography and magnetic resonance imaging: dynamic changes during the heart cycle in children. *Heart* 2000; 83(5):537–542.
40. Scharf A, Geka F, Steinborn A, et al. 3D real-time imaging of the fetal heart. *Fetal Diagn & Ther* 2000;15(5): 267–274.

41. Acar P, Marx GR, Saliba Z, et al. Three-dimensional echocardiographic measurement of left ventricular stroke volume in children: comparison with Doppler method. *Pediatr Cardiol* 2001;22(2):116–120.
42. Bega G, Kuhlman K, Lev-Toaff A, et al. Application of three-dimensional ultrasonography in the evaluation of the fetal heart. *J Ultrasound Med* 2001;20:307–313.
43. Deng J, Birkett AG, Kalache KD, et al. Conversion of umbilical arterial Doppler waveforms to cardiac cycle triggering signals: a preparatory study for online motion-gated three-dimensional fetal echocardiography. *Ultrasound Med & Biol* 2001;27(1):51–59.
44. Deng J, Yates R, Birkett AG, et al. Online motion-gated dynamic three-dimensional echocardiography in the fetus—preliminary results. *Ultrasound Med & Biol* 2001; 27:43–50.
45. Jurgens J. 3D-sonography as "2D-M-mode sonography in fetal echocardiography]. [German]. *Ultraschall in der Medizin* 2001;22:12–16.
46. Meyer-Wittkopf M, Cole A, Cooper SG, et al. Three-dimensional quantitative echocardiographic assessment of ventricular volume in healthy human fetuses and in fetuses with congenital heart disease. *J Ultrasound Med* 2001;20:317–327.
47. Nekkanti R, Nanda NC, Ansingkar KG, et al. Transesophageal three dimensional echocardiographic assessment of left main coronary artery fistula. *Echocardiography* 2001;18:305–308.
48. Nekkanti R, Mukhtar O, Nanda NC, et al. Transesophageal color Doppler three dimensional echocardiographic assessment of left circumflex coronary artery fistula. *Echocardiography* (In press, October 2002).

Chapter 7

Three-Dimensional Echocardiography in Adult Congenital Heart Disease

Jesus Vargas-Barron, MD, Angel Romero-Cardenas, MD, Nilda Espinola-Zavaleta, MD, Francisco Javier Roldan, MD, Clara Vazquez-Antona, MD, Fause Attie, MD, and Navin C. Nanda, MD

There is universal agreement that a segmental nomenclature for description and classification of congential heart disease (CHD) is necessary. Of the many disputed topics in pediatric cardiology, no issue is more controversial than approaches to a segmental nomenclature.

If we analyze the anatomical features of a normal heart and those with CHD, we conclude that cardiac segments are fundamental building blocks that connect together, forming a functional unit in both normal heart and congenital heart malformations. These functional units include three segments called the atria, the ventricles, and great arteries. Connection among these segments is informative; it is capable of describing any combination of cardiac malformation that might be encountered. Futhermore, the connection among atria, ventricle, and great arteries offers the understanding of the route of the circulation which is fundamental to the physiology, hemodynamics, and treatment of the patient with CHD.

With these criteria the heart can thus be divided into three distinct and fundamental segments which are identified by strict anatomic criteria. But it is essential and logical to incorporate the concept of the internal organization of the heart in terms of connection among these segments.

Three-dimensional (3D) echocardiography defines the cardiac segments in terms of their morphology and the characteristics of their proximal and distal connection; furthermore the procedure allows the definition of the internal organization of the heart.

In the following pages, we will present the cardiac segments in terms of their morphology and characterize their proximal and distal connection using material illustrative of 3D echocardiography. We will try to summarize the segmental nomenclature from an echocardiographic viewpoint, and also focus on the 3D recognition of normal and malformed hearts.

Atrial Situs

The atrial situs represents the assymetry pattern in relation to spatial position of the diverse organs and structures. It refers to nonpaired organs and structures, or to those that are paired but not equal. The appendages are the best guides for atrial morphology; their shape defines them as right or left. The anatomic references to precisely define the situs are the position of the liver, the suprahepatic portion of the inferior vena cava (IVC), and the anatomically right atrium, since they are very constant and interrelate to form the hepato-cava-atrial triad. When the organs are located on the right, then the situs is solitus (SS), which is the most common pattern found; when it is on the left, then the situs is inversus (SI). There are a group of individuals who do not present this asymmetry pattern and cannot be defined as SS or SI; they tend toward a bilateral isomerism that can be right (asplenia) or left (polysplenia).

Determination of the situs with echocardiography using subxiphoid approximations is based on the position of the IVC and the aorta in relation to the spinal cord.[1] In SS, the IVC is found on the right, the hepatic vein's connection is to the cava, following into the right atrium, and the aorta is to the left. Determination of the atrial situs is independent from the position of the heart within the thorax, and is the starting point for the analysis of the atrioventricular connection.

From Nanda NC and Sorrell VL: *Atlas of Three-Dimensional Echocardiography.* ©Futura Publishing Co., Inc, Armonk, NY, 2002.

The appendages of older children and adolescents are not easily identified with transthoracic or subxiphoid approximations. Transesophageal echocardiography[2] (TEE) and especially the multiplanar transducer facilitate definition of their morphology and, through them, the situs can be precisely established. Three-dimensional echocardiography eases reconstruction of the anatomical details of the structures,[3] allows to describe their morphology and, by orienting the cutplane, both atria can be visualized simultaneously. There are three possible variants: situs solitus, situs inversus, and isomeric situs (also called ambiguous), which can be either right or left.

Situs Solitus

Situs Solitus is determined by identifying the right atrial structures to the right, i.e., the right appendage with triangular morphology, a wide base and blunt contour (Figure 1), both right venae cavae connected to the right atrium, and the lateral wall of the atrium with pectinate muscles. The crista terminalis can be identified as a prominence separating the trabeculated portion of the appendage from the smooth atrial portion (Figure 2). The coronary sinus flows into the right atrium (Figure 3) and the Eustachian valve crosses the right atrial cavity. Injecting a contrast medium into a peripheral vein makes the right atrium opaque.

The left atrium is identified by its "finger-like" appendage, irregular, with a narrow base and gnarled edge or with lobulations. The atrial walls are smooth, and the pulmonary veins connect to it.

Situs Inversus

In this anomaly the anatomical and morphological indicators of the right atrium and appendages are spatially located to the left and vice versa (Figure 4).

Atrial Isomerism (Situs Ambiguous)

This condition is characterized by the tendency toward symmetry of usually asymmetric structures. It is always anomalous and associated with the presence of complex cardiac malformations. The term refers to the lack of atrial lateralization. Anomalies in systemic and pulmonary venous return are frequent in the presence of atrial isomerism. To precisely define the details is important for surgical correction.

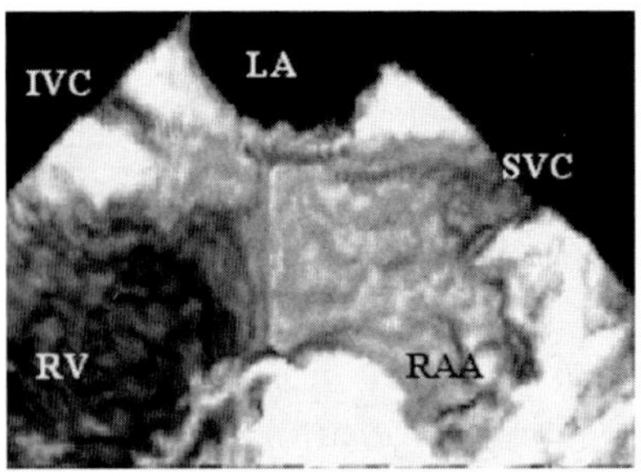

Figure 1. Situs solitus. Right atrium appendage has triangular morphology with a large implantation base connecting to the atrial cavity. IVC = inferior vena cava; LA = left atrium; RV = right ventricle; RAA = right atrial appendage; SVC = superior vena cava.

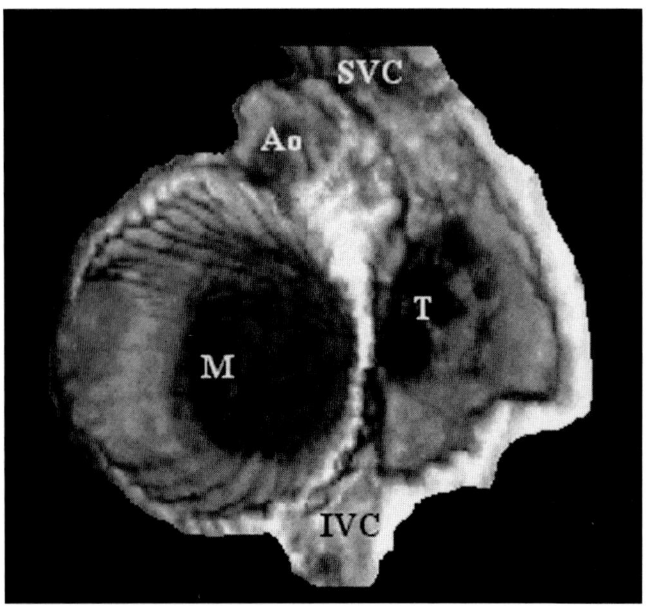

Figure 2. Situs solitus. The superior and inferior venae cavae enter the right atrium posteriorly. Ao = aorta; M = mitral valve; IVC = inferior vena cava; SVC = superior vena cava; T= tricuspid valve.

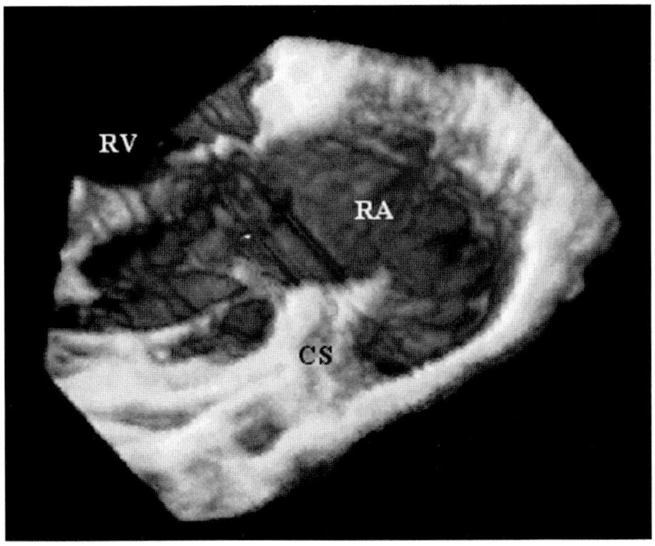

Figure 3. Situs solitus. The connection of the coronary sinus to the right atrium is shown. CS = coronary sinus; RA = right atrium; RV = right ventricle.

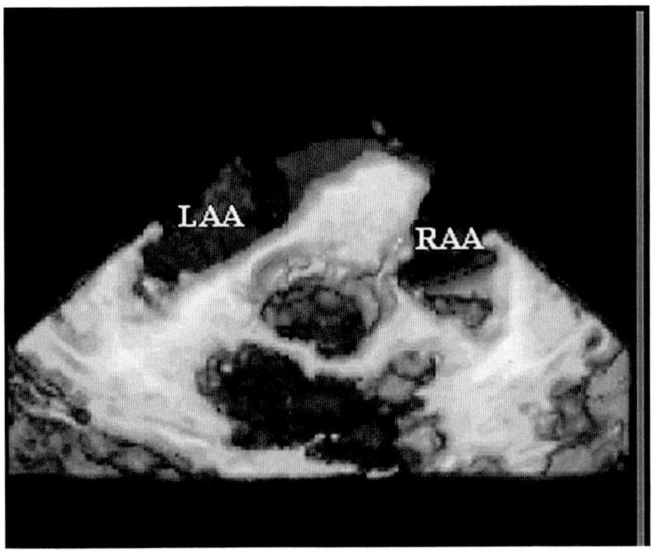

Figure 4. Situs inversus. The anatomic left atrial appendage is located on the right, the right atrial appendage to the left. LAA = left atrial appendage; RAA = right atrial appendage.

Right Atrial Isomerism (Dextroisomerism)

Both appendages depict right morphology, i.e., they are triangular with a wide base (Figure 5). In these cases, it is important to search for the connection of two venae cavae draining directly into both atrial cavities, as well as the anomalous connection of the hepatic veins to the inferior cava and anomalies in the pulmonary vein connection, among other alterations. Both the IVC and the aorta are located to the right of the spinal cord (aorto-cava juxtaposition).

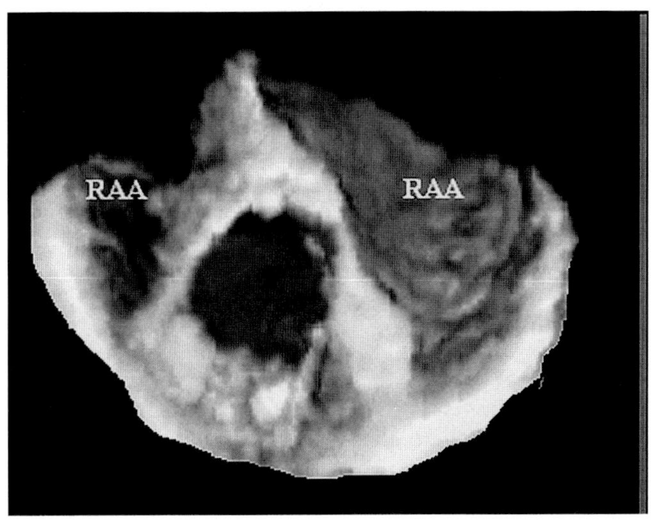

Figure 5. Right atrial isomerism. Both atrial appendages have a right morphology. RAA = right atrial appendage.

Left Atrial Isomerism (Levo-Isomerism)

Both appendages have a narrow base and elongated shape (Figure 6). It is common to find interruption of the IVC that proceeds with an azygos or hemiazygos vein, a bilateral superior vena cava, and pulmonary venous re-

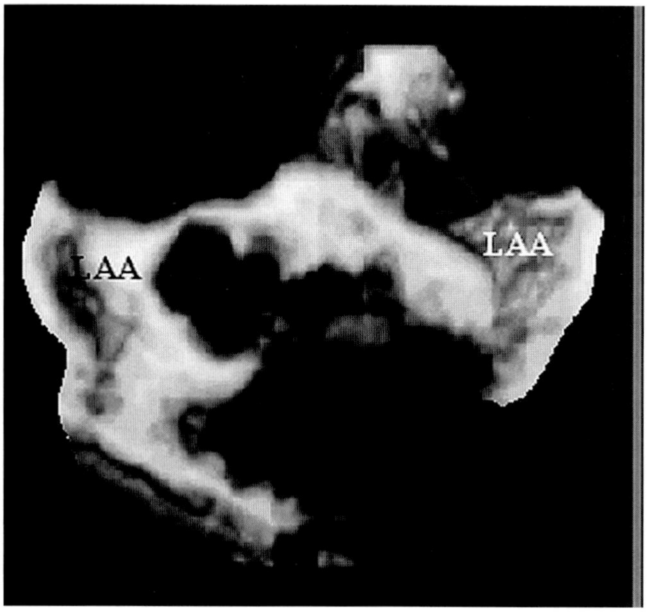

Figure 6. Left atrial isomerism. Both atrial appendages have a left morphology. LAA = left atrial appendage.

turn with two veins connected to the right-placed atrium and two with the left-placed atrium.

Embryonic Remnants of Right Atrium

Among the nonpathologic embryonic remnants found in the right atrium are the Eustachian and Tebesian valves. Persistence of other structures related to the right valve of the embryonic sinus venosus produces a large array of anomalies that range from prominent crista terminalis and the Chiari network to the cor triatriatum dexter.[4]

Up to the present, the best study to define the anatomy of the right atrium and its related structures used to be two-dimensional (2D) echocardiography; however, some limitations were encountered when only transthoracic images were used. Transesophageal echocardiography has allowed to define with greater precision the anatomic details[4] facilitating differential diagnosis regarding tumors and thrombi.[5–7]

Although the Eustachian and Tebesian valves can be visualized frequently with TEE studies[8] they are rarely big enough to be visualized with transthoracic imaging.[9]

The Eustachian valve is seen as a laminar structure projecting toward the atrial lumen from the junction of the IVC with the right atrium.[10] The Chiari network is visualized as a discontinuous structure formed by a set of interrelated echos depicting an undulatory movement.[11] The crista terminalis can be seen as a prominence at the posterior external region of the right atrium. Diagnosis of cor triatriatum dexter is established based on the observation of an intra-atrial structure that extends from the roof to the base of the right atrium. It can vary in size and can be observed in transversal sections as a nodular structure.

Three-dimensional echocardiographic studies of embryonic structures are closely related to current anatomical and embryological knowledge. Figure 7 depicts the crista terminalis as a longitudinal relief of the posterior external wall of the right atrium between both venae cavae. The Tebesian valve is seen as a laminar structure separating the anterior region of the IVC from the right atrial lumen (Figure 8). The quality of

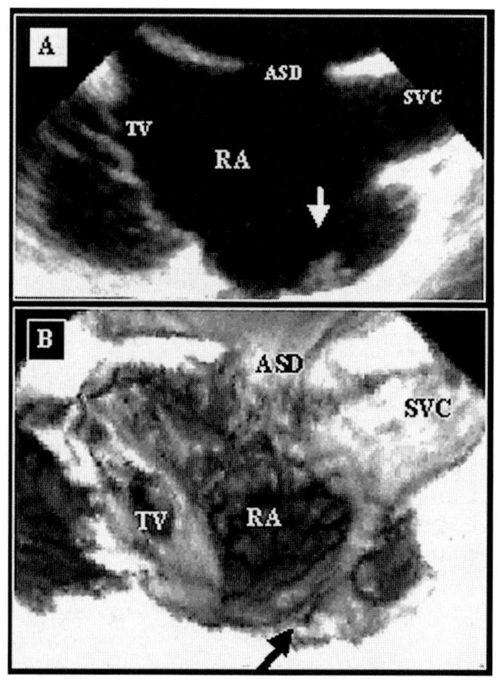

Figure 7. Crista terminalis. (**A**) Transesophageal two-dimensional study visualizes the crista terminalis as a prominence in the posterolateral region of the right atrium (RA) (white arrow). (**B**) The three-dimensional study reveals it as a band extending from the superior vena cava (SVC) to the lower regions of the right atrium (black arrow). RV = right ventricle; LA = left atrium; ASD= atrial septal defect. From *Am J Cardiol*, Roldán FJ, et al. Three-dimensional echocardiography of the right atrial embryonic remnants. (in press), reprinted with permission.

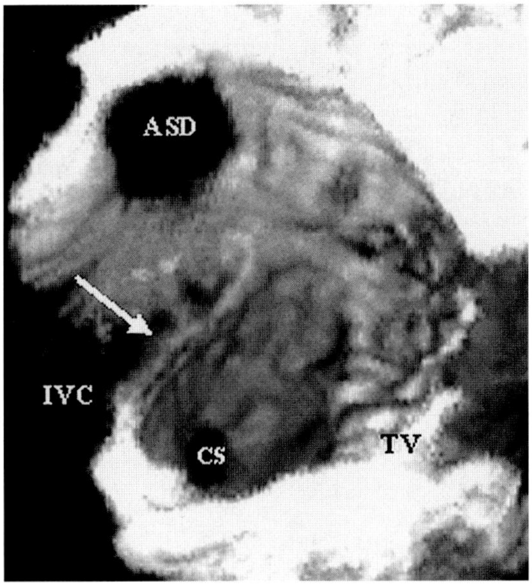

Figure 8. Prominent Eustachian valve. The three-dimensional image depicts the interatrial septum seen from the superior-lateral portion of the right atrium. An atrial septal defect (ASD) type ostium secundum type and the connection of the coronary sinus (CS) are depicted; between them and in front of the inferior vena cava (IVC) a prominent Eustachian valve is visualized. TV = Tricuspid valve. From *Am J Cardiol,* Roldán FJ, et al. Three-dimensional echocardiography of the right atrial embryonic remnants. (in press), reprinted with permission.

the 3D echocardiographic study of the Chiari network will depend on the synchrony of its movement with the cardiac cycle. In elongated structures, reconstruction can be incomplete, better defined at the basal portions that maintain a relatively synchronous movement with the electrocardiogram, and less defined, or even not visualized, at the distal portions, because the latter do not play a specific role in each cardiac cycle movement. Figure 9 depicts the reconstruction of a cor triatriatum dexter, an extreme case in which reabsorption of the right valve of the embryonic sinus venosus is minimal.

Other Atrial Malformations

Left Atrial Appendage

The left atrial appendage is a muscular extension of the left atrium that arises anterolaterally near the connection of the left pulmonary veins. Finding several accessory lobes in an echocardiographic study should not be considered a pathological finding, since in 80% of the cases this is a multilobulated structure. However, it is important to take into account when

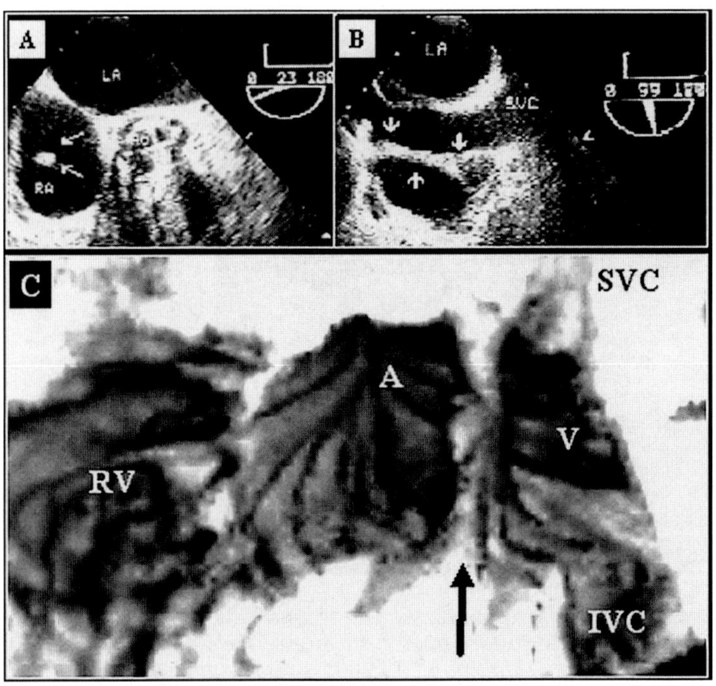

Figure 9. Cor triatriatum dexter. The upper part of the image depicts two orthogonal planes from a transesophageal study showing a structure inside the right atrium (RA) as a nodular image (**A**) in the transversal section and as a band (**B**) in the longitudinal section (white arrows). The lower part of the image (**C**) depicts the 3D reconstruction showing a tubular image (black arrow) that extends from the superior vena cava (SVC) to the base of the right atrium near the tricuspid valve (TV). LA = left atrium; IVC = inferior vena cava. From Roldán FJ, et al. Cor triatriatum dexter: Transesophageal echocardiographic diagnosis and three-dimensional reconstruction. *J Am Soc Echo* 2001;14: 634–636.

searching for the source of cardioembolism, since accessory lobes are known to produce intracavitary thrombosis.[12] Three lobes are found in 23% of the cases, and four are found in 3%; they are usually located at different planes.[13]

Transesophageal echocardiography is the study of choice to assess adequately these small structures.[14] It has been recently evidenced that 3D echocardiography obtained from transesophageal images yields an adequate correlation with the actual anatomy of the left atrial appendage.[15] Figure 10 shows how 3D echocardiography can depict the long axis of each of the main lumen in a bilobulated appendage, independently from its spatial location. On the other hand, as shown in Figure 11, by establishing its profile and volume it is possible to perform a complete dissection of the structure in the desired plane.

Idiopathic Atriomegaly

This condition is considered as an authentic malformation of the left atrial appendage. In this pathology, the atrial appendage depicts a disproportioned growth and micro-structural alterations.[16] In the absence of other cardiac malformations it can be a casual

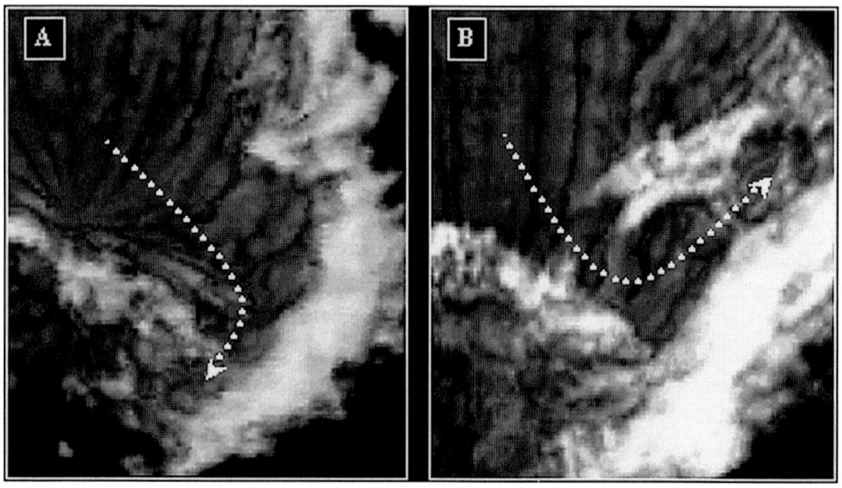

Figure 10. Bilobulated left atrial appendage. Three-dimensional echocardiography permits orientation of the cutplane to allow visualization of the long axis of both lobes (**A** and **B**), regardless of their spatial location.

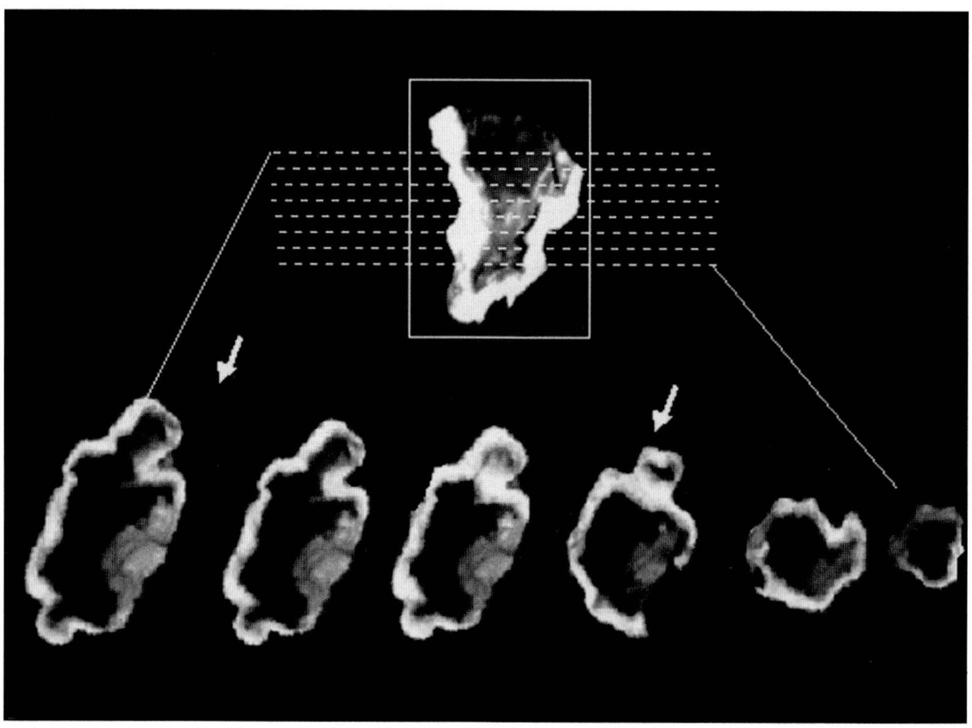

Figure 11. Dissection using three-dimensional echocardiography of a left atrial appendage. Arrows indicate an accessory lobe, its lumen can be seen separated from the main lobe as the cutplane is moved more distally. From Roldán FJ, et al. Anatomic correlation of left atrial appendage by three-dimensional echocardiography. *J Am Soc Echo* 2001;14:941–944.

finding. Although diagnosis can be established through standard echocardiographic approximations, 3D echocardiography has the advantage of allowing variation of the cutplane independently from the transductor position during imaging; hence, allowing depiction of the long axis of the atrial appendage in almost all patients leading to a closer anatomic vision. This method also allows calculating its volume without having to make anatomical inferences. Figure 12 depicts the 3D reconstruction of this pathology.

Unroofed Coronary Sinus

The syndrome of coronary sinus without roof is a cardiac anomaly in which the common wall separating the left atrium from the coronary sinus is either partially or totally absent. It is mainly associated to the atrioventricular (AV) canal, generally with a single atrium or atrial isomerism.[17] It is also closely related to persistent superior vena cava with or without inominated vein. Two-dimensional echocardiography is useful to diagnose this pathology and the associated malformations. By injecting microbubbles of saline solution it is possible to detect drainage of the left superior vena cava into an unroofed coronary sinus.[18] Three-dimensional echocardiography provides complementary morphological information and allows finding association of structures that might seem independent in the 2D. Figure 13 shows how the 2D study reveals a parallel membrane to the mitral ring, which actually corresponds to the floor of an unroofed coronary sinus as demonstrated by the three-dimensional study.

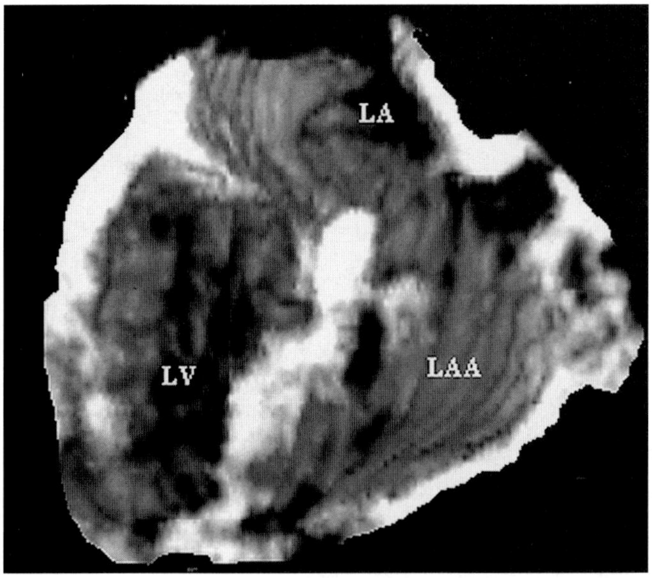

Figure 12. Disproportioned congenital growth of the left atrial appendage (idiopathic atriomegalia). The chosen three-dimensional cutplane allows comparison of the size of the atrial appendage with the left ventricle in diastole, LA = left atrium; LV = left ventricle; LAA = left atrial appendage.

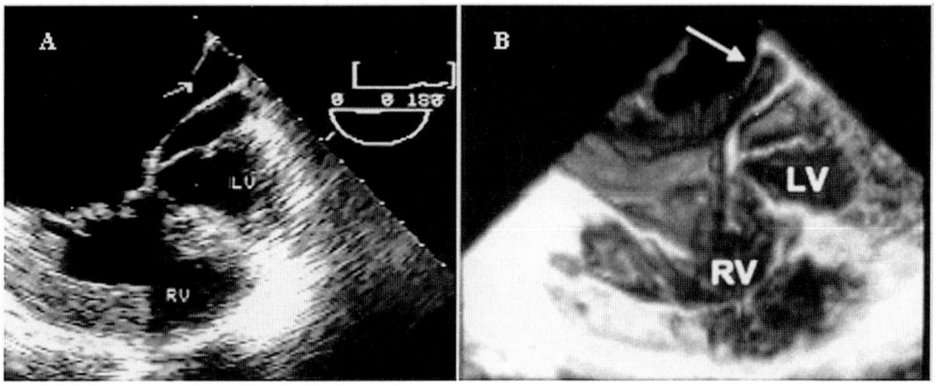

Figure 13. Congenital unroofed coronary sinus. (**A**) Two-dimensional transesophageal image demonstrating a common atrium and a small remnant corresponding to the roof of the coronary sinus (arrow). Above and parallel to the mitral valve, a membrane can be seen that corresponds to the floor of the unroofed coronary sinus in the three-dimensional study (**B**). LV = left ventricle; RV = right ventricle. From Vargas-Barrón, et al. Two and three-dimensional echocardiographic unroofed coronary sinus. *J Am Soc Echo* 2001;14:742–744.

Atrioventricular Connection

Echocardiographic diagnosis of AV connection requires a systemized study based on the sequential identification of the atrial situs and ventricles.

Three-dimensional reconstruction shows that atrial morphology can be identified correctly on the basis of the morphologic features of the appendages and the extent of pectinate muscles within the appendages.[19]

The ability of 3D echocardiography to identify the ventricles is based on the recognition of some morphologic features: a) The moderator band and coarse trabeculations of the right ventricle in contrast to the smooth septum and fine trabeculations of the left ventricle, b) a more apical insertion of the tricuspid septal leaflet in the interventricular septum than of the mitral septal leaflet, and c) tricuspid subvalvular apparatus with insertions into the interventricular septum.

The possible variations of AV connections include:

Concordant

In this condition a Doppler study from a four-chamber image shows that right atrial flow passes through the tricuspid valve into the anatomically right ventricle, and left atrial flow crosses the mitral valve into the anatomically left ventricle.

Discordant

In this condition, the 3D echocardiographic diagnosis can be established in both situs solitus and situs inversus, as well as in levocardia, mesocardia, and dextrocardia. In patients with discordant AV connection the ventriculo-arterial connection is also discordant; this condition corresponds to the anomaly known as corrected transposition of the great arteries (CTGA) (Figures 14–17). Occasionally the tricuspid valve is tethered to the ventricular wall, a finding known as left-sided Ebstein's anomaly, and one which is easily recognized in 3D TEE reconstruction.

In CTGA, 3D echocardiography and volumetry are focused not only on tricuspid valvular function, but also on concomitant ventricular septal defect, and subvalvular pulmonary obstruction, as well as on assessing adaptation of the morphologic right ventricle to systemic load.[20]

Ambiguous Atrioventricular Connection

In ambiguous AV connection, 3D reconstruction of the atrial appendages reveals that both have a right or left morphology, i.e., that there is right or left isomerism. Color Doppler shows that each atrium is connected to a different ventricle.

Univentricular Atrioventricular Connection

Double inlet ventricle and absence of right or left AV connection correspond to univentricular AV connection. The double inlet corresponds most commonly to the anatomically left ventricle; in the 3D TEE four-chamber plane, the two AV valves open into the same ventricular cavity, and their septal leaflets approximate each other during diastole due to the lack of septal tissue among them.

The rudimentary ventricular cavity can be identified with transgastric recordings in the transversal planes; these unique views, looking down through the tricuspid or mitral valve annulus into the main ven-

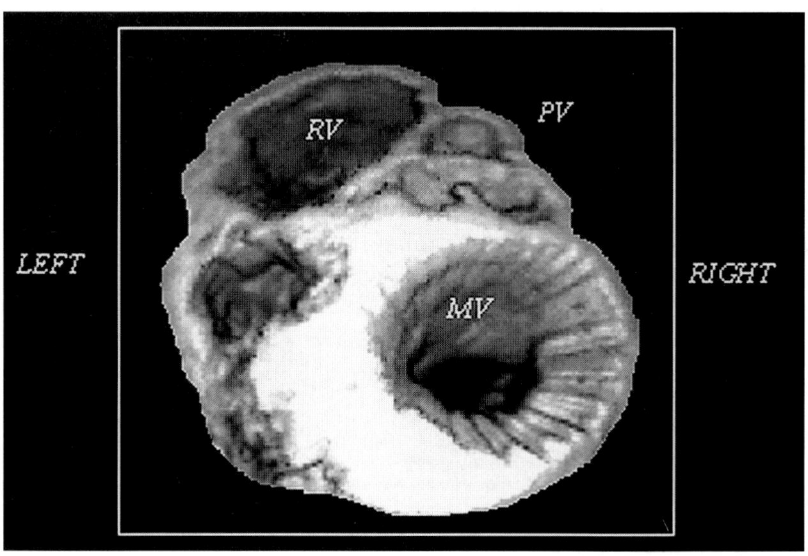

Figure 14. In the presence of discordant atrioventricular connection, the anatomically left ventricle located on the right is recognized by the two mitral leaflets (MV) identified from the right atrium; mitral-pulmonary continuity is also identified. RV = right ventricle; PV = pulmonary valve.

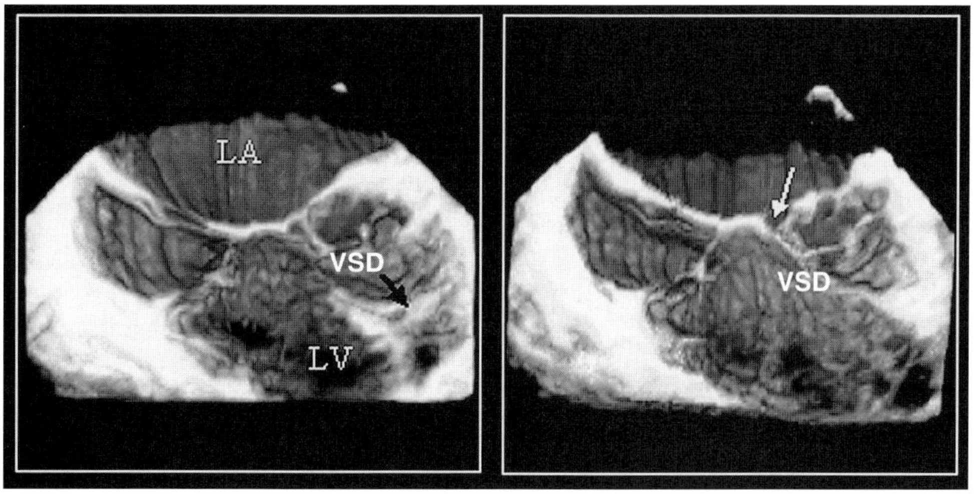

Figure 15. In situs solitus, the right ventricle connected to the atrium (LA) is recognized by the moderator band (left arrow) and by the more apical insertion of the tricuspid septal leaflet (right arrow). Besides, there is a ventricular septal defect (VSD). LV = left ventricle.

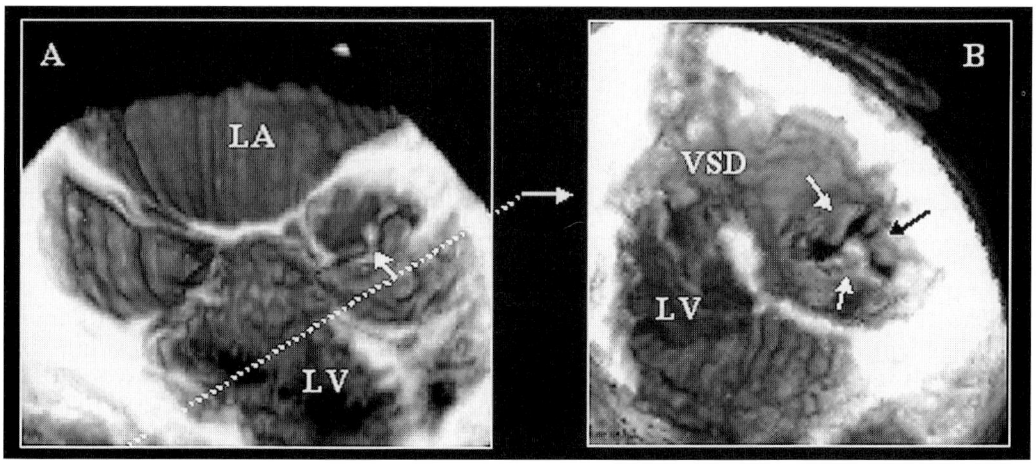

Figure 16. From the four chamber reconstruction (**A**) the transversal view from the right ventricle (**B**) allows identification of the right ventricle located to the left by the three cusps (leaflets) (arrows). VSD = ventricular septal defect; LA = left atrium; LV = left ventricle.

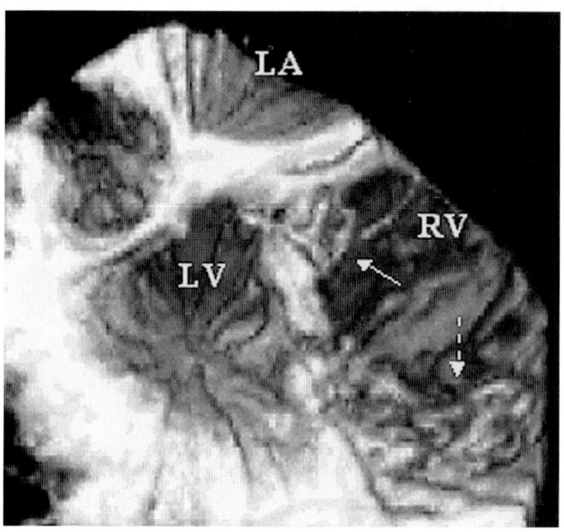

Figure 17. In a patient with dextrocardia and discordant AV connection, the anatomically right ventricle can be identified by the insertion of chordae tendinae into the interventricular septum (upper arrow) and by the moderator band (lower arrow). LA = left atrium; LV = left ventricle.

tricular chamber and looking up from the main ventricle into the atrial chambers, allow recognition of the position of the rudimentary ventricle in relation to the main ventricle.

Other features that can be detected by 3D echocardiography include a ventricular septal defect of variable size, the left AV valve may be dome-shaped owing to its insertion into a single papillary muscle (parachute valve), and overriding of the anterior AV valve over the interventricular septum. Vogel concluded that 3D echocardiography of complex heart defects could be valuable in surgical planning, as it offers diagnostic information superior to 2D echocardiography on the anatomy of straddling AV valves, particularly in cases where anomalous left ventricular tendons are present, which may mimic tensor apparatus if viewed only in one imaging plane.[21]

Absence of Atrioventricular Connection

Right sided absence or classic tricuspid atresia is characterized by a lack of continuity between the right cavities. The floor of the right atrium is muscular and is separated from the right ventricle by fibrous tissue from the AV sulcus; rare cases of true tricuspid atresia exist in which the right chambers have a potential connection through an imperforate valvular membrane.

In patients with absence of right AV connection (classic tricuspid atresia), absence of movement of the tricuspid valve with ample diastolic mobility of the mitral valve can be observed with 3D TEE. In the four-chamber plane, a line of dense echoes can be seen below the right atrial floor, which represents the fibrous tissue of the AV sulcus (Figure 18). The presence of a small right ventricle and a dilated and hypertrophied left ventricle is confirmed by multiplanar transgastric and TEE recordings.

Congenital Malformations of the Mitral Valve

Mitral Stenosis

Congenital malformations of the mitral valve are unusual. Among them, congenital stenosis occurs with greatest frequency, representing 0.21% of the cases of CHD at the Instituto Nacional de Cardiologìa and in the literature as much as 6%.[22] Congenital mitral stenosis presents with degrees of severity that vary from an obstruction of little significance, involving a structurally normal mitral valve, to severe mitral stenosis with extremely abnormal subvalvular apparatus.[23,24] Parachute mitral valve is the most common type of malformation causing obstruction, followed in order of frequency by supravalvular mitral ring, cor triatriatum, and mitral arcade. Other congenital anomalies of the mitral valve that are even more uncommon include double orifice of the mitral valve, unicuspid mitral valve, cleft mitral valve (as an isolated entity), and accessory mitral tissue.

The valvular apparatus is a complex structure. Its functional integrity depends on optimal interaction of the annulus, leaflets, chordae tendineae, papillary muscles, left atrium, and left ventricular free wall.[25] Consequently, precise evaluation of mitral pathology requires adequate visualization of all these elements.[26]

Echocardiography is the method of choice to analyze valve disease, particularly mitral valve disease. However, detailed anatomical analysis for reconstructive surgery on the mitral valve is not always possible with transthoracic images. Multiplane TEE technique has increased diagnostic precision,[27] but when mitral structures are shown in only two dimensions, cardiologists are forced to mentally reconstruct the complex 3D relationship of the different elements of the mitral valve. At present, it is possible to obtain direct visual-

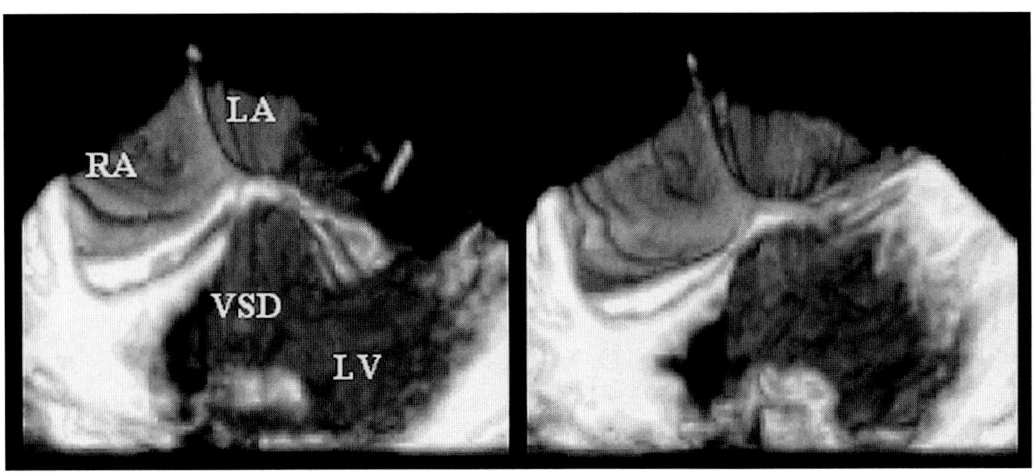

Figure 18. In a patient with tricuspid atresia, the four chamber reconstruction during diastole (**A**) and systole (**B**) reveals the lack of connection between the right atrium and ventricle. The hypoplastic right ventricle and an ample ventricular septal defect (VSD) are also shown. RA = right atrium; LA = left atrium; LV = left ventricle.

ization of the cardiac structures in movement with dynamic 3D echocardiography.[28–31] This technique has contributed significantly to the evaluation of morphologic abnormalities and to the understanding of complex spatial relationships in CHD.[32–34] It provides an opportunity for more comprehensive imaging of the mitral valve apparatus that aids in defining the location and extent of deformities due to congenital mitral anomalies. It can improve the surgical result of mitral valve repair or replacement in patients with significant mitral regurgitation and/or stenosis.

Mitral Arcade

Mitral arcade is a rare condition in which the mitral leaflets are thickened with shortened or absent chordae. As observed with 3D TEE, they appear to insert directly into the papillary muscles, which are often abnormal. In most cases limited coaptation of the valve leaflets causes predominant mitral insufficiency, however, mitral stenosis might also be present.[35–36] The 3D TEE examination of the four chambers allows viewing of the obstruction to left ventricular filling caused by an anatomical deformity of the mitral subvalvular apparatus (Figure 19).

Double Mitral Orifice

Double mitral orifice is defined as the presence of two orifices through the mitral valve, as a consequence of bridging tissue that connects the mitral valve leaflets. This bridging tissue may be only a small strand of tissue that connects the leaflets at their edges or a thickened fibrous bridge that divides the left AV orifice into equal or unequal parts. In addition, double mitral orifice may occur as a result of fusion of the subvalvular chordal apparatus, hindering complete opening of the valve with a resultant double-orifice appearance in diastole. Double mitral orifice may be an incidental echocardiographic finding or may be associated to valvular stenosis and/or insufficiency in approximately 50% of cases. More commonly, the orifices are unequal in size, with the smaller orifice directed toward the anterolateral commissure (41%) or the posteromedial commissure (44%).[37,38] The 3D TEE images at 30° show the double mitral orifice. Additional characteristics of the size and spatial relationship of the two valvular orifices can be obtained with transgastric images (Figure 20).

Accessory Mitral Tissue

In the most severe form, the interchordal spaces are obliterated by excessive valvular tissue. Occasionally, redundant mitral chordae may be present in the left ventricular outflow tract, with variable degrees of subaortic obstruction. Histopathology of such accessory valve leaflets reveals fibrous tissue and myxoid dysplasia.[39,40] Three-dimensional reconstruction of the left ventricular outflow tract may demonstrate partial obstruction of the subaortic area by mitral valve tissue and aid in dismissing a membrane or fibromuscular ring at approximately 120° (Figure 21).

Cleft of the Anterior Mitral Leaflet

Cleft of the anterior mitral leaflet is often associated with significant mitral insufficiency. The AV septum is intact. Less commonly the posterior leaflet is involved.[41] Mitral valve clefts may occur as isolated defects in asymptomatic individuals.[42,43] Three-dimensional images from the left atrium show a cleft of the anterior mitral leaflet with the vertex of the cleft directed toward the aorta (Figure 22).

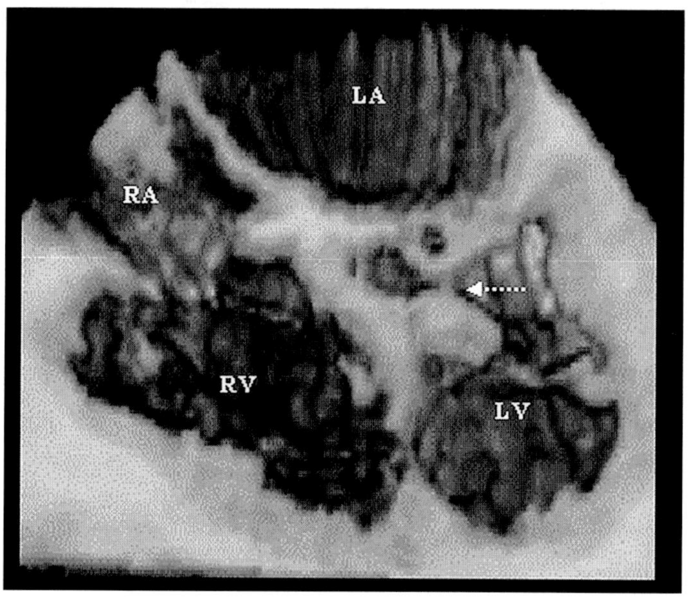

Figure 19. Three-dimensional image of a mitral arcade. Chordae tendineae are not present. The leaflets insert directly into the papillary muscles (arrow). RA = right atrium; RV = right ventricle; LA = left atrium; LV = left ventricle.

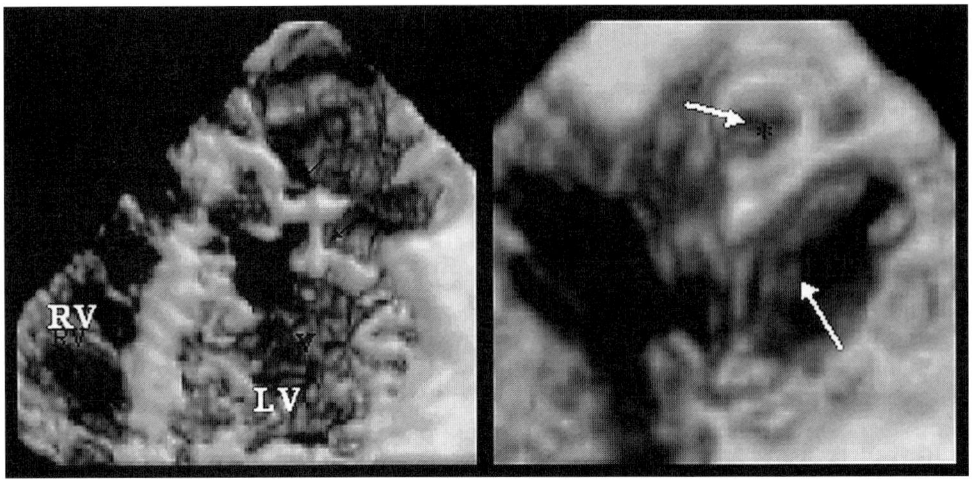

Figure 20. Three-dimensional study with transesophageal and transgastric images of a mitral valve with double orifice (arrows). LV = left ventricle; RV = right ventricle.

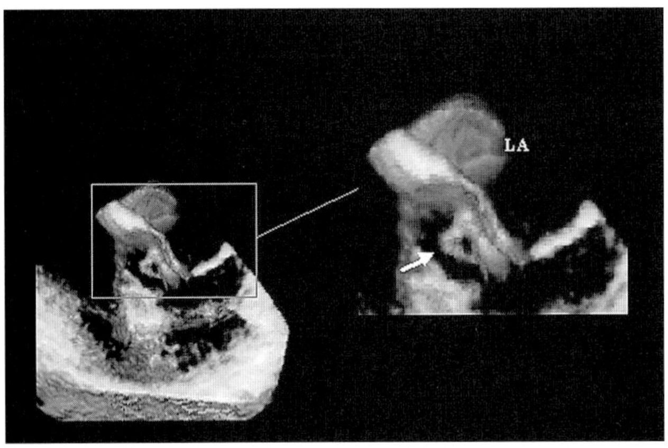

Figure 21. Three-dimensional image of accessory mitral tissue that partially obstructs the left ventricular outflow tract (arrow). LA = left atrium.

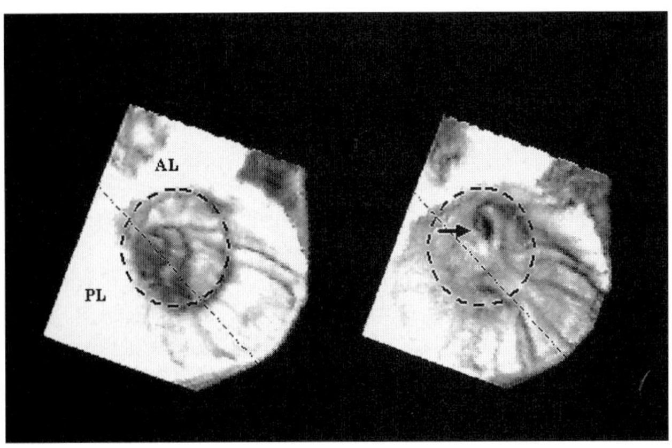

Figure 22. Three-dimensional reconstruction of a cleft mitral valve. The cleft in the anterior leaflet can be seen in systole (arrow). AL = anterolateral; OL = posterolateral.

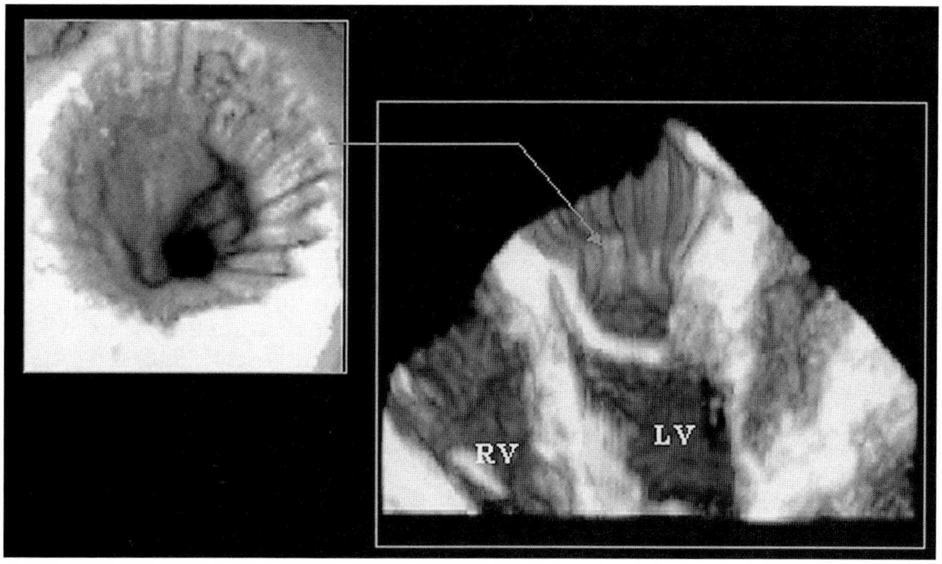

Figure 23. Three-dimensional image of a unicuspid mitral valve. View of four chambers and left atrium (arrow). RV = right ventricle; LV = left ventricle.

Unicuspid Mitral Valve

Unicuspid mitral valve is the rarest entity described here. It can be associated with mitral insufficiency. Three-dimensional reconstruction of TEE four-chamber views and of the left atrium ease identification of this anomaly. Three-dimensional reconstruction of a TEE four-chamber image demonstrates a single anterior leaflet with ample movement. The image from the left atrium helps to corroborate the diagnosis of unicuspid mitral valve (Figure 23).

Ebstein's Anomaly

This malformation is characterized by abnormal insertion of the tricuspid valve, which is tethered from the atrioventricular ring along the endocardium of the right ventricle, creating an atrialized portion of the right ventricle located between the true valve ring and the area corresponding to the abnormal attachment of the tricuspid leaflets. The degree of attachment is variable; in the mild form only the proximal portions of the septal and posterior leaflets are tethered to the interventricular septum and ventricular wall, respectively. Generally, the anterior leaflet is elongated and has an abnormal posterior insertion into the edge of the junction of the right ventricular inlet and trabecular portion.

The diagnosis of Ebstein's anomaly by 2D echocardiography has replaced angiocardiography as the procedure of choice. The advent of TEE has allowed creation of a more detailed evaluation of the heart in adults. The characteristics of each of the three tricuspid leaflets can be identified, a complete visualization of the interatrial septum is obtained, and all portions of the right ventricle can be defined using recordings with multiplane probes.[44]

The 3D reconstruction from TEE and transgastric 2D images allow precise identification of the size and movement of the anterior tricuspid leaflet: a long mobile anterior leaflet sets the stage for surgical repair. In few patients the leaflet has restricted motion as a result of thickening and shortening of the chordae tendinae. Three-dimensional images of the right ventricle in the longitudinal plane are particularly valuable to visualize the anterior leaflet's insertion to the right ventricular infundibulum.

Three-dimensional four-chambers image planes allows exploration of the septal leaflet and reveal that the leaflet is displaced into the ventricle. Displacement of the septal leaflet is measured in early systole as the distance from the tricuspid annulus to the distal point of the septal leaflet attachment. The percentage of displacement of the septal tricuspid leaflet is calculated as the ratio of this value to the total right ventricular dimension. The displacement percentage of the septal tricuspid leaflet is considered severe when larger than 50%.

The tricuspid annulus, with the atrialized ventricular chamber and functional right ventricle, can be explored through unique views looking down through the tricuspid valve annulus from the right atrium, or looking up from the functional right ventricle into the atrialized right ventricular portion. Three-dimensional reconstruction is useful to differentiate a small atrialized chamber with a thick contractile wall from a large chamber with a thin noncontractile wall (Figure 24). Right atrium, atrialized portion of right ventricle, and functional right ventricle volumes can be measured from 3D echocardiograms.[45]

Tricuspid regurgitation is usually severe and is not always proportional to the degree of anatomic abnormality. Color flow shows regurgitation emerging from the displaced septal and posterior leaflets. In few cases, tricuspid stenosis is diagnosed on the basis of

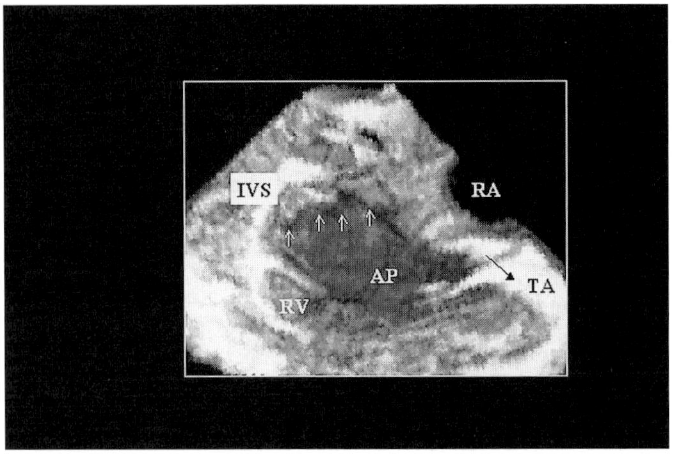

Figure 24. Reconstruction of right cavities reveals an extensive atrialized portion of the right ventricle (AP). Arrows indicate tethering of the tricuspid septal leaflet to the ventricular wall. IVS = interventricular septum; RV = right ventricle; TA = tricuspid ring; RA = right atrium.

significant thickening and diminished mobility of the leaflets.

The most frequently associated malformation is the atrial septal defect; 3D reconstruction displays the defect in numerous new projections and may allow measurement of the defect (Figure 25). Other associated malformations, like mild hypoplasia of the right ventricular outflow or ventricular septal defect, can be visualized in unique 3D echocardiographic image planes. This new technique provides spatial and volumetric information that will aid in planning surgical management of patients with Ebstein's anomaly.

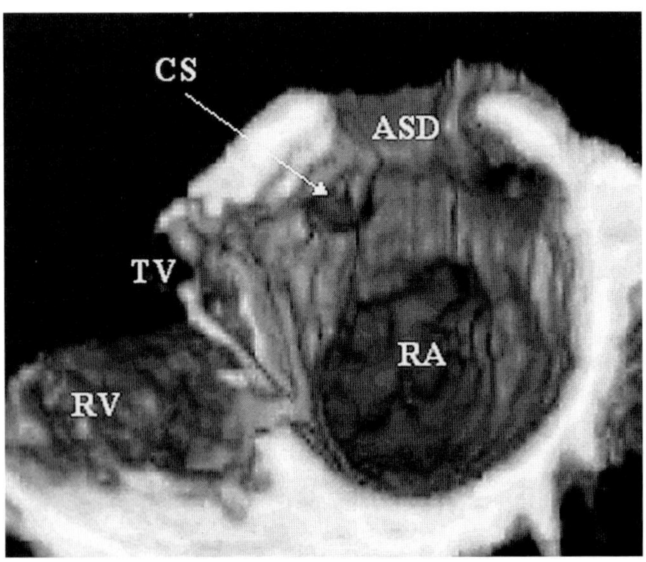

Figure 25. In a patient with Ebstein's anomaly, the view from the right atrium (RA) evidences an atrial septal defect (ASD). The right functional ventricle (RV) as well as the atrialized ventricular portion between the valvular ring close to the sinus (CS) and the tricuspid valves (TV) can be observed.

Ventriculo-Arterial Connections

Concordant Ventriculo-Arterial Connection

In this type of connection, the left ventricle is connected to the aorta and the right ventricle to the pulmonary artery. Transesophageal 3D echocardiography allows visualization of the outlet of the right ventricle and the pulmonary artery surrounding the aorta and the spatial relationships of the aortic and pulmonary valves (Figures 26A, B). The aorta normally lies posterior and to the right of the pulmonary artery. The number of semilunar cusps and the origin and distribution of the main coronary arteries can also be established.

Discordant Ventriculo-Arterial Connection

The term "complete transposition" describes an abnormal or discordant ventriculo-arterial connection in which the aorta arises from the morphologic right ventricle and the pulmonary artery from the morphologic left ventricle, but the AV connection is concordant.

In most cases of complete transposition of the great arteries, the aorta is spatially to the right and anterior, however, other spatial relationships are possible.[46,47]

Corrected transposition of the great arteries is a condition in which atrioventricular and ventriculo-arterial discordances coexist. The ventricular outflow tract and great arteries exit the heart in a parallel fashion and the right ventricle is usually to the left of the morphologic left ventricle. When situs is solitus, the aorta will be anterior and to the left, whereas the main pulmonary artery will be posterior and to the right (Figure 27A, B). Associated defects are frequent (70%–90% of the cases), especially ventricular septal defect, either isolated or with pulmonary stenosis (valvular or subvalvular), and/or Ebstein's anomaly of the left atrioventricular valve (tricuspid)[47] (Figures 28A, B).

Three-dimensional echocardiography has been proven valuable to elucidate some specific alterations in transposition of the great arteries, such as the internal morphologic characteristics of atria, the morphologic features, position and connection of the ventricles to the great arteries, and their spatial relationships (Figure 27A, B, C), as well as in showing atrioventricular valve anomalies (Figure 28A, B).[48] This technique can define the number, thickness, and pliability of the aortic and pulmonary valve leaflets; involvement of the subvalvular structures can be displayed with longitudinal and transverse views from different directions. This technique also allows delineating more precisely and in greater detail the most frequently associated defects, such as atrial and ventricular septal defects, either right- or left-sided. Three-dimensional echocardiography not only provides a "surgeon's view" of the defect before the heart is opened, but also enables accurate measurement of the dimensions of the defect directly on 3D images, and allows accurate quantification of ventricular performance.

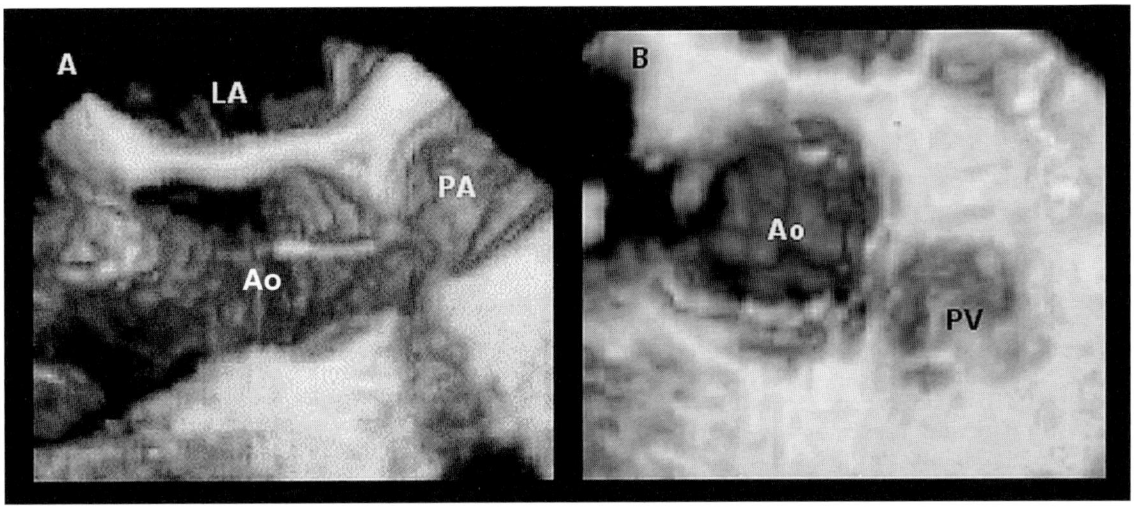

Figure 26. (**A**) Three-dimensional image showing the point at which the great arteries are crossed in longitudinal plane. (**B**) In transversal plane, the aorta is posterior and to the right of the pulmonary artery. Valvular pulmonary stenosis can be observed. LA = left atrium; PA = pulmonary artery; AO = Aorta; PV = Pulmonary valve.

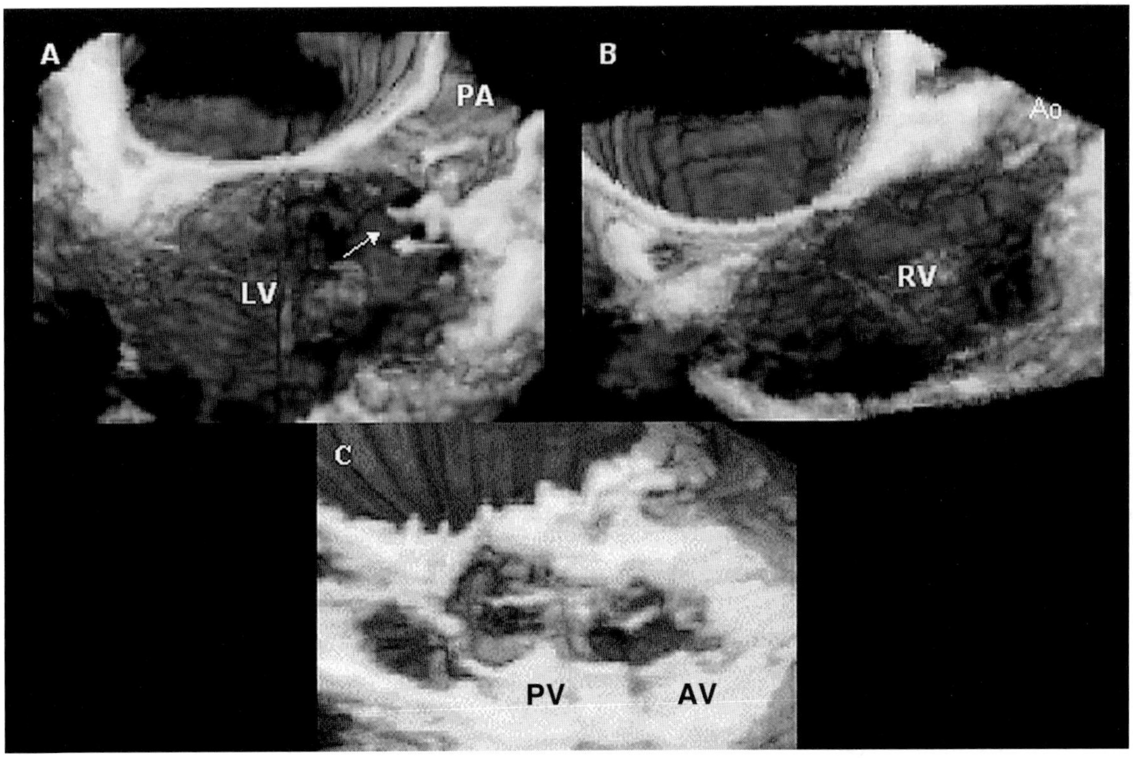

Figure 27. Three-dimensional volume-rendered display of corrected transposition. (**A**) The pulmonary artery arises from the left ventricle. Subpulmonary obstruction by a membrane is shown (arrow). (**B**) The aorta emerges from the right ventricle. (**C**) In transverse plane, the aorta is anterior and to the left of the pulmonary artery. The pulmonary valve is bicuspid and the cusps are thickened. RV = right ventricle; LV = left ventricle; PA =pulmonary artery; Ao = aorta; Av = aortic valve; PV = pulmonary valve.

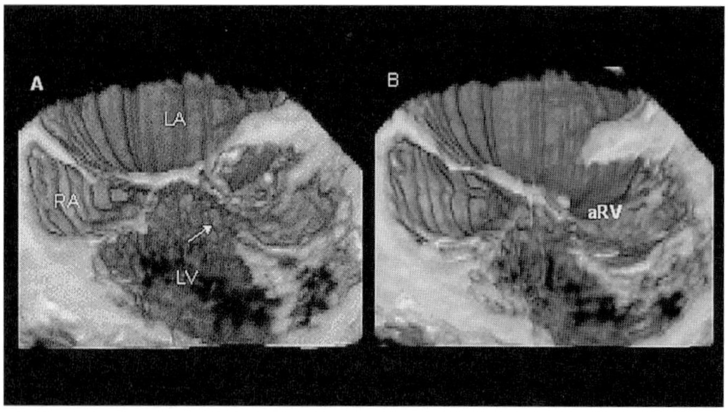

Figure 28. Three-dimensional four-chamber view of a patient with corrected transposition, demonstrating Ebstein's anomaly of the left (tricuspid) atrioventricular valve. The attachment of the septal leaflet is displaced from the tricuspid annulus toward the right ventricular apex. A ventricular septal defect is present (white arrow). (**A**) Systole. (**B**) diastole. LA = left atrium; RA = right atrium; LV =left ventricle; aRV = atrialized right ventricle.

Double-Outlet Right Ventricle

In this type of ventriculo-arterial connection, both great arteries connect mainly or completely to the right ventricle (Figure 29). The position of the vessels is variable. When they are side-to-side or the aorta is anterior, the emergence of the vessels is parallel (Figure 5), and when the aorta is posterior and to the right, the great arteries cross in space.[49]

The diagnostic method of choice is echocardiography.[50,51] Actually, 3D echocardiography can be used to define more precisely some morphologic aspects of this anomaly, such as the overriding degree of the posterior vessel over the interventricular septum (Figure 29), the connection of both vessels with the right ventricle, and the spatial relationship of the great arteries (Figure 30). The associated defects can be delineated in greater detail through excellent images, giving the surgeon an advance look of what to expect intraoperatively.

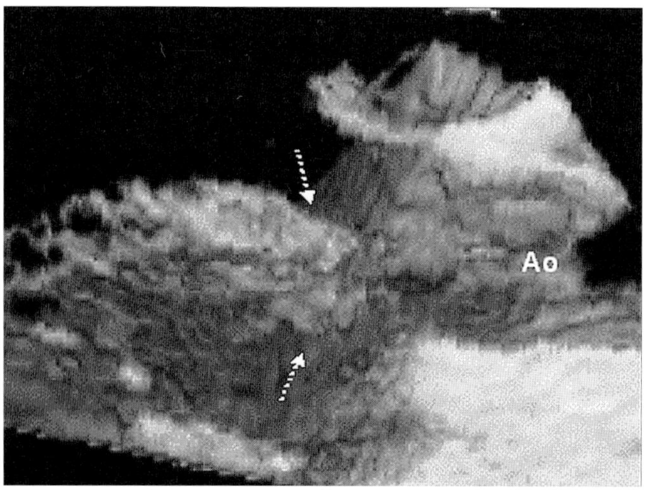

Figure 29. Three-dimensional image of a patient with tetralogy of Fallot and double-outlet right ventricle. Note that the aorta overrides the ventricular septum by more than 50% (arrows). Ao = aorta.

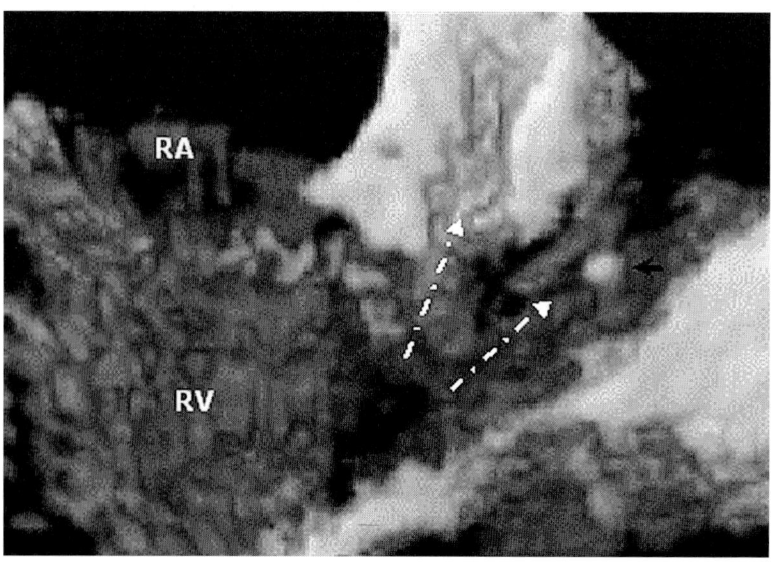

Figure 30. Three-dimensional reconstruction of double-outlet right ventricle with parallel emergence of the vessels in longitudinal plane (white arrows). The anterior vessel has subvalvular obstruction by membrane and the posterior one is hypoplastic.

Aortic Valve Stenosis

Aortic valve stenosis is a common form of CHD that can occur as an isolated defect or in combination with multiple left-sided obstructive lesions. It is caused by cusp deformities, either with or without narrowing of the fibrous annulus. Anatomic types of stenosis include unicuspid, bicuspid, tricuspid, quadricuspid, and undifferentiated aortic valves.[52]

Congenital bicuspid aortic valve occurs in about 2% of the population.[53] In the parasternal short axis view, the two cusps are usually equal or near equal in size. In rare cases, however, there is one large and another small cusp. In diastole, a raphe may or may not be present. When a raphe is not present, the valve has a single closure line in diastole, whereas in its presence, the valve appears to have three distinct closure lines in diastole. In systole, however, the valve cusps separate only along two of the closure lines, and the valve orifice is shaped like a fish-mouth.[54]

The congenitally stenotic tricuspid aortic valve has three aortic cusps. In some cases, the cusps are incompletely developed lumps of fibrous tissue. [52] The edges of the cusp are rolled and gnarled, and there are varying degrees of commissural fusion. This type of valve morphology tends to occur with a narrowed aortic annulus and to cause symptoms in the newborn. In other instances, three well-developed edges are present. The thickening of the edges of the valve leaflets makes the diastolic Y pattern easier to visualize in the parasternal short axis view. In systole, a distinct, restrictive triangular valve orifice is seen.

Congenitally quadricuspid aortic valves are extremely rare. These valves usually have three-normal sized cusps and one small accessory cusp.[55] In the parasternal short axis view, four diastolic closure lines are evidenced.[56]

In some newborn infants with critical aortic stenosis, the aortic valve cusps are not differentiated; instead a fibrous diaphragm or an immobile lump of tissue occupies the position of the normal valve leaflets. In parasternal long -or short- axis views, it is usually not possible to discern individual valve leaflets or a clear valve orifice.

Three-dimensional echocardiography allows display of any desired plane of the cardiac structure. Dynamic volume-rendered display may provide a spatial demonstration of the stenotic valve. Horizontal cross sections above the aortic valve, simulating a surgical aortotomy, provide information on the shape of the lesions and on their distance from the semilunar valve (Figure 31). Views looking to the left ventricular outflow tract, from below the obstruction, allow evaluation of their extension into the ventricle and their relation to the septum and the ventricular surface of the anterior mitral valve leaflet, providing a more accurate and realistic depiction of the complex lesions. Volume-rendered reconstructions display the opening patterns of the aortic valve and the movement of the cusps, allow visualization of their surface, provide better delineation of the cusp edges, and are advantageous for the diagnosis of bicuspid aorta (Figures 32A, B; 33A, B)[57,58]

Aortic valve stenosis constitutes the most common cause of left ventricular outflow obstruction. To determine the anatomic severity, a calculation of valve orifice can be obtained by invasive measurement or echocardiography, by either the continuity equation or the multiplane TEE planimetric technique. In cases of pinhole stenosis, severe valvular calcification or bi-

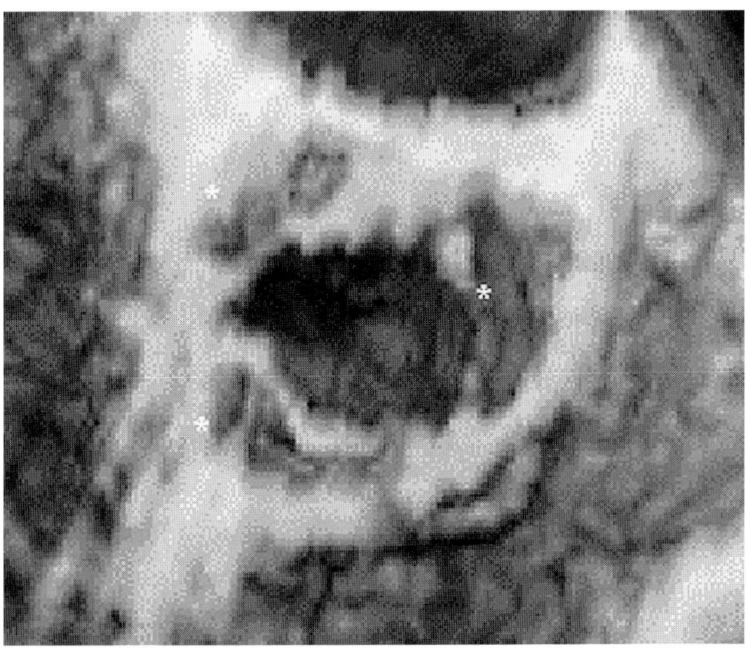

Figure 31. Three-dimensional image of tricuspid aortic valve with thickness of leaflet edges in transverse plane during systole (asterisks).

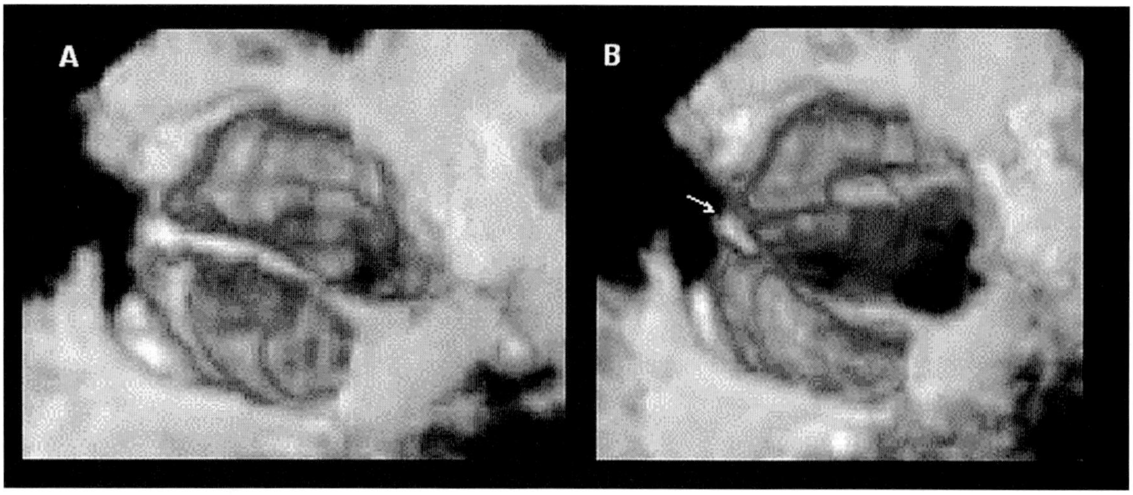

Figure 32. (**A**) Three-dimensional view of bicuspid aortic valve in diastole. The two leaflets have equal areas and their edges appear thickened. (**B**) In systole, fusion of anterior commissure associated with thickness of leaflet edges is observed (arrow).

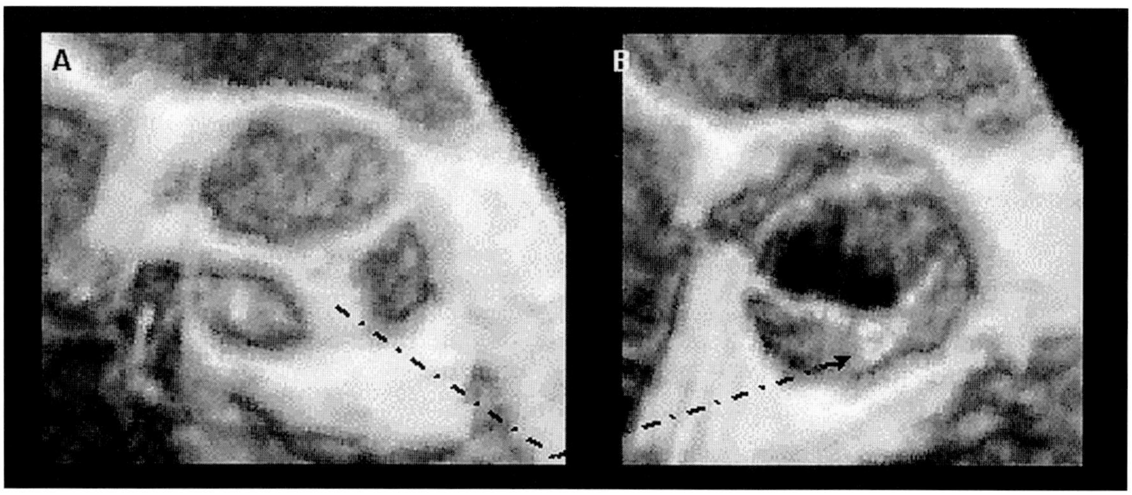

Figure 33. Three-dimensional views (**A** and **B**) of a bicuspid aortic valve. During systole, two fused leaflets are observed (arrow).

cuspid aortic valve, evaluation of aortic stenosis may be difficult, sometimes even impossible. Menzel et al.[57] found that in 42 (88%) of 48 patients, planimetric determination of aortic valve by 3D echocardiography was possible. Statistical analysis of data revealed a good correlation between 3D echocardiography and TEE (r = 95, mean difference +0.018 cm^2, SD ± 0.086) and between 3D echocardiography and the invasive technique (r = 0.88, mean difference +0.12 cm^2, SD ± 0.12). Additional information, including detailed anatomical findings, was achieved from a new perspective, and improved quantification was obtained in 31% of patients.[57]

Transesophageal 3D echocardiography may also provide a more comprehensive assessment of Lambl's excrescences on the aortic valve (valvular strands) than multiplane 2D imaging.[59]

Subvalvular Aortic Stenosis

Subvalvular aortic stenosis accounts for 10% to 20% of all forms of left ventricular outflow obstruction. Three types of subvalvular aortic stenosis have been described: In the discrete membranous type, a thin fibrous diaphragm encircles the left ventricular outflow tract. The membrane can be located a few millimeters below the aortic valve and, in this location, has attachments to the base of the anterior mitral leaflet and to the ventricular septum below the right aortic cusp. Alternatively, the membrane can be located 2 to 3 cm below the aortic valve and, in this location, usually has connections to the anterior mitral valve leaflet. A second type of subvalvular aortic stenosis is a thicker, fibromuscular obstruction that forms a collar-like obstruction around the left ventric-

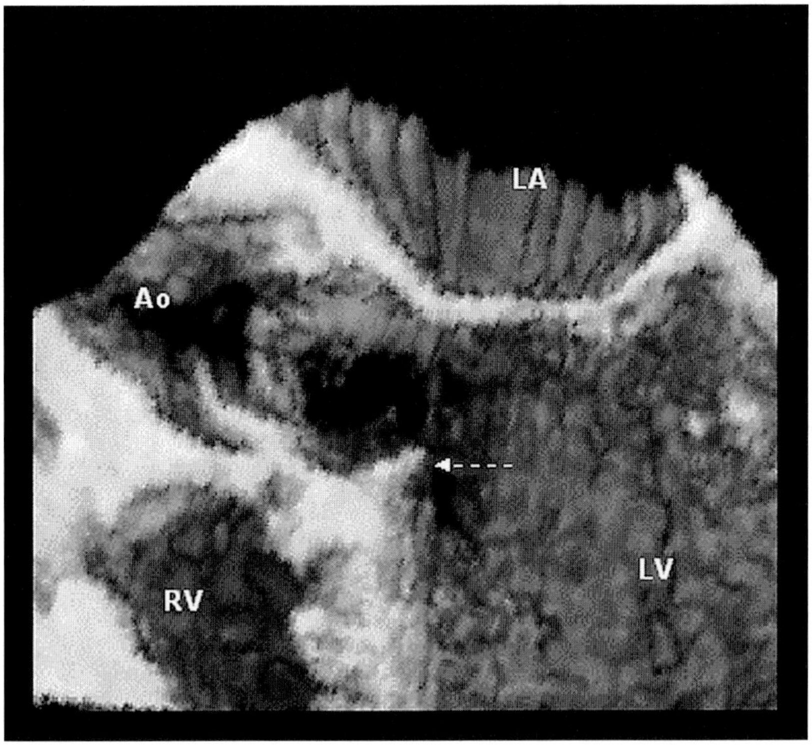

Figure 34. Three-dimensional reconstruction of subaortic membrane (arrow) in a transesophageal five chambers view. LA = left atrium; LV = left ventricle; RV = right ventricle; Ao = aorta.

ular outflow tract a few centimeters below the aortic valve. In the third and most severe form, a fibromuscular obstruction narrows the left ventricular outflow tract to several centimeters, thus forming a tunnel subaortic stenosis.[60,61]

The lesions were best imaged by using a 3D TEE-generated "aortotomy view" of the left ventricular outflow tract immediately below the plane of the aortic valve. The 3D images correlate well with surgical and pathological findings and are suitable for analysis in all cases. Three-dimensional echocardiography generates nonconventional cross sections and displays the left ventricular outflow tract in a realistic perspective, thereby providing additional information (Figure 34). This technique can accurately display and quantify subaortic stenosis and could be a new clinically useful tool to assess discrete subaortic stenosis and in guiding surgical and transcatheter interventions.[62] Both transthoracic and transesophageal echocardiography have been used to diagnose and evaluate discrete subaortic stenosis using long-axis view in the parasternal or apical window. However, these views may limit the detection of discrete subaortic stenosis, especially when it is not circumferential. The aortotomy view, just below the plane of the aortic valve, provides the optimal perspective for displaying the entire subaortic stenosis. Discrete subaortic stenosis is a dynamic lesion that may progress or recur after surgical excision. The morphology of discrete subaortic stenosis can influence the outcome of surgery and balloon dilation. Direct visualization and accurate quantification of subaortic stenosis with 3D TEE may provide a clinically useful tool for the diagnosis and management of these patients.[63]

Supravalvular Aortic Stenosis

Three specific anatomic types of supravalvular aortic stenosis have been described.[52] The membranous type consists of a simple fibrous diaphragm just above the sinuses of Valsalva, with minimal or no narrowing of the external aorta. In the second type, there is an internal structure above the aortic sinuses involving some length of the aorta and accompanied by an external narrowing of the aorta in the region of the structure (Figure 35). The external narrowing gives the aorta the appearance of an hourglass deformity. In the third type of supravalvular aortic stenosis, a severely narrowed and hypoplastic segment of the ascending aorta is present from immediately above the sinuses of Valsalva to the origin of the innominate artery. Blood flow to the arch vessels and descending aorta is usually by way of patent ductus arteriosus.[64–68] Three-dimensional reconstruction of supravalvular aortic stenosis is suitable for analysis in 100% according to the surgical findings.[63]

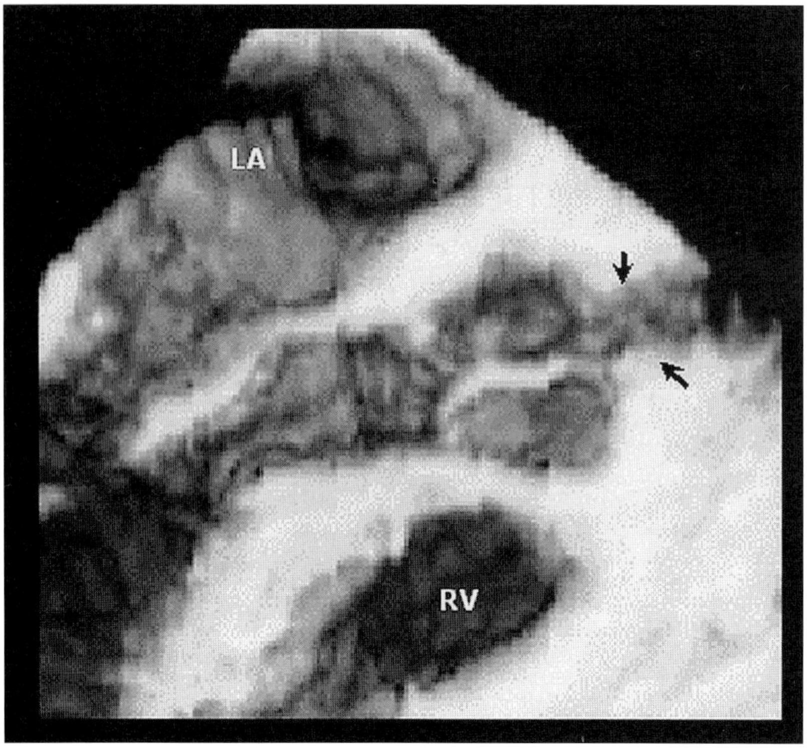

Figure 35. Three-dimensional long axis image of supravalvular obstruction (arrows) in a patient with Williams syndrome. LA = left atrium; RV = right ventricle.

Atrial Septal Defect

After bicuspid aorta and mitral prolapse, atrial septal defect (ASD) is the most frequently identified congenital cardiopathy in the adult, representing from 22% to 25% of all cases. It is found two times more often in women than in men.

The relevance of the defect depends on its hemodynamic repercussion and the latter, in turn, depends on the size of the ASD, magnitude of the left-to-right shunt, and the degree of pulmonary hypertension (PH). Usually the defect is well tolerated with few clinical manifestations, therefore it is often not noted until adult age and can be an incidental finding during a routine medical examination. If it follows its natural evolution it will induce PH after the third decade of life and atrial fibrillation in 25% to 50% of those patients over 50 years of age. It can course with severe cyanosis in the long-range as a consequence of severe PH and the inverted shunt.

The echocardiographic study of patients with ASD is aimed at defining the characteristics of the defect, its exact location, size and area, calculation of the shunt, connection site of the pulmonary veins, and the presence of associated defects.

Macroscopic Anatomy of the Interatrial Septum

The interatrial septum is a curtain that separates both atria; it develops from weeks 4 to 6 of gestation. A communication between atria, located in the anterior and superior portion of the fossa ovalis, is present during fetal life. At the time of birth, this communication closes physiologically, the anatomic closure can occur between 6 to 18 months after birth, or can remain patent for the rest of the patient's life in up to 30% of individuals without evidencing any cardiopathy. The septum, at its right atrial side, presents a thinning at the fossa ovalis level, which is surrounded by a well-defined annulus edge that separates it from the thicker muscular portion of the septum. Its left atrial side is smooth, uniform, and only presents a semilunar fold at its anterosuperior portion.

Types of Atrial Septal Defect

The spectrum of ASD goes from the patent fossa ovalis to the single atrium.

Patent Foramen Ovale

This defect is caused by the persistence of the communication between both atria after birth, in the anterosuperior region of the fossa ovalis (Figure 36). It can be present in up to 30% of subjects without presenting evidence of cardiopathy.

Defects of the Fossa Ovalis

Defects are located within the limbus of the fossa ovalis (Figure 37), and represent the most common type of ASD; among these, ostium secundum defects located at the medial part of the septum (Figure 38) are the most frequent (60% to 70% of cases). The valve can

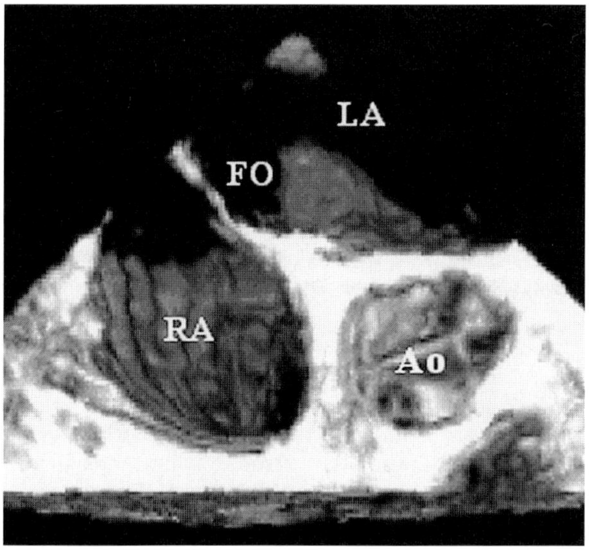

Figure 36. Patent foramen ovale. The fossa ovalis is a shallow depression that often has a prominent fold or limbus. Ao = aorta; FO = foramen ovale; LA = left atrium; RA = right atrium.

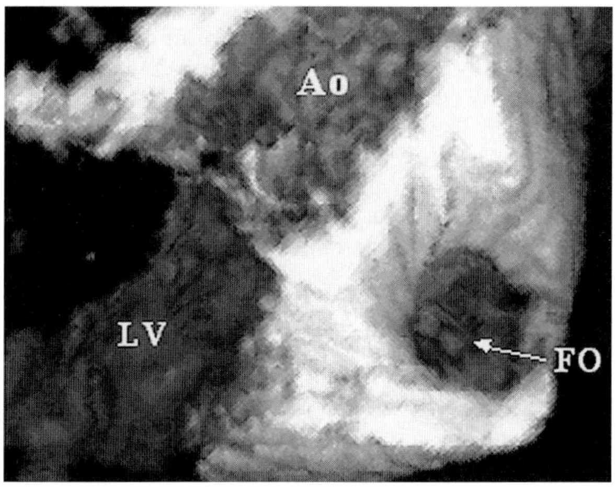

Figure 37. Atrial septal defect at the fossa ovalis level viewed from the left atrium. Ao = aorta; FO = fossa ovalis; LV = left ventricle.

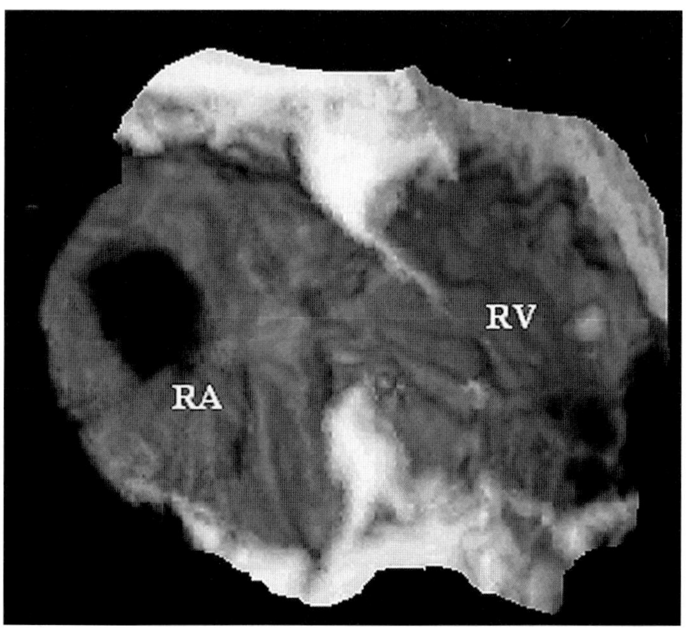

Figure 38. Ostium secundum atrial septal defect. This defect involves the region of the fossa ovalis. Atrial septal tissue separates the inferior edge of the defect from the atrioventricular valves.

be fenestrated by multiple orifices or can be partially absent. They can occur as an isolated entity or associated to other anomalies.

Sinus Venosus Type

This is a superior vena cava type or high ASD (Figure 39). This defect is located at the region of the embryonic septum secundum, outside the limbus of the fossa ovalis, close to where the superior vena cava and the right superior pulmonary vein empty. It is often accompanied by an anomalous connection of the right pulmonary veins to the superior vena cava or to the right atrium. It represents 5% to 15% of cases.

Ostium Primum

This defect is located outside the fossa ovalis at the lower part of the septum in relation to the atrioventricular valves (Figure 40). It can be an isolated entity, or associated to AV canal defects, to other anomalies of the endocardial cushions, and to trisomy 21. It is found in 15% to 20% of cases.

Inferior Vena Cava Type (Inferior ASD of the sinus venosus)

This defect is located outside the limbus of the fossa ovalis, close to where the IVC empties. It is not frequent.

Common Atrium or Single Atrium

This defect is due to large defects that compromise several regions of the septum. It is called common atrium when some remnants of the septum persist and single atrium when no septal remnant exists, and is usually associated to more complex cardiopathies with undetermined situs.

Atrial Septal Closure by Devices

At present it is possible to close the ASD by means of occluding devices during cardiac catheterism. To perform the closure it is indispensable to know the size, shape and variations of the defect, as well as its relations with neighboring structures.[69] It is necessary to establish precisely the distance between the edges of the ASD and the fixed references of the right atrium. The posterosuperior edge is in relation to the superior vena cava, the posteroinferior edge with the IVC, the anteroinferior with the tricuspid ring, and the aortic edge is anterosuperior. Ostium secundum type defects are ideal for closure with occluding devices (Figure 41).

Three-dimensional echocardiography can identify the anatomic details and the spatial resolution more precisely than 2D images. Transthoracic echo underestimates ASD dimensions in about 30%. The septal defect presents a dynamic behavior during the cardiac cycle, its perimeter is larger during ventricular systole and reduced during atrial systole, and the area of the defect can vary up to 70% (Figure 42).[70] Dimensions of the ASD are

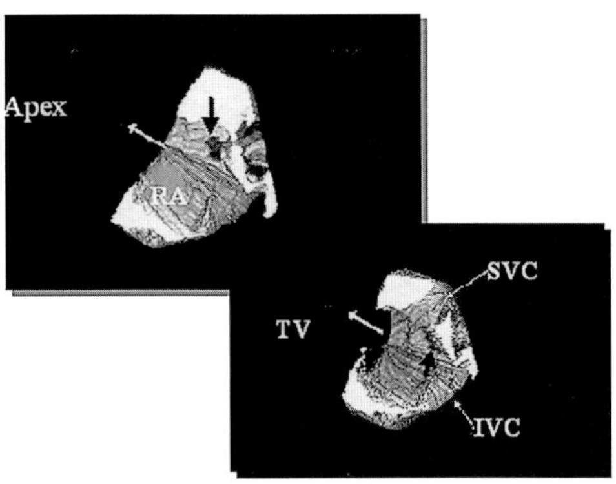

Figure 39. Sinus venosus defect (black arrows). It appears like a biatrial connection of the superior vena cava, frequently involving an anomalous connection of one or more of the right-sided pulmonary veins. IVC = inferior vena cava; RA = right atrium; SVC = superior vena cava; TV= tricuspid valve.

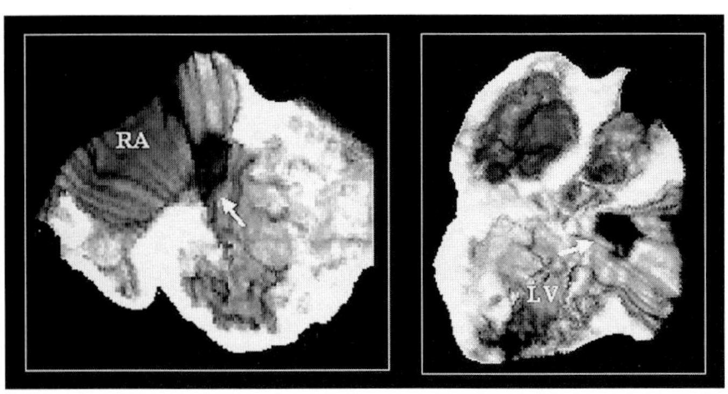

Figure 40. Ostium primum atrial septal defect (arrow). The defect lies inferior to the fossa ovalis. LV= left ventricle; RA = right atrium.

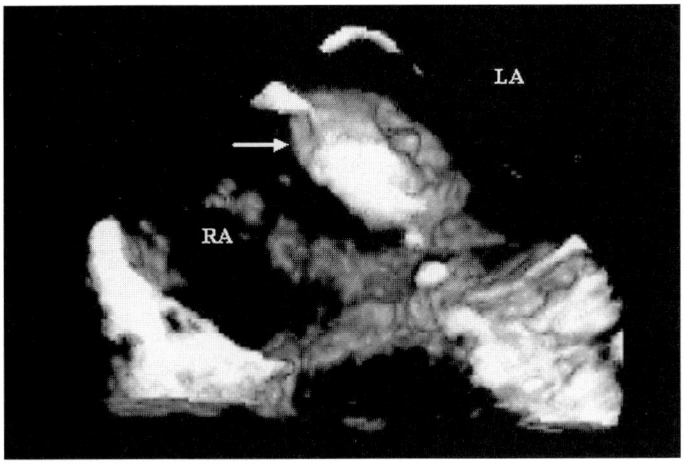

Figure 41. Amplatzer device (arrow) closing an atrial septal defect. RA = right atrium; LA = left atrium.

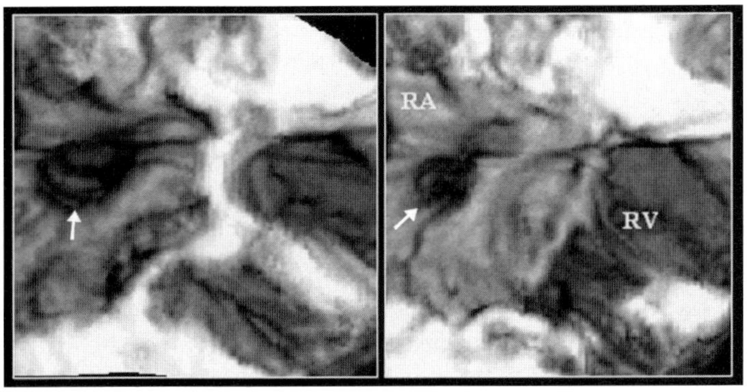

Figure 42. Ostium secundum atrial septal defect (arrows). The shape of the defect changes with the cardiac cycle. RA = right atrium; RV = right ventricle.

very important, since small defects can be occluded easily; those smaller than 13 mm can be closed completely, whereas those larger than 20 mm might be inadequate for closure. The size of the orifice and the dimensions of the anterosuperior edge (aortic edge) are independent predictors of the results obtained through the closure procedure.[71] In some instances, if defects are larger than 26 mm when extended (measured through the inflated balloon) they are not included for the procedure. The device is removed if it is unstable or compromises the function of the mitral valve.[72] Three-dimensional TEE allows better definition of the edges of the defect: the anterosuperior up to 90%, the inferoposterior up to 60% of cases, but even with this technique some additional small fenestrations cannot be identified.[73]

It is important to consider that after placement of the devices there might still be subtle changes in their position for up to 20 minutes, therefore they must be monitored continuously.[74]

Residual shunt might occur and varying degrees of occurrences have been reported. After surgical correction of the ASD, residual shunt has been found in 2% of patients, whereas immediately after closure with the device it has been found in 91%, which decreases to 53% at 10 months of follow-up. In these cases, no direct relation has been found between the shunt and the dimensions, location, or position of the device, nor with the location of the defect, or the size of the device in relation to the expanded diameter of the ASD.[75]

Although in most medical centers with adequate experience, the procedure is performed at an average time of 1 hour and 15 minutes for fluoroscopy, successful attempts have been made to perform the whole procedure only under TEE (without fluoroscopy). Under these conditions, the total time might be up to 100 minutes.[76] Closure of more complex defects is currently being tried, for example in multiple defects requiring more than one device[77] (Figure 43), as well as in more complicated pathologies, including mitral or pulmonary valvular defects, multiple or separated de-

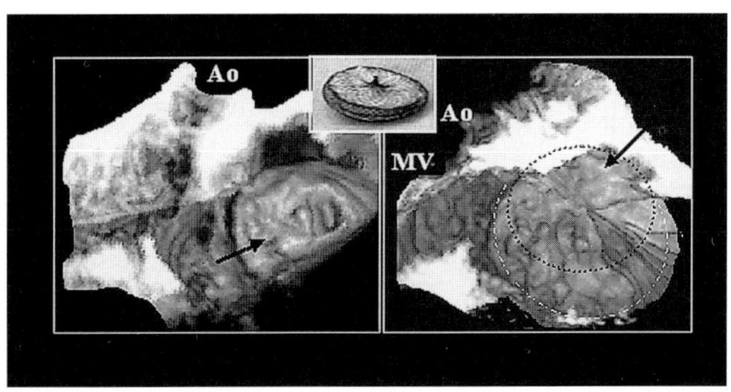

Figure 43. This atrial septal defect was too large and irregular, requiring the use of two Amplatzer devices (arrows). Ao = aorta; MV = mitral valve.

fects, single defects larger than 30 mm, or residual defects after partial closure with occluding devices.[78]

Closure with devices has been made in patients with aneurysms at the perforated interatrial septum,[79] as well as in patients with cerebrovascular event antecedents,[80] and to prevent recurrence of neurological decompression illness in divers or to correct patent foramen ovale (diagnosed through TEE).[81] Indications for the use of devices to close an ASD have extended beyond the simple defects, and its use has been reported in cases of abnormal locations in the fossa ovalis, with partially deficient septal edge, in cases of multiple defects, and aneurysms at the multiperforated interatrial septum.[82]

It is clear that closure of simple and complex septal defects in patients of any age is now a reality, and that 3D TEE is at present and for the near future a good tool for the adequate control of the procedure.

Ventricular Septal Defects

The most useful form to classify ventricular septal defects is through the anatomy of the interventricular septum. The latter is constituted by two portions, a muscular and a fibrous one. The muscular portion is made up by three regions: inlet, trabecular, and outlet. The membranous septum is a small structure divided in two parts by the fibrous ring of the tricuspid valve at the level of the septal leaflet, i.e., the AV and the interventricular regions. Based on the aforementioned, the ventricular septal defects can be classified in perimembranous, muscular, and subarterial. The first two can involve the inlet, trabecular, and outlet regions of the septum.

Two-dimensional echocardiographic assessment of septal defects presents limitations since it is necessary to perform diverse approximations to define their location and relation to other structures besides, evaluation of shape and size is sometimes difficult since borders cannot be defined clearly. The precise definition of the communication borders and their relation with other structures is at present important, since one of the treatment option is transcatheter closure with occluder devices. When closure is surgical, the technique offers advantages for the surgeon in planning the surgery.[83]

Reconstruction with 3D echocardiography has been proposed as a new technique able to simulate intraoperative visualization of cardiac structures, which allows understanding of their anatomy.[84,85] It also provides enough information on the morphology, size, location, and spatial relations of the different types of interventricular defects, allowing to select patients for device closure and to choose the size of the device. It also allows to define the defects' relation with the AV valves (i.e., whether overriding or straddling).

Evaluation can be performed from views of the right or left ventricle.[86,87] The right-sided view equals that of the surgeon, reproducing the surgical view of right ventriculotomy. The latter can be insufficient, since perimembranous defects are covered by the septal leaflet of the tricuspid or by remnants of the membranous septum. In muscular defects, thick trabeculae often hinder definition of the borders of the defect. When there are technical difficulties, such as a thickened, immobile valve partially covering and hindering visualization of the defect, the defect must be exposed electronically, eliminating the tricuspid valve or creating new cutplanes in which the tricuspid valve is not present.[88]

The view from the left ventricle allows a total view of the interventricular septum, determining the position, size, and shape of the defect.[87,89]

Membranous defects can be three-dimensionally observed from the view of the left ventricle immediately below the aortic valve. Their circumference is easily identified by the smooth surface of the interventricular septum on this side. In general, they are round- or oval-shaped, their structure is musculo-membranous, and they are located beneath the aorta always in relation to the tricuspid valve. There are three basic extensions, but there might be combinations in the more complex defects. When the extension is to the inlet, the main axis is directed to the cross of the heart, related to the fibrous ring of the tricuspid valve, the septal leaflet, and directly to the aortic sigmoid, away from the mitral valve. When the extension is trabecular, the main axis of the defect is toward the apex and is less related to the tricuspid valve. In the extension to the outlet, the main axis is directed to the front and has no relation with the tricuspid valve.

Septal defects of the inlet portion are better assessed from the right ventricle view (Figure 44), defining its distance with the apex and the state of the tricuspid valve.[85] Their edges can be muscular or musculo-membranous

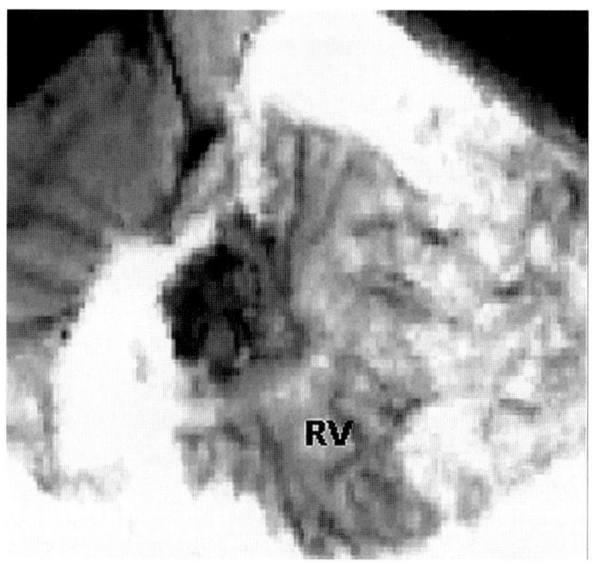

Figure 44. View of the interventricular septum from the right ventricle revealing a large perimembranous septal defect that extends to the inlet and is related to the fibrous ring of the tricuspid valve. RV = right ventricle.

and they are tightly related to the septal leaflet of the tricuspid. When the defects are musculo-membranous, they can produce a cleft in the tricuspid valve due to the flow of the shunt.

Muscular defects are better assessed from the view of the left ventricle,[87] which allows one to define their location in the anterior or posterior portion of the septum, their closeness to the apex, whether there are multiple defects, and the shape. Edges are exclusively muscular and are away from the valves (Figures 45 and 46).

Defects from the outlet portion can present exclusively muscular or musculofibrous edges. The muscular edges are located above the branches of the septomarginalis trabecula. When the communication edges are musculo-fibrous, a tight relation with the aortic and pulmonary valves exists, and therefore prolapse or aortic insufficiency can be produced. By 3D echocardiography the view of the right ventricle allows observation of the relation of the defect with the pulmonary valve and the aortic prolapse when present, as well as the conditions existing above the crista terminalis. From left ventricle, *en face* view, ventricular septal defects appeared subaortic in position. The left ventricular protection must include the aorta, but at a more anterior plane than for a perimembrenous defect. This allows defininition of the prolapse and the relation with pulmonary valvular plane.

In conclusion, some cutplanes have been standardized for a better evaluation of the different types of ventricular septal defects, considering their anatomy and spatial relations. For example, to assess membranous defects, the best way to visualize them is the three-chamber view, which includes the atrium, the left ventricle, and the aorta. For the muscular defects, the cutplane simulates the membranous defects with a parallel orientation to the left septal surface; however, this plane must be rotated in several directions for the best visualization of the muscular defects, depending on their location in the septum. A cutplane that includes the aorta allows defining the high muscular defects. The two-chamber view, including the atrium and the left ventricle, allows visualization of the posterior and inferior defects. For subarterial defects, the cutplane must be more anterior.

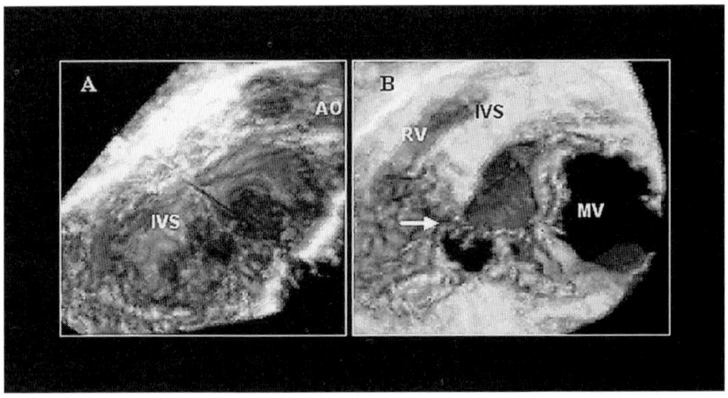

Figure 45. Sagittal and coronal sections of a wide muscular interventricular defect. (**A**) View of the interventricular septum from the left ventricle revealing the defect in the medial and posterior portion of the septum, with irregular borders and with insertion of chorda tendinae from the tricuspid valve (arrow). (**B**) Coronal section underneath the atrioventricular rings in which mild overriding of the tricuspid valve can be seen as well as tricuspid valve chordal insertions into the interventricular septum. AO = aorta; IVS = interventricular septum; RV = Right ventricle; MV = mitral valve. * = insertions of the tricuspid valve.

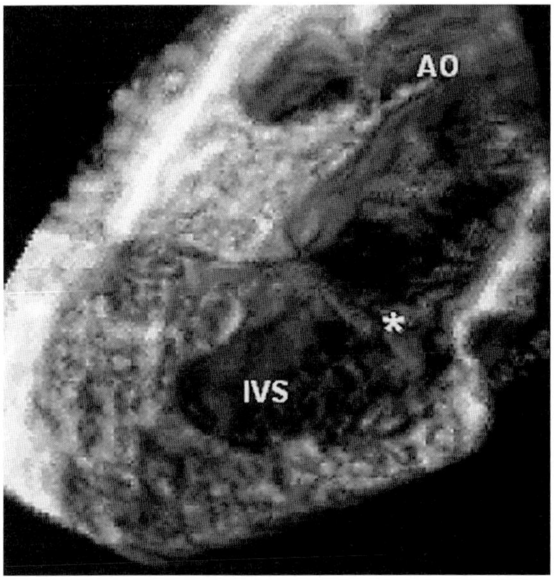

Figure 46. View of the interventricular septum from the left ventricle, showing a large muscular defect in the medial and posterior portion of the septum, divided by insertions of the tricuspid valve. AO = aorta; IVS = interventricular septum; * = chords of the tricuspid valve.

Atrioventricular Septal Defect

Atrioventricular septal defect is the extreme form of the defect of endocardial cushions, also called common AV canal. Common characteristics are a fibrous AV ring associated to one or two valvular rings, perimembranous inlet interventricular communication, geometric modification of the left ventricle, alterations in the fibrous skeleton of the heart, alterations of the atrioventricular valves and in the conduction system.

The common fibrous ring is due to the absence of the ventral and dorsal endocardial cushions. The interventricular communication lacks the tissue from the inlet septum and from the membranous septum that originates from the atrioventricular septum. The left ventricle is also modified. Under normal conditions, the AV rings are attached above and below, and the aorta lies in the center of the base of the heart. In common AV canal, the AV valve is not attached to the AV septum, and since it is absent, the fibrous ring dilates and displaces to the front, which, in turn, displaces the aortic root to the front, producing unwedging of the aorta. There are also modifications in the relation between the ring-apex and the outflow tract of the left ventricle, producing lengthening of the outlet portion, whereas the inlet portion shortens. There is only one fibrous ring that can have only one valve with five leaflets or two analog valves from left to right, found in one plane. Finally, the AV septum is absent.

When there are five leaflets, three correspond to the left ventricle in lateral, anterior, and posterior positions, and two correspond to the right ventricle, one anterior and the other lateral. The posterior leaflet crosses the interventricular septum toward the right ventricle and is called the "bridge valve." The left anterior forms the anterior "bridge valve" in type B and C Rastelli. When there are two valvular rings, the lack of attachment of this valve to the posterior one produces the "mitral cleft." The most relevant valve is the left anterior valve, since, depending on its insertion, the canal is classified in three types: In type A Rastelli the left anterior bridging leaflet crosses the interventricular septum and inserts in the medial papillary muscle and insertions are in the crest of the interventricular septum. In type B Rastelli, insertions are in the medial papillary muscle, which is shifted to the apex, between the septum and the free wall of the right ventricle. In type C Rastelli, insertions are to the medial papillary muscle located in the free wall of the right ventricle, fused to the anterior papillary muscle.

Other valvular anomalies include accessory orifices, parachute insertion, and right leaflets tethered to the interventricular septum (Ebstein's).

The recent echocardiographic techniques of three-dimensional reconstruction have shown to be particularly useful to define the morphology of the valve and its insertions, to determine the level of shunts, and to estimate the size of the ventricles. During presurgical evaluation, it allows to identify the atrial and ventricular components of the AV septum, the size of the atrial and ventricular defects, the insertions of the chorda tendinae, the distribution of the valve in the ventricles, the degree of valvular insufficiency, as well as the associated lesions. In patients with two valvular orifices, 3D echocardiography allows assessment of the bridges of the anterior and posterior left leaflets that are joined by a band of fibrous tissue dividing the common fibrous ring.

Atrioventricular septal defects can be defined in sagittal and coronal sections[90] in four-chamber views (Figure 47). Sometimes, reconstruction of the heart is not possible at the level of the AV valve, due to gray structures produced by valvular reverberations that hinder the view of the valve.

Three-dimensional echocardiography is useful for the evaluation of regurgitation flows after surgery of

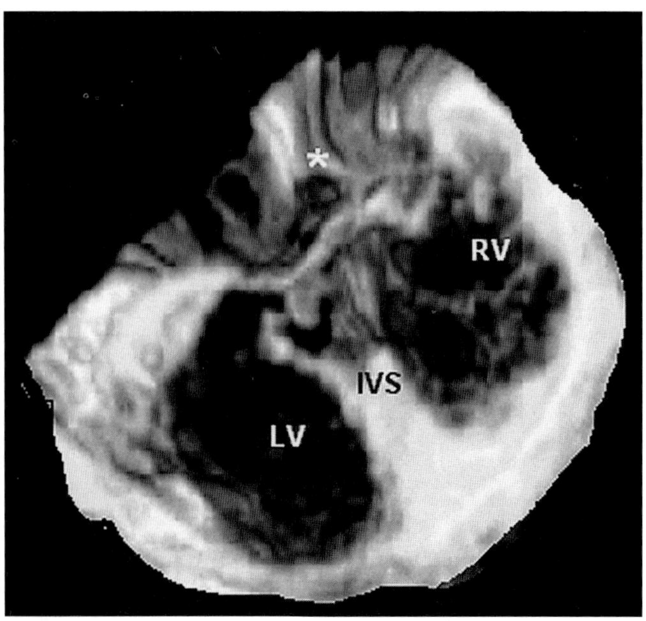

Figure 47. Sagittal section in four-chamber view showing the common atrioventricular valve. Note the insertion on the interventricular septum (Rastelli type A) that partially occludes the septal defect. The ostium primum atrial septal defect can also be observed (asterisk). RV = right ventricle; LV = left ventricle.

the left portion of the common valve (mitral). Recent studies have assessed these flows by relating them with the surface area of the superior, inferior, or mural leaflets.[91] Reconstruction was made from the view of the left atrium, which allows assessment of valvular function when closed, looking from the superior surface. Redundant or prolapsing valves require different angulations and hence the measurements of the leaflets surface can be modified. Color mapping can contribute to a better understanding of valvular morphology and function.

References

1. Huhta JC, Smalhorn JF, Macartney FJ. Two dimensional echocardiography diagnosis of situs. *Br Heart J* 1982; 48:97–108.
2. Stümper O, Sreram N, Elzenga NJ, et al. Diagnosis of atrial situs by transesophageal echocardiography. *J Am Coll Cardiol* 1990;16:442–446.
3. Salustri A, Spitaels S, McGhie J, et al. Transthoracic three-dimensional echocardiography in adult patients with congenital heart disease. *J Am Coll Cardiol* 1995;26:759–767.
4. Roldán FJ, Vargas-Barrón J, Espinola Zavaleta N, et al. Cor triatriatum dexter: Transesophageal echocardiographic diagnosis and three-dimensional reconstruction. *J Am Soc Echocardiog* 2001;14:634–636.
5. Battle-Díaz J, Stanley P, Kratz C, et al. Echocardiographic manifestation of persistence of the right sinus venous as valve. *Am J Cardiol* 1979;43:850–853.
6. Roldán FJ, Vargas-Barrón J, Espinola ZN, et al. Three-dimensional echocardiography of the right atrial embryonic remnants. *Am J Cardiol* (in press).
7. Chartier L, Bera J, Delomez M, et al. Free-floating thrombi in the right heart: Diagnosis, management, and prognostic indexes in 38 consecutive patients. *Circulation* 1999; 99;2779–2783.
8. Yodfat, UA. Right atrial membrane interfering with insertion of pulmonary artery catheter. *Anesthesiology* 2000;9:576–578.
9. Mahy I, Anderson R. Division of the right atrium. *Circulation* 1998;98:2352–2353.
10. Limacher MC, Gutgesell HP, Vick GW. Echocardiographic anatomy of the Eustachian valve. *Am J Cardiol* 1986;57:363–365.
11. Werner JA, Cheitlin MD, Gross BW, et al. Echocardiographic appearance of the Chiari network: Differentiation from right heart pathology. *Circulation* 1981;63: 1104–1109.
12. Vargas-Barrón J, Espinola-Zavaleta N, Roldán FJ, et al. Transesophageal echocardiographic diagnosis of thrombus in accessory lobes of the left atrial appendage. *Echocardiography* 2000;17:689–691.
13. Veniot JP, Harrity PJ, Gentile F, et al. Anatomy of the left atrial appendage. A quantitative study of age related changes in 500 autopsy hearts: Implications for echocardiographic examinations. *Circulation* 1997;96:3112–3115.
14. Agmon Y, Khandheria BK, Gentile F, et al. Echocardiographic assessment of the left atrial appendage. *JAAC* 1999;34:1867–1877.
15. Roldán FJ, Vargas-Barrón J, Loredo Mendoza L, et al. Anatomic correlation of left atrial appendage by three-dimensional echocardiography. *J Am Soc Echocardiogr* 2001;14:742–744.
16. Tomisawa M, Onouchi Z, Goto M, et al. Congenital left atrial enlargement. A case report with special reference to myocardial fine structure. *Jpn Circ J* 1975;39: 417–424.
17. Kirklin JW, Barrat-Boyes BG. Unroofed coronary sinus syndrome. In Kirklin JW, Barrat-Boyes BG (eds): *Cardiac surgery, 2nd edition.* New York, Churchill-Livingstone, 1993, 683–692.
18. Vargas-Barrón J, Espinola-Zavaleta N, Romero-Cárdenas A, et al. Two and three dimensional echocardiographic unroofed coronary sinus. *J Am Soc Echocardiogr* 2001; 14:742–744.
19. Vogel M, Ho S, Anderson RH. Comparison of three-dimensional echocardiographic findings with anatomical specimens of various congenitally malformed hearts. *Br Heart J* 1995;73:566–570.
20. Bartel T, Müller S. Corrected transposition of the great arteries: Dynamic three-dimensional echocardiography and volumetry. *Jpn Heart J* 1995;36:819–824.
21. Vogel M, Ho S, Ludomirsky A, et al. Transthoracic 3-dimensional echocardiography provides new information on straddling or overriding AV valves in complex heart defects. *Circulation* 1994;90 I-531 (Abstract).
22. Collins-Nakai RL, Rosenthal A, Castañeda AR, et al. Congenital mitral stenosis. *Circulation* 1977;56:1039–1047.
23. Davachi F, Moller JH, Edwards JR. Disease of the mitral valve in infancy. *Circulation* 1971;43:565–579.
24. Ruckman RN, Van Praagh R. Anatomic types of congenital mitral stenosis. Report of 49 autopsy cases with consideration of diagnosis and surgical implications. *Am J Cardiol* 1978;42:592–601.
25. Roberts WC. Morphologic features of the normal and abnormal mitral valve. *Am J Cardiol* 1983;51:1005–1008.
26. Perloff JK, Roberts WC. The mitral apparatus. Functional anatomy of mitral regurgitation. *Circulation* 1972;46: 227–239.
27. Fehske W, Grayburn PA, Omran H, et al. Morphology of the mitral valve as displayed by multiplane transesophageal echocardiography. *J Am Soc Echocardiogr* 1994;7:472–479.
28. Salustri A, Roelandt JRTC. Ultrasonic three-dimensional reconstruction of the heart. *Ultrasound Med Biol* 1995; 21:281–293.
29. Nanda NC, Pinheiro L, Sanyal R, et al. Multiplane transesophageal echocardiographic imaging and three-dimensional reconstruction. *Echocardiography* 1992;9: 667–676.
30. Levine RA, Handschumacher MD, Sanfilippo AJ, et al. Three-dimensional echocardiographic reconstruction of the mitral valve, with implications for the diagnosis of mitral valve prolapse. *Circulation* 1989;80:589–598.
31. Salustri A, Becker AE, Herwerden LV, et al. Three-dimensional echocardiography of normal and pathologic mitral valve: A comparison with two-dimensional transesophageal echocardiography. *J Am Coll Cardiol* 1996; 27:1502–1510.
32. Fulton DR, Marx GR, Pandian NG, et al. Dynamic three-dimensional echocardiographic imaging of congenital heart defects in infants and children by computed-controlled tomographic parallel slicing using a single integrated ultrasound instrument. *Echocardiography* 1994;11:155–164.
33. Bartel T, Müller S, Erbel R. Dynamic three-dimensional echocardiography using parallel slicing: A promising diagnostic procedure in adults with congenital heart disease. *Cardiology* 1998;89:140–147.
34. Belohavek M, Foley DA, Gerber TC, et al. Three-

dimensional ultrasound imaging of the atrial septum. Normal and pathologic anatomy. *J Am Coll Cardiol* 1993; 22:1673–1678.
35. Layman T, Edwards J. Anomalous mitral arcade. *Circulation* 1967;35:389–395.
36. Matushima A, Park J, Szulc M, et al. Anomalous atrioventricular valve arcade. *Am Heart J* 1991;121: 1824–1826.
37. Bano-Rodrigro A, Van Praagh S, Trowitzsch E, et al. Double orifice mitral valve: A study of 27 postmortem cases with developmental, diagnostic and surgical considerations. *Am J Cardiol* 1988;61:152–160.
38. Trowitzsch E, Bano-Rodrigo A, Burger B, et al. Two-dimensional echocardiographic findings in double orifice mitral valve. *J Am Coll Cardiol* 1985;6:383–387.
39. Khalil KG, Shapiro I, Kilman JW, Congenital mitral stenosis. *J Thorac Cardiovasc Surg* 1975;70:40–45.
40. Sono J, McKay R, Arnold R. Accessory mitral valve leaflet causing aortic regurgitation and left ventricular outflow tract obstruction: Case report and review of published reports. *Br Heart J* 1988;59:491–497.
41. McEnany MT, English TA, Ross DM. The congenitally cleft posterior mitral valve leaflet. *Ann Thoracic Surg* 1973;16:281–292.
42. Ranganathan M, Lam JHC, Wigle ED, et al. Morphology of the human mitral valve II: The valve leaflets. *Circulation* 1970;41:459–467.
43. Smallhorn J, DeLeval M, Stark J, et al. Isolated anterior mitral cleft: Two-dimensional echocardiographic assessment and differentiation from "clefts" associated with atrioventricular septal defect. *Br Heart J* 1982;48: 109–116.
44. Vargas-Barron J, Rijlaarsdam M, Romero-Cárdenas A, et al. Transesophageal echocardiographic study of Ebstein's anomaly. *Echocardiography* 1995;12:253–261.
45. Ludomirsky A, Vermilion R, Nesser J, et al. Improved anatomic delineation of Ebstein's anomaly from three-dimensional images obtained by echocardiography and magnetic resonance imaging. *Circulation* 1994;90:I530 (Abstract).
46. Kidd BSL. Complete transposition of the great arteries. In Keith JD, Rowe RD, Vlad P (eds): *Heart Disease in Infancy and Childhood. 3rd edition.* New York, Macmillan Publishing Co, 1978; pp 590–611.
47. Perloff JK. Congenitally corrected transposition of the great arteries. In: *Clinical Recognition of Congenital Heart Disease.* Philadelphia, PA, WB Saunders Co, 1988; pp 62–83.
48. Roelandt JRTC. Three-dimensional echocardiography: The future today! *Acta Cardiol* 1998;53(6):333–336.
49. Sridaromont S, Feldt RH, Ritte DG, et al. Double outlet right ventricle. Hemodynamic and anatomic correlations. *Am J Cardiol* 1976;38:85–94.
50. DiSessa TG, Hagan AD, Pope C, et al. Two-dimensional echocardiographic characteristics of double outlet right ventricle. *Am J Cardiol* 1979;44:1146–1154.
51. Thanopoulos BD, Dubrow JW, Fisher EA, et al. Double outlet right ventricle with subvalvular aortic stenosis. *Br Heart J* 1979;41:241–244.
52. Goor DA, Lillehei CW. *Congenital Malformation of the Heart.* New York, Grune and Stratton, 1975.
53. Nanda NC, Gramiak R, Manning J, et al. Echocardiographic recognition of the congenital bicuspid aortic valve. *Circulation* 1974;49:870–875.
54. Fowles RE, Martin RP, Abrams JM, et al. Two-dimensional echocardiographic features of bicuspid aortic valve. *Chest* 1979;75:434–440.
55. Fernicola DJ, Mann JM, Roberts WC. Congenitally quadricuspid aortic valve: Analysis of six patients. *Am J Cardiol* 1989;63:136–138.
56. Coeurderoy A, Biron Y, Laurent M, et al. Quadricuspid aortique congenitale. *Arch Mal Coeur* 1986;79:745–748.
57. Menzel T, Mohr-Hakaly S, Kolsch B, et al. Quantitative assesment of aortic stenosis by three-dimensional echocardiography. *J Am Soc Echocardiogr* 1997;10:215–223.
58. Kasprzak JD, Salustri A, Roelandt JRTC, et al. Three-dimensional echocardiography of the aortic valve: Feasibility, clinical potential, and limitations. *Echocardiography* 1998;15:127–138.
59. Samal AK, Nanda N, Thakur AC, et al. Three-dimensional echocardiographic assessment of Lambl's excrescences on the aortic valve. *Echocardiography* 1999;16:437–441.
60. Newfeld EA, Muster AJ, Paul MH, et al. Discrete subvalvular aortic stenosis in childhood. Study of 51 patients. *Am J Cardiol* 1976;38:53–61.
61. Reis RL, Peterson LM, Mason DT, et al. Congenital fixed subvalvular aortic stenosis. An anatomical classification and correlations with operative results. *Circulation* 1971;43(Suppl 1):1–18.
62. Ge S, Warner JG, Fowle KM, et al. Morphology and dynamic change of discrete subaortic stenosis can be imaged and quantified with three-dimensional transesophageal echocardiography. *J Am Soc Echocardiogr* 1997;10:713–716.
63. Dall'Agata A, Cromme-Dijkuis AH, Meijboom FJ, et al. Use of three-dimensional echocardiography for analysis of outflow obstruction in congenital heart disease. *Am J Cardiol* 1999;83:921–925.
64. Weyman AE, Caldwell RL, Hurwitz RA, et al. Cross-sectional echocardiographic characterization of aortic obstruction. 1. Supravalvular aortic stenosis and aortic hypoplasia. *Circulation* 1978;57:491–497.
65. Vogt J, Rupprath G, Grimm T, et al. Qualitative and quantitative evaluation of supravalvular aortic stenosis by cross-sectional echocardiography. A report of 80 patients. *Pediatr Cardiol* 1982;3:13–17.
66. Williams JCP, Barrat-Boyes BG, Lowe JB. Supravalvular aortic stenosis. *Circulation* 1961;64:1311–1318.
67. Beuren AJ, Schulze C, Eberle P, et al. The syndrome of supravalvular aortic stenosis, peripheral pulmonary stenosis, mental retardation, and similar facial appearance. *Am J Cardiol* 1964;13:471–483.
68. Johnson LW, Fishman RA, Schneider B, et al. Familial supravalvular aortic stenosis. Report of a large family and review of the literature. *Chest* 1976;70:404–500.
69. Magni G, Hijazi ZM, Pandian NG, et al. Two- and three-dimensional echocardiography in patients selection and assessment of atrial septal defect closure by the new DAS-Angel wing device. *Circulation* 1997;96:1722–1728.
70. Acar A, Piéchaud JF, Nonhoffer P, et al. Evaluation anatomique des communications interauriculaires de type ostium secundum par echocardiography trimensionalle. *Arch Mal Coeur* 1998;91:543–550.
71. Aeschbacher BC, Chaterjee T, Meier B. Transesophageal echocardiography to evaluate success of transcatheter closure of large secundum atrial septal defects in adults using the buttoned device. *Mayo Clin Proc* 2000;75:913–920.
72. Fisher G, Kramer HH, Stueh H, et al. Transcatheter closure of secundum atrial septal defect with the new self-centering Amplatzer septal occluder. *Eur Heart J* 1999;20:541–549.
73. Maeno YV, Benson LN, Boutin C. Impact of dynamic 3D transesophageal echocardiography in the assessment of atrial septal defects and occlusion by the double-umbrella device. *Cardiol Young* 1998;8:368–378.

74. Elzenga NJ. The role of echocardiography in transcatheter closure of atrial septal defects. *Cardiol Young* 2000;10:474–483.
75. Boutin C, Musewe NN, Smalhorn JF, et al. Echocardiographic follow-up of atrial septal defect after catheter closure by double-umbrella device. *Circulation* 1993;88:621–627.
76. Ewert P, Berger F, Daehnert I, et al. Transcatheter closure of atrial septal defect without fluoroscopy: Feasibility of a new method. *Circulation* 2000;101:847–849.
77. Cao Q, Radtke W, Berger F, et al. Transcatheter closure of multiple atrial septal defects. Initial results and value of two- and three dimensional transesophageal echocardiography. *Eur Hear J* 2000;21:941–947.
78. Suarez De Lezo J, Medina A, Pan M, et al. Transcatheter occlusion of complex atrial septal defects. *Catheter Cardiovasc Interv* 2000;1:33–41.
79. Ewert P, Berger F, Vogel M, et al. Morphology of perforated atrial septal aneurysm suitable for closure by transcatheter device placement. *Heart* 2000;84(3):327–331.
80. Cujec B, Mainra R, Johnson DH. Prevention of recurrent cerebral ischemic events in patients with patent foramen ovale and cryptogenic strokes or transient ischemic attacks. *Can J Cardiol* 1999;15:57–64.
81. Walsh KP, Wilmshurst PT, Morrison WL, Transcatheter closure of patent foramen ovale using the Amplatzer septal occluder to prevent recurrence of neurological decompression illness in divers. *Heart* 1999;81:257–261.
82. Kaulitz R, Paul T, Hausdorf G. Extending the limits of transcatheter closure of atrial septal defect with the double umbrella device (CardioSEAL). *Heart* 1998;80:54–59.
83. Tantengco MV, Bates JR, Ryan T, et al. Dynamic three-dimensional echocardiography reconstruction of congenital cardiac septation defects. *Pediatr Cardiol* 1997; 18:184–190.
84. Schwartz SL, Cao QL, Azevedo J, et al. Simulation of intraoperative visualization of cardiac structures and study of dynamic surgical anatomy with real-time three-dimensional echocardiography. *Am J Cardiol* 1994;73:501–507.
85. Rivera JM, Siu SC, Handschumacher MD, et al. Three-dimensional reconstruction of ventricular septal defects: Validation studies and in vivo feasibility. *J Am Coll Cardiol* 1994;23:201–208.
86. Vogel M, Ho SY, Lincoln C, et al. Three-dimensional echocardiography can simulate intraoperative visualization of congenitally malformed hearts. *Ann Thorac Surg* 1995;60:1282–1288.
87. Kardon RE, Cao QL, Massani N, et al. New insights and observations in three-dimensional echocardiographic visualization of ventricular septal defects: Experimental and clinical studies. *Circulation* 1988;98:1307–1314.
88. Dall'Agata A, Cromme-Dijkhuis AH, Meijboom FJ, et al. Three-dimensional echocardiography enhances the assessment of ventricular septal defect. *Am J Cardiol* 1999;83:1576–1579.
89. Pandian N, Cao QL, Erbel R, et al. A comprehensive approach for image segmentation, cutting planes and display projections in three dimensional echocardiography: Suggested guidelines for clinically useful projections based on multicenter experience in 300 adults and pediatric patients. *J Am Coll Cardiol* 1994;1 A-484:9A.
90. Vogel M, Pandian N, Marx G, et al. Transthoracic real-time three dimensional echocardiography in 100 pediatric and adult patients with heart disease: Clinical utility of unique new views unavailable in 2-dimensional echocardiography. *Circulation* 1993;88(Supl 1):1870.
91. Acar P, Laskari C, Rhodes J, et al. Three-dimensional echocardiography analysis of valve anatomy as a determinant of mitral regurgitation after surgery for atrioventricular septal defects. *J Am Cardiol* 1999;83:745–749.

Suggested Reading List

1. Magni G, Hijazi ZM, Pandian NG, et al. Two- and three-dimensional transesophageal echocardiography in patient selection and assessment of atrial septal defect closure by the new DAS-Angel Wings device: Initial clinical experience. *Circulation* 1997;96:1722–1728.
2. Bartel T, Muller S, Erbel R. Dynamic three-dimensional echocardiography using parallel slicing: A promising diagnostic procedure in adults with congenital heart disease. *Cardiology* 1998;89:140–147.
3. Maeno YV, Benson LN, Boutin C. Impact of dynamic 3D transoesophageal echocardiography in the assessment of atrial septal defects and occlusion by the double-umbrella device (CardioSEAL). [see comments]. *Cardiol in the Young* 1998;8:368–378.
4. Sadaniantz A, Burtt D, Nanda NC, et al. Three dimensional echocardiography of right heart pathology. *Echocardiography* 1998;15:795–806.
5. Bemurat L, Jimenez M, Roudaut R, et al. [Surgical evaluation of transthoracic tridimensional echocardiography in the anatomic study of atrial septal defect]. [French]. *Arch Mal Coeur et Vaisseaux* 1999;92:573–580.
6. Dall'Agata A, Cromme-Dijkhuis AH, Meijboom FJ, et al. Three-dimensional echocardiography enhances the assessment of ventricular septal defect. *Am J Cardiol* 1999; 83:1576–1579.
7. de Lemos JA, Delacretaz E, Piana RN, et al. Images in cardiovascular medicine. Ebstein's anomaly associated with an anomalous coronary artery, 2 myocardial bridges, and a mahaim fiber. *Circulation* 1999;100:1757–1759.
8. Zhu W, Cao QL, Hijazi ZM. Transcatheter closure of a large residual shunt after deployment of the Das-Angel Wings device using the Amplatzer septal occluder. *Cath .& Cardiovasc Intervent* 1999;48:184–187.
9. Acar P. Three-dimensional echocardiography in transcatheter closure of atrial septal defects. [Review] [17 refs]. *Cardiol in the Young* 2000;10:484–492.
10. Acar P, Saliba Z, Sidi D, et al. New insight into left ventricular function in tricuspid atresia after total cavopulmonary connection: a three-dimensional echocardiographic study. *Cardiol in the Young* 2000;10(2):83–89.
11. Cao Q, Radtke W, Berger F, et al. Transcatheter closure of multiple atrial septal defects. Initial results and value of two- and three-dimensional transoesophageal echocardiography. *Eur Heart J* 2000;21(11):941–947.
12. Maeno YV, Benson LN, McLaughlin PR, et al. Dynamic morphology of the secundum atrial septal defect evaluated by three dimensional transoesophageal echocardiography. *Heart* 2000;83(6):673–677.
13. Pedra CA, Pihkala J, Lee KJ, et al. Transcatheter closure of atrial septal defects using the Cardio-Seal implant. *Heart* 2000;84(3):320–326.
14. Zhu W, Cao QL, Rhodes J, et al. Measurement of atrial septal defect size: A comparative study between three-dimensional transesophageal echocardiography and the standard balloon sizing methods. *Pediatric Cardiology* 2000;21(5):465–469.
15. Cooke JC, Gelman JS, Harper RW. Echocardiologists' role

in the deployment of the Amplatzer atrial septal occluder device in adults. *J Am Soc Echocardiography* 2001;14(6):588–594.
16. Ishii M, Hashino K, Eto G, et al. Quantitative assessment of severity of ventricular septal defect by three-dimensional reconstruction of color Doppler-imaged vena contracta and flow convergence region. *Circulation* 2001; 103:664–669.
17. Miller A, Mukhtar O, Aaluri SR, et al. 2-D and 3-D TEE differentiation of lymphoma involving the atrial septum from lipomatous hypertrophy. *Echocardiography* 2001; 18:205–209.

Chapter 8

Cardiac Masses

Navin C. Nanda, MD and Vincent L. Sorrell, MD

Cardiac masses most commonly represent vegetations, clots, or tumors. The associated manifestations found with ultrasound help to determine the likelihood of pathology, since histopathology is not possible with echocardiography. Equally important is the location and extension of the mass. This latter important characteristic of cardiac masses is superior with three-dimensional (3D) data sets. The ability to provide cutplane (or anyplane) two-dimensional (2D) displays from any chosen location and direction within the 3D data is vitally important in confirming the location and extent of mass. We have included numerous examples of these benefits of 3D echocardiography.

Within this chapter, the reader will see both the common masses (left atrial thrombus; left atrial myxoma) and some uncommon masses (cardiac tumors). In each case, it is notable that the extent and exact location of the mass is most clarified when viewed from the 3D data set.

An additional advantage of 3D imaging is an enhanced ability to accurately obtain the truest mass volume and diameter. This is related to the artifactual measurement with 2D frequently obtained when the transducer alignment is from a nonparallel orientation. By viewing the object from multiple positions and creating a 3D data set, this problem is rectified. Direct comparisons with surgical confirmation have routinely revealed the superiority of 3D over 2D imaging sets.

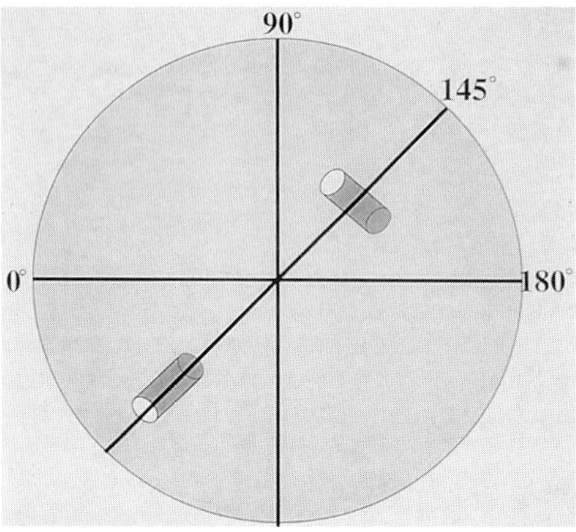

Figure 1. Schematic diagram demonstrating that the maximum dimension of an object (in this case, a cylinder) can be obtained only if the ultrasound beam cuts through its longest dimension (true long axis) when using a multiplane probe. However, when the two-dimensional planes (dotted lines) are stacked together to obtain a three-dimensional image, the object (cylinder), including its long axis, can be viewed completely, even though it is not oriented parallel to the ultrasonic beam as it is rotated from 0° to 180°. Reproduced with permission from Nanda NC et al. Incremental value of three-dimensional echocardiography over transesophageal multiplane two-dimensional echocardiography in qualitative and quantitative assessment of cardiac masses and defects. *Echocardiography* 1995;12:619–628.

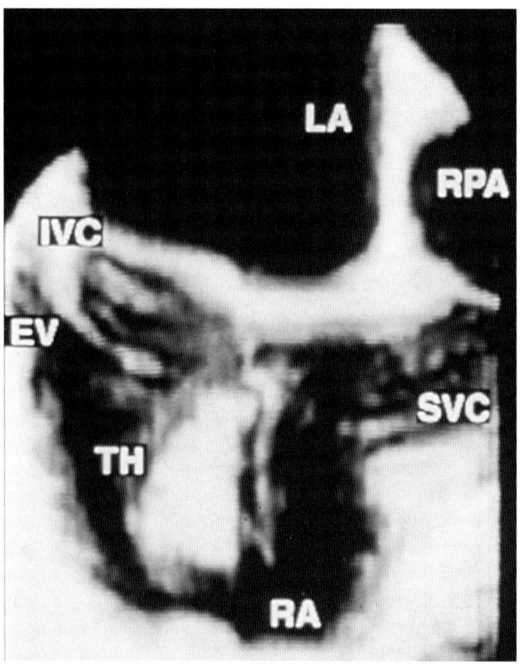

Figure 2. Three-dimensional view of a large thrombus (TH) in the right atrium (RA). EV = Eustachian valve; IVC = inferior vena cava; LA = left atrium; RPA = right pulmonary artery; SVC = superior vena cava. Reproduced with permission from Nanda NC et al. Incremental value of three-dimensional echocardiography over transesophageal multiplane two-dimensional echocardiography in qualitative and quantitative assessment of cardiac masses and defects. *Echocardiography* 1995;12:619–628.

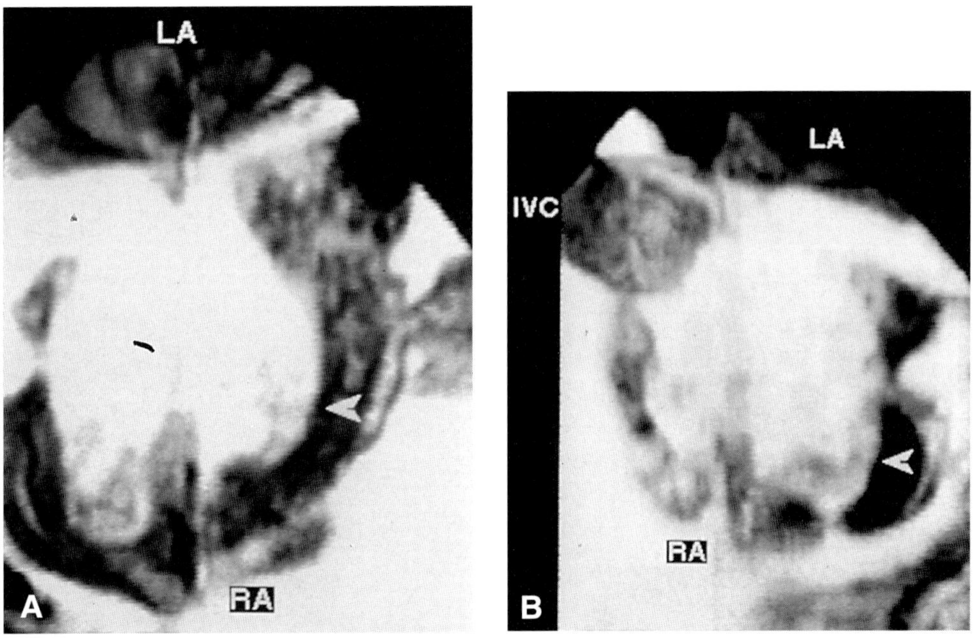

Figure 3. (**A**) Transesophageal, three-dimensional echo bicaval view, oriented with the superior vena cava on the right, in a patient with a very large, infected thrombus in the right atrium (arrow). (**B**) With a slightly different orientation, the relationship of the thrombus (arrow) to the inferior vena cava is more clearly delineated.

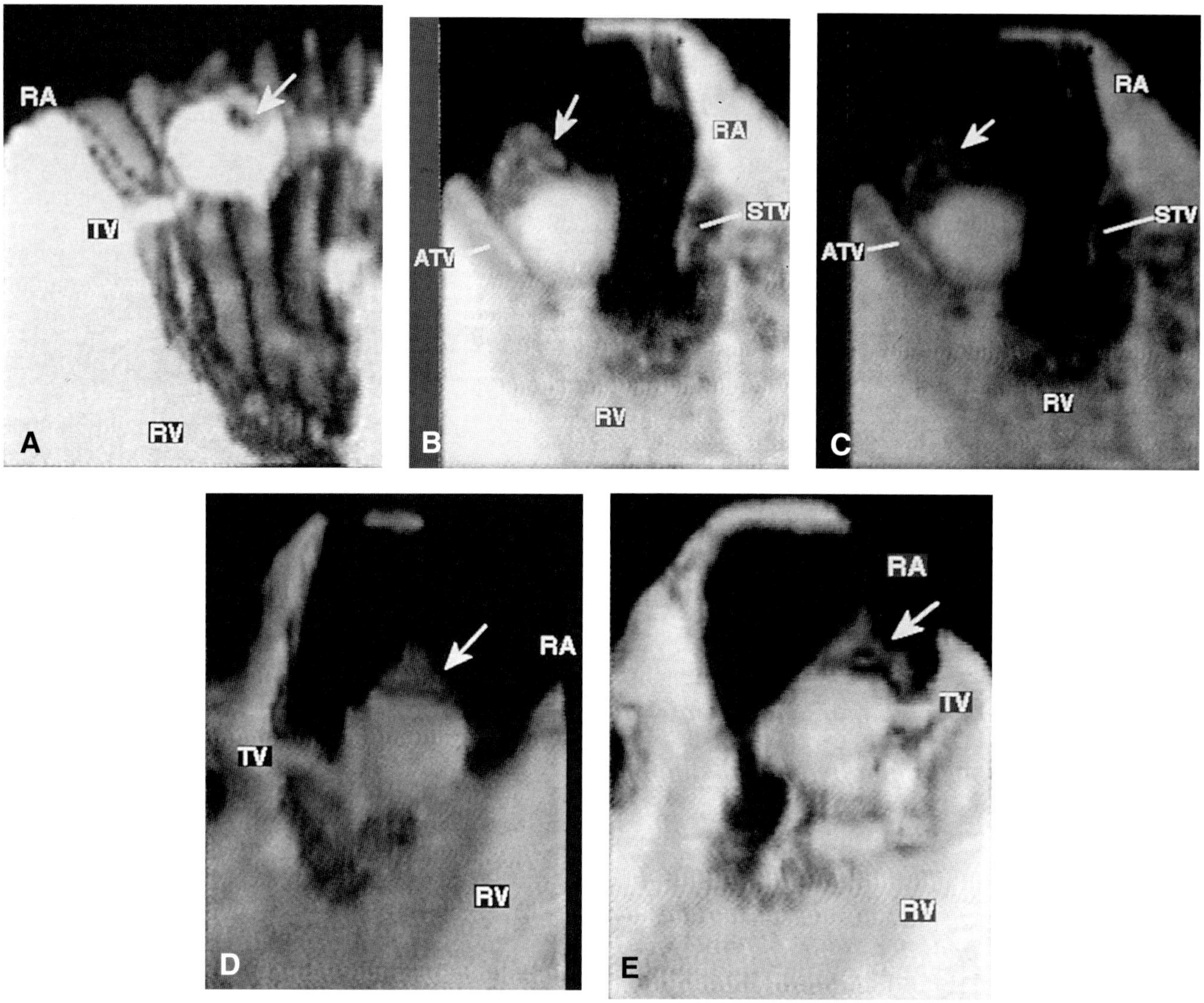

Figure 4. (**A**) Transesophageal echo (TEE) view highlighting the right atrium and right ventricle in a patient with a myxoma attached to the anterior tricuspid valve (TV) leaflet (arrow). (**B, C**) Three-dimensional (3D), TEE display oriented with a greater tilt concentrating on the TV apparatus and the myxoma (arrow). The shading is also adjusted for optimal characterization. Left = less shading; Right = more shading; ATV = anterior TV leaflet; STV = septal TV leaflet. (**D, E**) The orientation of the image is chosen and obtained through a detailed, retrospective review of the 3D data set. Two slightly different views are obtained and displayed so that each provides a different level of perspective regarding the morphology of the pathologic mass.

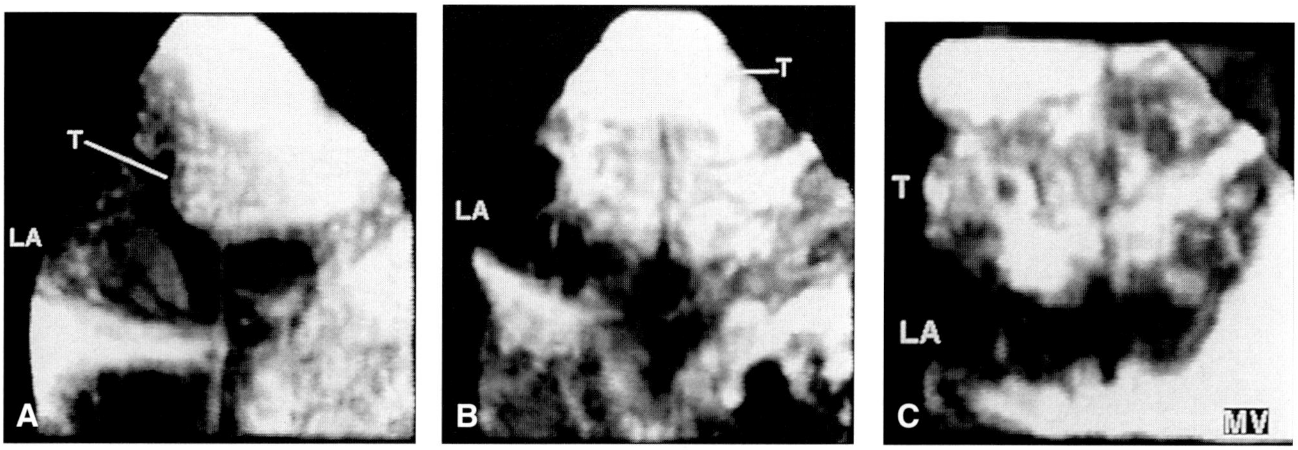

Figure 5. (**A**) Transesophageal echo image of the left atrium in a patient with a leiomyosarcoma (T = tumor). (**B, C**) Same patient is viewed from different perspectives to provide the greatest understanding of the relationship of this pathologic mass with the surrounding tissues.

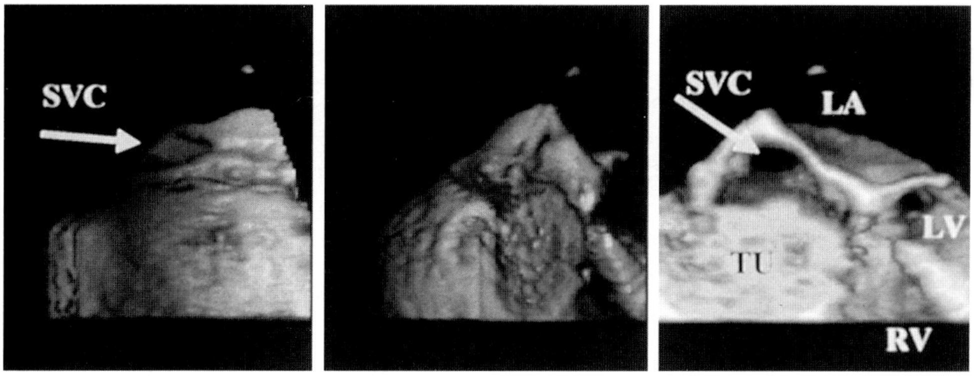

Figure 6. Recurrent angiosarcoma of the heart. A 32-year-old female, 5 months after surgical excision of the angiosarcoma from the right atrium. Three-dimensional calculation of the volume of the recurrent mass reveals 121 mL. Based on anyplane views from different angels (**left, middle,** and **right** panels) the detailed anatomical localization of the mass could be demonstrated, including exclusion of superior vena cava (SVC) obstruction. From Jaroslaw Drozdz, MD and Jaroslaw D. Kasprzak, MD.

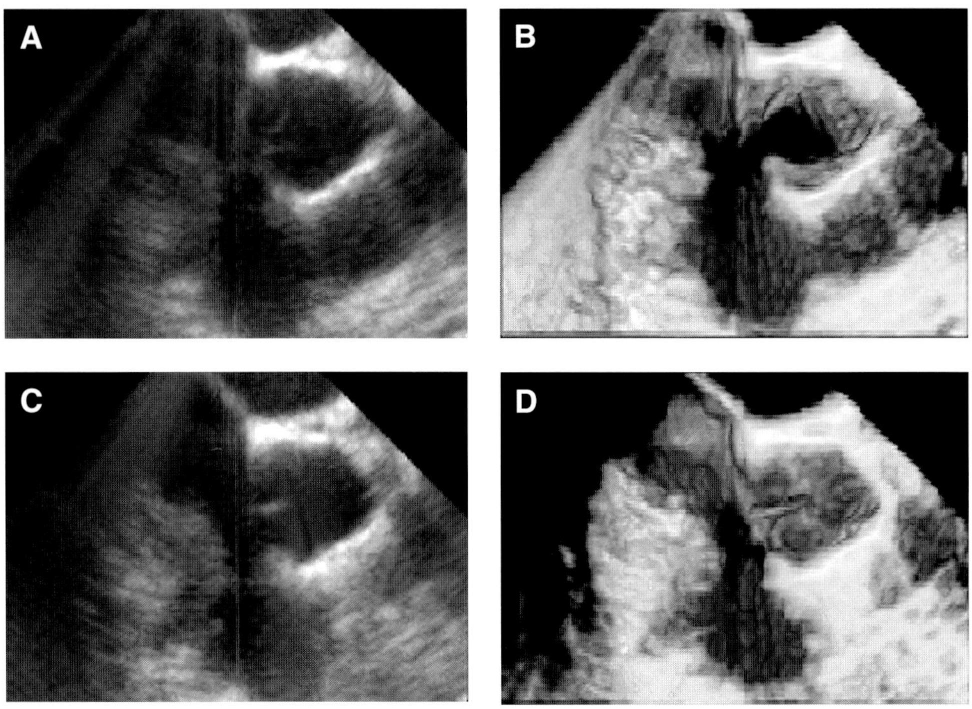

Figure 7. Right atrial angiosarcoma. (**A–D**) Transesophageal, three-dimensional (TEE 3D) and comparative two-dimensional short-axis images of the typical appearance of an angiosarcoma penetrating the right atrial (RA) wall and noted within the RA cavity in systole (**A, B**) and diastole (**C, D**). The aortic valve may be used to identify the cardiac cycle. This was confirmed at surgery. From Vincent L. Sorrell, MD.

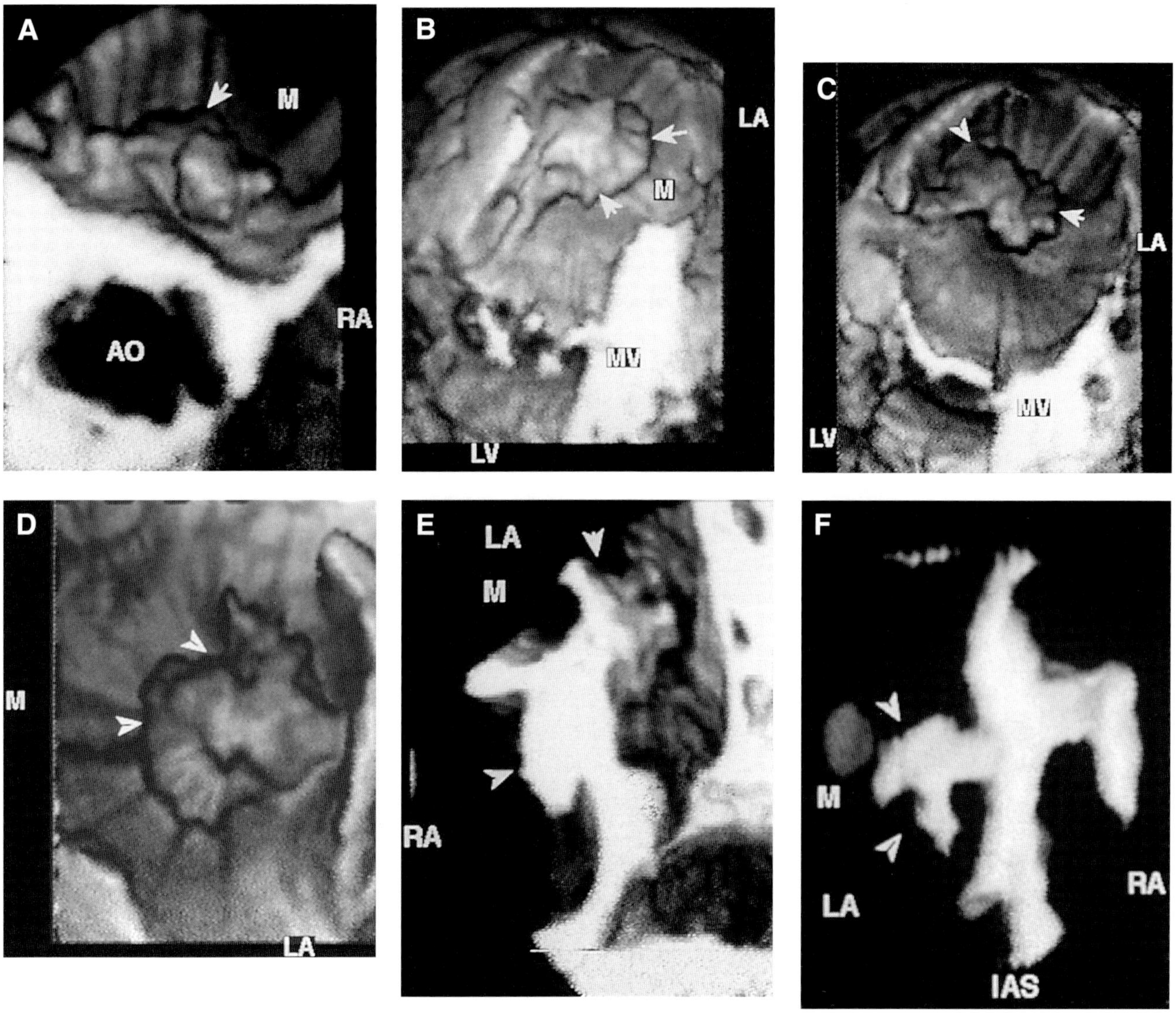

Figure 8. (**A**) Transesophageal (TEE) short-axis image of the left atrium (LA) in a patient with a mass (arrow) in the LA cavity. Note the excellent definition of the LA wall. (**B**) A TEE *en-face* image of the LA and mass (arrows) providing an excellent appreciation of the location and relationship of the mass (arrows) to the surrounding tissues. (**C, D**) A TEE short-axis image of the left atrium (**C**) with the mass (arrows) is noted and can be displayed as a zoomed image (**D**). (**E**) Pathologic masses can be displayed in many possible viewpoints. A long-axis image appears to show the mass (arrows) on the right atrium and the LA side of the atrium. (**F**) Also, the mass under review can be "extracted" and displayed independent of the surrounding tissues. Due to direct involvement with the atrial septum, this structure is also included in the extracted image (IAS). This may lead to greater preparation for surgery and enhanced opportunities for training as well as decision making.

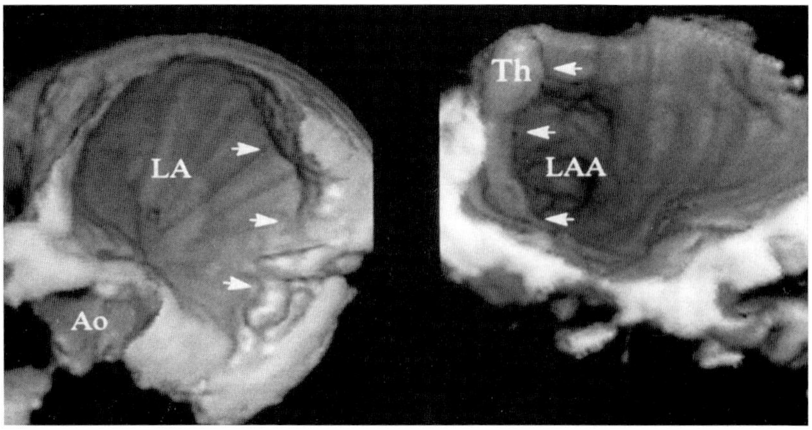

Figure 9. Mural thrombus in a patient with mitral valve stenosis. Information on the most common complications of mitral valve stenosis, such as left atrial clots, can be derived and displayed. It allows derivation of spatial relationships between thrombus and nearby structures. From Stefano De Castro, MD and Rachele Adorisio, MD.

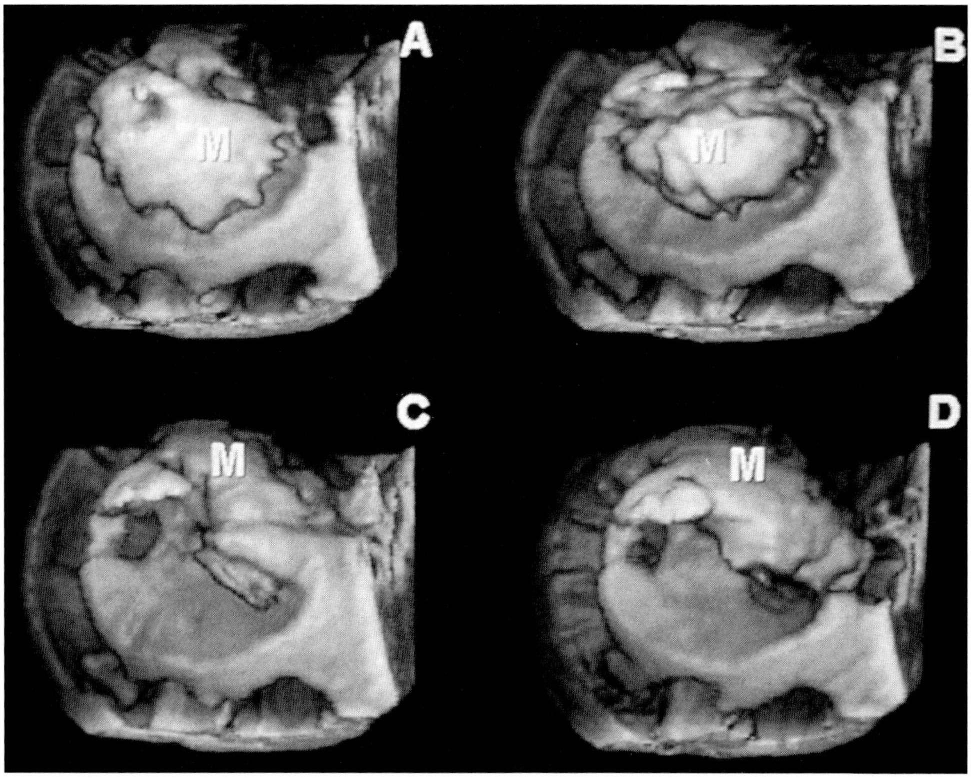

Figure 10. Myxoma of left atrium. (**A**) In systole, the mitral valve was closed and the myxoma (M) was situated in left atrium. (**B, C**) In early diastole, the mitral valve opened, and the myxoma moved into the left ventricle particularly. (**D**) In later diastole, the free end of the myxoma passed through the orifice from the left atrium into the left ventricle, but the base of the mass was still adhered to the interatrial septum. From Xin-Fang Wang, MD.

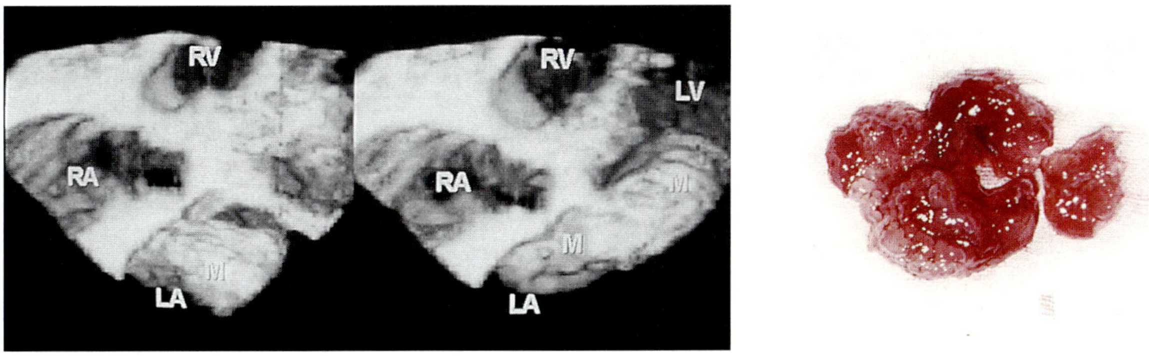

Figure 11. These dynamic three-dimensional pictures were taken from a patient with myxoma (M) of the left atrium by trans-esophaegeal echo. **Left:** In systole, the mitral valve was closed and there was nodular reflection of myxoma in the left atrium (LA). **Middle:** In diastole, the mitral valve was open and the free end of the myxoma passed through orifice from the left atrium into the left ventricle; the base of the mass was adherent to interatrial septum. **Right:** Pathologic changes confirmed echocardiographic findings. Figure 11 left and middle are reproduced with permission from Wang XF: Four-dimensional echocardiography: Methods and clinical application. *Am Heart J* 1996;132:672–84.

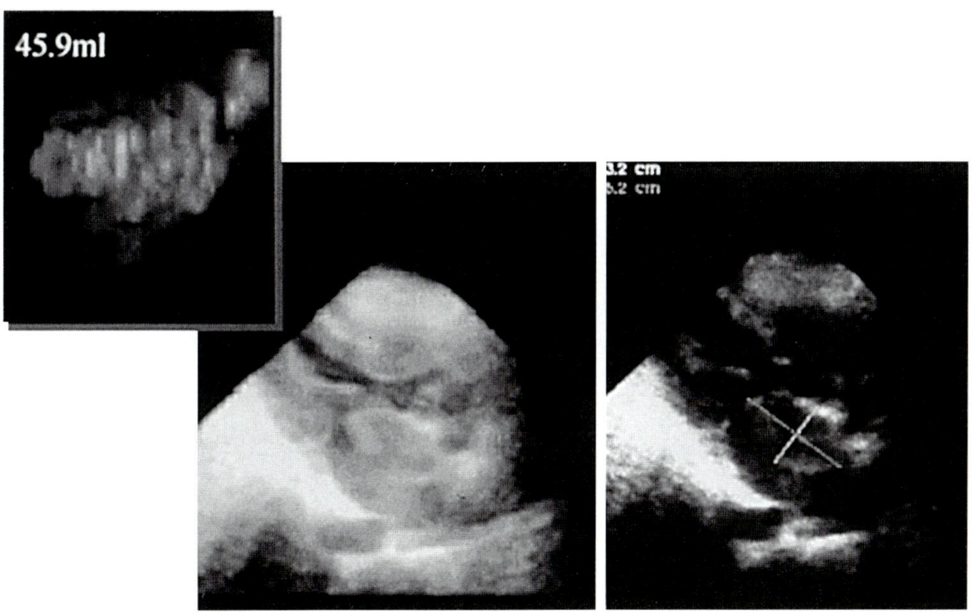

Figure 12. Recurrent leiomyosarcoma of the heart. A left atrial mass recurred 5 months after a surgical removal of cardiac leiomyosarcoma. Three-dimensional data set allowed an electronic excision (upper left panel) and detailed sizing (32 × 52 mm) and calculation of volume of the mass (46 mL). Anyplane reconstructed views allowed to assess the relationships of the tumor to the neighboring structures, including the exclusion of pulmonary vein obstruction. From Jaroslaw D. Kasprzak, MD and Jaroslaw Drozdz, MD.

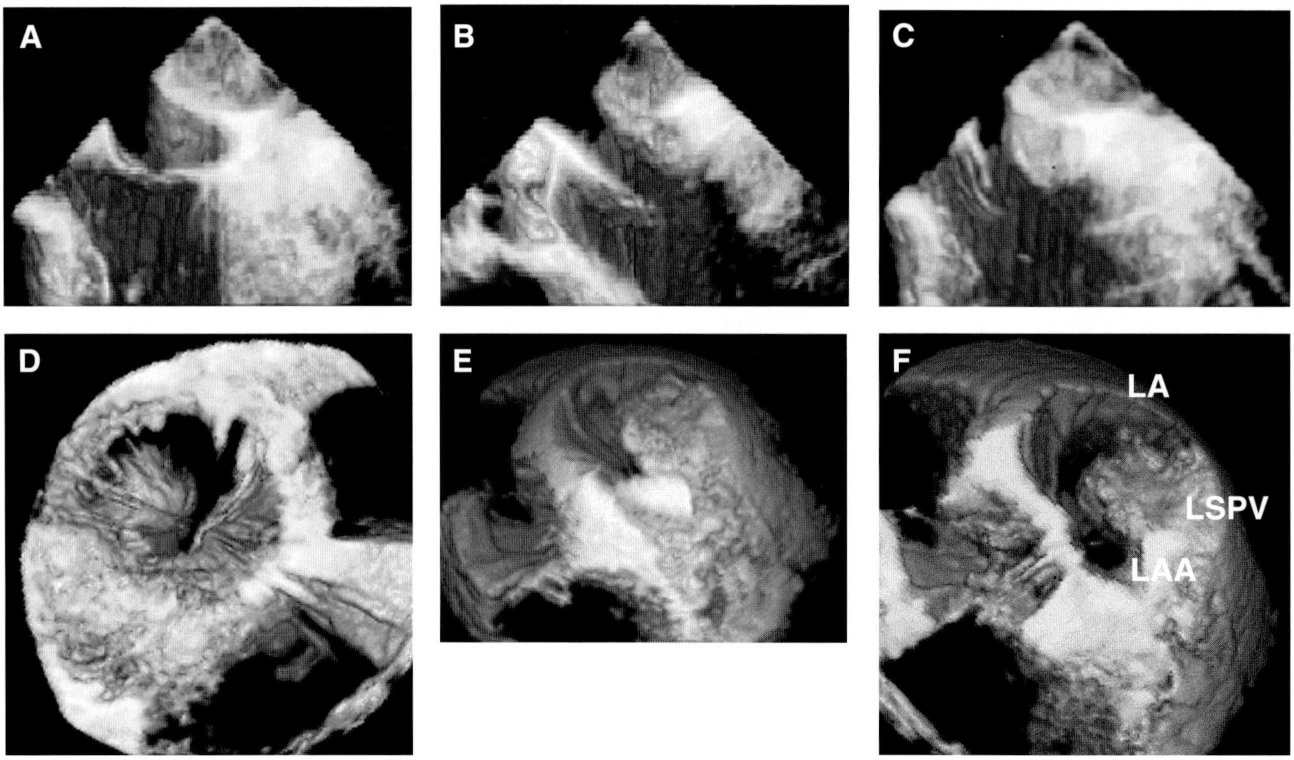

Figure 13. Metastatic renal cell carcinoma. (**A–C**) Transesophageal echo, three-dimensional (TEE 3D) horizontal imaging plane of a large, highly mobile mass seen within the left atrium (LA). Note the change in position throughout the cardiac cycle (**A** = systole; **B** = mid-systole; **C** = diastole). (**D**) This image was obtained during diastole from the perspective of the left ventricle. The mass can be seen within the LA. (**E**) With careful additional processing, a specific orientation obtained at the level of the left superior pulmonary vein (LSPV) allowed the origin of the tumor to be clarified and this was confirmed at surgery. (**F**) A similar image from a slightly more inferior position allowed the LSPV (and tumor mass) to be separated from the LA appendages. From Vincent L. Sorrell, MD.

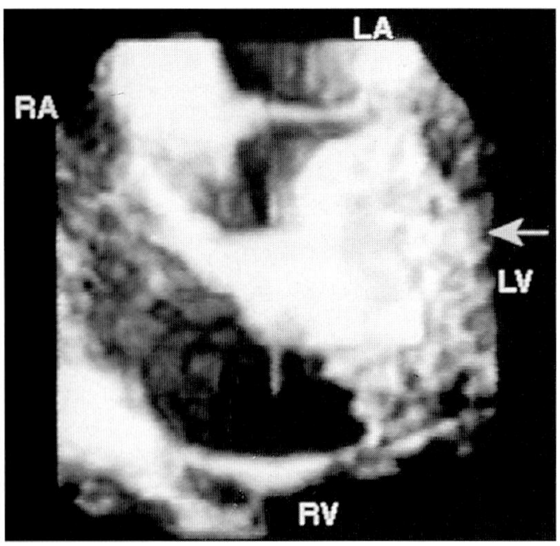

Figure 14. Transesophageal, three-dimensionally reconstructed image of a patient with an extremely large left ventricular (LV) thrombus (arrow) displayed in an apical four-chamber view. Note the well-defined, irregular contour of the border of this mass. This patient had severe LV dysfunction and a left ventricular assist device.

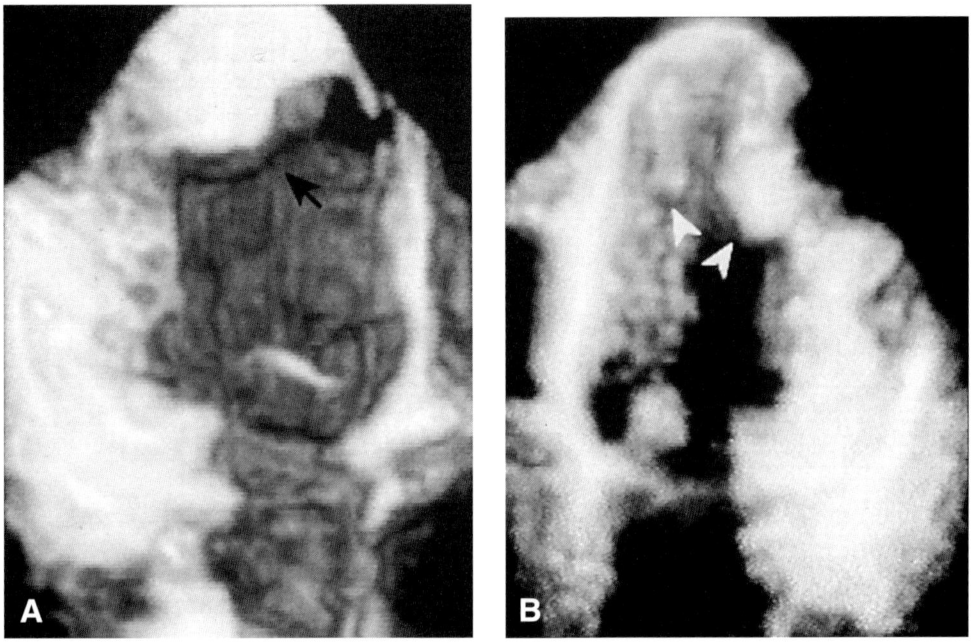

Figure 15. (**A**) Transthoracic three-dimensional reconstruction of an apical 2–chamber image of a patient with an apical thrombus (arrow). (**B**) Same patient with a slightly different orientation shows either two separate clots or two distinct protrusions of the same large clot (arrows).

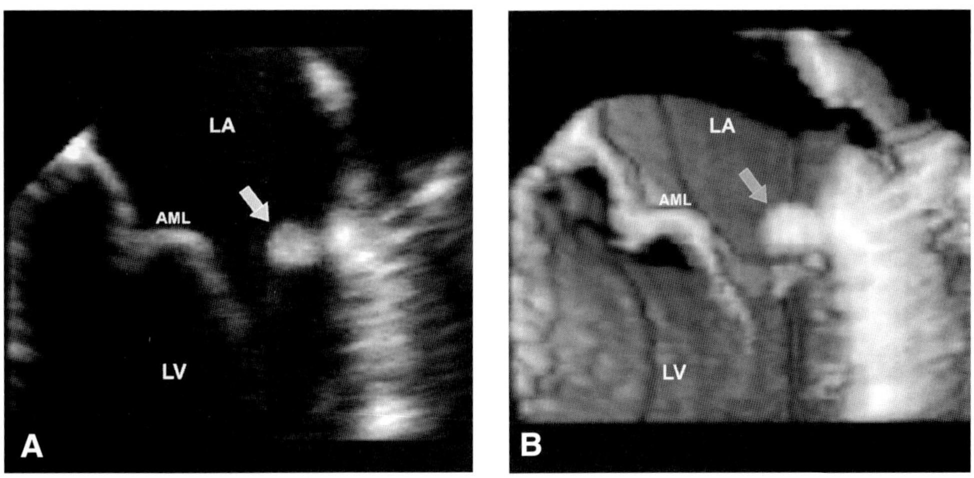

Figure 16. (**A**) Two-dimensional (2D) echocardiogram. A 39-year-old patient with myxoma located on the posterior mitral leaflet (arrow). The diagnosis was confirmed postoperatively by histological examination. (**B**) Three-dimensional echocardiographic reconstruction of the previous 2D image. AML = anterior mitral leaflet; LA = left atrium; LV = left ventricle. From Annette Geibel, MD, Michael Handke, MD, Dietrich Markus Schäfer, MD, Anja Schöchlin, MA, and Helmut Wollschläger, MD

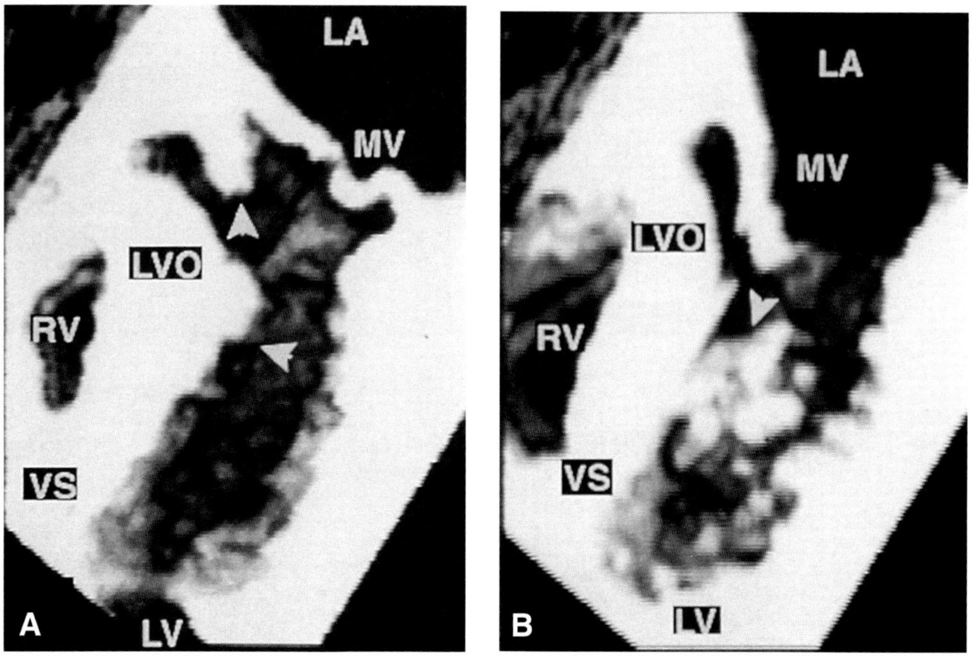

Figure 17. Transesophageal echo, apical long-axis orientation in a patient with left ventricular outflow tract mass (arrows) seen in both systole (**A**) and diastole (**B**).

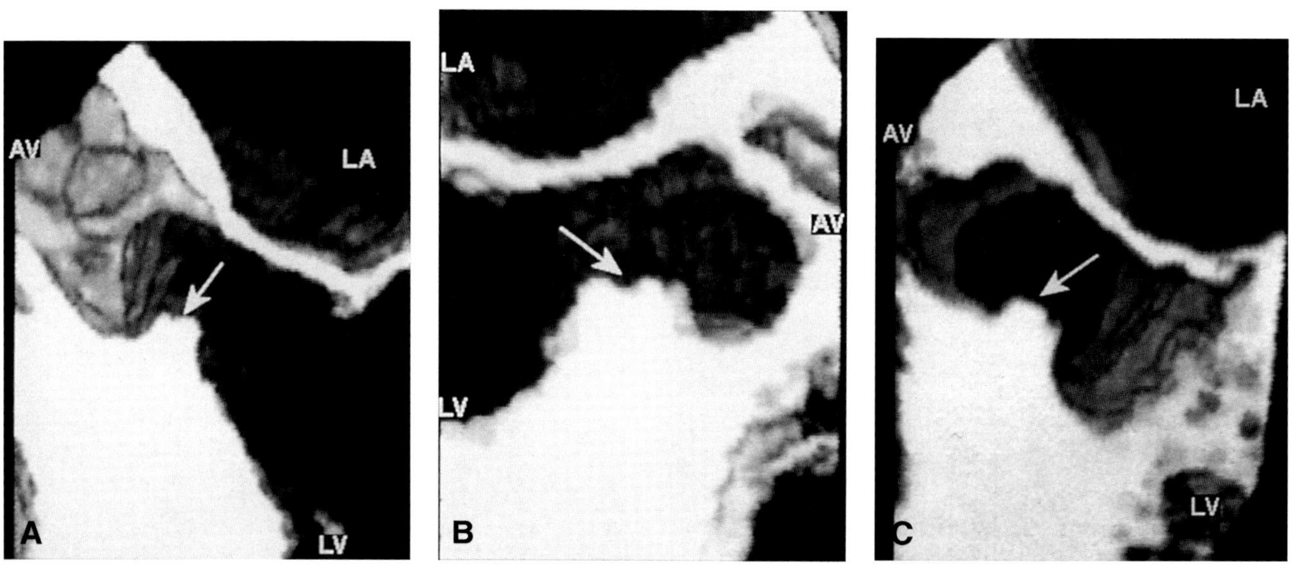

Figure 18. Transesophageal echo, three-dimesnional (TEE 3D) zoom image highlighting a left ventricular (LV) tumor (arrow) located in the LV outflow tract from distinctly different orientations. (**A**) An apical 5-chamber equivalent view with the left atrium (LA) and LV on the right side of the image. Note the anatomic detail of the aortic valve and root. (**B**) An apical 3–chamber (long-axis) view with the LA and LV on left side of the image. (**C**) TEE 3D short axis orientation of the same patient (arrow = LV outflow tract tumor).

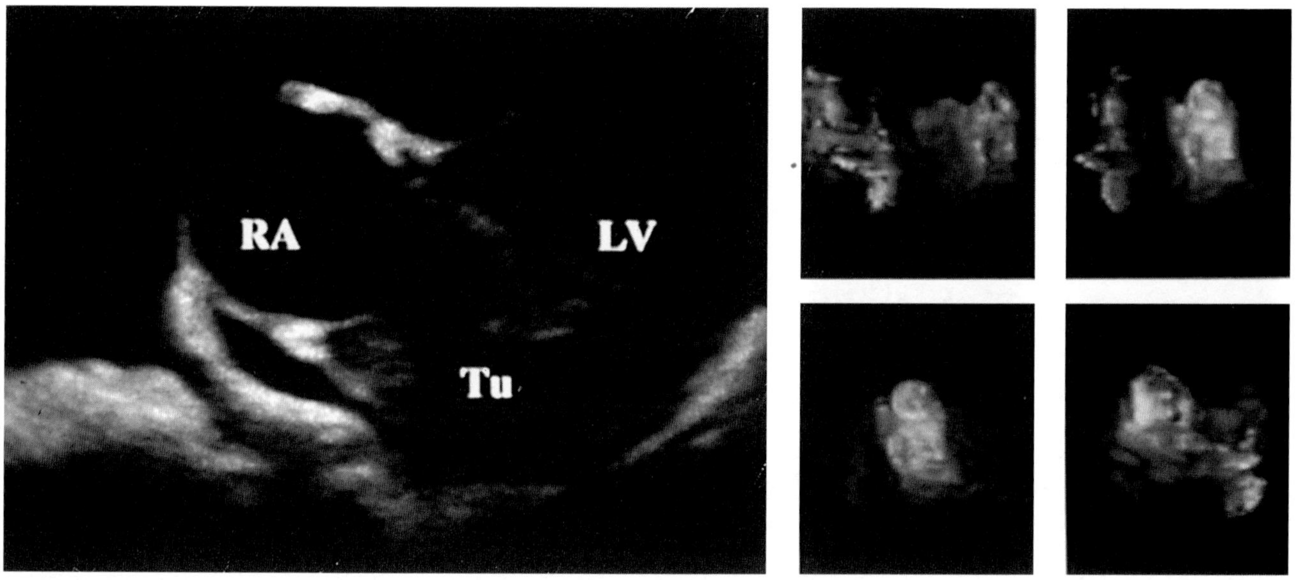

Figure 19. Rhabdomyoma of the heart. A 26-year-old male with clinical picture of congestive heart failure. Transesophageal echo, two-dimensional four-chamber view shows a nearly complete obstruction of the right ventricle by nonhomogeneous mass (**left panel**). Three-dimensional data set allowed an electronic excision and calculation of volume of the mass (89 mL). Right panels show the electronically excised mass from different angles, illustrating the complex structure of the mass. From Jaroslaw Drozdz, MD and Jaroslaw D. Kasprzak, MD

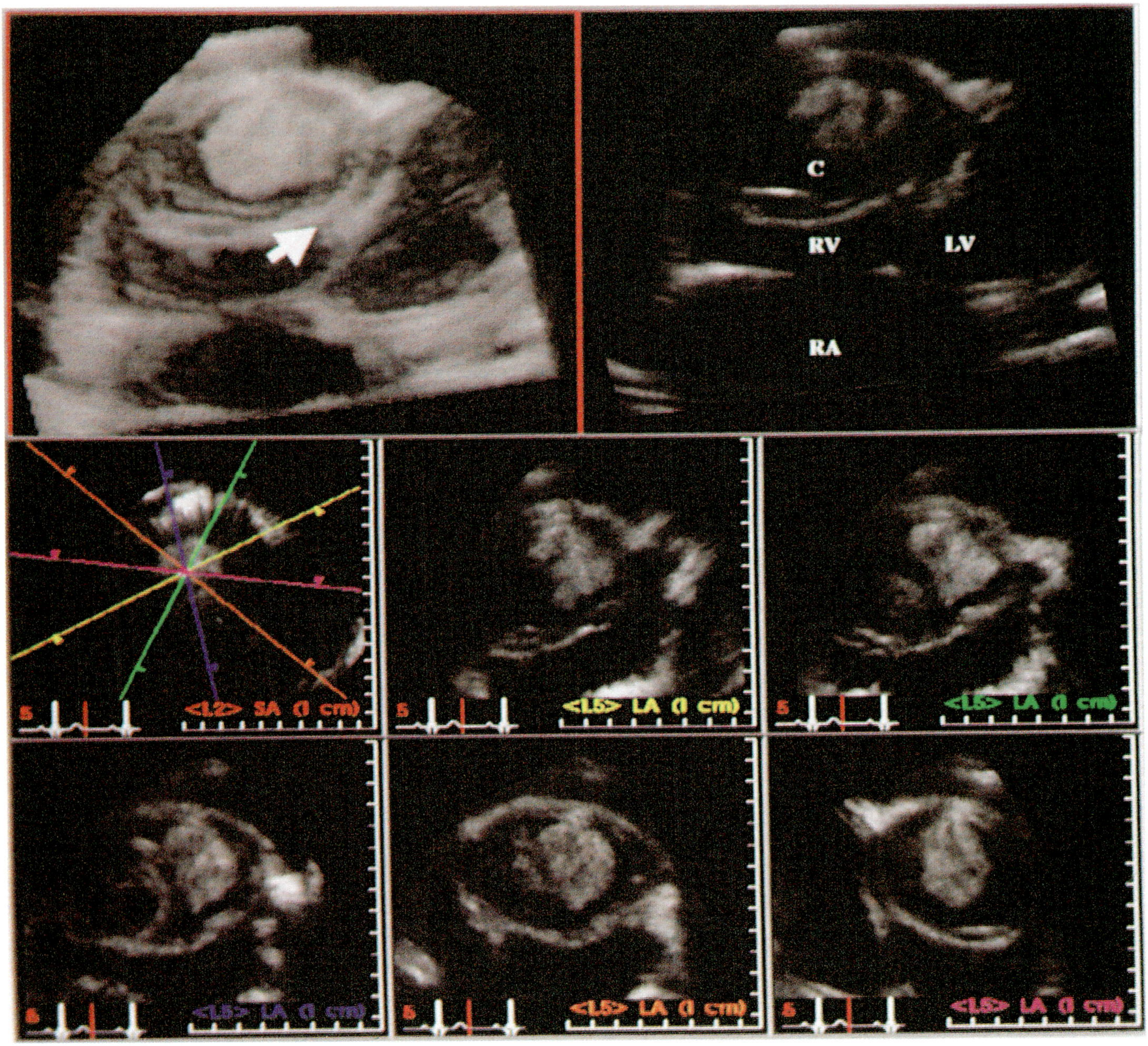

Figure 20. Echinococcal cyst. Upper panels show a volume-rendering of the mass attached to the right side of interventricular septum. A corresponding anyplane cut is shown with legends: C = cyst; LV = left ventricle; RA = right atrium; RV = right ventricle. Multiple cystic masses can be seen. The attachment to the septum, not visible in two-dimensional study, can be clearly displayed from a three-dimensional dataset. Middle and bottom row provide enhanced anatomical information in multiple meridional cuts across the cyst. From Jaroslaw D. Kasprzak, MD.

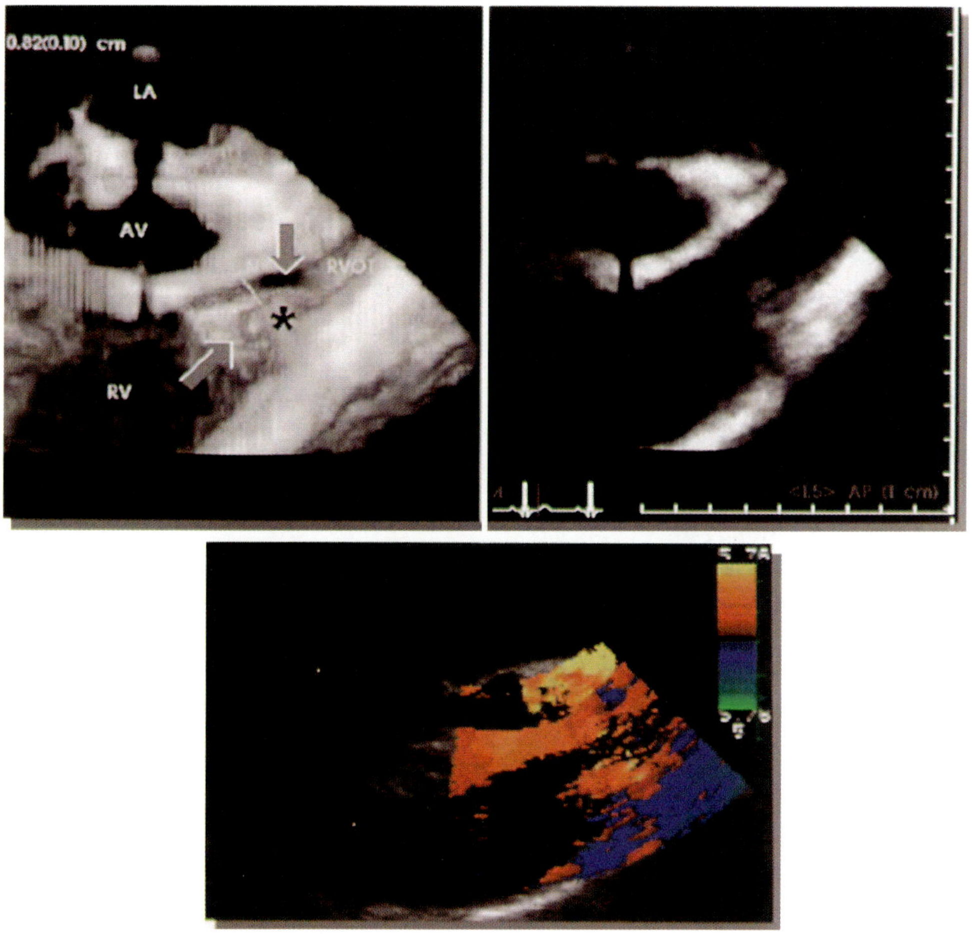

Figure 21. Right ventricular outflow tract mass (asterisk) in a patient with carcinoid disease. The mass resulted in the narrowing of the outflow tract (diameter 8 mm), with pressure gradient 36 mmHg. The mass was poorly visible in original (**left**) and reconstructed (**right**) two-dimensional views but more distinct in tissue Doppler mode (**bottom**). AV = aortic valve; LA = left atrium; RV = right ventricle; RVOT = right ventricular outflow tract. From Jaroslaw D. Kasprzak, MD and Jaroslaw Drozdz, MD.

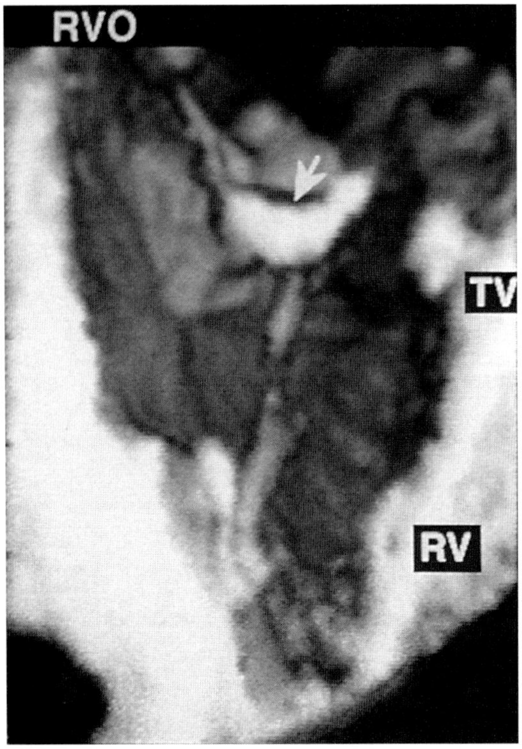

Figure 22. A mass (arrow) is noted in the right ventricle in this transesophageal three-dimensional echo reconstruction, longitudinal image shown during diastole (note the open tricuspid valve).

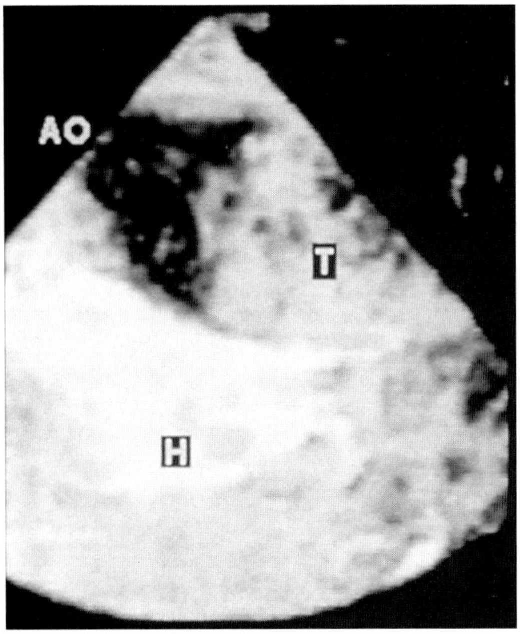

Figure 23. Transesophageal three-dimensional reconstruction of aortic leiomyosarcoma. The tumor (T) occupies most of the descending thoracic aortic (AO) lumen. H represents a hematoma resulting from tumor-induced rupture of the aortic wall. From Nanda NC et al. Three-dimensional echocardiographic assessment of aortic dissection. *Echocardiography* 1998;15;745–754.

Suggested Reading List

1. Jamil F, Nanda NC, Thakur AC, et al. Echocardiographic detection of intramyocardial coronary obstruction produced by pericardial hydatid cyst. *Echocardiography* 1997;14:459–460.
2. Melzer C, Bartel T, Baumann G. Dynamic 3-D-echo in the preoperative assessment of left atrial myxoma in a 51-year-old male. *Int J Cardiol* 1997;59:167–169.
3. Greco C, Romano P, Di Segni M, et al. Three-dimensional transesophageal echocardiographic evaluation of a left atrial myxoma. *Giornale Italiano Cardiologia* 1998; 28:193.
4. Handke M, Schochlin A, Schafer DM, et al. Myxoma of the mitral valve: Diagnosis by 2-dimensional and 3-dimensional echocardiography. *J Am Soc Echocardiography* 1999;12:773–776.
5. Mukhtar OM, Miller AP, Nanda NC, et al. Two and three dimensional transesophageal echocardiographic localization of a right atrial lipoma: Importance of orienting echocardiographic images to the surgeon's view. *Echocardiography* (In press, August 2001).

Chapter 9

Miscellaneous Lesions

Navin C. Nanda, MD and Vincent L. Sorrell, MD

Infiltrative cardiomyopathies are not common, but should be considered whenever the left ventricular (LV) myocardial wall is excessively thickened, and the electrical voltage on the ECG is paradoxically low. Hypertrophic obstructive cardiomyopathy (HOCM) also has a thickened myocardium, either globally, apically, or predominantly involving the septum, and the ECG is usually markedly abnormal. Examples of HOCM are included before and after myectomy procedures. Potential advantages of three-dimensional (3D) imaging in this setting include a more complete appreciation of the anterior motion of the mitral valve and the extent of the septal contact, thereby determining the exact location and extent of surgical resection of the ventricular septum required.

Another unusual finding illustrated with 3D imaging is a large hydatid cyst.

A large pleural effusion is also demonstrated and is noted to be highly complex with multiple adhesions and thrombi. Three-dimensional imaging allowed a much greater detail of the extensive latticework noted in this patient.

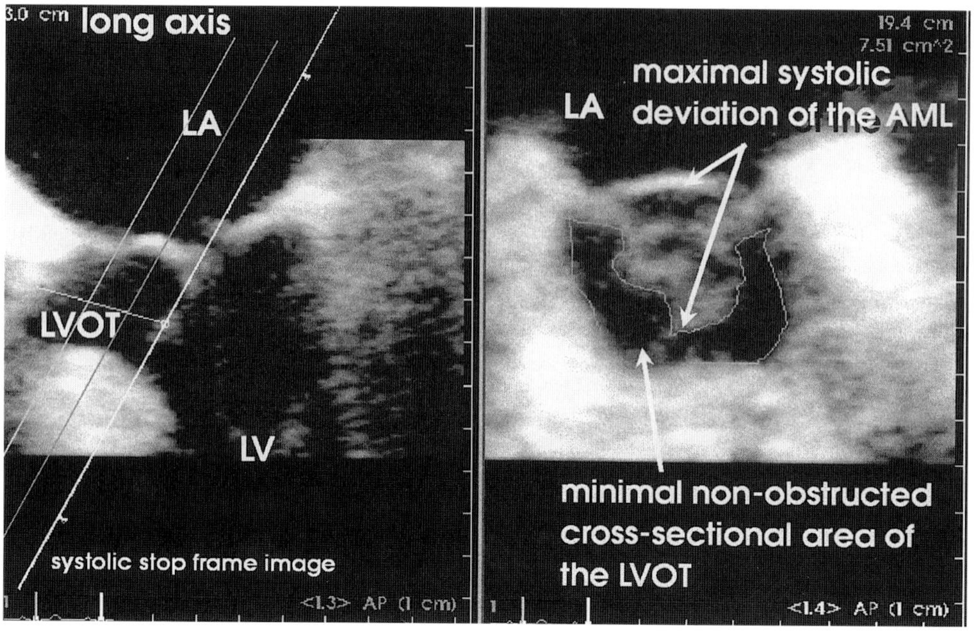

Figure 1. Cross-sectional area of the left ventricular outflow tract (LVOT) in hypertrophic obstructive cardiomyopathy (HOCM). Stop frame images during mid-systole in a patient with moderate obstruction of the LVOT at rest (no contact of the mitral leaflet to the septum). **Left:** Reconstructed long axis of the LV (LA = left atrium, AML/PML = anterior and posterior mitral leaflet). **Right:** Short axis cross-section of the LVOT taken at the position of the third line on the left image. Other parallel image planes in the three-dimensional data set are demonstrated by the first and the second lines on the left image. The maximal systolic deviation of the AML and the minimal cross-sectional area of the LVOT were quantified by manual planimetry (right image). From Andreas Franke, MD, Harald P. Kühl, MD, and Peter Hanrath, MD. Reprinted with permission from Franke A et al. Quantitative assessment of the operative results after extended myectomy and surgical reconstruction of the subvalvular mitral apparatus in hypertrophic obstructive cardiomyopathy using dynamic three-dimensional transesophageal echocardiography. *J Am Coll Cardiol* 1998; 31:1641–1649.

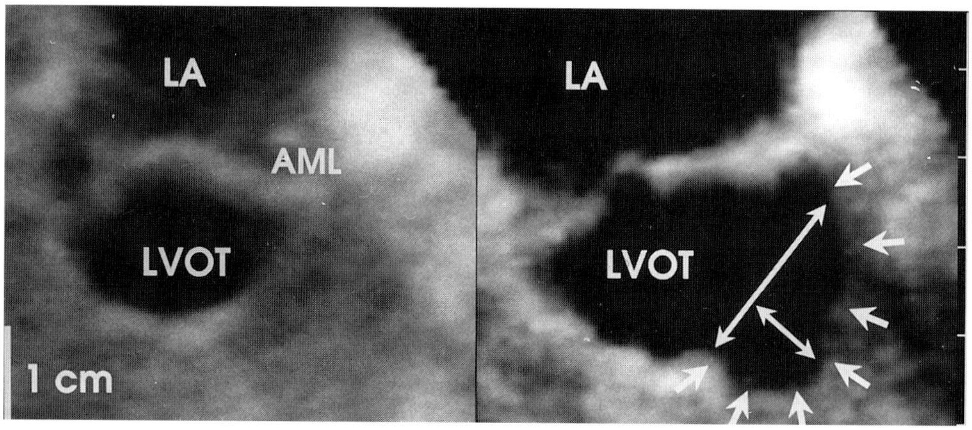

Figure 2. Left ventricular outflow tract area before and after myectomy in hypertrophic obstructive cardiomyopathy. Two corresponding stop frame cross-sections of the left ventricular outflow tract in a patient with hypertrophic obstructive cardiomyopathy generated from the 3D data set. On the left pre operatively, on the right after extended myectomy and surgical reconstruction of the subvalvular mitral apparatus. Maximal width and depth of the myectomy trough are marked by the large arrows. LA = left atrium; AML = anterior mitral leaflet; small arrows = limits of myectomy trough. From Andreas Franke, MD, Harald P. Kühl, MD, and Peter Hanrath, MD. Reprinted with permission from Franke A et al. Quantitative assessment of the operative results after extended myectomy and surgical reconstruction of the subvalvular mitral apparatus in hypertrophic obstructive cardiomyopathy using dynamic three-dimensional transesophageal echocardiography. *J Am Coll Cardiol* 1998;31:1641–1649.

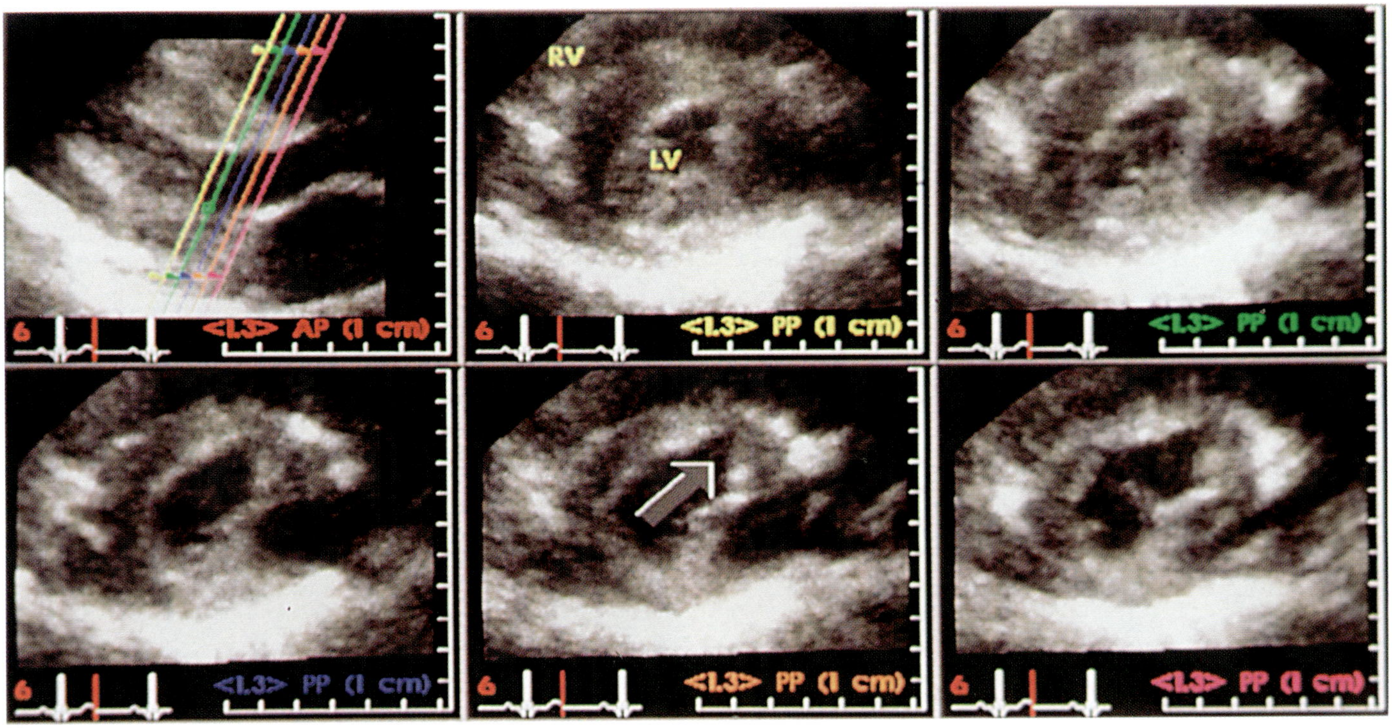

Figure 3. Hypertrophic obstructive cardiomyopathy after a myectomy procedure. **Upper left** panel is a reference long-axis view of the left ventricular outflow tract, displaying the position of five paraplane cutplanes. **Lower left** and **middle** panels clearly display the localization of excised septal tissue (arrow). LV = left ventricle; RV = right ventricle. From Jaroslaw D. Kasprzak, MD

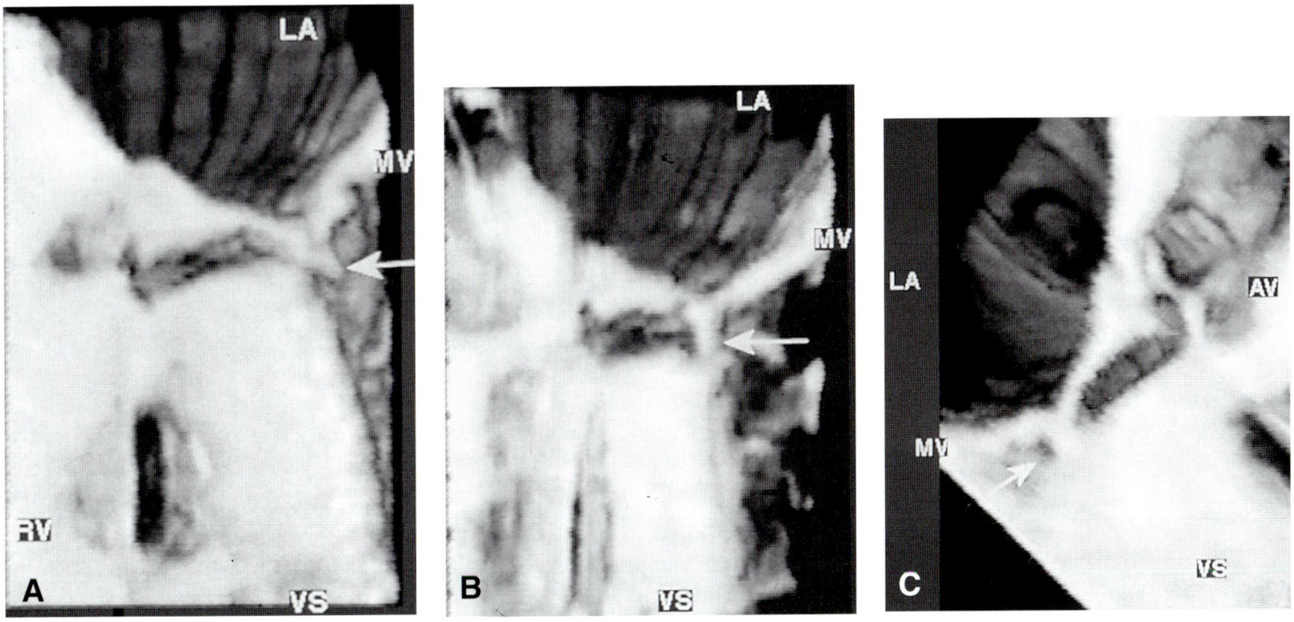

Figure 4A-C. Hypertrophic obstructive cardiomyopathy (HOCM) series. (**A**) Transesophageal echo (TEE) apical 4-chamber orientation in a patient with a markedly thickened interventricular septum (VS), narrow left ventricular outflow tract (LVOT) and systolic anterior motion (SAM; arrow) of the anterior mitral valve leaflet consistent with HOCM. (**B,C**) These two images are also obtained from the previous patient with TEE and displayed from different cutplanes, providing further insight into the structural orientation. The abnormal anterior position of the mitral valve apparatus is seen in the LVOT (arrow).

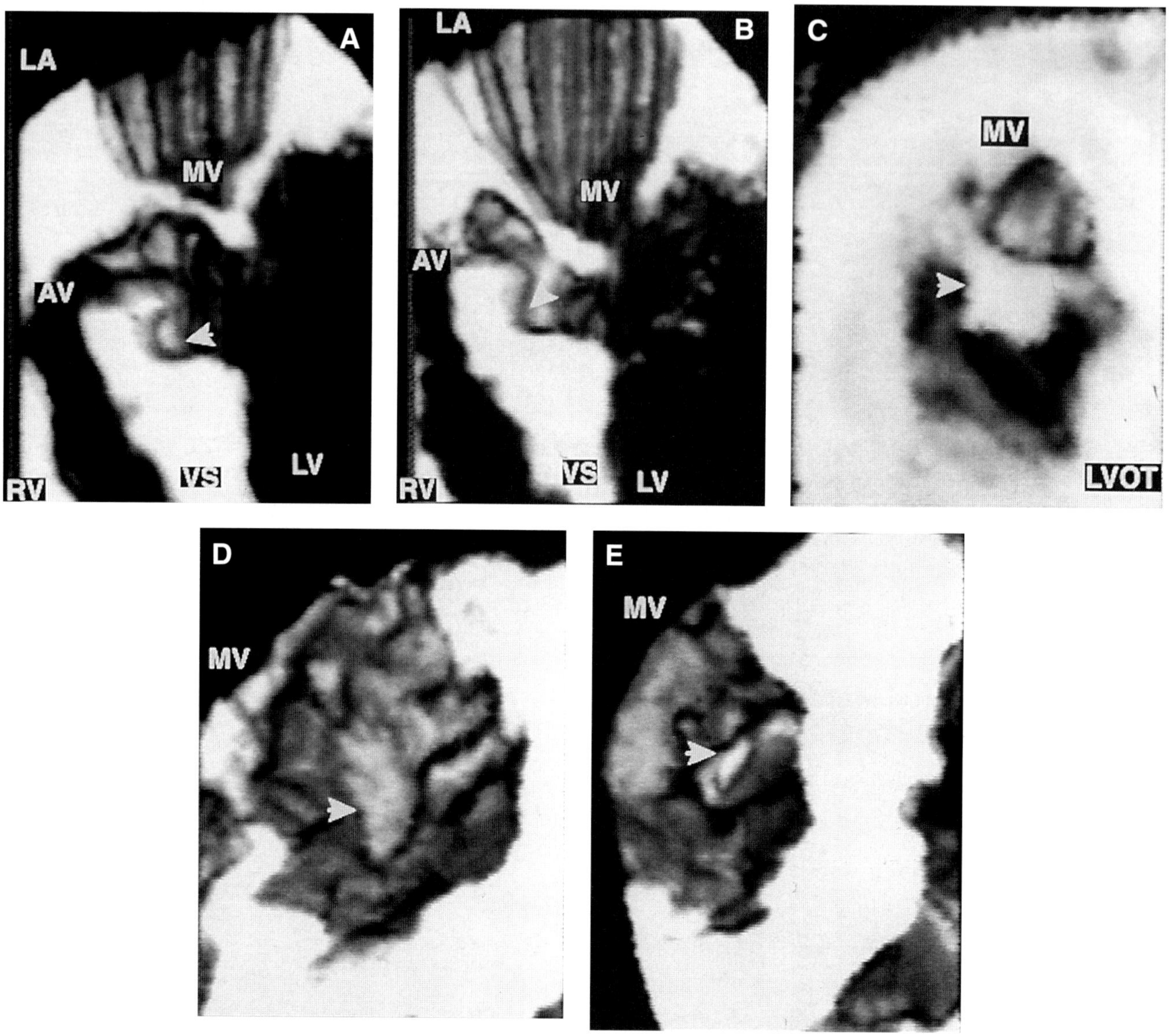

Figure 5A-E. (**A, B**) Transesophageal three-dimensional echo (TEE 3D) apical 4-chamber images, displayed with slightly different degrees of zoom in a patient with hypertrophic obstructive cardiomyopathy (HOCM) who received septal myectomy (arrow) to relieve the obstruction (VS = ventricular septum). (**C**) In this TEE short axis image of the patient in the previous figure, the exact area of the left ventricular outflow tract is determined and the degree of obstruction relief from surgery carefully assessed (arrow = systolic anterior motion [SAM]). Note the distance from the mitral valve position and the adjacent ventricular septum. (**D, E**) When viewed from the left ventricular perspective, the degree of SAM of the patient shown in the previous figures is well visualized from an *en-face* orientation (**D**) and slightly more off-axis. (**E**).

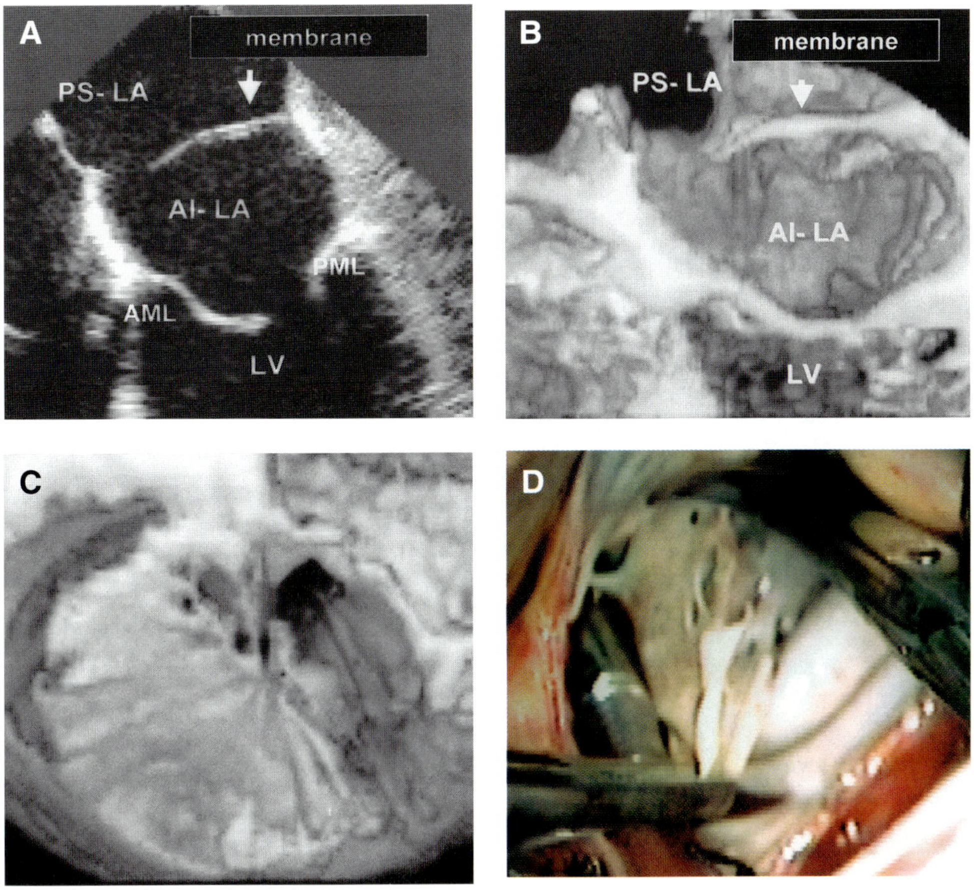

Figure 6. A 70-year-old woman was evaluated for worsening angina. Physical examination disclosed a harsh diastolic murmur. (**A**) Transesophageal echocardiography (TEE) showed a membrane (arrow) attached laterally to the junction of the left upper pulmonic vein and left atrial appendage. This membrane divided the left atrium into two chambers; (1) a posterosuperior chamber that received blood from the pulmonic veins (PS-LA) and (2) an anterointerior (AI-LA) chamber that contained the left atrial appendage and mitral valve. The presence of a large communicating orifice together with multiple fenestrations of the membrane was clearly visualized from the three-dimensional (3D) reconstruction of the TEE-acquired images (**B,** reconstructed left atrium and **C,** view from the roof of the posterosuperior chamber). The atrial membrane was excised during surgery, which was recommended because of the presence of associated significant coronary artery disease. **D** corresponds to the surgical view from the roof of the posterosuperior chamber showing the identical membrane perforations previously diagnosed by 3D echocardiography (**C**). AML = anterior mitral leaflet; LV = left ventricle; PML = posterior mitral leaflet. From Lissa Sugeng, MD, Ivan Godoy, MD, Kirk T. Spencer, MD, Jim Bednarz, BS, Lynn Weinert, BS, and Roberto M. Lang, MD

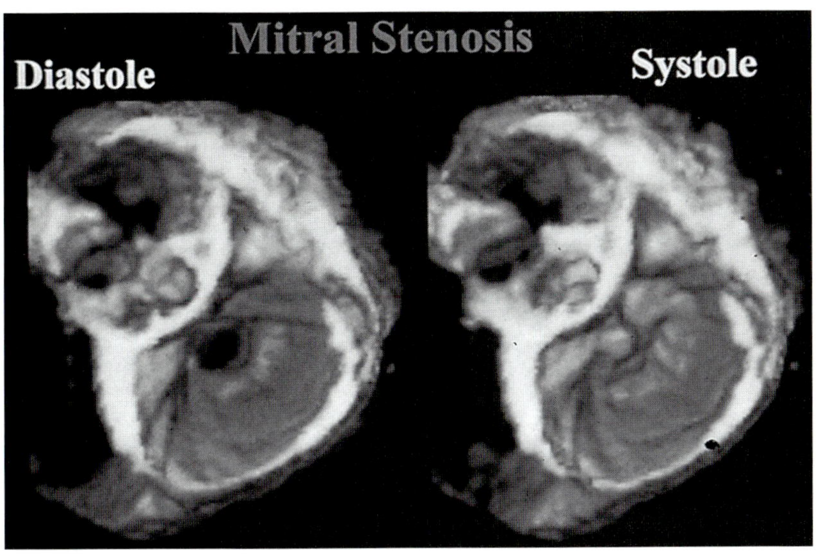

Figure 7. A stenotic mitral valve reconstructed from an atrial perspective during systole and diastole. Other cardiac structures such as left atrial appendage, aortic valve and pulmonary valve are well visualized. From Aleksandra Lange, MD

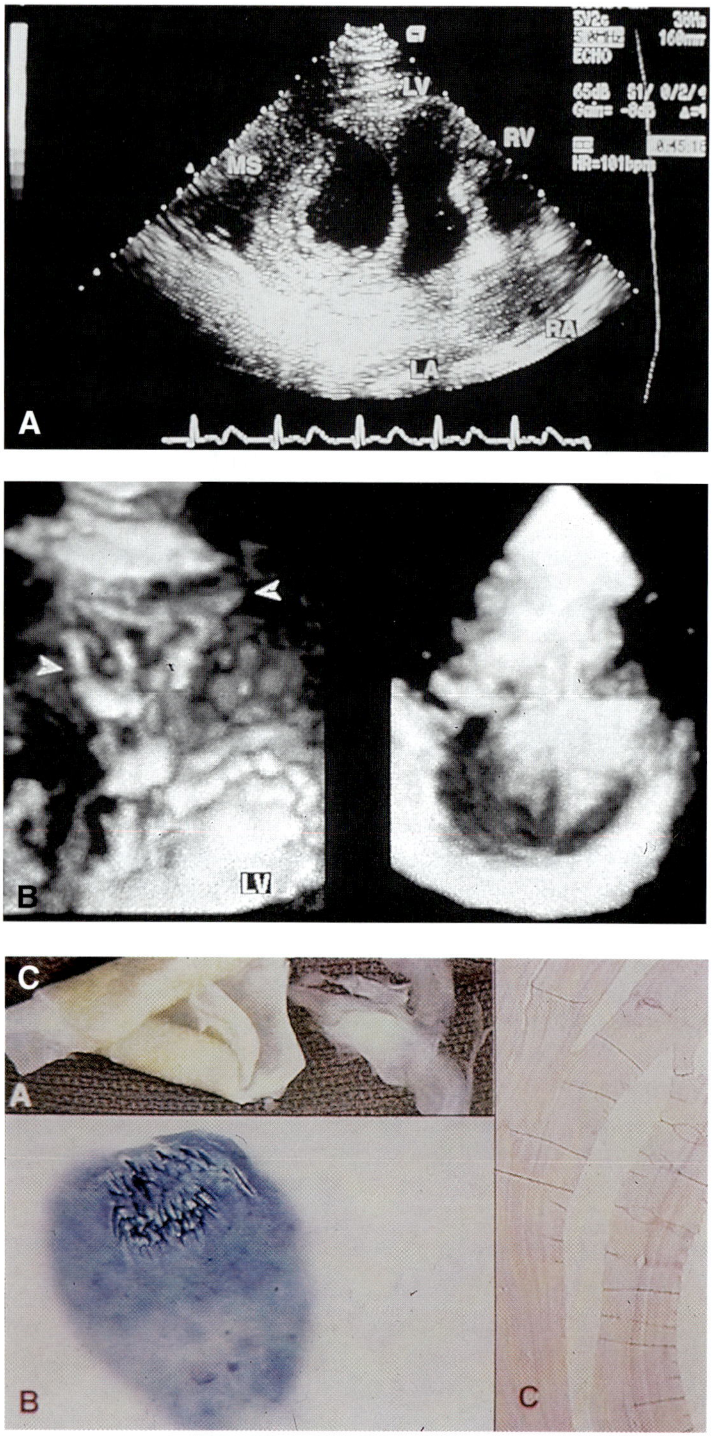

Figure 8. (**A**) Transthoracic echo shows a large pericardial hydatid cyst (MS) compressing the left ventricular (LV) lateral wall. It measures approximately 8 cm in diameter and appears to contain layered solid tissue. (**B**) Right: Three-dimensional (3D) reconstruction demonstrates membrane-like solid issue in the cyst. Left: 3D reconstruction of intramyocardial coronary vessels (arrows) in the compressed LV wall. (**C**) Left upper panel: Hydatid cyst wall and surrounding soft tissue. Left lower panel: Close up of hydatid scolex with double rows of hooklets (100x). Right panel: Laminated membrane. C = pericardial cyst; LA = left atrium; RA = right atrium; RV = right ventricle. Figures A-B: Reproduced with permission from Jamil F et al: Echocardiographic detection of intramyocardial coronary obstruction produced by pericardial hydatid cyst. Echocardiography;1997:14:456–460.

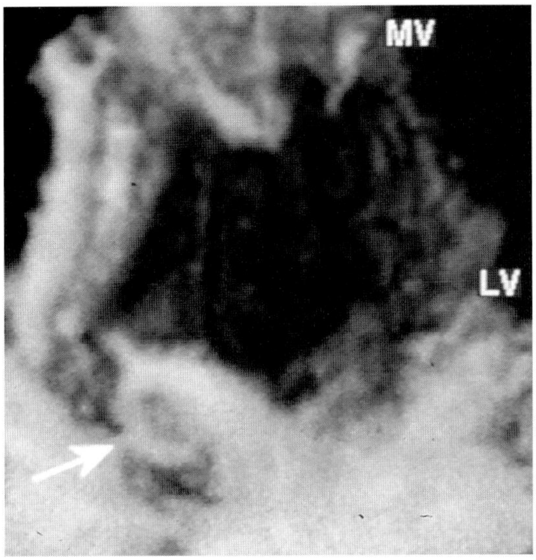

Figure 9. Transesophageallly-obtained three-dimensional echo image of a patient with a dilated left ventricle and an implanted left ventricular assist device (LVAD). Arrow = apical cannulation.

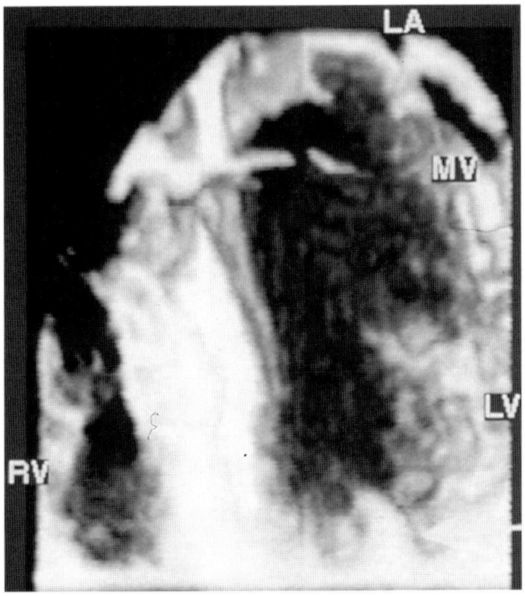

Figure 10. Another patient with a left ventricular assist device in the left ventricular apex is visualized and the apical cannulation is noted (arrow).

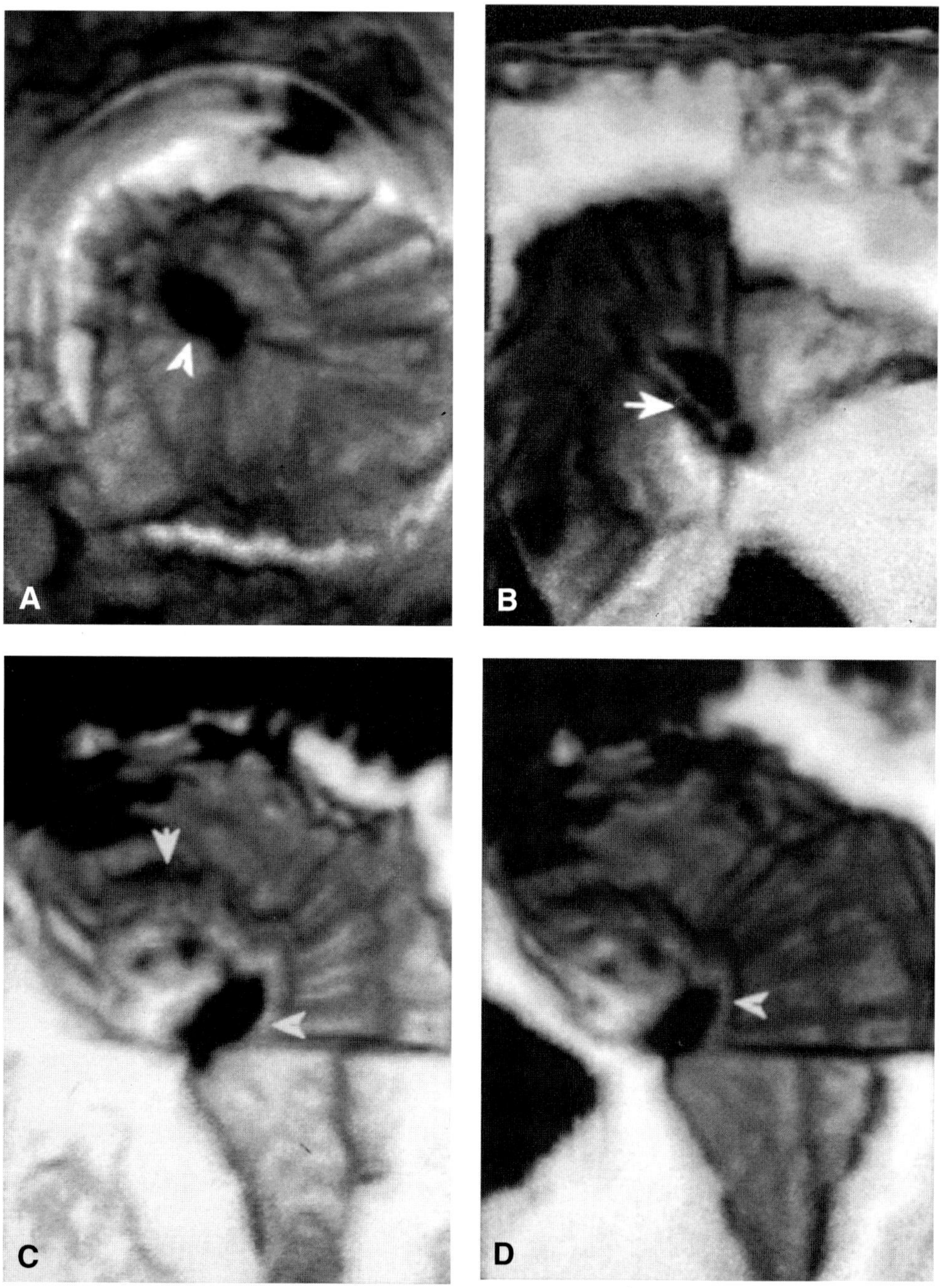

Figure 11. Secundum atrial septal defect with atrial septal aneurysm. (**A, B**) Transesophageally-obtained three-dimensional data set provides extraordinary information about the details of the atrial septum. A secundum atrial septal defect is readily seen (arrow) in an *en-face* orientation from the left atrium (**A**) and the right atrium (**B**). These types of images are impossible with conventional two-dimensional echo since the transducer can never be positioned for this orientation. (**C, D**) These two images are from the same patient and again show the defect (arrow) as viewed from slightly two different right atrial positions. Note the bulging of the atrial septum (observed from the right) with two or three small "perforations."

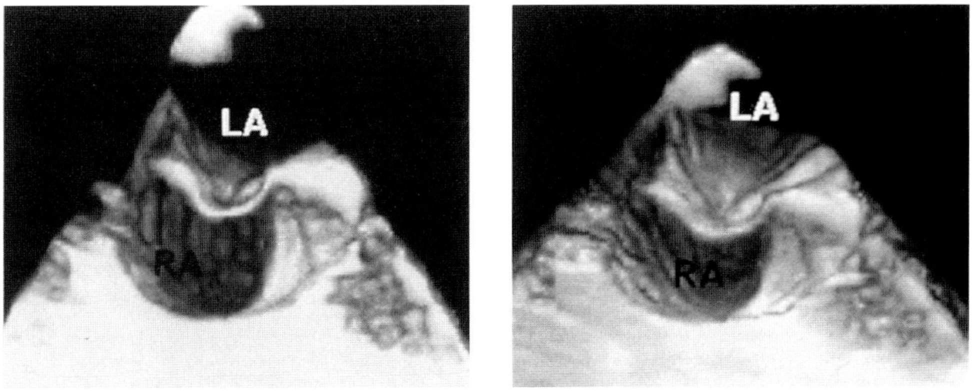

Figure 12. Atrial septal aneurysm without a shunt. Three-dimensional reconstruction of spatial structure of the lesion with tilted views (right) confirming the integrity of interatrial septum; no shunt flow was detected. LA = left atrium; RA = right atrium. From Jaroslaw D. Kasprzak, MD and Jaroslaw Drozdz, MD.

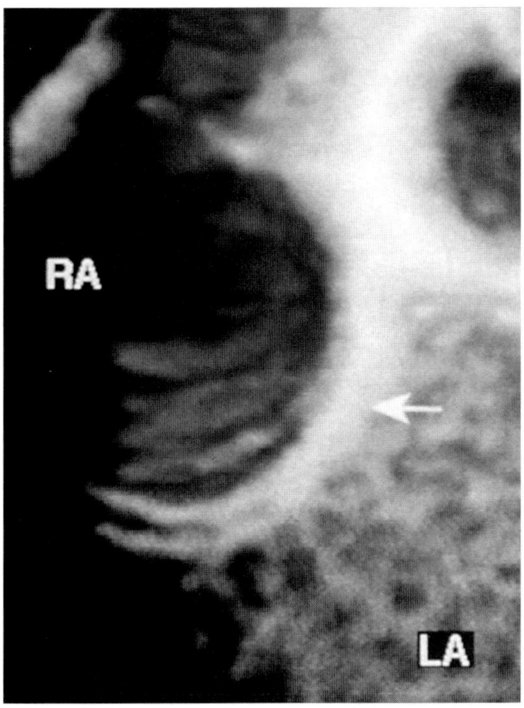

Figure 13. An atrial septal aneurysm (arrow) is noted in this transesophageal image obtained with transesophageal echo. Note the excessive bowing of the septum towards the left atrial cavity.

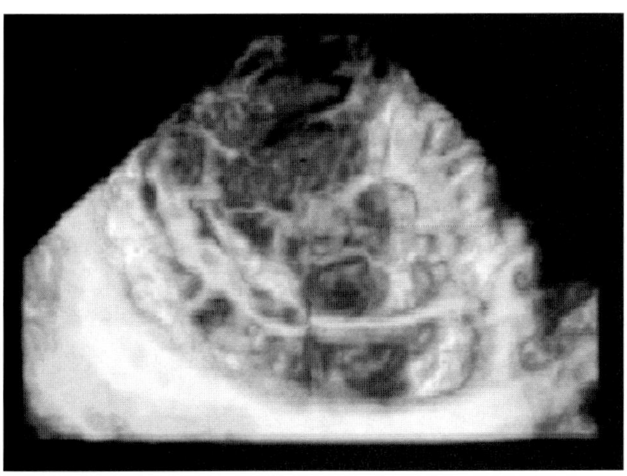

Figure 14. Pleural effusion. Transesophageal, three-dimensional echo image of a large hemothorax in an elderly patient with an acute, type A aortic dissection. Multiple adhesions, which likely represent thrombus in this clinical situation, were seen in greater detail than was noted with two-dimensional imaging alone. From Vincent L. Sorrell, MD.

Suggested Reading List

1. Buck T, Schon F, Baumgart D, et al. Tomographic left ventricular volume determination in the presence of aneurysm by three-dimensional echocardiographic imaging. I: Asymmetric model hearts. *J Am Soc Echocardiography* 1996;9:488–500.
2. Buck T, Hunold P, Wentz KU, et al. Tomographic three-dimensional echocardiographic determination of chamber size and systolic function in patients with left ventricular aneurysm: Comparison to magnetic resonance imaging, cineventriculography, and two-dimensional echocardiography. *Circulation* 1997;96:4286–4297.
3. Melzer C, Bartel T, Muller S, et al. Dynamic three-dimensional echocardiography in the assessment of cor triatriatum. *Clin Cardiol* 1997;20:82–83.
4. Valocik G, Allaart CP, Kamp O. Anterior mitral valve aneurysm: Evaluation by three-dimensional echocardiography. *J Am Soc Echocardiography* 1998;11:673–676.
5. Xiaokui T, Schwartz GA, Rusk RA, et al. A digital 3-dimensional method for computing great artery flows: In vitro validation studies. *J Am Soc Echocardiography* 2000;13(9):841–848.
6. Yu TH, Fu M, Chua S. Three-dimensional echocardiographic image of atrial septal aneurysm: Report of two cases. *Changgeng Yi Xue Za Zhi* 2000;23(11):701–705.
7. Van Langenhove G, Vermeersch P, Serruys PW. Thrombus overlying the main stem crista: A three dimensional reconstruction. *Heart* 2001;85(2):178.
8. Keberle M, Jenett M, Wittenberg G, et al. [Comparison of 3D power doppler ultrasound, color doppler ultrasound and digital subtraction angiography in carotid stenosis]. [German]. *Rofo Fortschritte Gebiete Rontgenstrahlen Neuen Bildgebenden Verfahren* 2001;173(2):133–138.
9. Khan GN, Dairywala IT, Liu Z, et al. Three-dimensional echocardiography of left atrial appendage thrombus. *Echocardiography* 2001;18(2):163–166.
10. Vargas-Barron J, Roldan FJ, Romero-Cardenas A, et al. Two- and three-dimensional transesophageal echocardiographic diagnosis of intramyocardial dissecting hematoma after myocardial infarction. *J Am Soc Echocardiography* 2001;14(6):637–640.

Chapter 10

Three-Dimensional Color Doppler

Navin C. Nanda, MD and Vincent L. Sorrell, MD

An exciting area that is rapidly evolving within the development of three-dimensional (3D) echocardiography is the ability to image color flow Doppler signals with three dimensions. The reasons for wanting to be able to image valvular regurgitation in multidimensions are obvious—to minimize significant over- and underestimation of severity. Since valve regurgitation is frequently eccentric and follows the contour of the receiving chamber, the full extent of the regurgitant jet is not imaged in any single imaging plane. With multiplane imaging, echocardiographers 'mentally' reconstruct this color flow to gain a greater understanding of the severity. This requires vigilance and skill to image and record in many various planes. With the advent of 3D color flow Doppler, the complete Doppler flow signal is imaged in its entirety and may be displayed by rotating the image through 360°. Furthermore, there are frequently less reverberation artifacts from prosthetic valves with this display compared with two-dimensional (2D) imaging.

Another advantage is the ability to image the flow acceleration proximal to the regurgitation (PISA) and ascertain if this is hemispheric. If so, then routine formulas apply and one can readily quantitate the effective regurgitant orifice (ERO) and the regurgitant volume using the radius of this flow acceleration. If, however, the shape of the alias velocity is noted *not* to represent a hemisphere, then standard calculations would be incorrect, and using them would at times overestimate and other times underestimate the severity of the lesion. This also applies to the most narrow region of regurgitation within the receiving chamber—the vena contracta. With 3D imaging, this should represent the ERO, and research in this area is continuing.

Finally, novel display algorithms are also frequently revealing. Since the complete 3D data set is available for post-processing, one can select between the antegrade or retrograde Doppler flow signals and highlight the interested flow while suppressing the other. This provides a Doppler jet with only the chosen signals shown, and should thereby further eliminate misinterpretation of the degree of regurgitation. For example, we choose to image mitral regurgitation with only the 'red' (transesophageal echo) color flow Doppler signals displayed. We also eliminate the surrounding tissue by removing the grey scale and are left with the mitral regurgitation as the only image. We have found this to be useful in clarifying the exact origin and direction of the jet and at times this is useful in confirming the etiology of the valve pathology. Removing the grey scale has also allowed unrecognized color jets to become visible within anatomic structures that were previously obscured, such as the more distal regions of the pulmonary veins.

At this time, due to the technique of 3D data acquisition, many of the reconstructions are suboptimal. Many regions of 2D flow turbulence result in zero color on 3D, since there is currently no algorithm for adequate display of color mosaics (with TomTec imaging, TomTec Imaging Systems GMBH, Munich, Germany). As this capability improves, it is likely that regurgitant volumes will become as simple as tracing the area of the color Doppler signals. Already, some investigators have begun to use wireframe displays in an effort to volume-render the regurgitation.

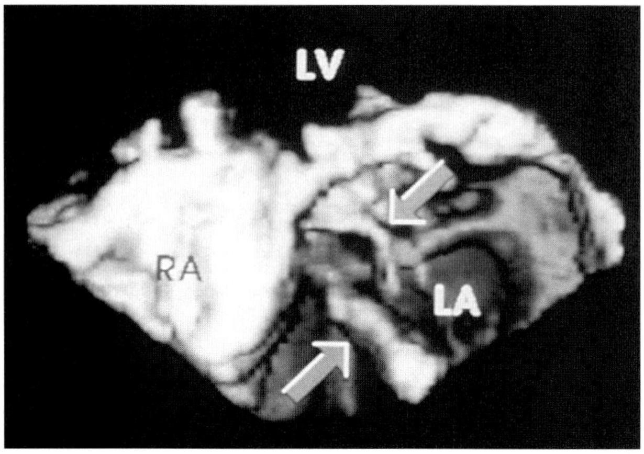

Figure 1. Dynamic three-dimensional images of prosthetic valvular regurgitation. Two regurgitant jets (arrows) originating from the large and small orifices, respectively, shown in the left atrium (LA). LV = left ventricle. Reproduced with permission from Li Z et al. Dynamic three-dimensional reconstruction of abnormal intracardiac blood flow. *Echocardiography* 1997;14:375–381.

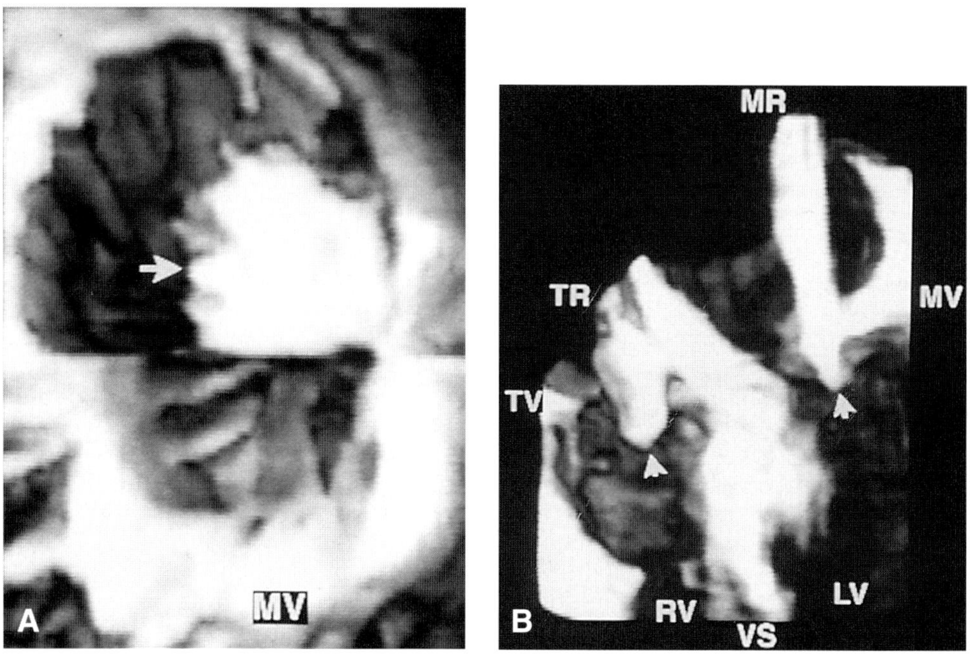

Figure 2. (**A**) Transesophageal, three-dimensional echo (TEE 3D) short axis image, viewed from the left atrial (LA) side of the mitral valve in systole with color flow Doppler also reconstructed in 3D. Mitral regurgitation (arrow) is visualized entering the LA. (**B**) TEE apical 4-chamber orientation with 3D reconstructed color flow Doppler highlighting tricuspid regurgitation (TR) within the right atrium during systole. Mitral regurgitation is also noted, as well as proximal flow acceleration of both regurgitant jets within the respective ventricles (arrows).

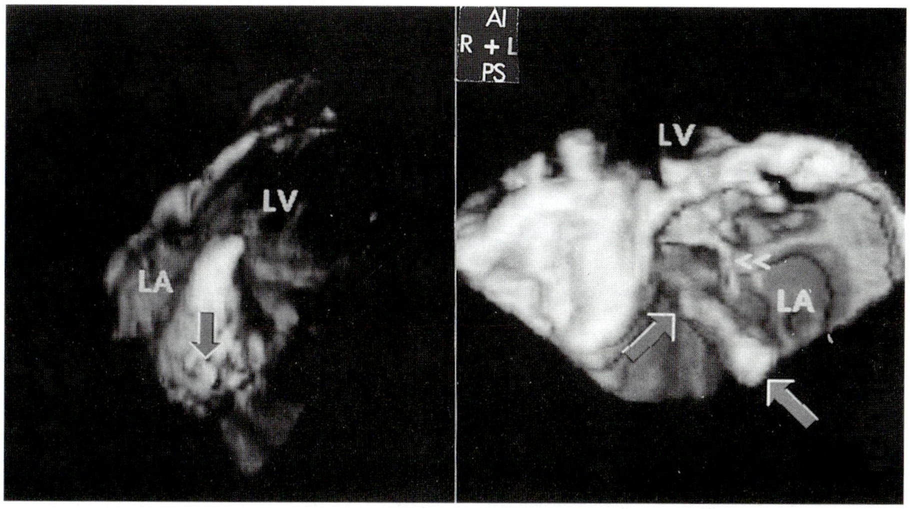

Figure 3. Four-dimensional Doppler flow imaging. **Left:** Mitral regurgitation (arrow). **Right:** Prosthetic valve at mitral position taken during operation. In early systole, two flow jets, one small and another large (arrows), pass through the prosthetic valve (arrowheads) from the left ventricle (LV) into the left atrium (LA), conforming to the dynamics of a prosthetic disc valve. Reproduced with permission from Wang XF. Four-dimensional echocardiography: Methods and clinical application. *Am Heart J* 1996;132:672–684.

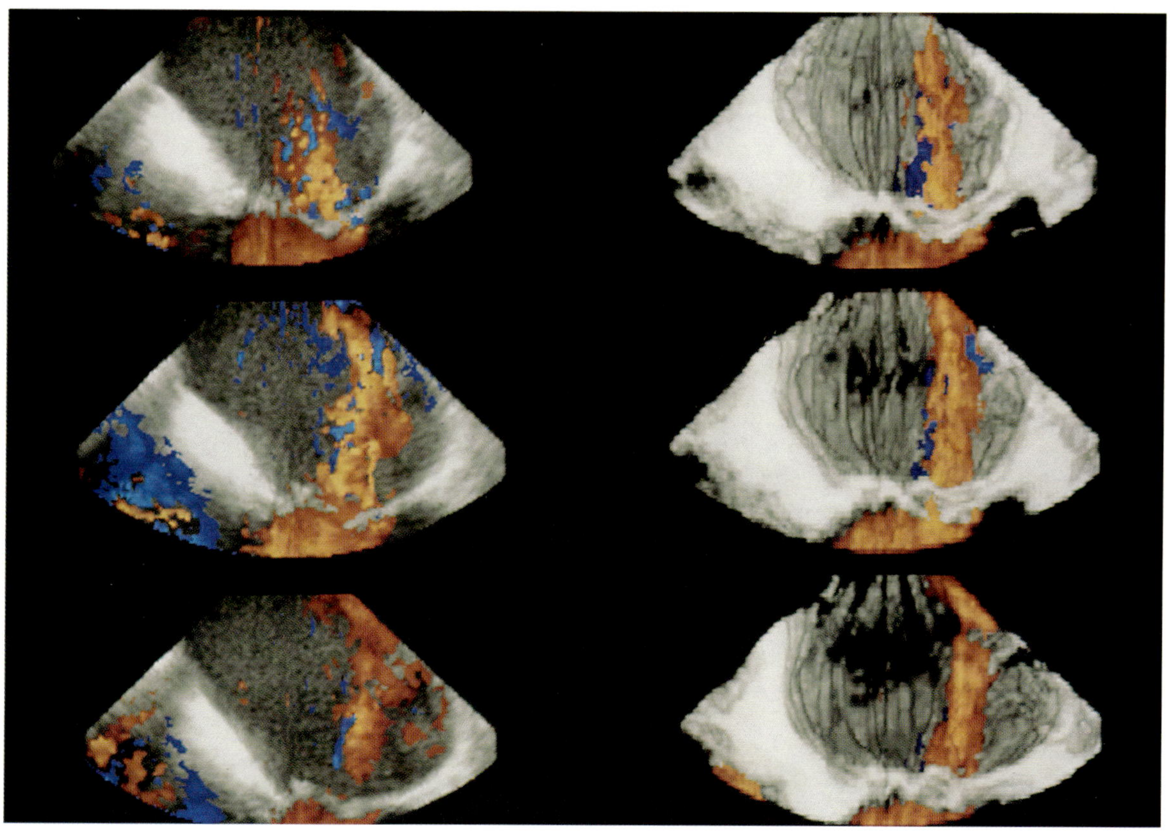

Figure 4. Serial frames from a moderate mitral regurgitant jet is observed in these two-dimensional images and corresponding three-dimensional reconstruction. From Lissa Sugeng, MD, Ivan Godoy, MD, Kirk T. Spencer, MD, Jim Bednarz, BS, Lynn Weinert, BS, and Roberto M. Lang, MD

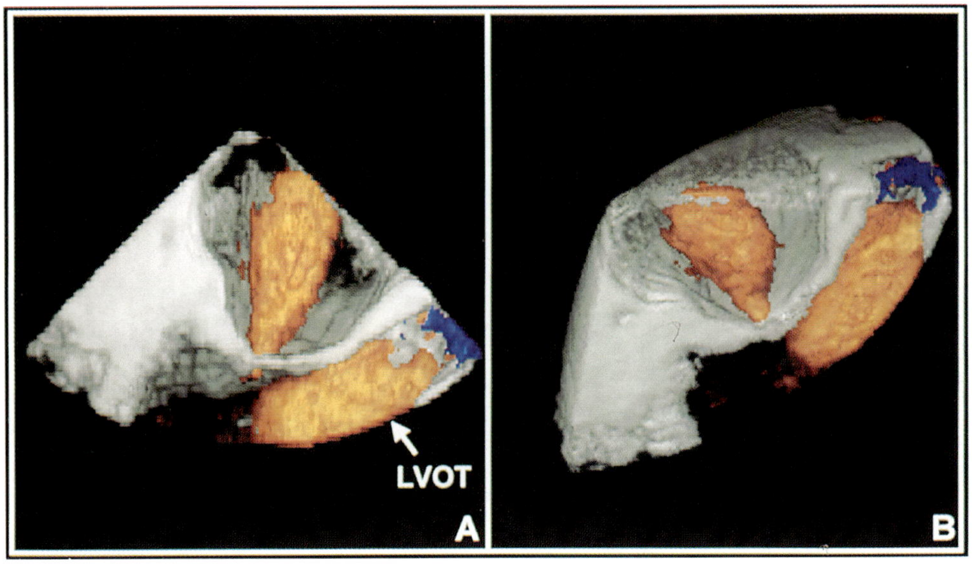

Figure 5. (**A,B**) A jet of mild mitral regurgitation, identified by two-dimensional echocardiography, is reconstructed in a long axis cut. The jet appears to be oriented anteriorly. The jet was only seen in one frame. The width at its origin is narrow; the jet spreads and reaches to roof of the left atrium. Flow is also observed in the left ventricular outflow tract. From Lissa Sugeng, MD, Ivan Godoy, MD, Kirk T. Spencer, MD, Jim Bednarz, BS, Lynn Weinert, BS, and Roberto M. Lang, MD.

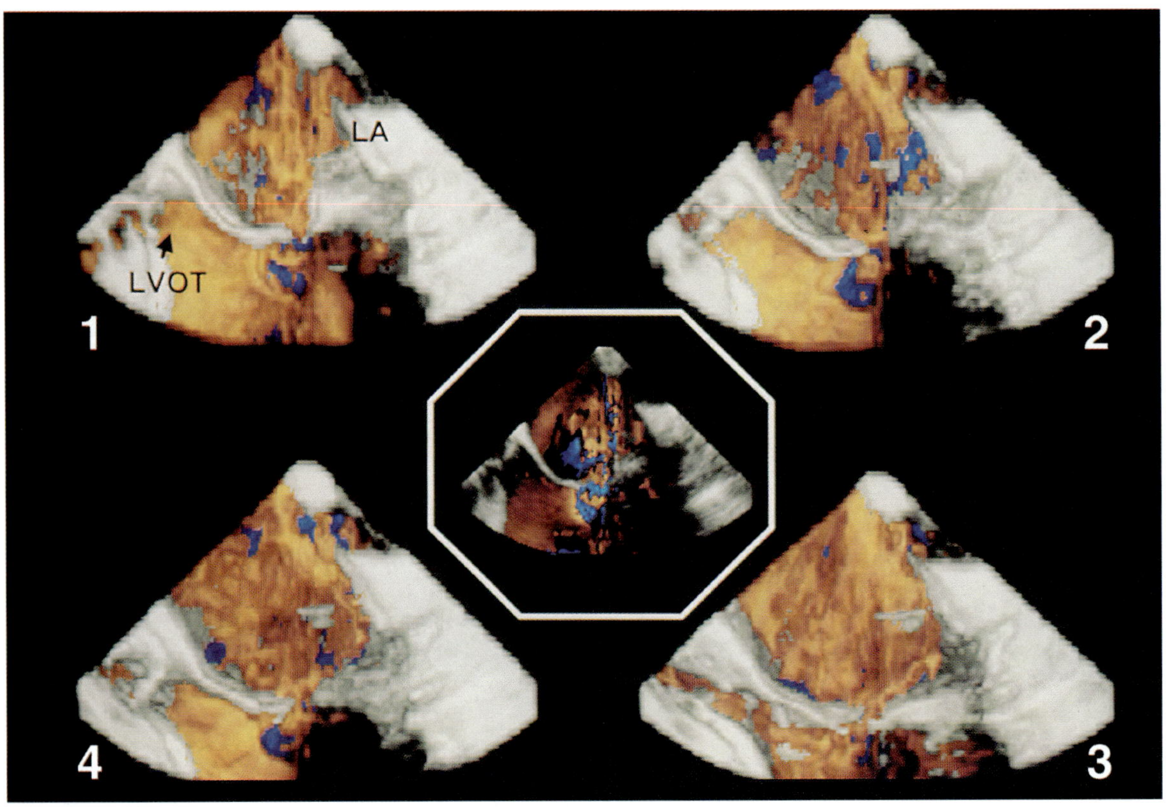

Figure 6. A patient with a flail mitral valve had moderate mitral regurgitation by two-dimensional echocardiography (center image). Three-dimensional reconstruction of a long axis view looking towards the posterior aspect of the heart was performed. Serial frames (**1–4**) demonstrate the regurgitant jet in sequence as it initially penetrates the left atrium (**1** and **2**) and curls against the lateral and posterior aspect of the left atrium (**3** and **4**). From Lissa Sugeng, MD, Ivan Godoy, MD, Kirk T. Spencer, MD, Jim Bednarz, BS, Lynn Weinert, BS, and Roberto M. Lang, MD.

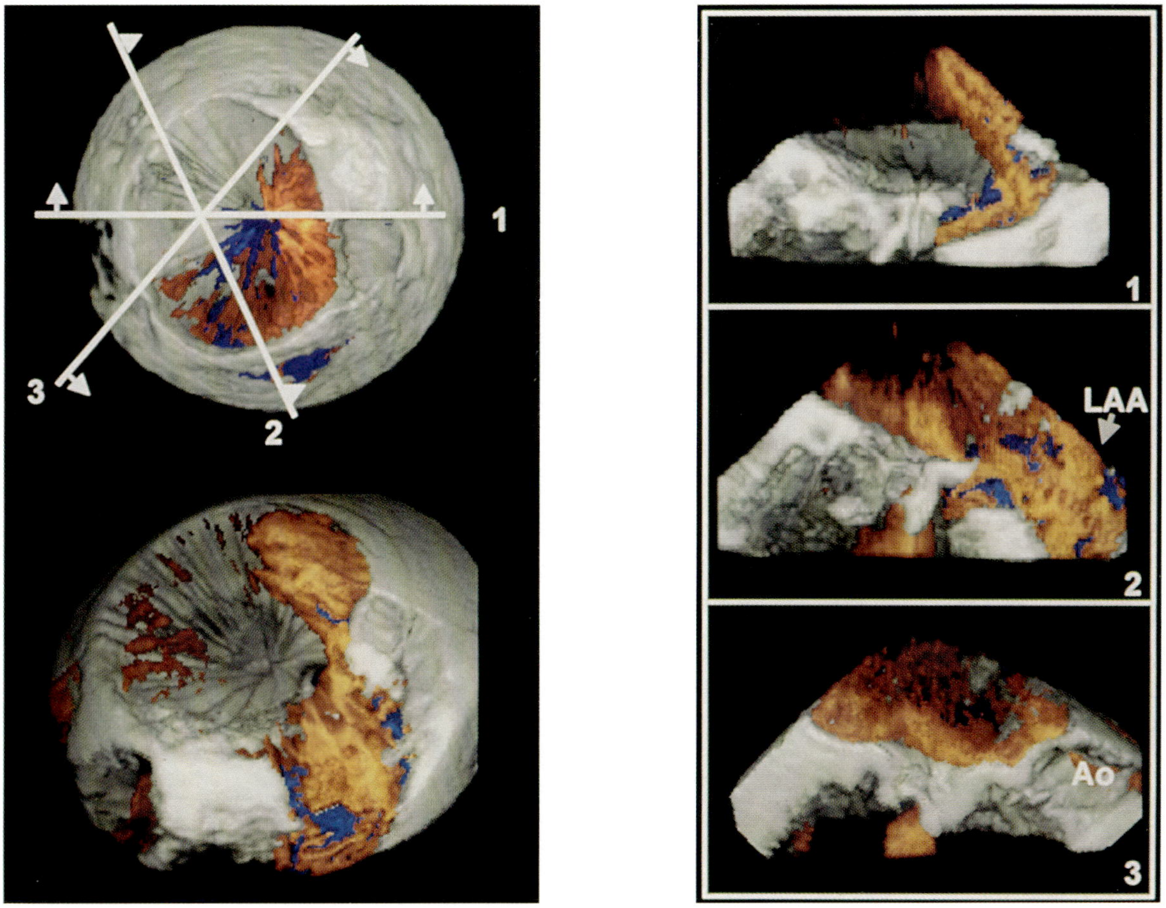

Figure 7. Severe mitral regurgitation in a patient with a mitral bioprosthetic valve. On two-dimensional echo, the patient had an eccentric jet that hugged the wall of the left atrium. In the top left corner, a view of the jet (in red) from the left atrium is observed. Several cutplanes were positioned to visualize the jet from different vantage points. The direction of the view is indicated by the arrows. From various points, the jet is seen originating from a paravalvular space (**1** and **2**). The jet fills the left atrial appendage (**2**). A long axis cut (**3**) demonstrates the extent of the eccentric regurgitant jet. The height and width of this eccentric jet and filling of the left atrial appendage can be observed in the lower left corner panel. From Lissa Sugeng, MD, Ivan Godoy, MD, Kirk T. Spencer, MD, Jim Bednarz, BS, Lynn Weinert, BS, and Roberto M. Lang, MD.

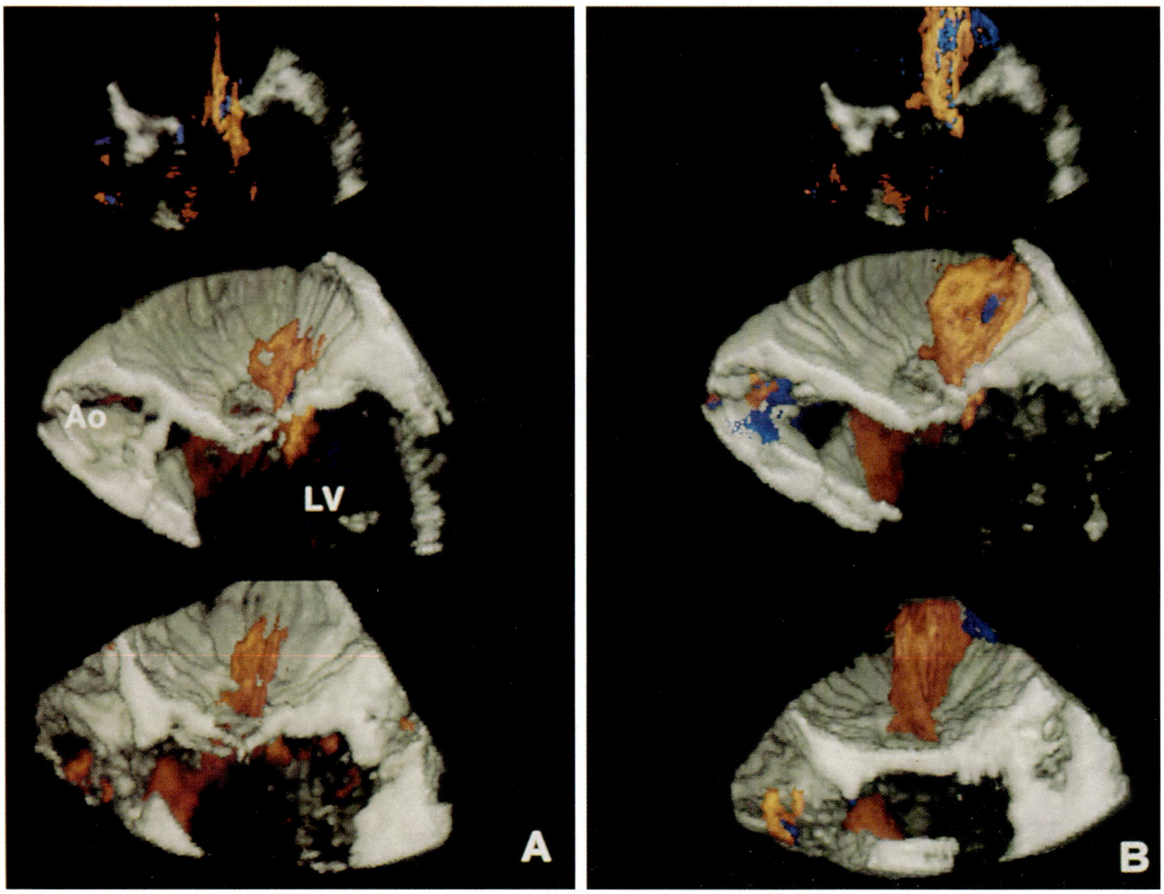

Figure 8. (**A-D**) Patient with a bioprosthetic mitral valve had severe central valvular mitral regurgitation. The regurgitant jet can be seen through four phases during systole (**A–D**). The corresponding two-dimensional cutplane can be seen on the top row. The middle row demonstrates a long axis cut, viewing the aortic valve and cross section of the mitral valve. On the bottom row, a different cutplane is used to see more mitral valve details. The origin of the jet can be identified from these images. The dimensions and direction of the regurgitation jet are also appreciated through various phases and orientations. From Lissa Sugeng, MD, Ivan Godoy, MD, Kirk T. Spencer, MD, Jim Bednarz, BS, Lynn Weinert, BS, and Roberto M. Lang, MD.

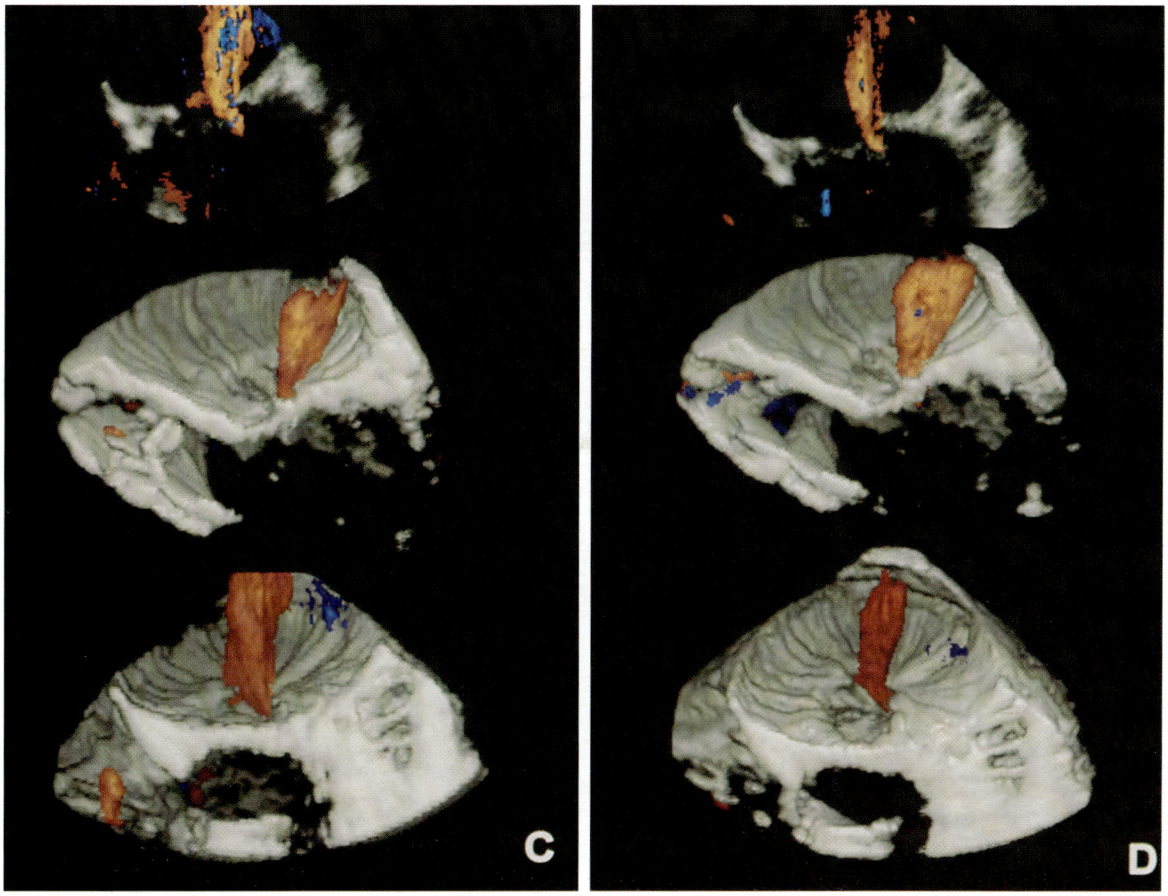

Figure 8. (**C-D**) Continued.

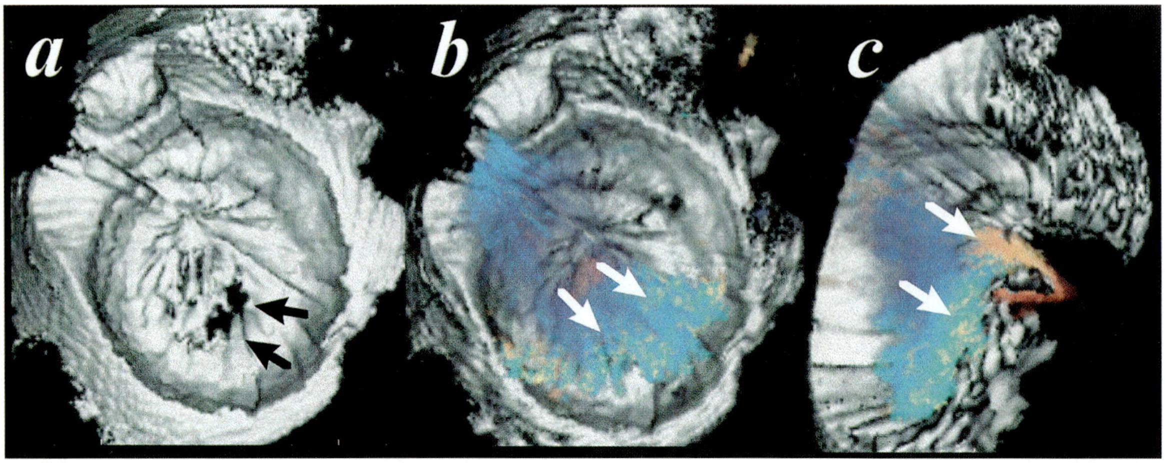

Figure 9. Bioprosthesis in mitral valve position with flail leaflet and severe transvalvular regurgitation. (**A**) Black-and white view from the left atrium on the mitral valve, stop-frame during mid-systole. The flail leaflet and the regurgitation orifice can easily be recognized (black arrows). (**B**) Same image with three-dimensional reconstruction of the color Doppler jet. The broad turbulent regurgitation jet (yellow and cyan color, white arrows) is wall adherent and the origin is difficult to recognize. (**C**) Longitudinal cutplane of the prosthesis at the same mid-systolic stop frame. Now origin and excentric shape of the jet can be demonstrated. (Transparent color reconstruction software: MedCom, Darmstadt, Germany). From Andreas Franke, MD, Harald P. Kühl, MD, and Peter Hanrath, MD.

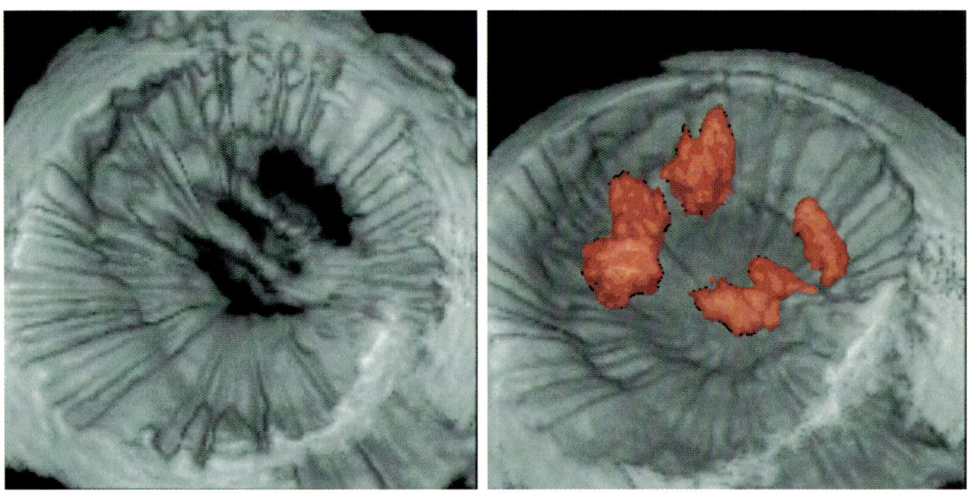

Figure 10. Bileaflet mechanical prosthesis in mitral valve position (St.Jude-Medical, St. Paul, MN), surgical view from the left atrium. **Left:** Black-and-white reconstruction during mid-diastole. Opened leaflets and valve ring are clearly visible. **Right:** Mid-systolic stop frame. Closed prosthesis with typical flame-like transvalvular regurgitation jets at the hinge points of both leaflets. (Color reconstruction software: TomTec Imaging Systems GMBH, Munich, Germany.) From Andreas Franke, MD, Harald P. Kühl, MD, and Peter Hanrath, MD.

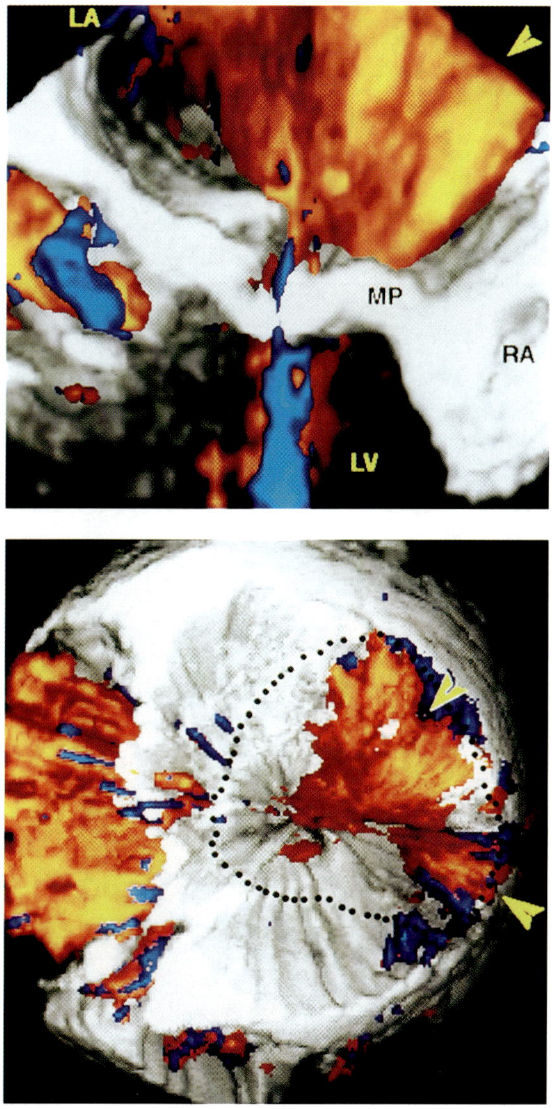

A

B

Figure 11. Transesophageal three-dimensional color Doppler reconstruction of mitral prosthetic regurgitation. (**A**) Arrowhead points to a large jet of mitral regurgitation, which originates within the confines of the heterograft mitral prosthesis (MP). This is consistent with valvular regurgitation. (**B**) Transverse section of the regurgitation jet (arrowheads) at the level of the mitral prosthesis (dotted line) demonstrating valvular origin. The color signals on the left represent tricuspid regurgitation jet in the right atrium. LA = left atrium; LV = left ventricle; RA = right atrium. Reproduced with permission from Anskingar K et al. Transesophageal three-dimensional color Doppler echocardiographic assessment of valvular and paravalvular mitral prosthetic regurgitation. *Echocardiography* 2000;17:579-583.

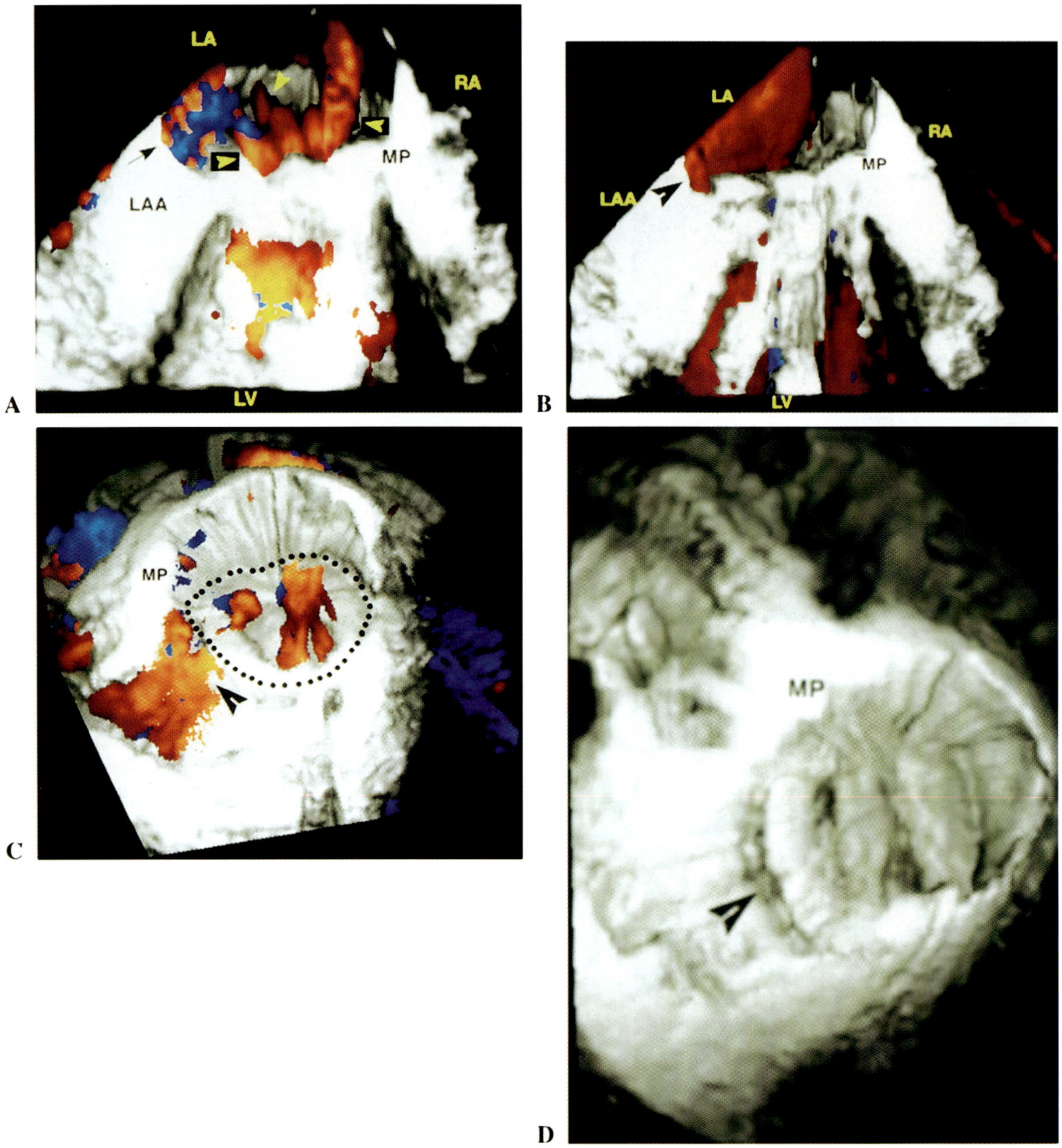

Figure 12. Transesophageal three-dimensional color Doppler reconstruction of mitral prosthetic regurgitation. (**A**) Arrowheads point to three jets of "normal" valvular regurgitation originating within the confines of the Carbomedics mitral prosthesis (MP). (**B**) Paravalvular regurgitation is well seen (arrowhead). (**C**) Oblique transverse section at the level of the prosthesis (dotted line) shows the paravalvular regurgitation (arrowhead) originating at the 7 to 8 o'clock position. This corresponded with the site of dehiscence found at surgery. Color signals within the prosthesis represent "normal" valvular regurgitation. Flow signals at the top represent right atrial flow. (**D**) Arrowhead shows the site of dehiscence located at 7 to 8 o'clock positions. It measured 1.4cm in circumferential length comparable to 1 cm estimated at surgery. LA = left atrium; LV = left ventricle; RA = right atrium; LAA = left atrial appendage. Reproduced with permission from Anskingar K, et al. Transesophageal three-dimensional color Doppler echocardiographic assessment of valvular and paravalvular mitral prosthetic regurgitation. *Echocardiography* 2000;17:579-583.

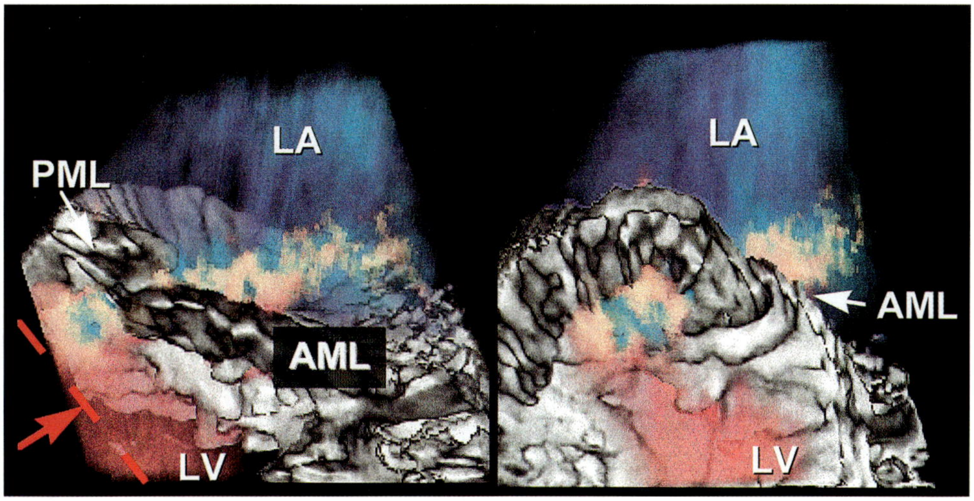

Figure 13. Systolic stop-frame images of an eccentric mitral regurgitation jet. Semi-transparent reconstruction of the color Doppler images (Reconstruction software: MedCom, Darmstadt, Germany) with two different views at the same time-point. **Left:** Longitudinal cutplane, view of the mitral regurgitation jet from the side. LA = left atrium; LV = left ventricle; AML = anterior mitral leaflet; PML = posterior mitral leaflet. **Right:** View of the ventricular surface of the mitral valve; cutplane and perspective are orientated as shown by the red line and the red arrow in the left image. On the ventricular side of the mitral valve the orange-cyan colored proximal convergence zone is clearly visible. Note the nonhemispherical shape of the proximal convergence zone, where geometrical assumptions of a hemisphere would lead to a wrong estimation of the mitral regurgitation. From Andreas Franke, MD, Harald P. Kühl, MD, and Peter Hanrath, MD. Reprinted with permission from Frank A et al: Dreidimensionale rekonstruktion echokardiographischer schnittbilder—methodik, klinischer stellenwert und sukunftsperspektiven. *Dtsch Med Wochenschr* 1998;123:1245–1249. Georg Thieme Verlag Stuttgart.

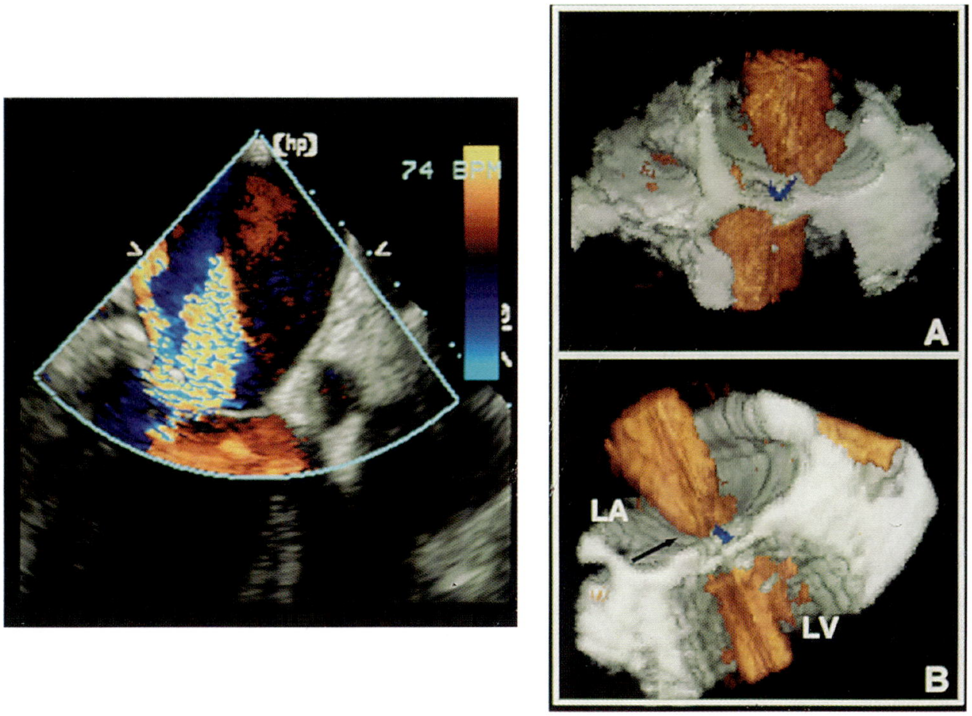

Figure 14. A color flow Doppler three-dimensional reconstruction was performed from the two-dimensional (2D) image on the left. By 2D echo, it was difficult to determine whether the jet was para-ring or valvular. (**A**) Three dimensional reconstructions from a 4-chamber orientation looking posteriorly demonstrates the jet originating from around the ring. (**B**) A 2-chamber orientation also visualized this jet arising from the outside perimeter of the ring. From Lissa Sugeng, MD, Ivan Godoy, MD, Kirk T. Spencer, MD, Jim Bednarz, BS, Lynn Weinert, BS, and Roberto M. Lang, MD.

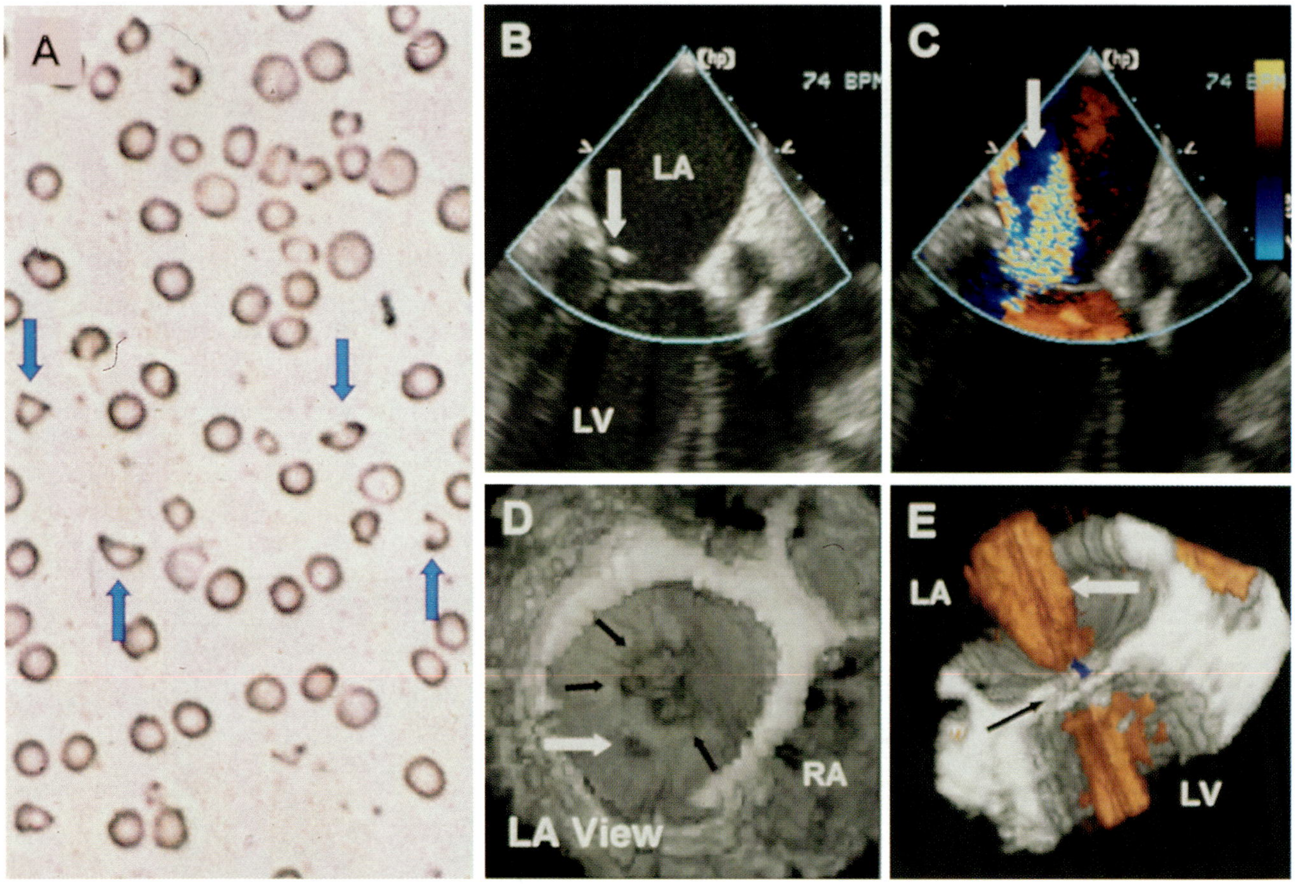

Figure 15. (**A**) Peripheral blood smear revealing schistocytes and red cell fragmentation due to mechanical shearing of red blood cells. (**B, C**) Transverse plane transesophageal images of the mitral valve. (**B**) Partial dehiscence (arrow) of the annuloplasty ring from the native mitral valve annulus. (**C**) Color Doppler imaging reveals fragmentation of the regurgitant flow into a valvular and a para-ring regurgitant jet. (**D**) Three-dimensional (3D) echocardiographic images of the mitral valve from left atrial (LA) view demonstrating an area of dehiscence (white arrow) of the annuloplasty ring from the native valve annulus. (The black arrows outline the medial border of the annuloplasty ring). (**E**) Long axis 3D color Doppler images of mitral valve and posterior LA wall demonstrate a high velocity regurgitant jet (white arrow) outside the annuloplasty ring. The lower velocity valvular regurgitant jet has been suppressed. (The black arrow identifies the posterior aspect of the annuloplasty ring.) From Lissa Sugeng, MD, Ivan Godoy, MD, Kirk T. Spencer, MD, Jim Bednarz, BS, Lynn Weinert, BS, and Roberto M. Lang, MD.

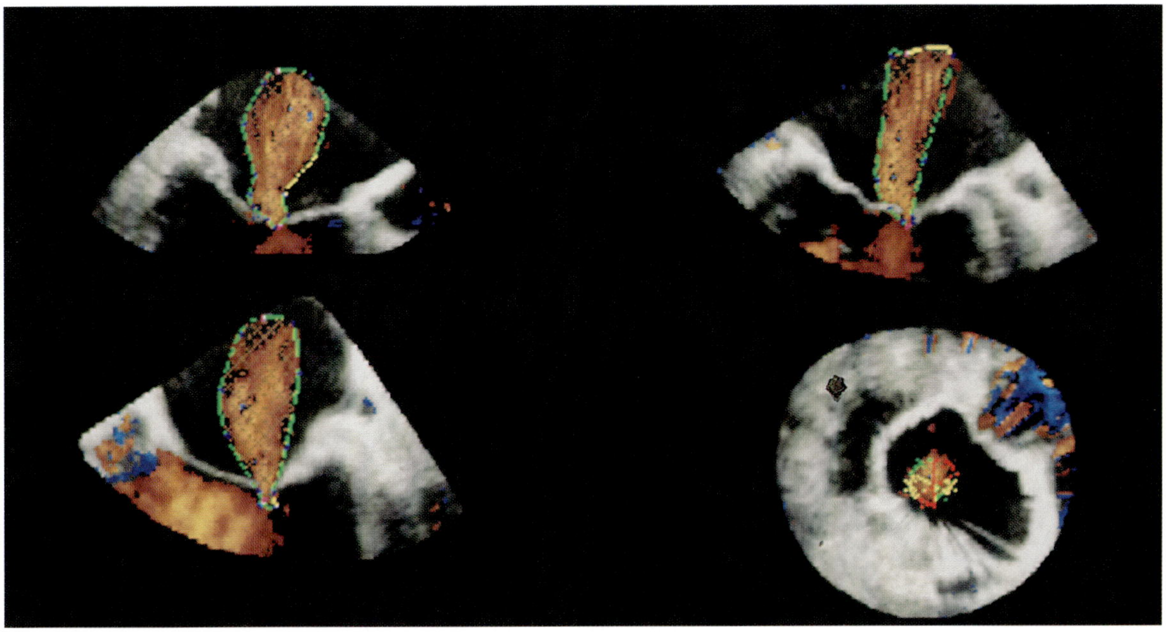

Figure 16. Reconstructed central jet of mitral regurgitation shown in three views. The outer contour of the jet is manually identified in order to obtain a dynamic wireframe display of the jet. This enables quantification of the volume of the regurgitant volume. From Lissa Sugeng, MD, Ivan Godoy, MD, Kirk T. Spencer, MD, Jim Bednarz, BS, Lynn Weinert, BS, and Roberto M. Lang, MD.

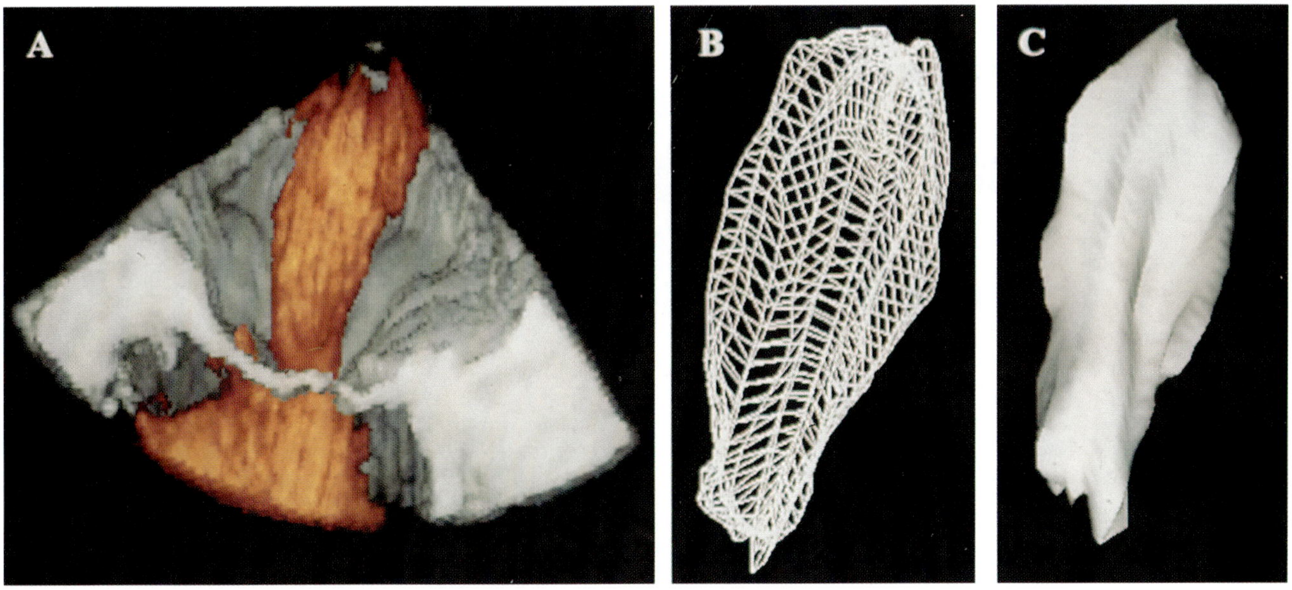

Figure 17. (**A**) Reconstructed central jet of mitral regurgitation. (**B**) Wireframe display of the jet. (**C**) Surface reconstructed jet. From Lissa Sugeng, MD, Ivan Godoy, MD, Kirk T. Spencer, MD, Jim Bednarz, BS, Lynn Weinert, BS, and Roberto M. Lang, MD.

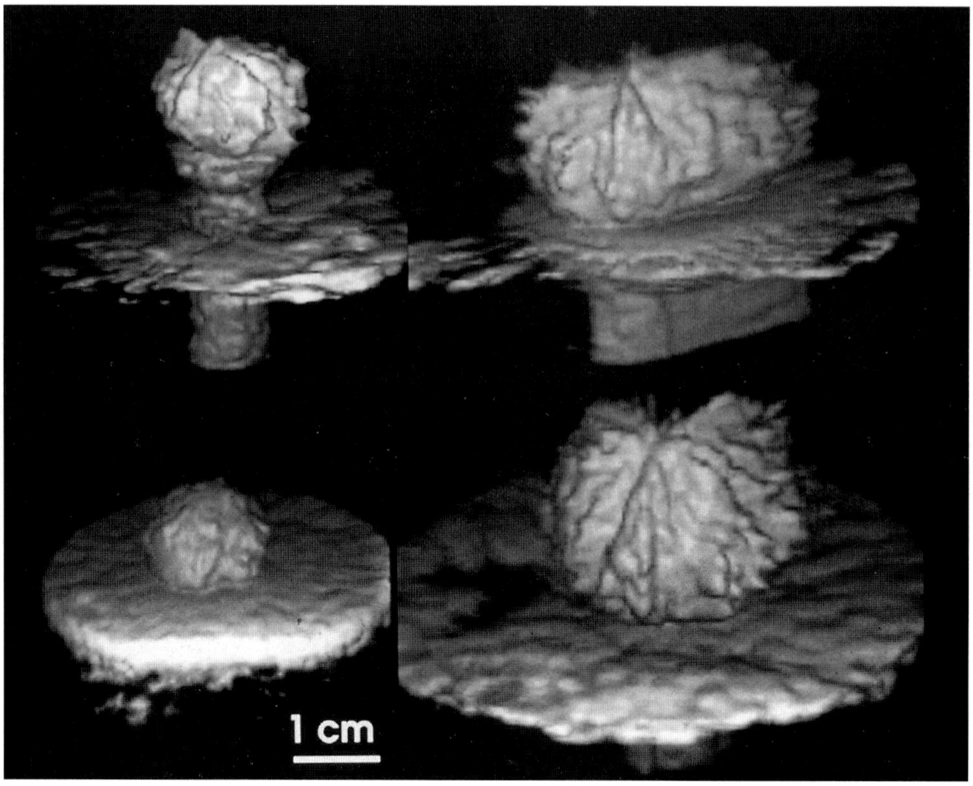

Figure 18. Volume-rendered reconstructions of proximal convergence zones. Black-and-white reconstruction of color Doppler images acquired in vitro. Flow direction from above to below. **Upper left:** Proximal isovelocity surface area (PISA) zone through a pyramidal orifice. **Lower left:** PISA zone at a small circular orifice. **Upper right:** PISA zone at a slit-like orifice. **Lower right:** PISA zone at a large circular orifice. Note the nonhemispherical shape of both upper PISA zones. From Andreas Franke, MD, Harald P. Kühl, MD, and Peter Hanrath, MD.

Suggested Reading List

1. Schott JR, Moos S, Raqueno R, et al. 4-dimensional reconstruction from 2-dimensional echocardiograms. (Abstract) *Circulation* 1986;74:11–144.
2. Wixson SE, Nanda NC. Display of 4-dimensional ultrasound data. (Abstract) *J Ultras in Med* 1986;5:(9)136.
3. Wixson SE, Nanda NC, Iliceto S, et al. Evaluation of aortic dissection by color Doppler echocardiography. (Abstract) Annual Scientific Assembly of Southern Medical Association, Nov. 1986, Atlanta, GA.
4. Ghosh A, Schott JR, Moos S, et al. Merging color Doppler imaging with 4-dimensional echocardiogram reconstruction. (Abstract) *J Am Coll Cardiol* 1987;III-A.
5. Schott JR, Moos S, Raqueno R, et al. Feasibility analysis of 3-dimensional reconstruction of color Doppler flow velocities. (Abstract) *J Am Coll Cardiol* 1987;III-214A.
6. Schott JR, Raqueno R, Moos S, et al. Successful merging of 3-dimensional color flow velocities and 3-dimensional reconstruction of the left ventricle. (Abstract) *Circulation* 1987;76:IV-527.
7. Schott JR, Raqueno R, Ghosh A, et al. Four-dimensional cardiac blood flow analysis using color Doppler echocardiography. In: Nanda NC (Ed), Textbook of Color Doppler Echocardiography. Philadelphia: Lea and Febiger 1989, pp. 332–341.
8. Li A, Wang XF, Xie M, et al. Dynamic three-dimensional reconstruction of abnormal intracardiac blood flow. *Echocardiography* 1997;14:375–381.
9. De Simone R, Glombitza G, Vahl CF, et al. Three-dimensional Doppler. Techniques and clinical applications. [letter; comment]. *Eur Heart J* 1999;20:619–627.
10. Ansingkar K, Nanda NC, Aaluri SR, et al. Transesophageal three dimensional color Doppler echocardiographic assessment of valvular and paravalvular mitral prosthetic regurgitation. *Echocardiography* 2000;17:579–583.
11. De Simone R, Glombitza G, Vahl CF, et al. Three-dimensional color Doppler flow reconstruction and its clinical applications. [Review] [18 refs]. *Echocardiography* 2000;17(8):765–771.
12. De Simone R, Glombitza G, Vahl CF, et al. Three-dimensional color Doppler reconstruction of intracardiac blood flow in patients with different heart valve diseases. *Am J Cardiol* 2000;86(12):1343–1348.
13. Irvine T, Li XN, Rusk R, et al. Three dimensional colour Doppler echocardiography for the characterisation and quantification of cardiac flow events. [Review] [37 refs]. *Heart* 2000;84(Suppl.2):II2–6.
14. Guo Z, Boughner DR, Dietrich JM, et al. Quantitative assessment of in vitro jets based on three-dimensional color Doppler reconstruction. *Ultrasound Med & Biol* 2001;27(2):235–243.
15. Mukhtar O, Horton Jr. CJ, Nanda NC, et al. Transesophageal color Doppler three dimensional echocardio-

graphic detection of prosthetic aortic valve dehiscence: Correlation with surgical findings. *Echocardiography* 2001;18:393–397.
16. Orta RG, Garcia-Fernandez MA, Moreno M, et al. Dynamic three-dimensional evaluation of intracardiac flow. *Revista Portuguesa Cardiologia* 2001;20(Suppl.1):I57–63.
17. Ansingkar KG, Nanda NC, Nekkanti R, et al. Transesophageal three dimensional color Doppler echocardiographic reconstruction of the left vertebral artery. *Echocardiography* (In press, October 2001).
18. Miller AP, Aaluri SR, Mukhtar OM, et al. Three-dimensional color Doppler transpharyngeal echocardiographic reconstruction of the left common, internal and external carotid arteries. *Echocardiography* (In press, May 2002).
19. Horton Jr. CJ, Nanda NC, Nekkanti R, et al. Prosthetic aortic valve abscess producing total right coronary artery occlusion: Diagnosis by transesophageal three-dimensional echocardiography. *Echocardiography* (In press, August 2002).

Chapter 11

Three-Dimensional Color Doppler Imaging

Raffaele De Simone, MD, Gerald Glombitza, PhD, Ivo Wolf, PhD, Christian Friedrich Vahl, MD, Hans Peter Meinzer, PhD, and Siegfried Hagl, MD

Introduction

Three-dimensional (3D) echocardiography[1–4] has been mainly used for assessing intracardiac anatomy[5–8] and for measuring heart chamber volumes.[9–15] Recently, the 3D visualization of Doppler flow signals has been performed by using Doppler data in digital format prior to converting them into colors.[16–18] This chapter includes the basics of the acquisition methods and the procedure for 3D color Doppler reconstruction. The examples include examinations covering the most important heart pathologies causing blood flow disturbances. The case studies compare the conventional multiplanar examinations at different rotation angles and the 3D color Doppler reconstructions visualized from different angle views.

The visualization and quantification of intracardiac blood flow has always been a challenging task for the cardiologist. The advent of cardiac angiography into clinical practice, which allowed for the study of intracardiac blood flow abnormalities, greatly improved the understanding of valvular disease.[19] The advent of color Doppler flow imaging substantially improved the clinical diagnosis of cardiovascular diseases by providing the physician with a sort of noninvasive angiography for assessing blood flow abnormalities.[20–21] Today color Doppler flow imaging is the most widely used diagnostic tool for assessing intracardiac blood flow although most cardiac valve diseases produce asymmetrical flow jets which are so complex geometrically that they cannot be entirely visualized and measured by conventional two-dimensional (2D) imaging.[22–24] We have developed a new technique for 3D reconstruction of color Doppler flow signals from the digital data directly derived from the echo scanner.[16–18] The possibility of processing digital data allowed us to separately visualize the Doppler signals and the cardiac structures. This approach also made it possible to display 3D color Doppler images in original color coding, and suggested new methods for the quantitative assessment of regurgitant flows.[25]

Three-dimensional color Doppler enhances the diagnostic value of color Doppler by overcoming the spatial limitation of 2D imaging techniques. Three-dimensional Doppler provides unique information about the actual extension, direction, origin, and size of intracardiac flows. In addition, new patterns of intracardiac blood flow, not yet described previously, can be observed and studied by this technique.[25]

Methods

The echocardiographic data were acquired by transesophageal and transthoracic multiplanar examinations with two commercially available scanners: Sonos 2500 and 5500 (Hewlett-Packard, Andover, MA). A multiplane transesophageal probe (5 MHz) and a conventional transthoracic probe (2.5 MHz) were used for the study (Figures 1 and 2). The rotation of the transducer was accomplished with 2° increments. The digital data from 2D echocardiography, which are displayed as a gray scale, and the data from 2D Doppler flow signals, displayed as a color palette, were separately stored on magneto-optical disks in their original formats for further processing and 3D reconstruction. The data obtained by rotational acquisition were first rearranged in a cartesian system according to their temporal and spatial coordinates. The Doppler data, stored on magneto-optical disks, contains information

Acknowledgments. This project discussed in this chapter is part of the "Sonderforschungsbereich 414—Teilprojekt H1," supported by the German National Foundation for Scientific Research.

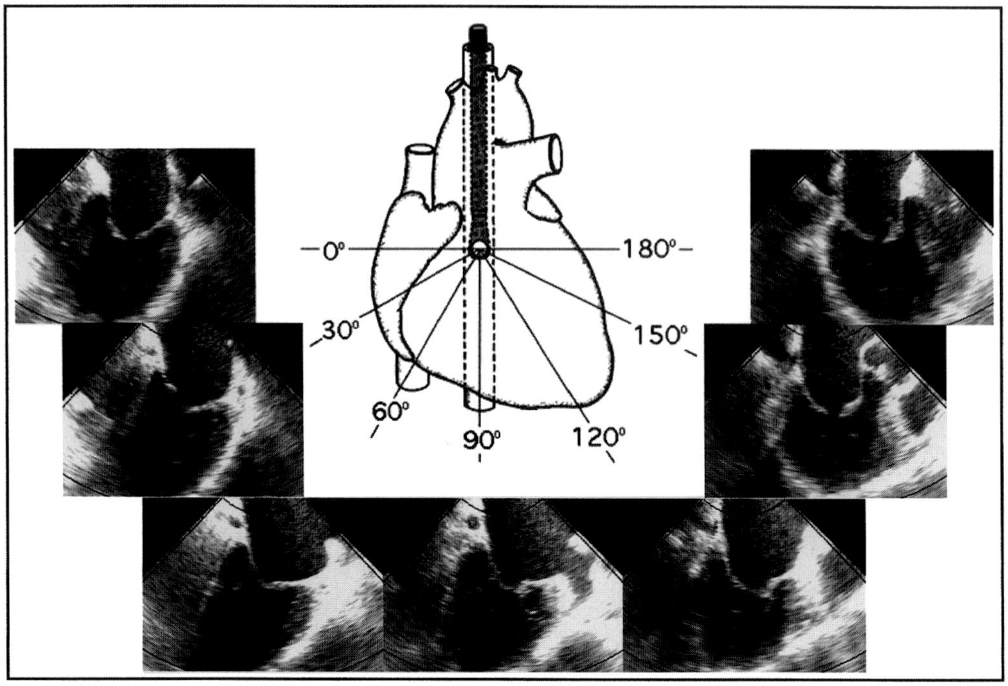

Figure 1. Multiplanar transesophageal echocardiography. Today almost all transesophageal probes are equipped with multiplanar transducers with which a complete series of intermediate planes from 0° to 180° can be viewed. This figure shows the left ventricle and the mitral valve viewed from each rotation angle at 30° steps.

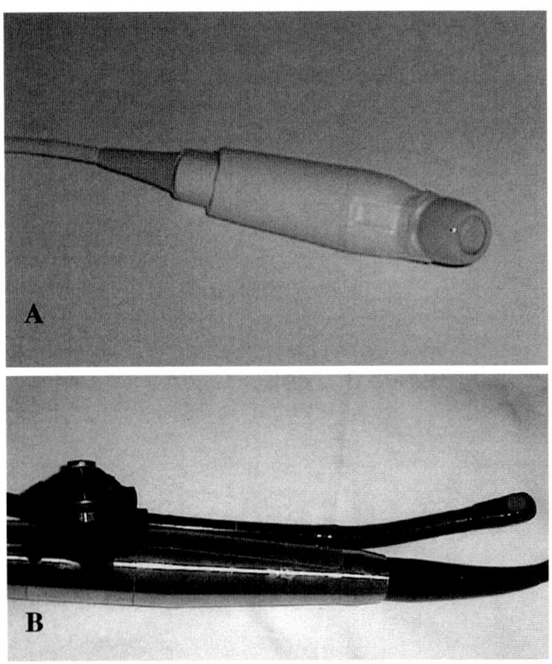

Figure 2. Multiplane transthoracic (**A**) and transesophageal (**B**) transducers. The rotation of the imaging plane is steered directly by the echo scanner (Hewlett-Packard, Andover, MA).

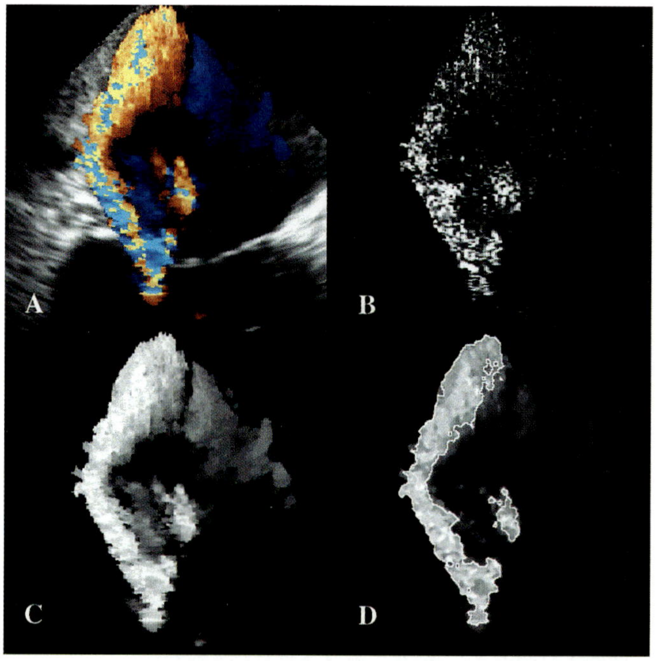

Figure 3. Different steps of the segmentation procedure. **(A)** Two-dimensional Doppler showing a typical, turbulent, high-velocity regurgitant jet. **(B)** Extraction of turbulence data (variance). **(C)** Display of velocity data. **(D)** The regurgitant jet has been automatically segmented and displayed.

on velocity and variance separately. The two values are stored together in 1 byte: the resolution for these values was 5-bit for the velocity and 3-bit for the variance. This 1-byte value is used by the echo machine for encoding Doppler data in colors. The transformed data set was post-processed by a median filtering. An entropy-minimizing algorithm[26] that separates turbulent and high-velocity components by setting a threshold value was used for segmenting the abnormal turbulent intracardiac flows, i.e., the "jets." This transformation was automatically performed over the whole 3D data set (Figure 3).

The 3D reconstructions of Doppler data were obtained by means of the "Heidelberg Raytracing Model" (HRM),[27–28] an algorithm initially developed for computer tomography and magnetic resonance images. Compared to other algorithms, such as maximum intensity projection or surface shading, this method enhances the 3D perception because two light sources are used for the virtual illumination. Finally, the Doppler data were visualized with the color encoding as presented by conventional 2D Doppler, by using the same color map used by the echo machine.

This chapter shows extensive examples covering the most important heart pathologies causing blood flow disturbances. The figures compare the conventional multiplanar examinations at different rotation angles and the 3D color Doppler reconstructions visualized from different angle views. In addition, the clinical application of 3D color Doppler for quantitative assessment of mitral regurgitation will be discussed.

The acquisition time of the echocardiographic data ranged from 50 seconds to 4 minutes, 15 seconds (mean acquisition time was 1 minute, 54 seconds). Adequate reconstructions of Doppler signals were achieved in all patients. The 3D reconstructions and jet volume measurements were obtained in 3 to 5 minutes according to the different angle resolutions.

Examples of Three-Dimensional Color Doppler

Mitral Regurgitation.

Three-Dimensional color Doppler allowed for the 3D and four-dimensional (4D) visualization of mitral regurgitant flows and for a classification according to their spatial distribution. The regurgitant jets were visualized in 3D by showing the systolic frame with the largest jet volume. In patients with central jets, the spatial distribution and the degree of mitral regurgitation can also be assessed by 2D imaging since its geometry is well predictable. In contrast, the 3D reconstruction of more complex mitral regurgitant jets renders 3D images that cannot be "mentally" conceived even by the most experienced examiner. In patients with eccentric jets due to mitral valve prolapse, two main patterns of regurgitant jets can be distinguished according to the 3D Doppler images: (1) those deriving from the posterior leaflet prolapse, and (2) those arising from the anterior leaflet prolapse. The regurgitant jets coming out from the posterior leaflet were directed along the atrial surface of the anterior leaflet and could be compared to a "cylinder" or to a "tongue" of flow oriented parallel to the main mitral annulus plane, according to the shape of the regurgitant orifice. A circular regurgitant orifice generates jets with a "cylinder" pattern (Figure 4); elliptical regurgitant orifices produce jets with the "tongue" pattern. The regurgitant jets coming out from the anterior leaflet also showed two different patterns.

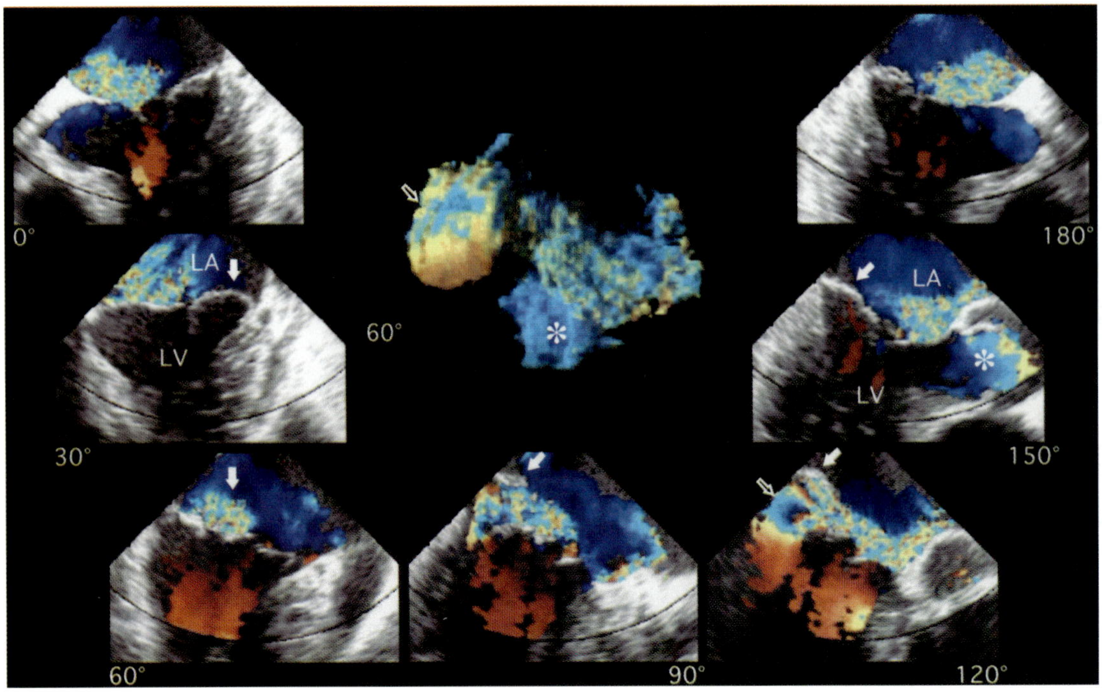

Figure 4. Three-dimensional reconstruction of color Doppler flow data. Mitral regurgitant jet in a patient with posterior mitral valve prolapse. This jet shows a "cylindrical" pattern. The prolapse of the posterior leaflet can be clearly observed at the multiplanar examinations from 30° to 150° (arrows). The main direction of the jet can be visualized at 120°, since this view cuts the jet longitudinally. The multiplanar view at 60° allows for an indirect estimation of the roughly circular shape of the regurgitant orifice, since it intersects the regurgitant jet transversally close to its origin. The shape of the proximal isovelocity region of the jet proximal to the regurgitant orifice can be clearly observed (open arrows). LA = left atrium; LV = left ventricle; * = left ventricular ejection flow.

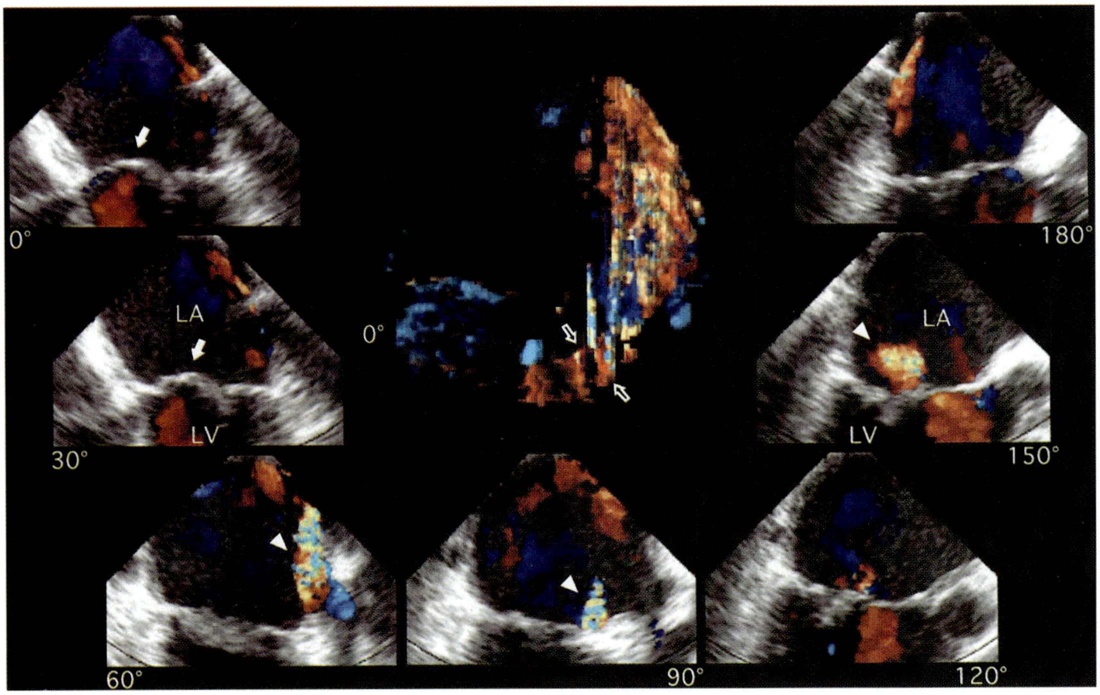

Figure 5. Anterior mitral valve prolapse. The regurgitant jet has a "spiral" pattern: it is directed perpendicular to the mitral annulus, then it forms an arch according to the curvature of the left atrial wall. The prolapse of the anterior mitral leaflet can be observed at 0° and 30° (arrows). The initial portion of the jet, immediately distal to the regurgitant orifice, is thin (open arrows) and reveals a small degree of regurgitation. The transversal section of the jet proximal to its origin has a circular shape. There is no single multiplanar examination that can visualize this jet in its entirety: only small portions of the jet (arrowheads) can be observed at 60°, 90°, and 150°. LA = left atrium; LV = left ventricle.

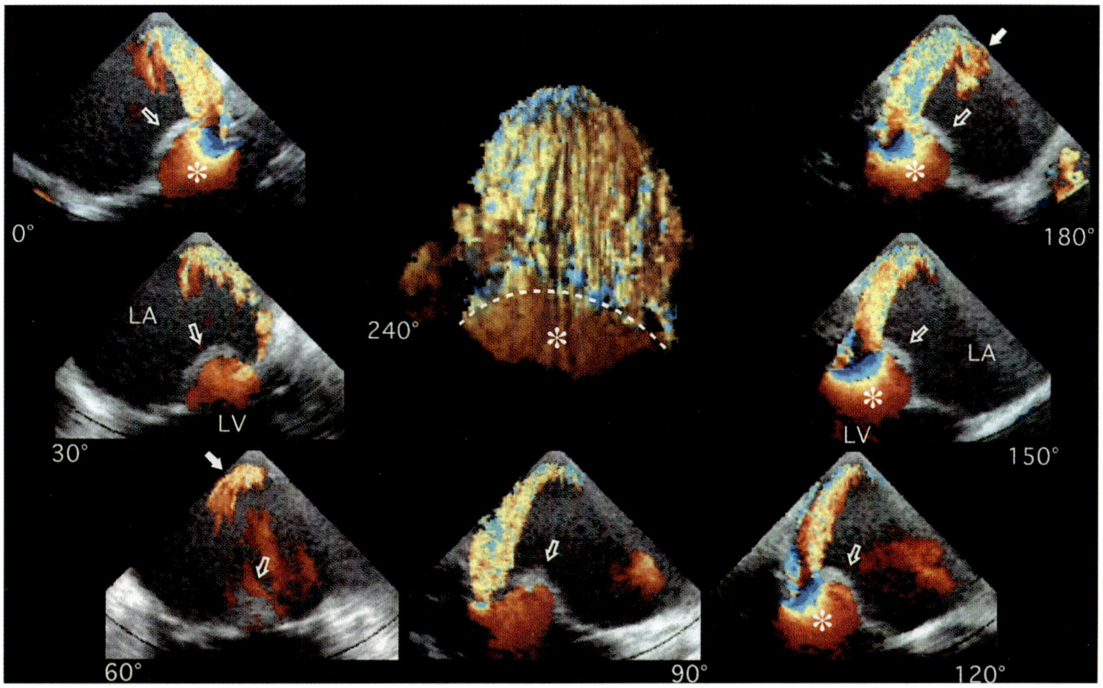

Figure 6. Severe mitral regurgitation in a patient with anterior mitral valve prolapse. The regurgitant jet has a "spoon" shape. The three-dimensional views at 240° show the concave face of the spoon. The origin of the jet can be clearly seen in the three-dimensional view at 240°. The dashed line separates the edge between the proximal isovelocity flow region (*) from the turbulent regurgitant jet, and hence, it also delineates the shape of the regurgitant orifice. The origin of this jet, which can be also observed in almost all multiplanar views, is approximately elliptical with a wide longitudinal diameter, and the regurgitant volume is accordingly large. The regurgitant jet spreads laterally against the atrial wall and hits the roof of the left atrium (arrows). The prolapse of the anterior mitral leaflet can be observed in all multiplanar views from 0° to 180° (open arrows). LA = left atrium; LV = left ventricle.

The first, due to a circular regurgitant orifice, appears like a "spiral" with a thin initial portion perpendicular to the annulus plane; these jets impinge the roof of the left atrium and curve their directions to form an arch according to the curvature of the atrial wall (Figure 5). The second pattern, due to elliptical regurgitant orifices, includes jets with a wide and relatively short initial portion, parallel to the annulus plane; they strike the posterior atrial wall and spread laterally, like a "fan" or a "spoon," according to the lateral curvature of the atrial walls (Figure 6). Other irregular shapes of the regurgitant orifice produce different patterns of regurgitant jet flows. Despite these 3D images have been obtained during a time delay, they are still able to provide unique geometrical information and reveal origin, direction, shape, extension and size of regurgitant jets. They provide a powerful tool for semiquantitative assessment of mitral regurgitation. In addition, although the relevance of the regurgitant jet volume as an indirect index of mitral regurgitation has been demonstrated in a clinical study,[16–18] this issue remains controversial and deserves further in vitro investigations.

Tricuspid Regurgitation

Tricuspid valve regurgitation is mostly due to the right ventricular enlargement and to the consequent dilatation of the valve annulus, generally secondary to left heart myocardial or valvular dysfunction (Figure 7). The tricuspid regurgitant jets arise from the incomplete systolic coaptation of the leaflets according to the degree of right ventricular or annular dilatation. The 3D reconstruction of color Doppler flow signals from the tricuspid valve requires particular transesophageal views that specially align the direction of the ultrasound beam to the direction of the regurgitant flow. The rotation axis of the multiplanar examinations should be set so that it intersects perpendicularly the tricuspid valve annulus as close as possible to the center. Nonetheless, due to the greater depth of the ultrasound signals originating from the tricuspid valve, the quality and intensity of the Doppler data is worse than those obtained from the mitral valve.

Mitral Stenosis

The diastolic left ventricular filling flow through the mitral and tricuspid valve is normally displayed as laminar flow at color Doppler. It consists of slow velocity flow with minimal variance. The obstruction to the left ventricular filling, caused by the inadequate diastolic separation of the mitral valve leaflets and/or by thickening of the subvalvular apparatus, produces acceleration of the diastolic blood flow and consequently

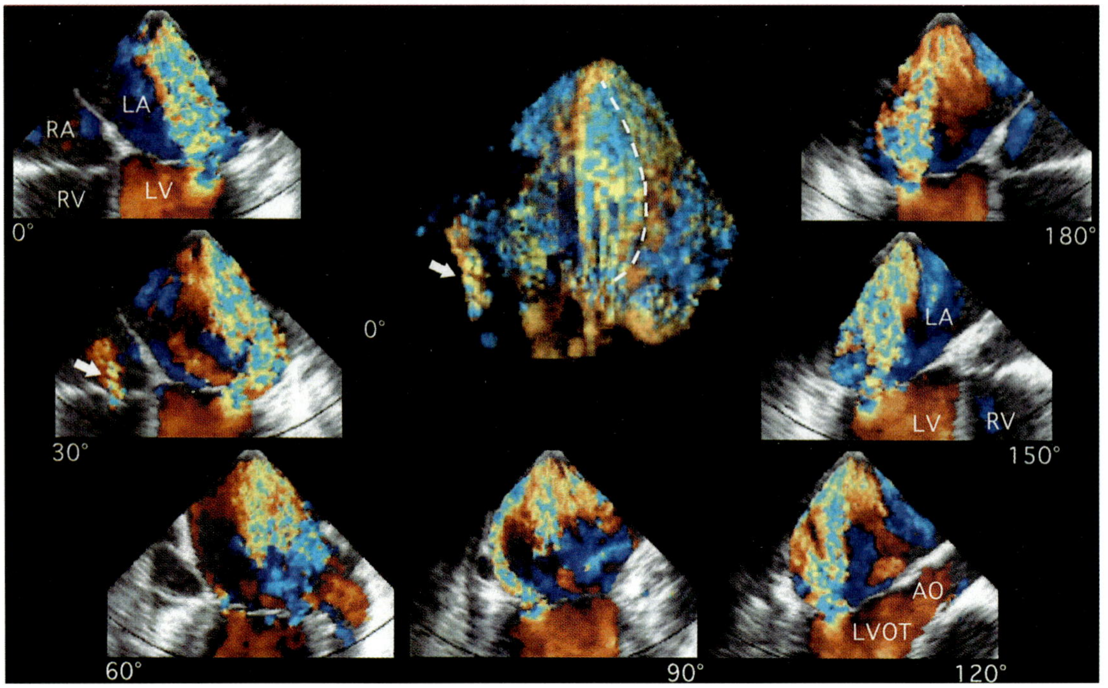

Figure 7. Small tricuspid valve regurgitation in a patient with severe mitral regurgitation. The tricuspid regurgitant jet (arrows) can only be observed in the view at 30°, since the rotation axis is not perfectly oriented towards the tricuspid valve during the multiplanar examination. The mitral regurgitant flow jet has a "spoon" pattern. The left atrium is enlarged. The three-dimensional views at 0° and 90° show the convex face (dashed lines) of the mitral jet. The origin of the mitral jet and the proximal isovelocity flow region (*), which can be clearly observed in the multiplanar views from 0° to 30° and from 90° to 180°, is approximately elliptical with a wide longitudinal diameter, and the regurgitant volume is accordingly large. The regurgitant jet spreads laterally against the atrial wall and hits the roof of the left atrium. LA = left atrium; LV = left ventricle; RA = right atrium; RV = right ventricle; LVOT = left ventricular outflow tract; AO = aortic valve.

a turbulent flow pattern distal to the mitral orifice (Figure 8). The flow proximal to the stenotic orifice also shows the typical "proximal isovelocity region," due to the blood flow acceleration. Three-dimensional color Doppler may be helpful for estimating the degree and for disclosing the location of the diastolic flow obstruction.

Aortic Regurgitation

The assessment of the aortic regurgitant flow by conventional color Doppler does not provide any reliable quantitative parameter for evaluating the degree of aortic regurgitation. The length, the width and the size of the regurgitant jet have been proposed for assessing the degree of aortic regurgitation, but the clinical value of these parameters has never been validated. Three-dimensional color Doppler imaging only allows for a more accurate visualization of the spatial spreading of the aortic regurgitation into the left ventricle. Higher degrees of aortic regurgitation may hinder the left ventricular diastolic filling, causing functional mitral stenosis (Figure 9). The extent to which the diastolic filling of the left ventricle is hindered by the regurgitant jet can be clearly studied by 3D color Doppler. The degree of diastolic obstruction may be a useful index for the severity of aortic regurgitation.

Aortic Stenosis

The study of the blood flow dynamics distal to a stenotic aortic valve has been the object of numerous investigations aiming to assess the effective aortic valve opening orifice. The planimetry of the "vena contracta", i.e., the area of a section of the flow immediately distal to the stenotic orifice, has been proposed as an index of the aortic opening area. However, since the leaflet separation of a highly calcified stenotic aortic valve has a very irregular shape, the clinical application of these experimental studies has not been yet validated. Three-dimensional color Doppler has a big potential for studying this issue, but the theoretical limitations regarding the quantitative assessment of the severity of the aortic stenosis still need further investigations. Three-dimensional color Doppler allows for a more accurate visualization of the spatial spreading of the turbulent post-stenotic flow in the ascending aorta (Figure 10).

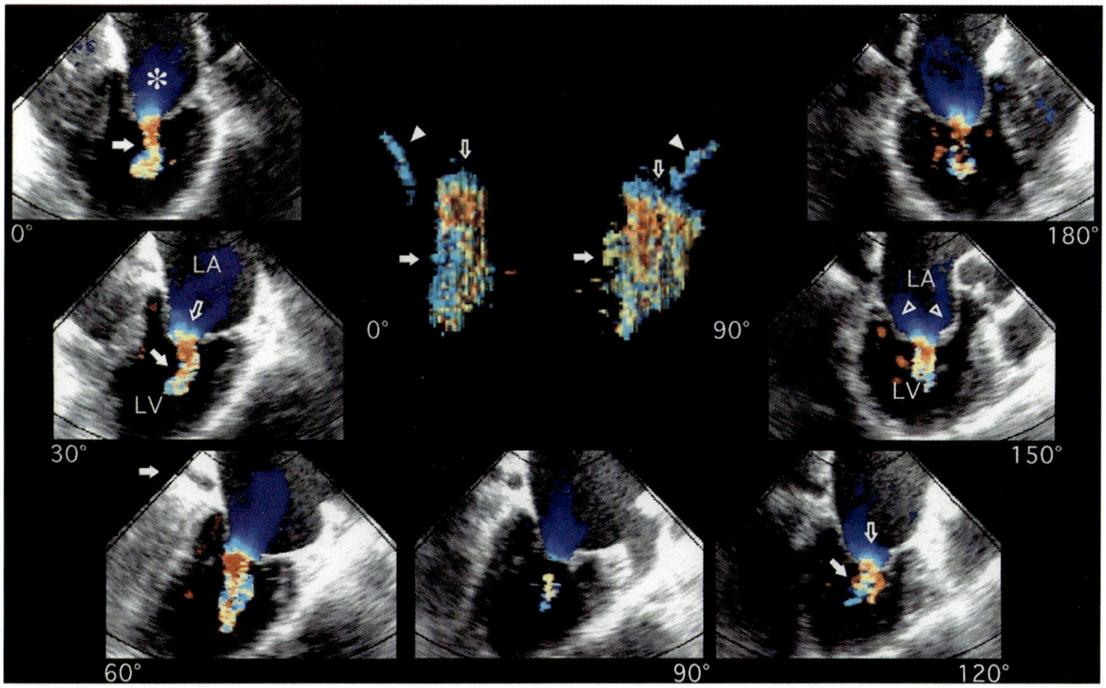

Figure 8. Diastolic filling flow through a stenotic mitral valve. The laminar flow (*) in the left atrium, proximal to the mitral orifice, turns into turbulent flow (arrows) after the obstruction. The proximal isovelocity region (open arrows) can be observed in the three-dimensional images. The "laminar" diastolic flow has been cut off by the segmentation procedure, which exclusively displays the high velocity and the turbulent portions of the flow. A small aortic regurgitation can be observed in the three-dimensional Doppler recontructions (arrowheads). The left atrium is enlarged. The multiplanar view at 150° shows the typical "doming" of the mitral leaflets (open arrows), which appear only moderately thickened. The shape of the diastolic jet suggests that the flow obstruction also occurs at the level of the subvalvular apparatus. LA = left atrium; LV = left ventricle.

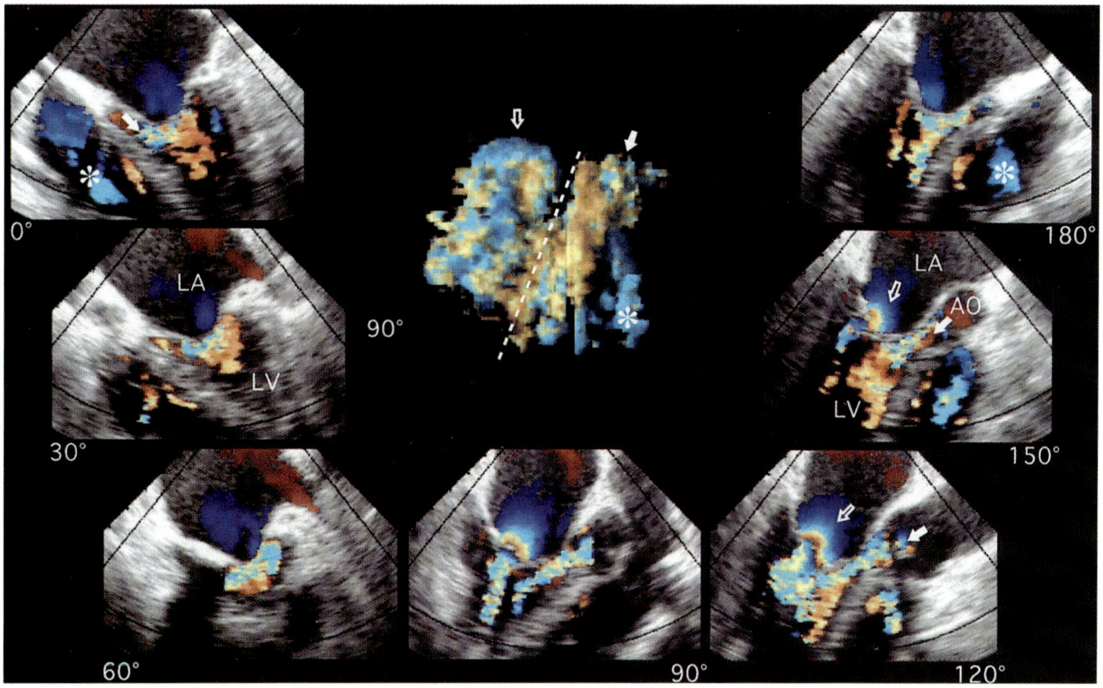

Figure 9. Aortic valve regurgitation and diastolic obstruction to left ventricular filling. The aortic regurgitant jet (arrows) spreads into the left ventricular outflow tract in diastole; it is directed toward the anterior mitral leaflet and causes obstruction to left ventricular filling flow. The extent to which the diastolic filling of the left ventricle is hindered by the regurgitant jet is an index for the severity of aortic regurgitation. This phenomenon corresponds to the "Austin Flint" murmur on auscultation, described by clinical cardiologists as a useful prognostic sign of aortic regurgitation. With three-dimensional color Doppler the spatial relationship and the degree of interference between the two diastolic flows (dashed line) can be appreciated. The diastolic filling of the left ventricle shows a proximal flow acceleration before the mitral valve (open arrows); the flow is laminar in the left atrium and becomes turbulent just distal to the mitral valve obstruction. The diastolic ventricular filling of right ventricle is laminar (*). LA = left atrium; LV = left ventricle; AO = aortic valve.

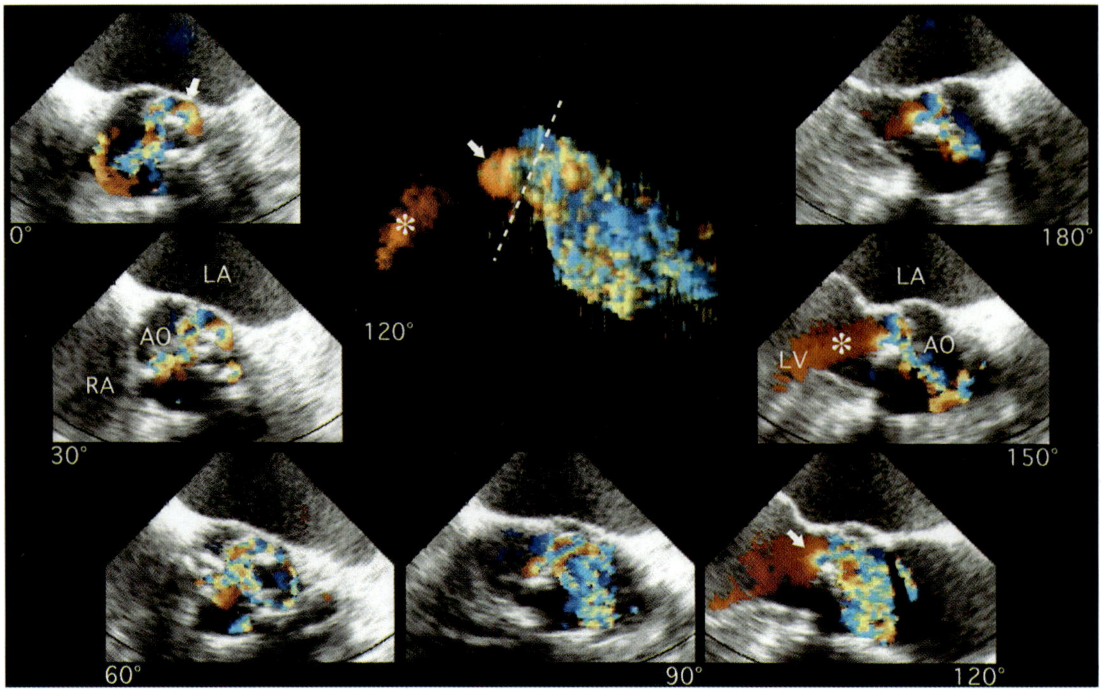

Figure 10. Aortic valve stenosis. The multiplanar acquisition has been obtained from a basal transesophageal view at the level of the aortic valve. The ejection flow in the left ventricular outflow tract is laminar (*), becoming turbulent distal to the stenotic aortic valve. The "vena contracta" is very short due to the lateral spreading into the aorta immediately after the stenosis. The cross-sectional area of the vena contracta can be assessed at the level indicated by the dashed line. The multiplanar examinations from 120° to 180° show the proximal flow acceleration (arrow). The transversal view of the aortic valve clearly shows the calcification of the aortic leaflets and the highly irregular shape of the opening orifice (multiplanar views at 30° and 60°). LA = left atrium; RA = right atrium; LV = left ventricle; AO = aortic valve; ASC = ascending aorta.

Other Flow Patterns

Reverse Pulmonary Venous Flow

Moderate mitral valve regurgitation with reverse systolic venous pulmonary flow is shown in Figure 11. The assessment of mitral regurgitation severity includes the examination of the flow in the pulmonary veins by pulsed wave Doppler. The finding of systolic flow inversion in the pulmonary veins has been considered a sign of a severe degree of mitral regurgitation. Nonetheless, if a regurgitant jet is directed specifically towards the entry of the pulmonary veins into the left atrium (LA), it may cause reverse pulmonary flow even in moderate degrees of mitral regurgitation. With 3D color Doppler the direction of these complex regurgitant jets and the flow in the pulmonary veins (*) can be studied and directly visualized. (LV = left ventricle).

Left Ventricular Outflow Obstruction

Left ventricular outflow tract obstruction due to systolic anterior motion (SAM) of the mitral valve is shown in Figure 12. The arrows show the point where the systolic motion of the anterior mitral leaflet causes obstruction to the left ventricular (LV) ejection flow. The anterior motion of the mitral leaflet also produces mitral valve regurgitation (open arrows). Mitral valve regurgitation due to the SAM has a high beat-to-beat variability and strongly depends on the loading conditions of the LV. The distal narrowing of the flow (arrowheads) shows impaired opening of the aortic valve (AO). The full extension of the ejection flow obstruction in the left ventricular outflow tract (LVOT) could not be entirely visualized by conventional two-dimensional color Doppler. (LA = left atrium).

Multiple Valvular Disease

A patient with multiple combined valvular diseases: aortic stenosis, mitral regurgitation and stenosis, pulmonary valve regurgitation, and tricuspid valve regurgitation, is shown in Figure 13. The aortic ejection flow (AS) after the stenosis can be observed in the 3D reconstruction from the view at 300°. The pulmonary ejection flow (PF) is turbulent and overlays the aortic ejection flow in the 3D view at 120°. Two thin tricuspid regurgitant jets (TR) can be observed in the multiplanar views at 0°. A small mitral regurgitant jet (MR) can be observed in the multiplanar examination at 150° and in the 3D reconstructions at 300°. The left and right atria are enlarged.

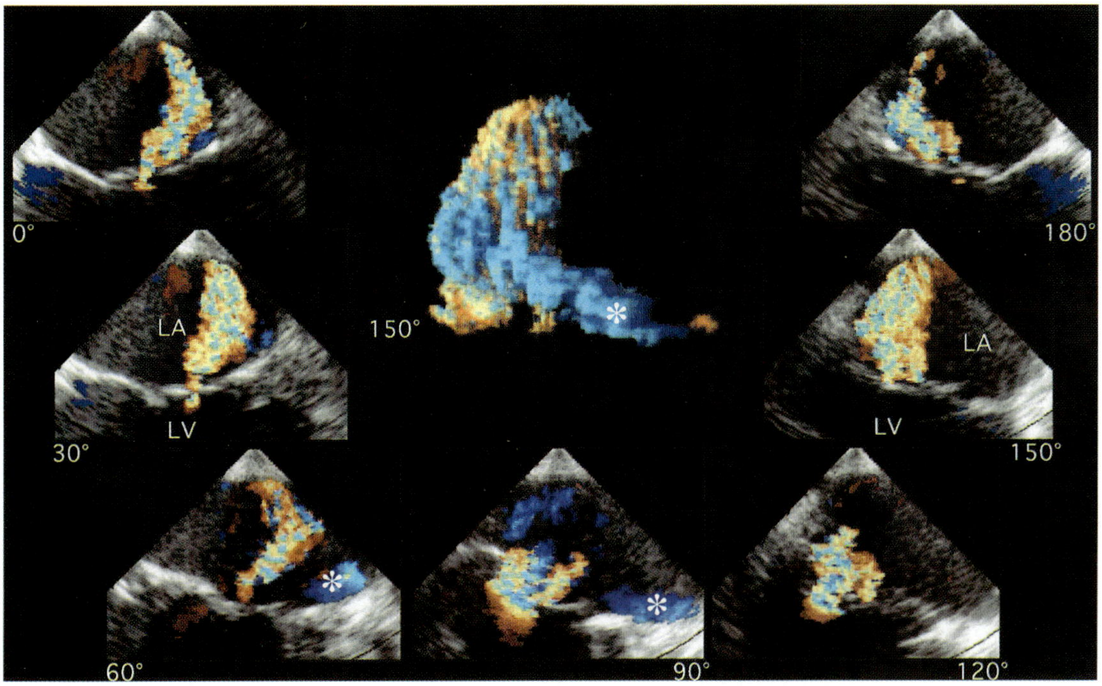

Figure 11. Moderate mitral valve regurgitation with reverse systolic venous pulmonary flow. See text for discussion.

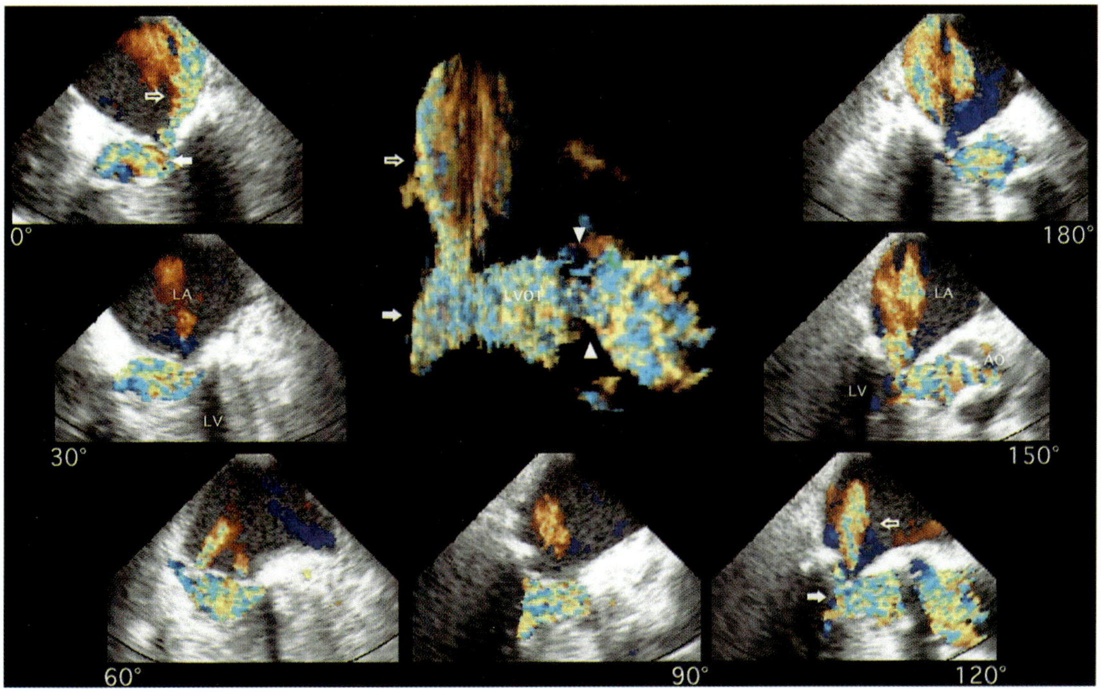

Figure 12. Left ventricular outflow tract obstruction due to systolic anterior motion (SAM) of the mitral valve. See text for discussion.

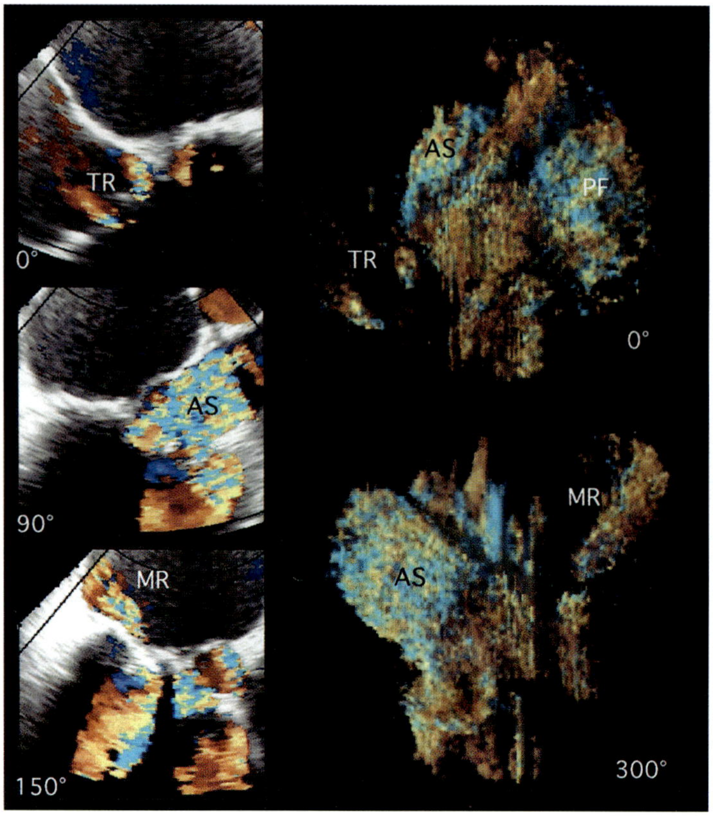

Figure 13. Patient with multiple combined valvular diseases: aortic stenosis, mitral regurgitation and stenosis, pulmonary valve regurgitation, and tricuspid valve regurgitation. See text for discussion.

Quantification of Regurgitation Jet Volumes

We have developed a technique for reconstructing color flow images in 3D by using Doppler data in digital format prior to converting them into colors. This approach allowed us to study the usefulness of a new automated procedure for segmentation and measurement of the turbulent portion of the jets. In addition, a new index of mitral regurgitation, 3D jet volumes, was compared to other clinical parameters for assessing mitral regurgitation. The segmentation technique used in this study is a fundamental step for objective measurements of the jet size. Two fully automated procedures are used for jet volume measurements: (1) the jet segmentation, based on the selection of turbulence and high-velocity components; and (2) the computation of all volume units (voxels) containing the selected Doppler information. Both procedures are independent of manual planimetry or subjective estimation and allow more precise measurements of 3D jet volumes.

The methods for assessing mitral regurgitation based on jet size at color Doppler assume that the spatial distribution of the jet velocities reflects or at least is proportional to the regurgitant volume. Although this is theoretically incorrect, almost all quantitative methods based on color Doppler incorporate this general assumption. Chen et al.[29] showed that the values of jet area in patients with asymmetrical jets were not correlated to regurgitant fractions as assessed by pulsed Doppler, and that the assessment of mitral regurgitation based on the systolic jet area underestimates the severity of valve regurgitation.

We studied 69 patients with isolated mitral regurgitation who underwent echocardiographic examinations during cardiac surgery. The severity of mitral regurgitation was assessed by left ventricular angiography on a scale from I to IV according to Sellers et al.[30] In addition, jet areas were measured by conventional planimetry of 2D color Doppler and mitral regurgitant volumes and fractions were measured by echocardiography and pulsed Doppler (Table 1). In all patients (n = 69), regression analysis of jet area did not show significant correlations with the regurgitant volume (r = 0.65), the regurgitant fraction (r = 0.62), and the angiographic grade of regurgitation (r = 0.63) (Table 1). In contrast, the jet volume showed significant correlations with the regurgitant volume (r = 0.92), the regurgitant fraction (r = 0.83), and the angiographic grade of regurgitation (r = 0.90) in all patients. In the group of patients with central jets (n = 30) both jet areas and jet volumes significantly correlated with the regurgitant volume (r = 0.84 and r = 0.87), the regurgitant fraction (r = 0.75 and r = 0.79), and the angiographic grade of regurgitation (r = 0.90 and r = 0.96). In the patients with eccentric jets (n = 39) no significant correlations between the jet area and the regurgitant volume (r = 0.50), the regurgitant fraction (r = 0.50), and the angiographic grade of regurgitation (r = 0.57) were found. In contrast, in the group of patients with eccentric jets the volume of regurgitant jets showed significant correlations with the regurgitant

Table 1.
Linear Regression Relations Between Mitral Regurgitation and Color Doppler Indexes.

Reg. Vol. vs. JA	*Reg. Vol. vs. JV*	*Reg. Fract. vs. JA*	*Reg. Fract. vs. JV*	*Angio vs. JA*	*Angio vs. JV*
All jets (*n*=*69*)					
r=0.65	r=0.92*	r=0.62	r=0.83*	r=0.63	r=0.90*
SEE=1.8	SEE=8.6	SEE=2.2	SEE=11.0	SEE=1.9	SEE=4.22
y=2.2+0.1x	y=−2.8+0.93x	y=2.4+9.2x	y=−2.0+98x	y=0.8+1.8x	y=−4.4+10.3x
Central jets (*n*=*30*)					
r=0.84*	r=0.87*	r=0.75*	r=0.79*	r=0.90*	r=0.96*
SEE=0.70	SEE=5.5	SEE=1.1	SEE=6.5	SEE=0.58	SEE=3.0
y=1.5+0.12x	y=−0.9+0.6x	y=2.8+7.0x	y=2.1+63.3x	y=1.5+1.5x	y=−4.7+10.1x
Eccentric jets (*n*=*39*)					
r=0.50	r=0.91*	r=0.50	r=0.77*	r=0.57	r=0.90*
SEE=2.78	SEE=9.67	SEE=2.69	SEE=12.9	SEE=2.2	SEE=10.7
y=3.3+0.09x	y=−1.4+0.91x	y=4+8.8x	y=0.7+94.2x	y=1.2+1.54x	y=−16.8+16x

Angio = Angiographic degree of mitral regurgitation; Reg. Fract. = regurgitant fraction (%); Reg. Vol. = Regurgitant Volume (mL); JA = jet area (cm2); JV = 3D jet volume (cm3); r = linear correlation coefficient.
SEE=standard error of estimate
*$p<0.01$; otherwise, p=NS.

volume (r = 0.91), the regurgitant fraction (r = 0.77), and the angiographic grade of regurgitation (r = 0.90).

Discussion

Until now, the 3D reconstruction of color Doppler signals in original color coding was still under investigation.[31–34] The regurgitant jets and cardiac structures have only been visualized in a gray-scale format,[32] and previous efforts to obtain 3D reconstructions of intracardiac flow jets in color coding required manual digitizing of Doppler flow signals.[33] The previous techniques used the video signals from the scanners, which did not allow a separate visualization of cardiac structures and flow. In addition, the analysis of single flow components and the differentiation of slow velocities from turbulent flows could not be performed. An additional limitation of these procedures include the fact that slow-velocity components and "displacement flow" cover the underlying jets and prevent the immediate visualization of the actual regurgitant flow. The advantages of the procedures based on the digital data include the possibility of processing velocity and turbulence data independently, which allowed to selectively visualize the flows with definite velocity patterns.

Three-dimensional Doppler enhances the diagnostic value of color Doppler by providing unique information about the actual extension, direction, origin, and size of intracardiac flow disturbances. In addition, new blood flow patterns of regurgitant jets, not yet described previously, can be observed and studied. Despite the fact that the issue regarding the correlation between the imaging of flow velocity, obtained by color Doppler, and the actual regurgitant flow volume remains unresolved, the clinical impact of 3D Doppler for the assessment of mitral regurgitant jets appears evident. The volume of mitral regurgitant jet provides a useful new parameter for quantitative assessment of mitral valve regurgitation, which is independent of manual planimetry or subjective estimation.

This chapter showed the first clinical applications of 3D color Doppler in patients with different heart valve disease. Although this technique is still under investigation, the new insights derived from the 3D study of intracardiac blood flow dynamics revealed a great impact on the clinical management of these patients. Three-dimensional color Doppler is the first noninvasive technique that not only provides unique new information on the spatial spreading of intracardiac flow disturbances, but also allows for a new quantitative assessment of mitral regurgitation.

References

1. Ghosh A, Nanda N, Maurer G. Three-dimensional reconstruction of echocardiographic images using the rotation method. *Ultrasound Med Biol* 1982;6:655–661.
2. Sheikh KH, Smith SW, von Ramm OT, et al. Real time three-dimensional echocardiography: Feasibility and initial use. *Echocardiography* 1991;9:677–687.
3. Pandian NG, Nanda N, Schwartz S, et al. Three-dimensional and four-dimensional transesophageal echocardiographic imaging of the heart and aorta in humans using a computed tomographic imaging probe. *Echocardiography* 1992;9:677–687.
4. Levine RA, Weyman AE, Handschumacher MD. Three-dimensional echocardiography: Techniques and applications. *Am J Cardiol* 1992;69:121H–130H.
5. Marx GR, Fulton DR, Pandian NG, et al. Delineation of site, relative size and dynamic geometry of atrial septal defects by real-time three-dimensional echocardiography. *J Am Coll Cardiol* 1995;25:482–490.
6. Vogel M, Ho SY, Anderson RH. Comparison of three dimensional echocardiographic findings with anatomical specimens of various congenitally malformed hearts. *Br Heart J* 1995;73:566–570.

7. Schwartz SL, Cao QL, Azevedo J, et al. Simulation of intraoperative visualization of cardiac structures and study of dynamic surgical anatomy with real-time three-dimensional echocardiography. *Am J Cardiol* 1994;73: 501–507.
8. Salustri A, Spitaels S, McGhie J, et al. Transthoracic three-dimensional echocardiography in adult patients with congenital heart disease. *J Am Coll Cardiol* 1995;26:759–767.
9. Gopal AS, Shen Z, Sapin PM, et al. Assessment of cardiac function by three-dimensional echocardiography compared with conventional noninvasive methods. *Circulation* 1995;92:842–853.
10. Jiang L, Siu SC, Handschumacher MD, et al. Three-dimensional echocardiography. In vivo validation for right ventricular volume and function. *Circulation* 1994; 89:2342–2350.
11. Siu SC, Rivera JM, Guerrero JL, et al. Three-dimensional echocardiography. In vivo validation for left ventricular volume and function. *Circulation* 1993;88:1715–1723.
12. Nosir YF, Fioretti PM, Vletter WB, et al. Accurate measurement of left ventricular ejection fraction by three-dimensional echocardiography. A comparison with radionuclide angiography. *Circulation* 1996;94:460–466.
13. Buck T, Schon F, Baumgart D, et al. Tomographic left ventricular volume determination in the presence of aneurysm by three-dimensional echocardiographic imaging. I: Asymmetric model hearts. *J Am Soc Echocardiogr* 1996;9:488–500.
14. Sapin PM, Schroeder KD, Smith MD, et al. Three-dimensional echocardiographic measurement of left ventricular volume in vitro: Comparison with two-dimensional echocardiography and cineventriculography. *J Am Coll Cardiol* 1993;22:1530–1537.
15. Sapin PM, Schroder KM, Gopal AS, et al. Comparison of two- and three-dimensional echocardiography with cineventriculography for measurement of left ventricular volume in patients. *J Am Coll Cardiol* 1994;24:1054–1063.
16. De Simone R, Glombitza G, Albers J, et al. Three-dimensional reconstruction and quantitative analysis of color Doppler jets in original color coding. *Echocardiography* 1997;14(6):S31.
17. De Simone R, Glombitza G, Vahl CF, et al. Three-dimensional Doppler. Techniques and clinical applications. *Eur Heart J* 1999;20:619–627.
18. De Simone R, Glombitza G, Vahl CF, et al. Three-dimensional color Doppler. A clinical study in patients with mitral regurgitation. J Am Coll Cardiol 1999;33: 1646–1654.
19. Sellers RD, Levy MJ, Amplatz L, et al. Left retrograde cardioangiography in acquired cardiac disease. *Am J Cardiol* 1964;14:432–442.
20. Stevenson JG, Kawabori I, Brandestini MA. Color-coded visualization of flow within ventricular septal defects. Implications for peak pulmonary artery pressure. *Am J Cardiol* 1982; 49:944 (Abstract).
21. Omoto R, Yokote Y, Takamoto S, et al. The development of real-time two-dimensional Doppler echocardiography and its significance in acquired valvular diseases with specific reference to the evaluation of valvular regurgitation. *Jpn Heart J* 1984;25:325–340.
22. Sahn DJ. Real-time two dimensional echocardiographic flow mapping. *Circulation* 1985;71:849–853.
23. Helmcke F, Nanda NC, Hsiung MC, et al. Color Doppler assessment of mitral regurgitation with orthogonal planes. *Circulation* 1987;75:175–183.
24. Miyatake K, Izumi S, Okamoto M, et al. Semiquantitative grading of severity of mitral regurgitation by real-time two-dimensional Doppler flow imaging technique. *J Am Coll Cardiol* 1986;7:82–88.
25. De Simone R, Glombitza G, Vahl CF, et al. Three-Dimensional Color Doppler: An Atlas of Intracardiac Flow Imaging. Armonk NY, Futura Publishing Company, 1999.
26. Pal NR, Pal SK. Entropic thresholding. Signal Processing 1989;16:1053–1058.
27. Meinzer HP, Meetz K, Scheppelmann D, et al. The Heidelberg Raytracing Model. *IEEE—Computer Graphics and Applications* 1991;6:34–43.
28. Vahl CF, Meinzer HP, Hagl S. Three-dimensional presentation of cardiac morphology. *J Thorac Cardiovasc Surg* 1991;39:198–204.
29. Chen C, Thomas JD, Anconina J, et al. Impact of impinging wall jet on color Doppler quantification of mitral regurgitation. *Circulation* 1991;84:712–720.
30. Sellers RD, Levy MJ, Amplatz L, et al. Left retrograde cardioangiography in acquired cardiac disease. *Am J Cardiol* 1964;14:432–442.
31. Yao J, Masani ND, Cao QL, et al. Clinical application of transthoracic volume-rendered three-dimensional echocardiography in the assessment of mitral regurgitation. *Am J Cardiol* 1998;82:189–196.
32. Delabays A, Sugeng L, Pandian NG, et al. Dynamic three-dimensional echocardiographic assessment of intracardiac blood flow jets. *Am J Cardiol* 1995;76:1053–1058.
33. Belohlavek M, Foley D, Gerber T, et al. Three-dimensional reconstruction of color Doppler jets in the human heart. *J Am Soc Ecocardiogr* 1994;7:553–560.
34. Bohs LN, Friemel BH, Kisslo J, et al. Three-dimensional flow images by reconstruction from two-dimensional vector velocity maps. *J Am Soc Echocardiogr* 1995; 8:915–923.

Suggested Reading List

1. De Simone R. Three-dimensional color Doppler. An atlas of intracardiac flow imaging. (Book and CD-ROM) Futura Publishing Co., Inc., Armonk, NY Armonk, New York, 1999.
2. De Simone R. Glombitza G, Vahl CF, et al. Three-dimensional Color Doppler Reconstruction of Intracardiac Blood Flow in Patients With Different Heart Valve Diseases. *Am J Cardiol,* 2000:86:1343–1348.
3. Lange A, Palka P, Nowicki A, et al. Three-dimensional echocardiographic evaluation of left ventricular volume: Comparison of Doppler myocardial imaging and standard gray-scale imaging with cineventriculography—an in vitro and in vivo study. *Am Heart J* 1998;135: 970–979.
4. Feigenbaum H. Three-dimensional ultrasonic imaging of blood flow. [letter; comment]. [Review] [9 refs]. *Eur Heart J* 1999;20:551–552.
5. Li X, Shiota T, Delabays A, et al. Flow convergence flow rates from 3-dimensional reconstruction of color Doppler flow maps for computing transvalvular regurgitant flows without geometric assumptions: An in vitro quantitative flow study. *J Am Soc Echocardiography* 1999;12: 1035–1044.
6. Berg S, Torp H, Haugen BO, et al. Volumetric blood flow measurement with the use of dynamic 3-dimensional ultrasound color flow imaging. *J Am Soc Echocardiography* 2000;13(5):393–402.

Chapter 12

Real-Time Three-Dimensional Echocardiography

John Oxaal

Concepts

Real-time volumetric imaging is "the acquisition and display of pulse echo information from a three-dimensional (3D) volume in real time without cardiac or respiratory gating" (Figure 1). Phased array principles are used in conjunction with receive mode parallel processing to rapidly steer the ultrasound beam over three dimensions (Figures 2A,B).

The two-dimensional (2D) phased array is used to steer and focus the ultrasound beam in both elevation and azimuth. This type of system scans a pyramidal volume that typically contains about 4100 lines at a rate of 30 volumes per second. Some of the more challenging problems in the development of real-time volumetric imaging are: the transducer, the enormous data acquisition rate, and the display of 3D data on a 2D screen. These problems are discussed below.

Transducers

Figure 3 depicts a typical transducer. The arrays are 2D phased arrays rather than the linear phased arrays of conventional systems. Some people call these 2D arrays "matrix arrays." Two-dimensional arrays allow electronic steering and focusing in both elevation and azimuth. These 2D arrays consist of approximately 2000 elements, 512 of which are connected. Two hundred fifty-six of the 512 elements are used to transmit and 256 are used to receive. This means that the cable connecting the transducer array to the system contains roughly 512 coaxial cables. The arrays measure approximately 14 mm on a side, so that they match the standard acoustic windows for cardiac applications.

The elements in the 2D (matrix) arrays are chosen so that the aperture is circularly symmetric. Circularly symmetric apertures, like annular arrays, have the unique property that the resolution is the same in all dimensions. So, unlike conventional 2D phased array ultrasound systems, the resolution is the same in elevation and azimuth.

Real-time volumetric ultrasound systems have 2.5 MHz matrix arrays, 3.5 MHz matrix arrays and a conventional 3.5 MHz phased array. New arrays, such as 5 MHz matrix arrays and 5 MHz TEE arrays, are in various phases of commercialization.

Beamformer

Remember that a conventional phased array uses all of the elements of the array to focus a beam of sound into the body. At every interface (e.g., the myocardium/blood interface or the valve/blood interface), a small percentage of the sound is reflected back toward the array and the rest of the sound is propagated still further into the body. The system uses sound that is echoed back to the transducer to produce a dot on the screen. The intensity of this dot is proportional to the difference in the acoustic impedences of the tissue structures at the interface. The phased array ultrasound system tracks the beam as it propagates through the body. By this mechanism a line with dots on it is produced. After echoes return from the periphery of the scan line, the system produces another scan line in a different direction. Over time, a number of lines with dots on them are produced. The eye fuses these lines with dots into an image. The eye also fuses images formed at a rate of 30 per second into smooth motion.

Since sound travels about 1540 meters per second in tissue about 200 ms are required to form each line of the scan. Therefore about 130 lines of the image can be formed about 30 times per second. Thus, it is the speed of sound that limits the rate at which lines of the image can be formed.

From Nanda NC and Sorrell VL: *Atlas of Three-Dimensional Echocardiography.* ©Futura Publishing Co., Inc, Armonk, NY, 2002.

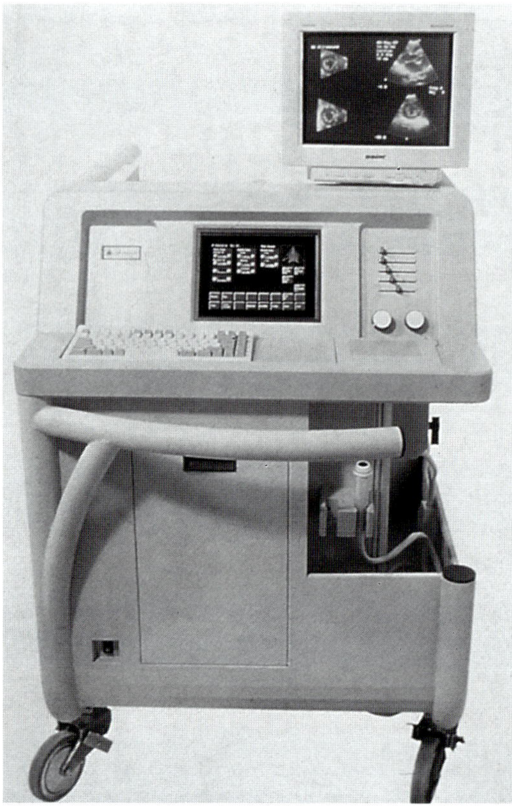

Figure 1. This is the ultrasound system developed to provide real-time, "on-line" three-dimensional imaging. Due to the advanced parallel processing responsibilities, this system is slightly larger than conventional ultrasound systems that only provide two-dimensional data.

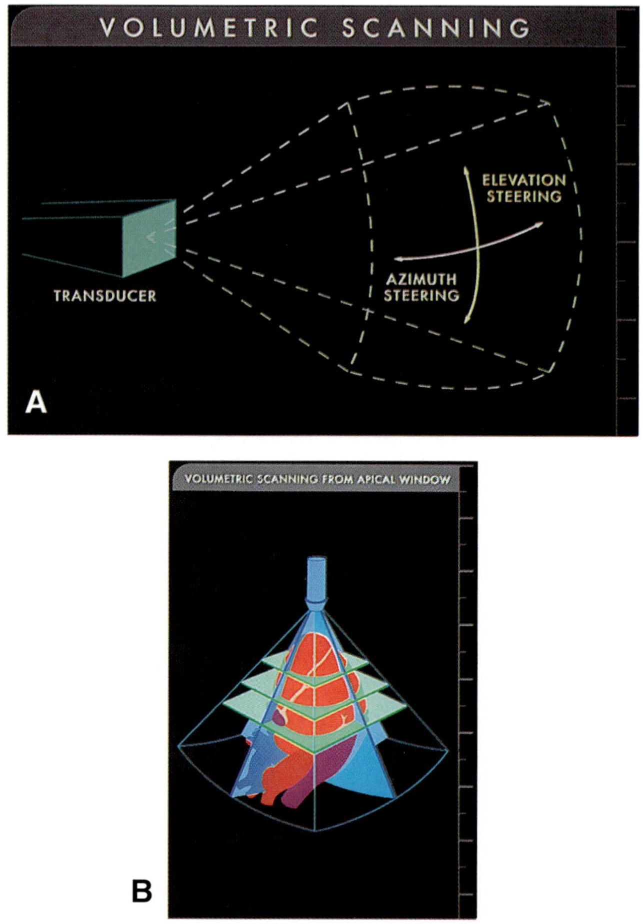

Figure 2. Receive mode parallel processing allows real-time scanning in both elevation (**A**) and azimuth (**B**) planes.

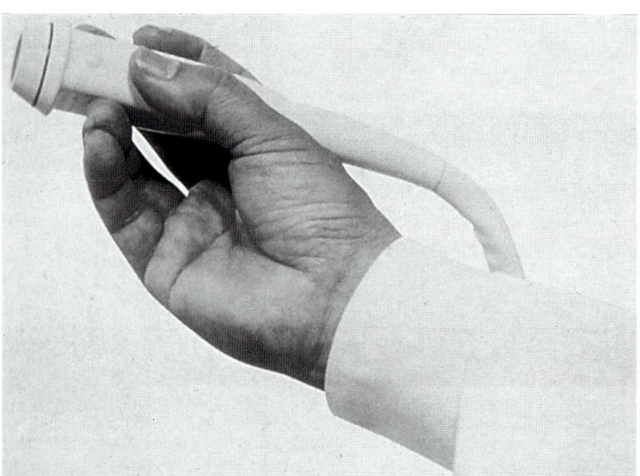

Figure 3. Note the slightly large transducer and cable, as well as the circular footprint.

Clearly, some way around the limitation imposed by the speed of sound is required to produce the 4100-line pyramidal volume of Figure 1 in real-time. A novel ultrasound signal processing approach for volumetric imaging, receive mode parallel processing, was pioneered at Duke University. Refinements of this technique are now available in commercial systems.

In the receive mode of parallel processing systems, a broader angular area of the body is illuminated in transmittal and in receive mode 16 lines of the image are formed. That is, the system looks in 16 different directions simultaneously in receive mode. Therefore, with each transmit a broader angular area of the image is formed. This allows a 4100-line pyramidal volume to be scanned in real-time.

The implementation of real-time volumetric scanning requires a separate beamformer for each of the 16 lines of the image that are formed in parallel. Thus current real-time volumetric imaging systems have 16 parallel beamformers. Since 256 elements from the matrix array are used for receive mode, and each of these elements are used to help form each of 16 lines of the image that are produced with each transmit, the systems have a 4096-channel beamformer (256 channels × 16 beamformers). In other words, real-time volumetric imaging systems require from 8 to 32 times more signal processing power than the highest-end conventional 2D systems on the market. With the continued advances in microchip technology and with the years of refinements of their circuits, these systems have become a commercial reality.

Display

Volumetrics Medical Imaging (Durham, NC) developed and marketed the world's first commercial real-time, volumetric ultrasound system. The system is based upon the concept of receive mode parallel processing. It scans twenty-two 64 × 64 degree pyramidal volumes per second at 15 cm. Each volume contains 4096 scan lines that are spaced approximately 1 degree apart in azimuth and in elevation. The scan rate scales linearly with depth. Therefore, at an 8-cm. depth over 40 volumes per second are scanned.

One of the most significant issues for real-time volumetric imaging is the display of the pyramidal scan. Clinical utility must be retained while at the same time, good use of the vastly larger data set must be made. To maintain clinical utility the real-time volumetric display must give sonographers the features that they are familiar with today. These include: B-Scans, real-time response to movements of the transducer, ECG display, and more. Before discussing the scan formats, however, it is necessary to introduce the concept of the real-time "C-Scan" and the "I-Scan".

As shown in Figure 4, C-Scans are scan planes parallel to the face of the transducer. They are by definition orthographic (correct or nondistorted) projections of the scan planes parallel to the face of the transducer. Sometimes C Scans are called "helicopter views" because these are the views an observer would have if he flew over a pyramid of data that had the top cut off at the level of the C-Scan. C-Scans provide an entirely different view of the anatomy than B-Scans would provide. For example, in Figure 5 you see two C- Scan planes that are displaying cross sections of the left ventricle (LV) obtained from an apical acquisition.

If B-Scans are displayed simultaneously with C-Scans, an instantaneous appreciation of the geometry of the internal structure is obtained. For example, in Figure 5 you have orthogonal B Scan planes shown together with the C Scan planes. The upper B-Scan displays an apical 4-chamber view while the lower B-

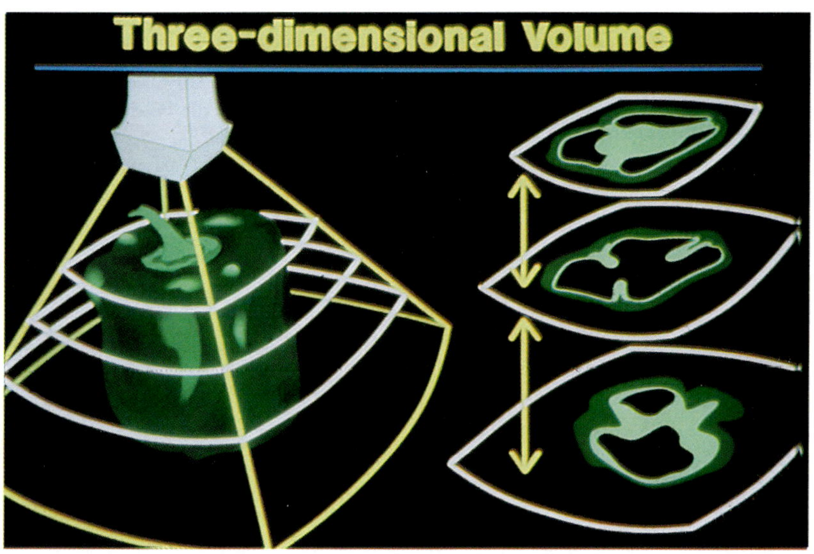

Figure 4. C-scans represent computer generated coronal sections obtained at any chosen location and are unique to three-dimensional data sets. Courtesy Duke University Medical Center.

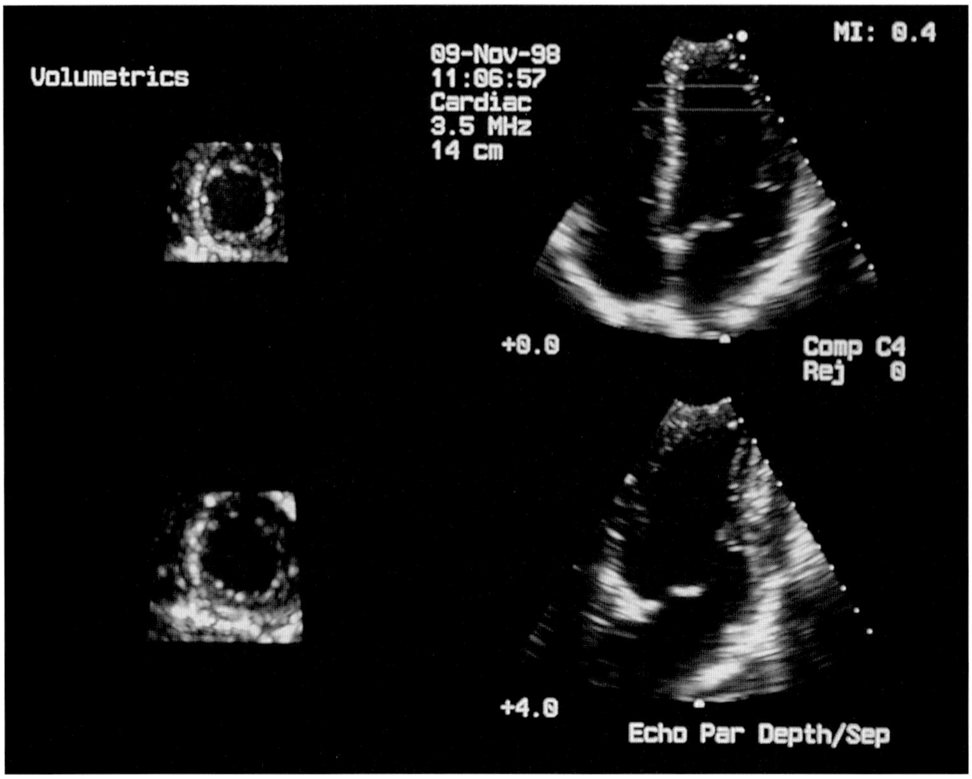

Figure 5. Simultaneous apical four-chamber (**top right**) and two-chamber (**bottom right**) images with two anatomically correct short axis slices displayed on the left. The location of the "C-scans" (short axis images) can be individually selected, and in this image, two adjacent apical "slices" were chosen.

Scan plane displays the apical 2-chamber view. All of these views come from a single volume that was acquired in a 1/30th of a second.

Not all internal structures of the body, however, line up so that planes parallel to the face of the transducer are useful for viewing them. Therefore, real-time volumetric imaging systems include inclined scans (I-Scans). I-Scans are the same in concept to the MRI oblique scans. Scan planes can be tilted in both azimuth or elevation, or in any combination thereof.

To make use of the volumetric data set as well as to provide the clinical utility of conventional 2D ultrasound, real-time volumetric imaging systems display, in real time, multiple simultaneous planes from the volume while scanning. Nominally, two orthogonal B-scans perpendicular to the transducer and 2 C-Scan planes, parallel to the face of the transducer, are displayed simultaneously, in real time. While scanning or in review, these scan planes can be moved around in the volume in real time.

The display of many simultaneous views of an organ in real time allows the clinician to see more of the internal anatomy at once. In Figure 6 for example, a simultaneous long axis (top right view) and short axis view (bottom right view) of an LV from a parasternal position are presented. On the left side of the figure, two anatomically correct short axis views of the LV at different depths are shown. Another example is provided in Figure 7.

Commercial real-time volumetric scanners acquire 22 volumes per second (at 15 cm) that consist of 4096 scan lines each. The system will also store 6 consecutive seconds of volumes (128 MB) at that rate. These 6 seconds of volumetric data can be subsequently stored on a removable optical disk. A patient's scan can later be recalled for interactive review of the data. Interactive review of real-time volumetric scans allows clinicians to replay in a real-time loop 6 seconds of stored volumes. The system will replay the stored data in real-time; during the replay the clinician will be able to change the location in the volumes of the various scan planes that are being displayed. In other words, anatomical dissection of the heart while it is beating in real time on the display is performed.

Since the entire volumetric data set is acquired in real time, the display possibilities are virtually limitless. On one hand, any slice from the volume (up to 16 can be viewed simultaneously) can be viewed from any orientation in real-time. In the future, volume rendered views from any viewpoint (inside or outside of the organ) will be possible, as well as stereo volume rendered views. Some of these more advanced review options are currently available as software that runs on standard PC platforms. Real-time volumetric ultrasound systems also support the standard single B-Scan display format of conventional 2D systems. When running in the Single B-Scan mode, the system scans at 60 frames per second. Each frame contains 332 lines of the image.

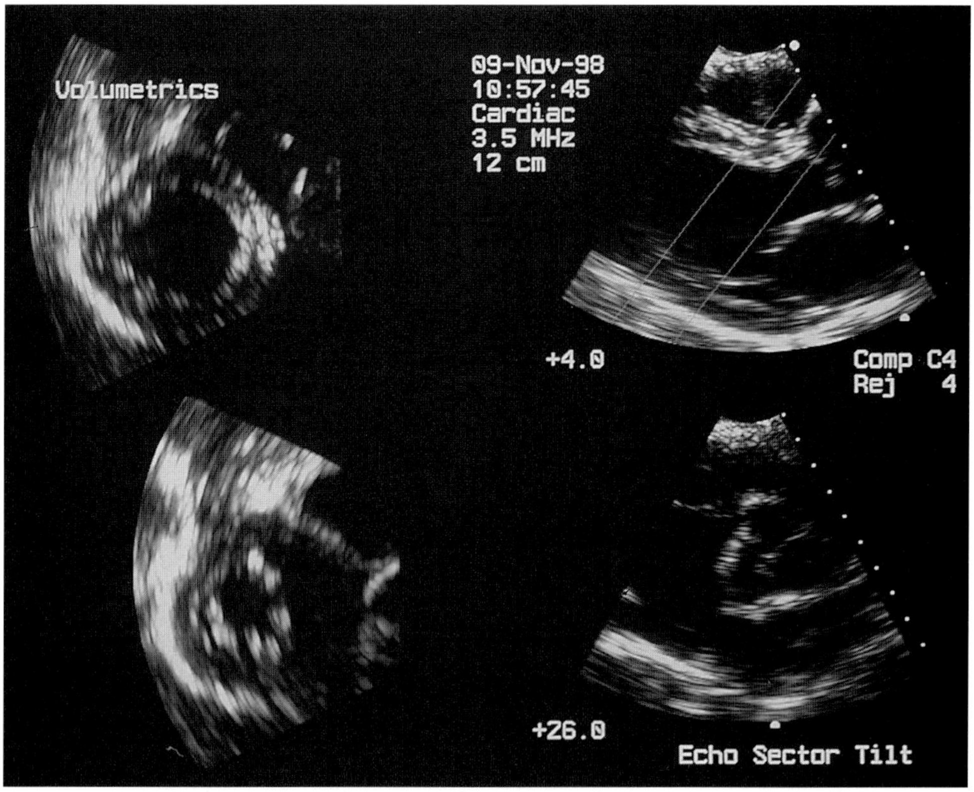

Figure 6. Standard, usual display provides real-time, simultaneous imaging of the parasternal long axis with three chosen short-axis images.

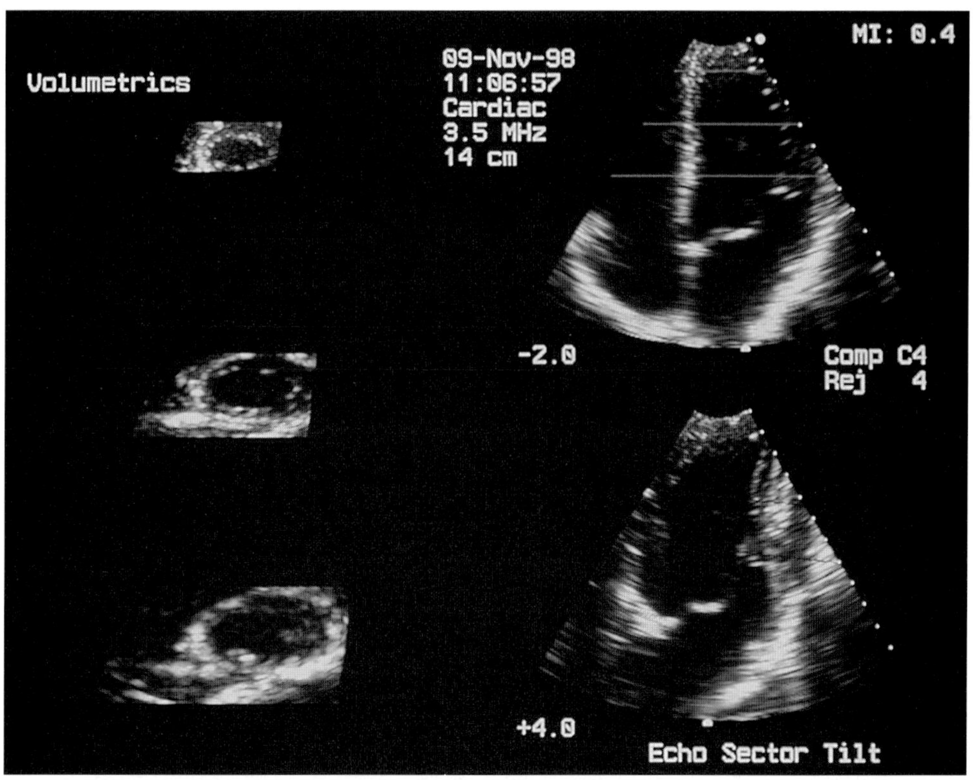

Figure 7. Same apical four- and two-chamber images as displayed in Figure 5, however, the displayed short axis images are now different.

Color Flow and Doppler

Real-time volumetric color flow is just now becoming available on real-time volumetric scanning systems. Real-time volumetric color flow is the acquisition and display of color flow information from a 3D volume in real-time without cardiac or respiratory gating. Phased array principles are used in conjunction with 2D (matrix) arrays, receive mode parallel processing, and 16 parallel color flow processors to rapidly produce a 3D volume of color data. As shown in Figure 8, the volumetric flow is comprised of a 20° by 20° pyramid within the 60° by 60° degree B-Mode pyramidal data set. Real-time volumetric scanners produce pyramidal color flow data sets at a rate of 15 volumes per second. Once the pyramidal data sets are acquired they can be interrogated in the B-Scan and C-Scan images in real time (Figures 9 and 10).

The principles of operation for the real-time volumetric color flow are the same as those for the real-time volumetric imaging. The same transducers are used, the same beamforming technology is used and the displays are similar. Color flow data is always acquired and coded as "toward or away" from the transducer. The color flow data is displayed by selecting the B-Scan or C-Scan images that best show the region of interest. For example, if the question is to evaluate an aortic jet, the use of a C-Scan plane in the LV outflow tract could be used to evaluate the jet as well as the simultaneous B-Scan planes.

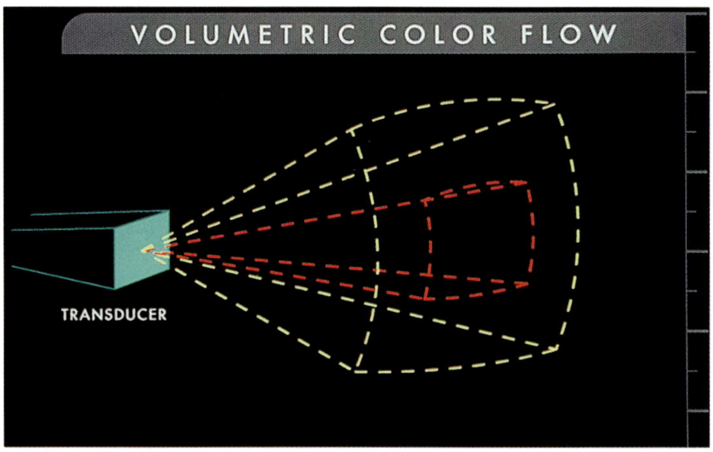

Figure 8. Real-time three-dimensional color flow Doppler is possible using a 20° × 20° pyramidal volume set within the conventional 60° × 60° B-mode pyramidal data set.

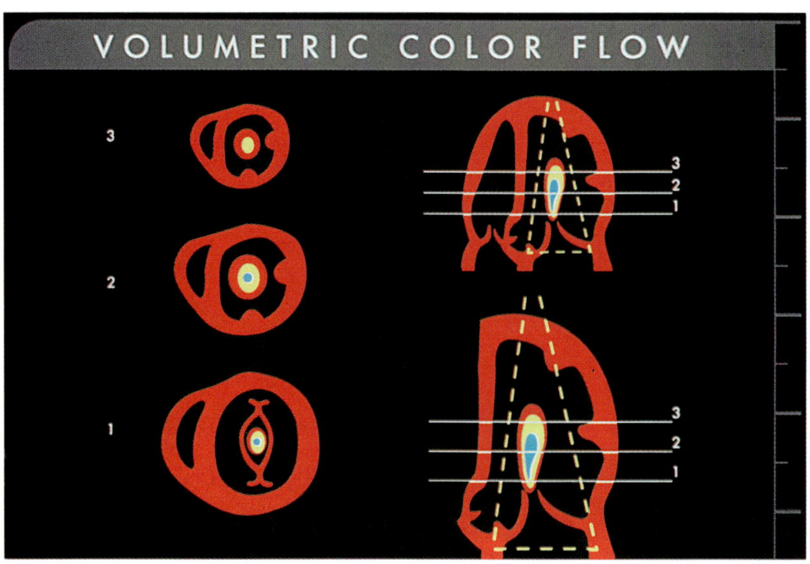

Figure 9. Schematic display of the potential of three-dimensional real-time color flow Doppler.

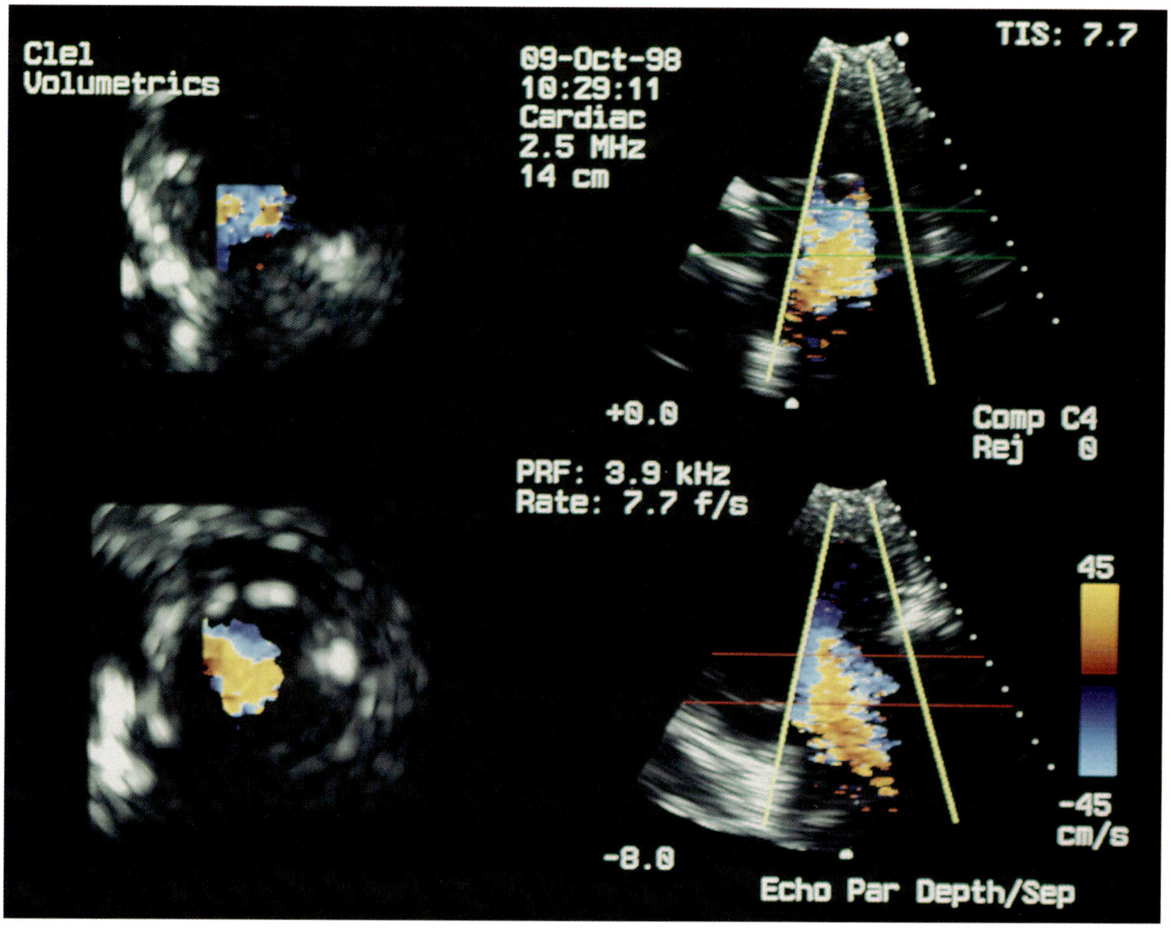

Figure 10. Example of simultaneous imaging in multiple planes using three-dimensional real-time color flow Doppler in a patient with mitral regurgitation.

Significance

The clinical importance of diagnostic ultrasound has grown in direct proportion to major improvements in the instrumentation. The integration of gray scale imaging, real-time imaging, high resolution imaging, and most recently, real-time flow (velocity) imaging have combined to make ultrasound both more specific and easier to use. Therefore, ultrasound has become a dominant medical imaging modality.

Real-time volumetric scanners have received FDA 510k clearance and have been installed for clinical work at institutions worldwide. These systems have been used in adult cardiology, radiology, pediatric cardiology and surgery settings. Over 50 abstracts have been given and approximately 15 manuscripts have been submitted for publication. These clinical investigations have focused on the following applications.

Left Ventricular Function

Huge proportions of the ultrasound studies performed are directed toward the evaluation of the health of the LV. These studies typically involve four measures of ventricular performance: LV volume (ejection fraction), LV Mass, LV wall motion, and LV perfusion. In this section, we will examine 2D and real-time volumetric imaging relative to these measures.

Left Ventricular Volumes (Ejection Fractions)

Left ventricular volumes have been determined using 2D phased array systems for some time. All techniques to measure volumes have a similar procedure: several views (e.g., long axis and short axis or apical 4-chamber and apical 2-chamber) are obtained, dimensions are extracted, and the volume is calculated with an assumed geometry. Unfortunately, many patients (e.g., those with ventricular aneurysms, post myocardial infarction expansion or ventricular hypertrophy) have irregular geometries, which negatively affect the accuracy and reproducibility of LV volume measurements by 2D echo. Therefore, studies have shown that the interobserver variability of ejection fraction measurements made by 2D echo using the apical biplane summation-of-disks method recommended by the American Society of Echocardiography is around 30%.[1–3] In fact, subjective visual assessment by conventional 2D echocardiography has been shown to yield the same accuracy as 2D quantitative methods.[4] The low accuracy and reproducibility in the estimation of the LV ejection fraction by 2D echo often results in duplicate testing by alternate imaging modalities. Moreover, because of the variability attendant to each measurement of the ejection fraction, the serial assessment of patients for the timing of therapeutic interventions becomes impractical.

To eliminate this problem, the entire LV volume must be captured instantaneously so that more measurements can be made and so that the geometric relationships between the measurements are fixed. As discussed earlier, the Model 1 images the entire LV at a rate of 22 volumes per second. These volumes are stored on disk and can be recalled to measure systolic and diastolic volumes. Volumes are measured by an on system utility which uses a modified Simpson's method that essentially sums the areas of slices of the lumen of the ventricle. Several studies have be performed to assess the accuracy of these measurements performed with the Model 1.[5–7]

Combining real-time 3D imaging with exercise or pharmacologic stress allows rapid acquisition of regional wall motion analysis and may increase the likelihood of detecting ischemic changes (Figures 11 and 12).

Myocardial Mass

The mass of the myocardium is an important measure in the management of hypertensive patients. Two-dimensional echocardiographic measurement of LV mass has similar procedural problems as 2D echocardiographic measurements of LV ejection fractions. Therefore, the accuracy of LV mass measurements with 2D echo suffers.[8] Early animal experiments have shown that real-time volumetric imaging has the possibility of significantly improving the measurement of LV mass.[5]

Myocardial Perfusion

With improved contrast media that passes from the right to the left side of the heart and that has some persistence, myocardial perfusion can be directly visualized throughout the ventricular volume. This holds the promise of correlating infarcted myocardium with the perfusion. While these measurements are possible with nuclear cardiography, the procedure is expensive (approximately $1,200 vs. $300 for an ultrasound), requires about 6 hours to perform, and has limited accuracy. Animal studies have shown a good correlation between the myocardial risk volume as measured by real-time volumetric ultrasound imaging and nuclear cardiology.[9]

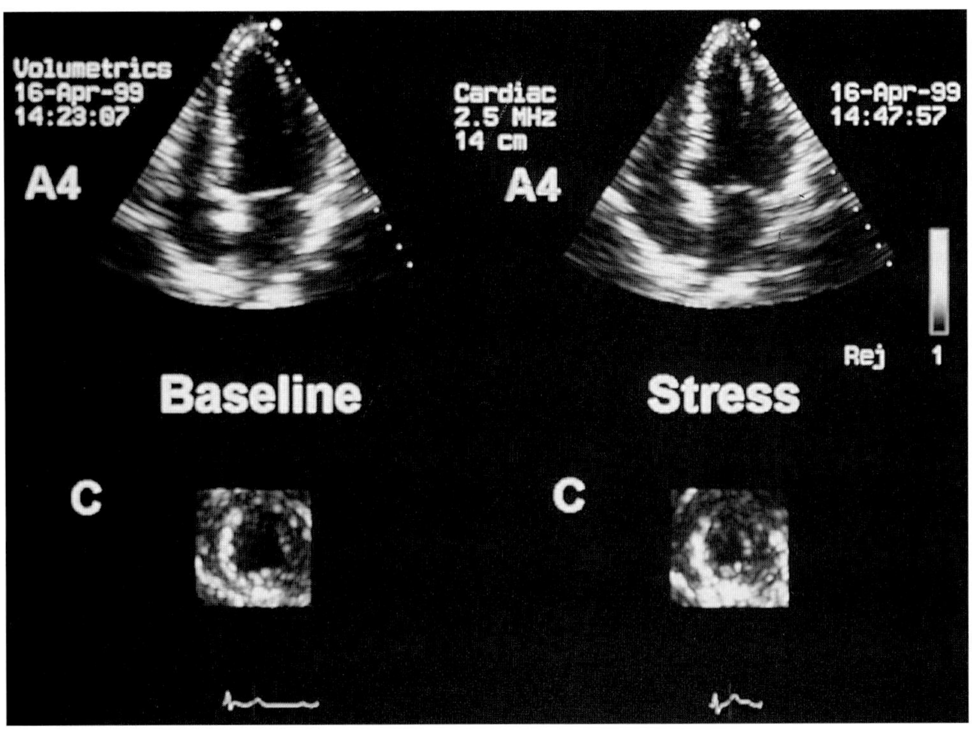

Figure 11. Left ventricular (LV) systolic frames from an apical 4-chamber view (A4) and simultaneous apical C-scans (cross sectional slices parallel to the face of the transducer) at baseline and at peak dobutamine induced stress in a patient with normal left ventricular (LV) wall motion. A uniform decrease in LV cavity size during stress is evident in the C-scan. Courtesy of Masood Ahmad, MD, Galveston, Texas.

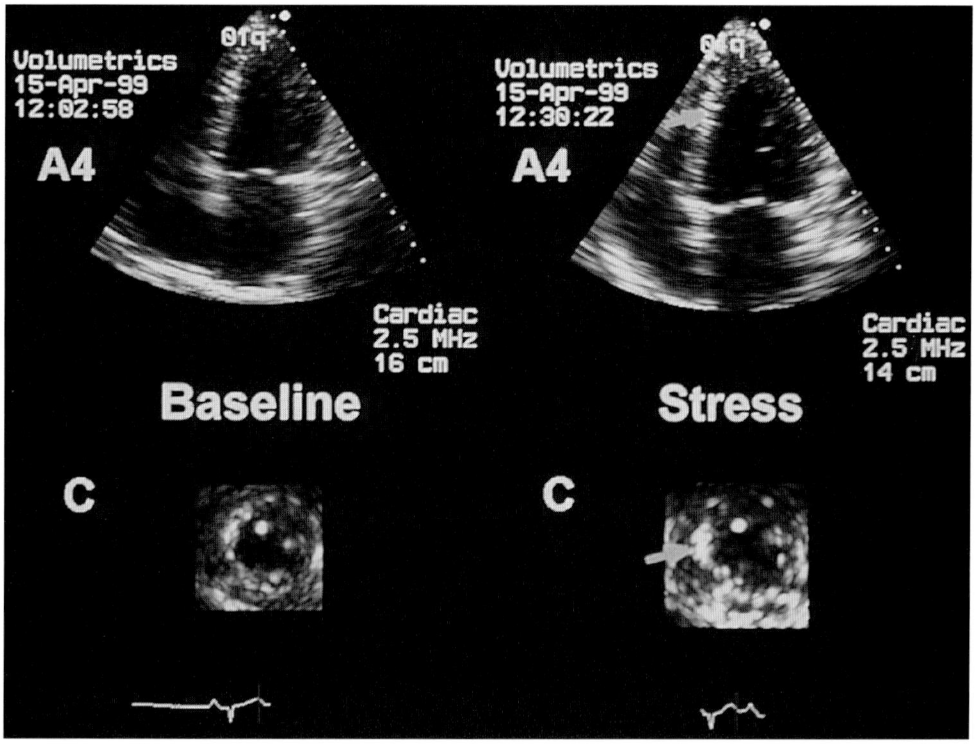

Figure 12. Left ventricular (LV) systolic frames from an apical 4-chamber view (A4) and simultaneous apical C-scans at baseline and at peak dobutamine induced stress in a patient with inducible ischemia. Arrows point to the LV wall abnormality in the inferoseptal segments in A4 and C-scan views. The region of inducible ischemia is well appreciated in the C-scan. Courtesy of Masood Ahmad, MD, Galveston, Texas.

Right Ventricular Function

Right ventricular (RV) performance is a critical issue in the management of patients with congestive heart failure,[10] acute inferior myocardial infarction,[11] routine open heart surgery,[12] long-term aortic or mitral insufficiency and obstructive lung disease,[13] congenital heart disease,[14] and heart transplantation.[13] Furthermore, *because of its geometry,* no good method for evaluating RV function exists, including 3D reconstructions from 2D scanners.[13,15–18] Moreover, important aspects of the pathophysiology of RV failure are not understood due to the inability to assess RV stroke volumes.[18–22]

Real-time volumetric ultrasound holds the possibility that RV systolic and diastolic volumes can be determined. From the apical view, the entire right ventricle can be seen and cross sectional areas can be measured in the scan planes parallel to the face of the transducer. By summing the areas in these scan planes, RV volumes can be calculated. Volumes can thus be calculated in both systole and diastole without any assumptions about the shape of the ventricle.[23] Work is ongoing to assess the accuracy of the measurements.[24]

Economic Implications

A lingering problem with ultrasound is that very highly trained people are required to perform the studies, the studies often require multiple views (which consumes time), and getting the same view on a sequential study is problematic. Real-time volumetric imaging addresses all of these problems. Once the organ or blood vessel that is to be studied is within the volume, the sonographer need only capture the volume. Later, off-line, the physician can position the multiple scan planes to obtain the precise view or set of views that is required to make the diagnosis. This saves time in the scan room and should decrease the sonographer-to-sonographer variability.

Even a 20% increase in throughput is a big benefit to both large and small practices. In small practices, an increase in throughput can delay a large capital outlay for a year or more by more efficient utilization of an existing system. In a large tertiary care institution with six or eight systems, higher throughput means fewer technicians, less space, and lower capital outlays. Improved repeatability leads to fewer rescans and fewer scheduling complications.

Valvular Assessments

Ultrasound is often used to determine the area of the mitral orifice. This requires that the 2D plane be located at the minimum extent of the orifice during diastole. This is often not easy to do reliably and repeatedly. Model 1.0 has the potential to measure the mitral orifice size in an accurate and repeatable manner. Since the entire volume is captured and since the scan planes can be moved in 1° increments during review of the data, a plane can be located repeatedly in the mitral orifice at its minimum extent.

References

1. Gopal AS, Shen Z, Sapin PM, et al. Assessment of cardiac function by three-dimensional echocardiography compared with conventional Noninvasive Methods. *Circulation* 1995;92(4):842–853.
2. King DL, Harrison MR, King DL Jr. et al. Ultrasound beam orientation during standard two dimensional imaging: Assessment by three-dimensional echocardiography. *J Am Soc Echocardiogr* 1992;6:569–576.
3. King DL, Harrison MR, King DL Jr, et al. Improved reproducibility of left atrial and left ventricular measurements by guided three-dimensional echocardiography. *J Am Coll Cardiol* 1992:20:1238–1245.
4. Amico AF, Lichtenberg GS, Reiser SA, et al. Superiority of visual versus computerized echocardiographic estimation of radionuclide left ventricular ejection fraction. *Am Heart J* 1989;118:1259–1265.
5. Ota T, Fleishman CE, Ohazama CJ, et al. Measurement of left ventricular volume by real-time, three-dimensional echocardiography in dogs. *Circulation* 1996;94(Suppl 1):379 Abstract.
6. Ota T, Fleishman CE, Li J, et al. Accuracy of manual and semiautomated methods for volume determination by real-time, three-dimensional echocardiography. *Circulation* 1996;94(Suppl 1):212 Abstract.
7. Ota T, Johes M, Fleishman CE, et al. Accuracy of left ventricular stroke volume measurement using real-time three-dimensional echocardiography and electromagnetic flow probe. *Circulation* 1997;96(Suppl 1):328 Abstract.
8. Sapin PM, Gopal AS, Clarke GB, et al. Three-dimensional echocardiography compared to two-dimensional echocardiography for measurement of left ventricular mass anatomic validation in an open chest canine model. *Am J Hypertens* 1996:9(5):467–474.
9. Fleishman CE, Ota T, Lewis, et al. Quantitative assessment of LV ischemic risk volume using real-time three-dimensional echocardiography. *Circulation* 1996;94(8) Suppl:
10. Schulman D, Mathay RA. The right ventricle in pulmonary disease. *Cardiol Clin* 1992;10:111–135.
11. Setaro JF, Cabin HS. Right ventricular infarction. *Cardiol Clin* 1992:10:69–90.
12. Fisk RL, Guilbeau EJ. Perioperative right heart failure: Etiology and pathophysiology. *Cardiovasc Clin* 1987;17: 219–229.
13. Jain D, Zaret BL. Assessment of right ventricular function. *Cardio Clin* 1992;10:23–39.
14. Hijazi ZM, Hellenbrand WE. The right ventricle in congential heart disease. *Cardiol Clin* 1992;10:01–110.
15. Boxt LM, Katz J. Magnetic resonance imaging for quantitation of right ventricular volume in patients with pulmonary hypertension. *J Thorac Imaging* 1993;8:92.
16. Spinale FG, Zeliner JL, Mukherjee R, et al. Thermodilution right ventricular ejection fraction. Catheter positioning effects. *Chest* 1990;98:1259–1265.
17. Jiang L, Siu SC, Handschumacher MD, et al. Three-dimensional echocardiography. In vivo validation for right ventricular volume and function. *Circulation* 1994; 89:2342–2350.
18. Wranne B, Pinto FJ, Siegel LC, et al. Abnormal postoperative interventricular motion: New intraoperative transesophagael echocardiographic evidence supports a novel hypothesis. *Am Heart J* 1993;126:161–167.
19. Konstam MA,Cohen SR, Salem DN. Comparison of left and right ventricular end systolic pressure-volume relations in congestive heart failure. *J Am Coll Cardiol* 1985; 5:1326.
20. Setari JF, Cleman MW, Remetz MS. The right ventricle in disorders causing pulmonary venous hypertension. *Cardiol Clin* 1992;10:185–193.
21. Lee FA. Hemodynamic of the right ventricle in normal and diseased states. *Cardiol Clin* 1992;10:59–67.
22. Schulman D, Biondi J, Zohgbi S. Coronary flow limits right ventricular performance during positive end-expiratory pressure. *Am Rev Respir Dis* 1990;141:1531.
23. Ota T, Fleishman CE, Strub M, et al. Real-time, three-dimensional echocardiography: Feasibility of dynamic right ventricular volume measurement with saline contrast. *Am Heart J* 1999;137:958–966.
24. Shiota T, Jones M, Chikada M, et al. Real-time three-dimensional echocardiography for determining right ventricular stroke volume in an animal model of chronic right ventricular volume overload. *Circulation* 1998;97: 1897–1900.

Suggested Reading List

1. Ota T, Fleishman CE, Strub M, et al. Real-time, three-dimensional echocardiography: feasibility of dynamic right ventricular volume measurement with saline contrast. *Am Heart J* 1999;137:958–966.
2. Stetten GD, Pizer SM. Medial-node models to identify and measure objects in real-time 3-D echocardiography. *IEEE Transactions Medical Imaging* 1999;18:1025–1034.
3. Takuma S, Zwas DR, Fard A, et al. Real-time, 3-dimensional echocardiography acquires all standard 2-dimensional images from 2 volume sets: A clinical demonstration in 45 patients. *J Am Soc Echocardiography* 1999; 12:1–6.
4. de Groot N, Bootsma M, Schalij MJ, et al. Three-dimensional catheter positioning during radiofrequency ablation in patients: First application of a real-time position management system. [see comments]. *J Cardiovasc Electrophysiol* 2000;11(11):1183–1192.
5. Kisslo J, Firek B, Ota T, et al. Real-time volumetric echocardiography: the technology and the possibilities. [Review] [0 refs]. *Echocardiography* 2000;17(8): 773–779.
6. Takuma S, Cardinale C, Homma S. Real-time three-dimensional stress echocardiography: A Review of current applications. [Review] [12 refs]. *Echocardiography* 2000; 17(8):791–794.
7. Ahmad M: Real-time three-dimensional echocardiography in assessment of heart disease. [Review] [11 refs]. *Echocardiography* 2001;18(1):73–77.
8. Chamoun AJ, Lenihan DJ, McCulloch M, et al. Resynchronization therapy in dilated cardiomyopathy: Confirmation of hemodynamic improvement with real-time three-dimensional echocardiography. *Circulation* 2001; 103(19):E98.

9. Ota T, Kisslo J, von Ramm OT, et al. Real-time, volumetric echocardiography: Usefulness of volumetric scanning for the assessment of cardiac volume and function. *J Cardiol* 2001;37(Suppl.1):93–101.
10. Schmidt MA, Freidlin RZ, Ohazama CJ, et al. Anatomic validation of a novel method for left ventricular volume and mass measurements with use of real-time 3-dimensional echocardiography. *J Am Soc Echocardiography* 2001;14(1):1–10.
11. Tsujino H, Jones M, Shiota T, et al. Real-time three-dimensional color Doppler echocardiography for characterizing the spatial velocity distribution and quantifying the peak flow rate in the left ventricular outflow tract. *Ultrasound Med & Biol* 2001;27(1):69–74.

Chapter 13

Future Directions

Navin C. Nanda, MD and Vincent L. Sorrell, MD

This atlas serves as a bridge to the future of traditional echocardiography. The rapid advancement of digital technology provides the framework to expand these imaging devices into a more clinically useful state-of-the-art system. Technical research will continue to improve the rapidity with which the three-dimensional (3D) data set is acquired, while also providing an adequate transthoracic transducer. Real-time 3D echocardiography has already revealed the potential of parallel processing techniques that will again allow rapid, multiplanar data acquisition from a single cardiac cycle.

Additionally, surface-rendering techniques and other post-processing capabilities will further enhance our display capabilities. The most comprehensive 3D-display format would, of course, be a virtual reality model. Advancements in this area have evolved, but it remains less likely that the current physicians practicing echocardiography today would be willing to don the additional headgear to be expected with this type of technology. Potentially, future echocardiographers, raised in an even greater digital society, may not only be willing, but may encourage this type of technology.

This chapter pays witness to many of these post-processing capabilities and provides numerous examples of the potential of 3D echocardiography. The reader is encouraged to also evaluate examples in the overview chapter.

From Nanda NC and Sorrell VL: *Atlas of Three-Dimensional Echocardiography.* ©Futura Publishing Co., Inc, Armonk, NY, 2002.

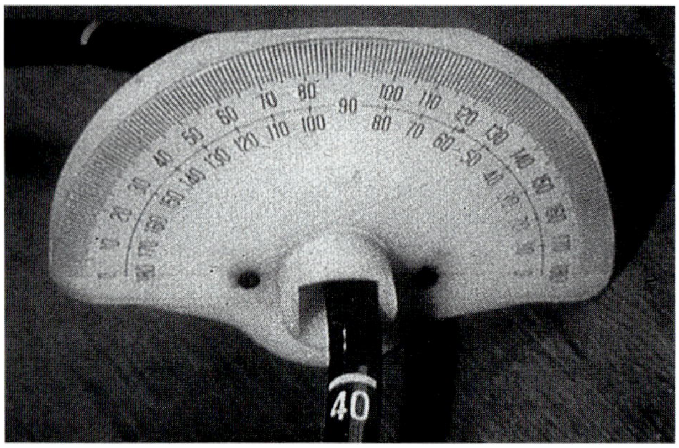

Figure 1. This device is used to lock the probe in the longitudinal plane prior to manual rotation. The three-dimensional data set derived from this method provides many of the following images.

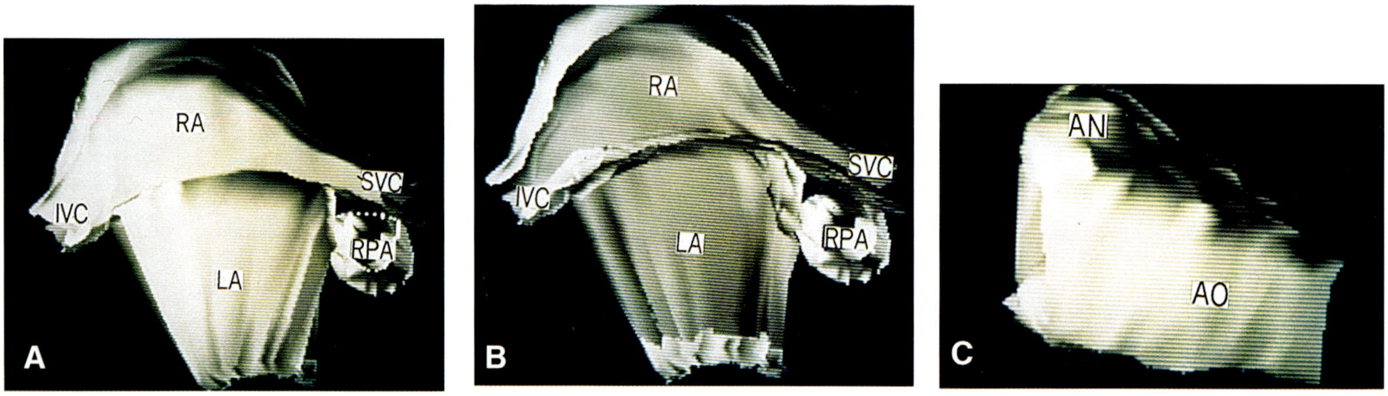

Figure 2. Regional display of a three-dimensionally (3D) reconstructed image. (**A**) 3D image of superior vena cava (SVC) zone showing 3-D reconstructed longitudinal structures of SVC, inferior vena cava (IVC), right atrium (RA), left atrium (LA), and right pulmonary artery (RPA). (**B**) Stereo-sectional display of the structures shown in **A.** (**C**) 3D image of ascending aorta zone, displaying the stereo-structure of longitudinal ascending aorta (AO) and the aneurysm (AN) of right sinus of Valsalva.

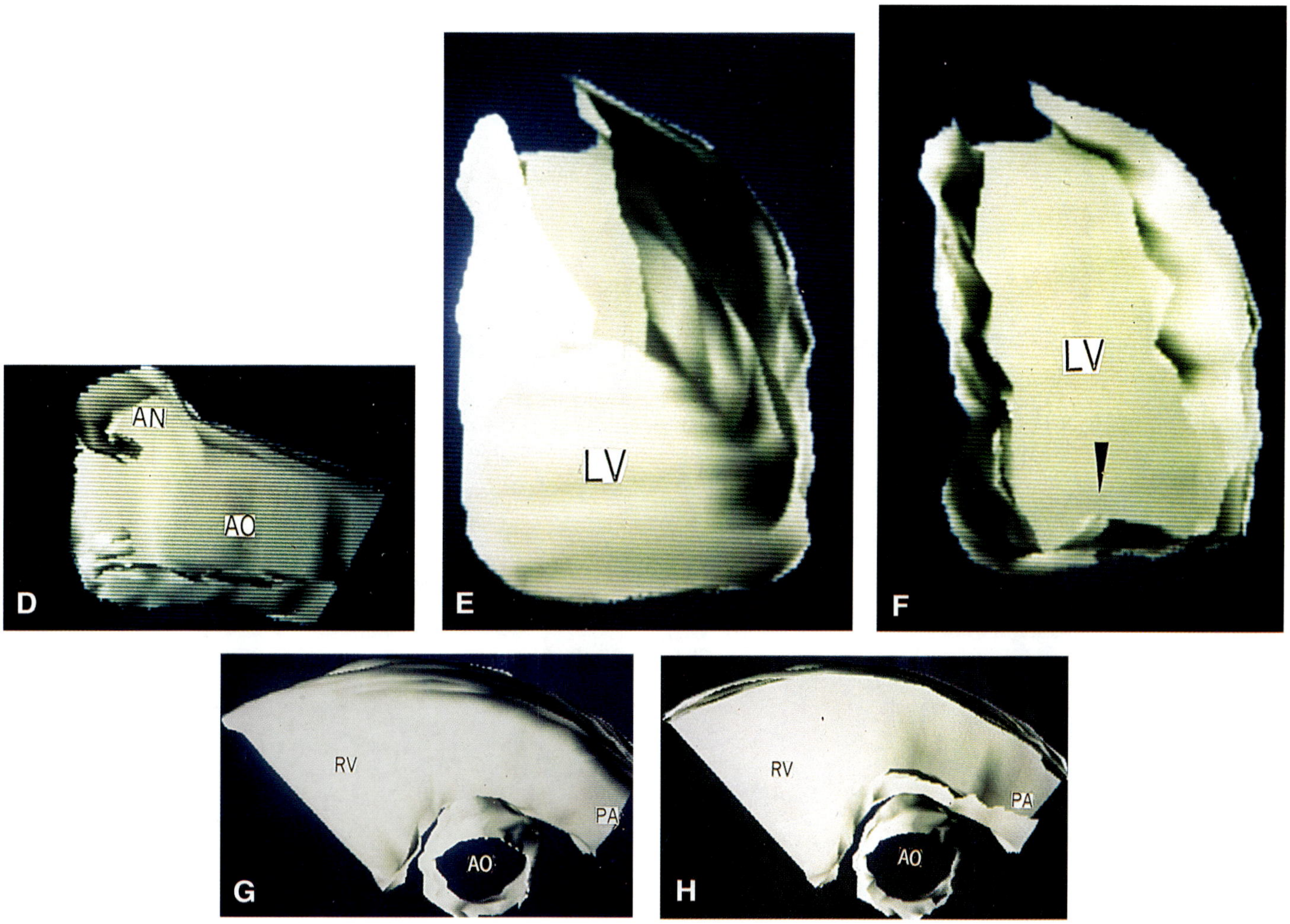

Figure 2. Continued. (**D**) Stereo-sectional display of the structures shown in **C.** (**E**) 3D image of the left ventricle (LV), showing its outline. (**F**) 3D display of a cut-open left ventricle (LV). The arrow points to normal closure of the mitral valve in systole. (**G**) 3D image of right ventricular (RV) outflow tract/ pulmonary artery (PA) zone, showing the longitudinal outline of these structures which are oriented perpendicular to the aortic root (A). (**H**) Display of cut-open structures shown in **G** (stereo-sectional display). Reproduced with permission from Zhian Li et al. Three dimensional reconstruction of transesophageal echocardiographic longitudinal images. *Echocardiography* 1995;12:367–375.

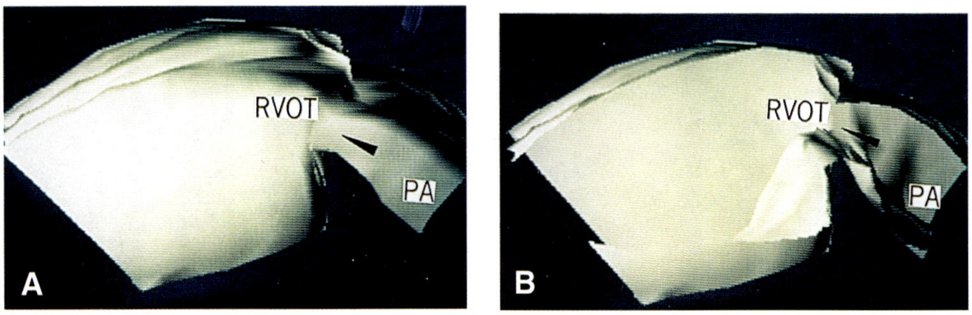

Figure 3. Three-dimensional (3D) image of obstructed right ventricular outflow tract (RVOT). (**A**) 3D outline imaging of the obstructed RVOT. The arrow points to the obstruction. (**B**) Cut-open image of the obstructed RVOT. The arrow points to the obstruction. Reproduced with permission from Zhian Li et al: Three dimensional reconstruction of transesophageal echocardiographic longitudinal images. *Echocardiography* 1995;12:367–375.

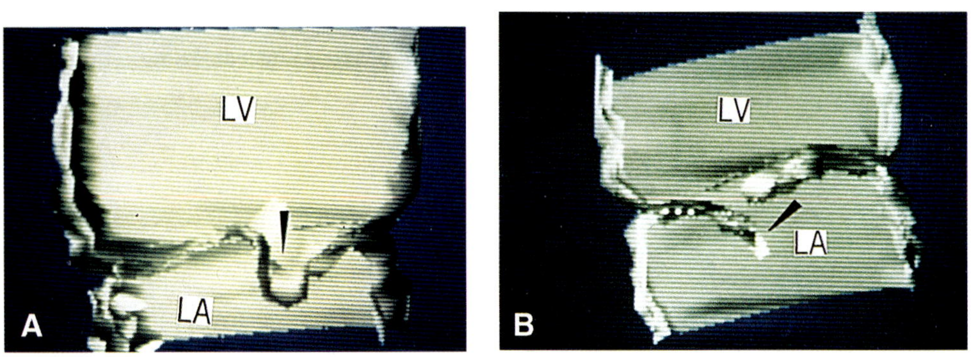

Figure 4. Three-dimensional (3D) imaging of mitral valve prolapse. (**A**) Stereo-sectional display of left heart zone, identifying prolapse (arrow) of the anterior mitral leaflet into the left atrium (LA) in systole. LV = left ventricle. (**B**) Stereo-sectional display of the left heart zone, identifying prolapse (arrow) of the posterior mitral leaflet into the LA in systole. Reproduced with permission from Zhian Li et al. Three dimensional reconstruction of transesophageal echocardiographic longitudinal images. *Echocardiography* 1995;12:367–375.

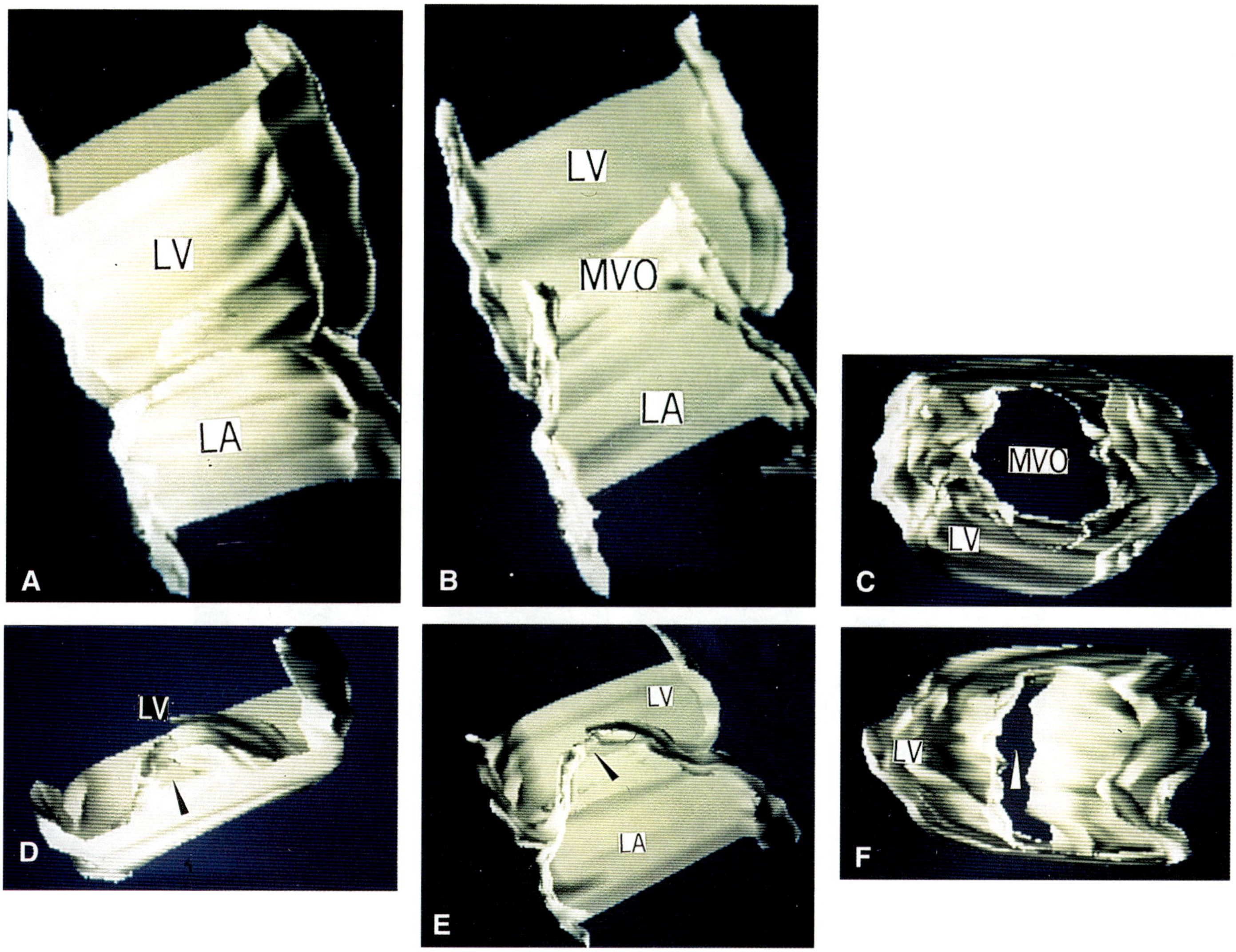

Figure 5. Three-dimensional (3D) imaging of mitral valve in diastole. (**A**) Normal 3D outline of the left ventricle (LV) and the left atrium (LA). (**B**) Normal diastolic opening of the mitral valve (MVO). (**C**) Bird's eye view of normal diastolic MVO, looking from the LV into the LA. (**D**) 3D outline of mitral stenosis, indicating the dome-like mitral valve (arrow). (**E**) Stereo-sectional display of mitral stenosis. The arrow points to the dome-shaped opening of the mitral valve. (**F**) Bird's eye view of the stenotic mitral valve (arrow), looking from the LV into the LA. Reproduced with permission from Zhian Li et al. Three dimensional reconstruction of transesophageal echocardiographic longitudinal images. *Echocardiography* 1995;12:367–375.

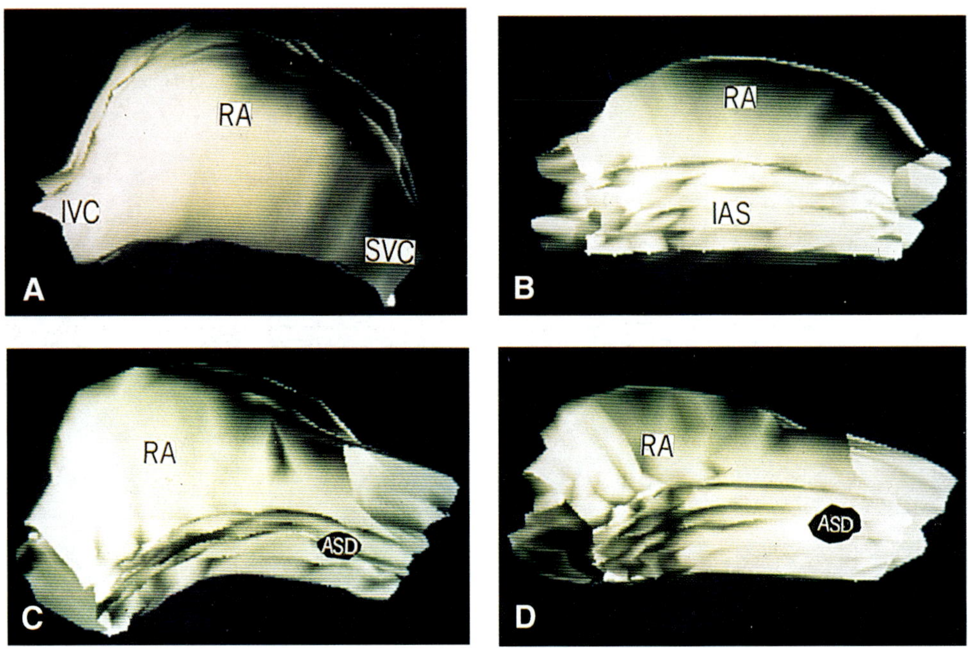

Figure 6. Three-dimensional (3D) imaging of atrial septum and sinus venus atrial septal defect (ASD). (**A**) 3D imaging of normal superior vena cava (SVC) zone, showing SVC, right atrium (RA) and inferior vena cava (IVC). (**B**) Vertical rotation (90°) of the structures shown in **A** displaying the full extent of the interatrial septum (IAS) without any defect. This was a normal subject. (**C, D**) 3D imaging in another patient with sinus venus ASD, showing the defect at different levels of vertical rotation. Reproduced with permission from Zhian Li et al. Three dimensional reconstruction of transesophageal echocardiographic longitudinal images. *Echocardiography* 1995;12:367–375.

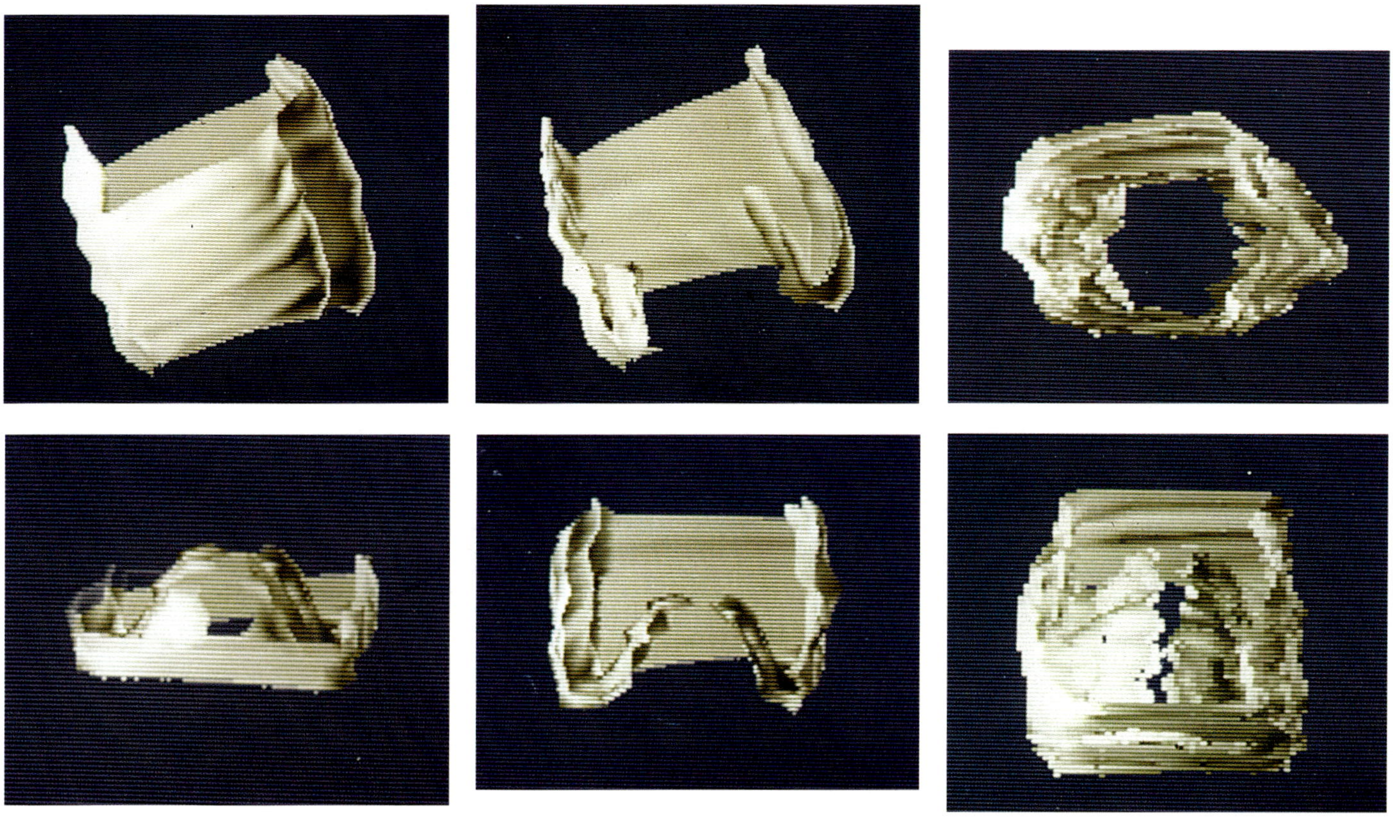

Figure 7. Static three-dimensional pictures of mitral valve during diastole taken by transesophageal echo (TEE). **Upper left:** Contour of the left ventricle (LV) in normal subject. **Upper middle:** After cutting away the front structure, the wide-open mitral valve orifice is clearly shown leading into the LV. **Upper right:** After vertical rotation, the wide-open, circular-like mitral valve orifice with smooth edges is seen leading into LV. **Lower left:** Contour of the stenotic mitral valve leading into LV. **Lower middle:** After cutting away the front, the stenotic mitral valve orifice is better visualized with anterior mitral leaflet ballooning into the LV. **Lower right:** On bird's-eye view from the LV side, the stenotic mitral valve orifice is seen as a crevice (arrow) with ragged edges. Reproduced with permission from Wang XF et al. Clinical application of three-dimensional transesophageal echocardiography. *Am Heart J* 1994;128:380–388.

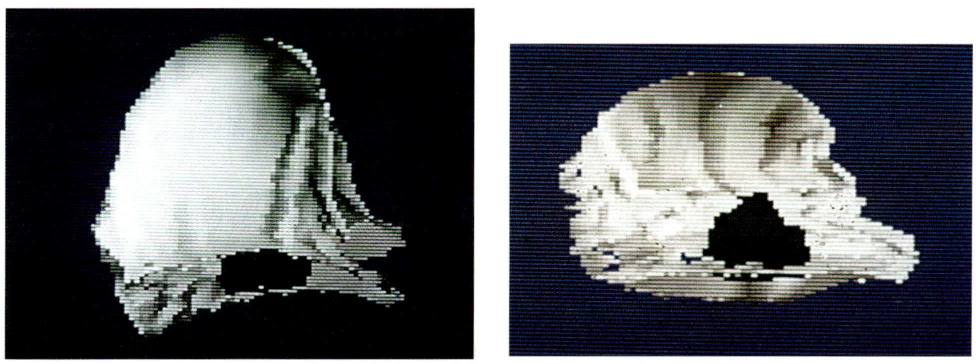

Figure 8. Right atrium and interatrial septum. **Left:** Patient with atrial septal defect (ASD). An elliptical defect is presented in the interatrial septum. **Right:** When rotated 90° vertically, image shows atrial septal defect to be classified to secondum-type defect. Reproduced with permission from Wang XF et al. Clinical application of three-dimensional transesophageal echocardiography. *Am Heart J* 1994;128:380–388.

Suggested Reading List

1. Binder T, Baumgartner H: Future trends in echocardiography. Contrast echocardiography and 3-dimensional echocardiography. [Review] [16 refs]. *Acta Anaesthesiol Scandinavica Supplementum* 1997;111:286–289.
2. Delabays A. [Three-dimensional echocardiography: curiosity or method of the future]. [Review] [10 refs] [French]. *Revue Medicale Suisse Romande* 1999;119:383–387.
3. Bruining N, Lancee C, Roelandt JR, et al. Three-dimensional echocardiography paves the way toward virtual reality. [Review] [63 refs]. *Ultrasound Med & Biol* 2000;26(7):1065–1074.
4. Gunasegaran K, Yao J, De Castro S, et al. Three-dimensional transesophageal echocardiography (TEE) and other future directions. [Review] [111 refs]. *Cardiology Clinics* 2000;18(4):893–910.
5. Salustri A, Roelandt JR. Three-dimensional echocardiography: Where we are, where we are going. [Review] [49 refs]. *Italian Heart J* 2000;1(1):26–32.

Index